Wavefront Customized Visual Correction

The Quest for Super Vision II

Ronald R. Krueger, MD, MSE
Medical Director, Department of Refractive Surgery
Cleveland Clinic Foundation
Cole Eye Institute
Cleveland, Ohio

Raymond A. Applegate, OD, PhD
Professor and Borish Chair of Optometry
College of Optometry
University of Houston
Houston, Tex

Scott M. MacRae, MD
Director of Refractive Surgery
Professor of Ophthalmology
Professor in the Center for Visual Science
University of Rochester Medical Center
Rochester, NY

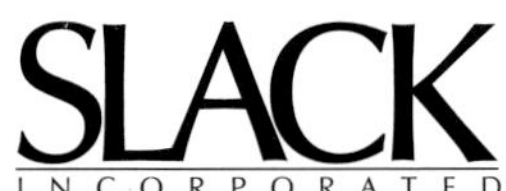

An innovative information, education, and management company
6900 Grove Road • Thorofare, NJ 08086

DEDICATION

To the Glory of God through the person of Jesus Christ,
To whom I owe everything, and without whom I am nothing,
He is my life, hope, and joy, now and forever...
....And to my loving mother, Lucie Krueger, God Bless You on your 80th Birthday Year!
Ronald R. Krueger, MD,MSE

I dedicate this book to my father, K. Edwin Applegate, and mother, Elizabeth Dilts Applegate,
for their unwavering love, support, and faith in my ability. Happy 60th anniversary.
Raymond A. Applegate, OD, PhD

I dedicate this book to my 6-year-old daughter, Morgan, whose energy, curiosity, and creativity will bless the world for many years to come. To my wife, Abby, whose loving support and thoughtful reflection lift my wings and feed my soul. To my mom, Bets, whose gentle spirit teaches me grace and appreciation.
Scott M. MacRae, MD

Front cover: Image courtesy of Dan Topa at WaveFront Sciences, Inc, Albuquerque, NM.
Back cover: The editors, hard at work on their edits. Photo courtesy of Bernadine Ursell.

The procedures and practices described in this book should be implemented in a manner consistent with the professional standards set for the circumstances that apply in each specific situation. Every effort has been made to confirm the accuracy of the information presented and to correctly relate generally accepted practices. The authors, editor, and publisher cannot accept responsibility for errors or exclusions or for the outcome of the application of the material presented herein. There is no expressed or implied warranty of this book or information imparted by it.

Care has been taken to ensure that drug selection, dosages, and treatments are in accordance with currently accepted/recommended practice. Due to continuing research, changes in government policy and regulations, and various effects of drug reactions and interactions, it is recommended that the reader review all materials and literature provided for each drug use, especially those that are new or not frequently used.

The work SLACK Incorporated publishes is peer reviewed. Prior to publication, recognized leaders in the field, educators, and clinicians provide important feedback on the concept and content that we publish. We welcome feedback on this work.

Any review or mention of specific companies or products is not intended as an endorsement by the authors, editors, or publisher.

Printed in the United States of America.
Wavefront customized visual corrections : the quest for super vision II
/ [edited by] Ronald R. Krueger, Raymond A. Applegate, Scott M. MacRae.
p. ; cm.
Rev. ed. of: Customized corneal ablation. c2001.
Includes bibliographical references and index.
ISBN 1-55642-625-9 (alk. paper)
1. LASIK (Eye surgery) 2. Corneal topography.
[DNLM: 1. Corneal Topography. 2. Cornea--surgery. 3. Ophthalmologic
Surgical Procedures--methods. 4. Refractive Errors--therapy. WW 220
W355 2004] I. Krueger, Ronald R. II. Applegate, Raymond Alan. III.
MacRae, Scott. IV. Customized corneal ablation.
RE336 .W386 2006
617.7'19059--dc22 2003023442

Published by: SLACK Incorporated
6900 Grove Road
Thorofare, NJ 08086 USA
Telephone: 856-848-1000
Fax: 856-853-5991
www.slackbooks.com

Contact SLACK Incorporated for more information about other books in this field or about the availability of our books from distributors outside the United States.

Last digit is print number: 10 9 8 7 6 5 4 3 2 1

Contents

Section IV Wavefront Customized Lenses

Section V Nonwavefront Customized Corrections

Basic Science Section

Clinical Science Section

Section VI The Future of Customization

Acknowledgments

I wish to acknowledge all those who contributed tirelessly to the completion of this book:

To our authors, the experts in their respective fields, who took their time and energy to write yet another book chapter, and yet make it the best chapter they've ever written,

To our editors at SLACK Incorporated—Amy McShane, Lauren Biddle Plummer, and April Billick—who believed in us and our novel ideas in compiling this book and its cover, and who kept pushing us to its completion, even when we were past our deadlines,

To my coeditors, Ray and Scott, who each play such a unique role in the editorial process, and who keep challenging me and pushing me to pursue excellence, even when we don't always agree (see the photo on the back cover),

To my Refractive Surgery Clinical Team at CCF, to Amy, Kelly, Ann, Regina, Jenny, Alan, Kim, and Sharon, and to my secretary, Bobbi, for keeping my clinical and professional life organized and running efficiently, so I have time to travel and pursue noble educational goals, such as the writing of this book!

Finally, to Stephen Trokel, MD, who 20 years ago (December 1983) wrote the first article on excimer laser photoablation of the cornea. Without that article, his mentorship, and input, I would not have entered into this field in the first place.

Ronald R. Krueger, MD, MSE

I wish to acknowledge scholars before my time; my mentors, coeditors, colleagues, students, and family; and the financial support of the National Eye Institute.

My work, like that of others, is built upon the shoulders of scientists and clinicians who took the time to write down their findings and observations in archival journals for future students to study, learn, and use as a foundation in their own work. I am routinely amazed and embarrassed to find that my "unique contributions" have already been published. Gerald Westheimer first brought this obvious and often overlooked truth to my attention. He kindly reminded me that I could save weeks and months of work in the laboratory with an hour or so in the library.

I am fortunate to have had many mentors, a fraction of whom I list here. I thank and acknowledge Lee Guth for taking this green undergraduate into his lab; Jim Huff for letting me build equipment and participate in his experiments as an undergraduate; Gordon Heath for taking the time to encourage; and my graduate advisor Tony Adams for providing me academic and scientific freedom uncommon for a graduate student—his contribution to my career is unsurpassed. Thanks also to Russ DeValois for his evening seminars and for expertly modeling critical thinking; Gerald Westheimer for the one-on-one interactions that gave final root to my love of ocular optics; Jay Enoch for modeling scientific integrity by retracting a paper; and Bob Massof for offering scientific opportunity and friendship at Wilmer during my early days as an assistant professor when I was starving for scientific opportunity.

I am honored to be able to work with two exceptionally talented coeditors. I thank and acknowledge Ron Krueger for his creative energy, his ability to quickly absorb, and his faith in God—it rubs off—and Scott MacRae for balance, insight, and the shared desire to create an academic balance between clinical and basic science that communicates to both. As editors, we have built the rare trust that withstands disagreements, confrontations, and the shared joy of accomplishment. It is a treasure I value deeply.

My colleagues, students, and postdoctoral fellows make every day a day of discovery and a scientific challenge. I am compelled to acknowledge a few individuals and apologize to those I should have listed. I wish to thank and acknowledge Larry Thibos, Arthur Bradley, Howard Howland, Ed Sarver, Joe Harrison, Wick van Heuven, Gene Hilmantel, Austin Roorda, David Williams, Bill Donnelly, Jason Marsack, and Konrad Pesudovs for helping to make my scientific life fun and challenging.

I wish to acknowledge my children—Aaron, Ryan, Camille, and Olivia—for their love, support, and faith in my abilities. Most of all I wish to acknowledge Rachel—my best friend, companion, and the love of my life.

Finally, I acknowledge my grant reviewers and the dedicated people at the National Eye Institute for funding my research efforts through most of my career, beginning with a postdoctoral fellowship (F32 EY05201), an AREA grant (R15 EY008005), R01 grant funding (RO1 EY10097 and R01 EY08520), and a CORE grant (P30EYO7551-15) to the College of Optometry. Without this support, it would have been difficult—if not impossible—to establish the scientific position allowing me to serve as a coeditor.

Raymond A. Applegate, OD, PhD

I am fortunate to work with many generous and talented individuals who have mentored, supported, and inspired me over the years. I am grateful for the mentorship of Mathew Davis, MD; Hank Edelhauser, PhD; and Fritz Fraundfelder, MD, who nurtured me in my early quest as a clinician and scientist. Each gave me room to grow in their own unique ways. I'm deeply grateful to Larry Rich, MD, my former partner who I worked with for 17 years in Oregon at the Casey Eye Institute. Larry introduced me to the field of refractive surgery as well as the works of the great Jose Barrequer, MD, and taught me the fine art of lamellar surgery.

I have worked with and enjoyed the professional inspiration of many exceptionally talented individuals, including George Waring, MD; Doug Koch, MD; Dan Durrie, MD; Steve Slade, MD; Marguerite McDonald, MD; Paolo Vinciguerra, MD; Roberto Zaldivar, MD; Arturo Chayet, MD; Howard Gimbel, MD; Jay Pepose, MD; Cindy Roberts, PhD; and Jim Schwiegerling, PhD. There are many more gifted friends too numerous to mention who also have enriched my journey in ophthalmology and on a personal level.

I am extremely fortunate to work with the very talented University of Rochester staff of Joseph Stamm, OD; Gary Gagarinas; Gina Crowley; Brenda Houtenbrink; and Jennifer Anstey, whose careful, diligent hours of hard work and careful observation helped generate important data that thrust the field forward, while keeping it fun for patients and staff alike. I am also very grateful to be able to work with an exceptionally talented team of basic scientists, including Jason Porter, MS; Guenyoung Yoon, PhD; Krystal Huxlin, PhD; Ian Cox, PhD; and David Williams, PhD. They are a great scientific team to work with and just a great group of people as well.

I am indebted to Peter Slack for taking a chance and encouraging us to pursue writing the first volume of this book. Who would have guessed that the field would have exploded so quickly to warrant a second volume of this series? We are lucky to have the thoughtful editing and wonderful support of Amy McShane, April Billick, and Lauren Biddle Plummer, who have persevered to make this second volume a reality.

I also want to thank my coauthors, Ron Krueger and Ray Applegate, who share their tremendous passion and insight into the field of wavefront correction of refractive errors that inspires and excites me. I am grateful to all the authors who have taken time from their busy schedules to share their important observations, the glue that holds this field together. We are indebted to those refractive surgeons who have gone before us and those who follow in our footsteps. May their path be blessed by the joy I have experienced encountering the many wonderful people mentioned as well as countless others.

Scott M. MacRae, MD

About the Editors

Ronald R. Krueger, MD, MSE, is the first of two children born to Arthur and Lucie Krueger, German immigrants and Godly, Christian parents. He was born in Elizabeth, NJ in 1960, and at a young age committed his life to a relationship with Jesus Christ.

Professionally, Dr. Krueger received his MD degree from the University of Medicine and Dentistry of New Jersey (1987). Prior to that, he received a BS in Electrical Engineering from Rutgers University and an MSE in Biomedical Engineering from the University of Washington, Seattle. He completed his ophthalmology residency at the Columbia-Presbyterian Medical Center, New York, NY. He also completed two fellowships in cornea and refractive surgery from the University of Oklahoma, Oklahoma City, Okla and the University of Southern California, Los Angeles, Calif. In 1993, he joined the department of ophthalmology at the University of Missouri—St. Louis, St. Louis, Mo where he was an associate professor of ophthalmology. He then joined the Cleveland Clinic Foundation in 1998 and serves as the medical director of the department of refractive surgery, overseeing a large department of six surgeons and support staff as well as maintaining his own full schedule of patients. He is on the program planning committee of the American Academy of Ophthalmology and the International Society of Refractive Surgery and is an associate editor for the *Journal of Refractive Surgery*. He is cofounder and organizer of the International Congress on Wavefront Sensing and Aberration-Free Refractive Correction. He has 20 years of experience in excimer laser research, and currently is investigating the causes of presbyopia and restoration of accommodation, as well as wavefront imaging of the eye for customized laser vision correction. He is an international lecturer and is widely published.

Raymond A. Applegate, OD, PhD, is the second of four children born to K. Edwin Applegate and Elizabeth Dilts Applegate. He was born in Bloomington, Ind in 1949 and attended Indiana University from Kindergarten through his Bachelor of Arts (1971), Doctor of Optometry (1975), and his Master of Science in Physiological Optics (1976). He practiced optometry in Galesburg, Ill before continuing his graduate education in Physiological Optics at the University of California, Berkeley where he received his PhD (1983). Dr. Applegate joined the University of Texas Health Science Center faculty in 1988 from the School of Optometry, University of Missouri—St. Louis where he served as an assistant professor of optometry. He rose through the faculty ranks quickly to become a tenured professor of ophthalmology in 1993. In January 2002, Dr. Applegate joined the College of Optometry at the University of Houston as Professor and Borish Chair in Optometry to direct the Visual Optics Institute. Dr. Applegate has served on the editorial board of *Optometry and Visual Science* and currently serves on the editorial boards for the *Journal of Refractive Surgery* and the *Journal of Cataract and Refractive Surgery*. He has been a feature editor on several occasions for the *Journal of the Optical Society of America-A, Applied Optics, Optometry and Vision Science*, and the *Journal of Refractive Surgery*. He is a cofounder of the International Congress on Wavefront Sensing and Aberration-Free Refraction Correction, is widely published in leading journals, and is a sought-after consultant and international lecturer whose National Institutes of Health-supported research interests center on the optics of the normal and clinical eye and early ocular disease detection and prevention.

Scott M. MacRae, MD, did his undergraduate, medical school, and residency program at the University of Wisconsin, Madison. He did three corneal fellowships including a cornea and external disease fellowship and a NEI-sponsored corneal physiology research training fellowship both at the Eye Institute, Medical College of Wisconsin, Milwaukee. He then did a brief contact lens and light toxicity fellowship at Emory University in Atlanta (1983).

In 1983, Dr. MacRae joined the faculty of Oregon Health Sciences University, Casey Eye Institute, in 1983 through 2000. He served as a panel member and consultant to the FDA Ophthalmic Devices Panel from 1986 to 2000, chaired the American Academy of Ophthalmology Public Health Committee from 1991 to 1994, and ran the American Academy of Ophthalmology Clinical Alert Program. He was an advisor to the White House in 1993 on two separate panels on health care delivery and served as a congressional advisor as well.

He has received an Honor Award in 1991 and the Senior Honor Award in 2000 from the American Academy of Ophthalmology. He has won numerous awards, including the Illinois Society to Prevent Blindness Young Researcher Award, The Kambara Award, The Amini Award (2003), and The Oregonian Citizen Winners Award. In 2003, he received the Lans Lectureship Award, which is an international award given to an outstanding young clinician researcher in the field of refractive surgery by the International Society of Refractive Surgery and the American Academy of Ophthalmology.

Author of over 100 published articles and book chapters, Dr. MacRae has turned his attention increasingly to refractive surgery and the development of new technology. He has spoken at over 300 meetings both in the United States and internationally. He has a special interest in customized ablation, the biomechanics of laser in-situ keratomileusis, laser subepithelial keratomileusis, astigmatism design, and interface keratitis. He has trained hundreds of clinicians, residents, and fellows and has participated and helped lead several Food and Drug Administration clinical trials in the United States, including the Nidek Oregon Kansas Study and the University of Rochester Zyoptix Customized Ablation Study. He holds a patent on the excimer laser treatment of astigmatism and has two other patents pending in the field of laser refractive surgery.

On the editorial board of three ophthalmic journals, he is currently senior associate editor for the *Journal of Refractive Surgery*, has coedited three special editions of the *Journal of Refractive Surgery*, and has chaired numerous international refractive symposiums. He is senior editor of a best-selling book in ophthalmology, *Customized Corneal Ablation: The Quest for SuperVision*, which is the first volume of this series.

In 2000, Dr. MacRae accepted an appointment as Professor of Ophthalmology and Professor of Visual Science at the University of Rochester, NY, where with the Center for Vision Science at the university and private industry he promotes research and development of new refractive surgery techniques and technology.

Contributors

Noel Alpins, FRACO, FRCOphth, FACS
Medical Director
New Vision Clinics
Melbourne, Australia

David J. Apple, MD
John A. Moran Eye Center
University of Utah
Salt Lake City, Utah

Pablo Artal, PhD
Laboratorio de Optica
Departamento de Física
Universidad de Murcia
Campus de Espinardo (Edificio C)
Murcia, Spain

Dimitri T. Azar, MD
Cornea and Refractive Surgery Service
Department of Ophthalmology
Massachusetts Eye and Ear Infirmary
Boston, Mass

Harkaran S. Bains
Nidek Clinical Director
Freemont, Calif

Sergio Barbero, MSc
Instituto de Optica
Consejo Superior de Investigaciones Científicas
Madrid, Spain

Michael Bergt, PhD
Carl Zeiss Meditec AG
Jena, Germany

Arthur Bradley, PhD
School of Optometry
Indiana University
Bloomington, Ind

Stephen A. Burns, PhD
Schepens Eye Research Institute
Boston, Mass

Philip M. Buscemi, OD
President
Battleground Eye Care
Greensboro, NC
Vice President/General Manager
Nidek Technologies America
Greensboro, NC

Charles E. Campbell, BS
Consultant, Ophthalmic Optics and Instrumentation
Berkeley, Calif

John A. Campin, BSc
Alcon Orlando Technology Center
Orlando, Fla

Jonathan D. Carr, MD, MA, FRCOphth
Emory Vision
Atlanta, Ga

Maria Regina Chalita, MD
Study Coordinator/Research Fellow
Cole Eye Institute
The Cleveland Clinic
Cleveland, Ohio

Shiao Chang, PhD
Calhoun Vision, Inc
Pasadena, Calif

Puwat Charukamnoetkanok, MD
Cornea and Refractive Surgery Service
Department of Ophthalmology
Massachusetts Eye and Ear Infirmary
Boston, Mass

Arturo Chayet, MD
Codet Eye Institute
Tijuana, Mexico

Li Chen, PhD
Center for Visual Science
University of Rochester
Rochester, NY

James Copland, MS
Wavefront Sciences
Albuquerque, NM

Ian Cox, PhD
Research Clinic
Bausch & Lomb
Rochester, NY

Arthur Cummings, MBChB, MMed, FCS(SA) FRCSEd
Wellington Ophthalmic Laser Clinic
Dublin, Ireland

Daniel S. Durrie, MD
Clinical Associate Professor
University of Kansas Medical Center
Durrie Vision
Kansas City, Kan

Jose Garcia, BS
Emory Vision
Atlanta, Ga

Harilaos Ginis, PhD
University Hospital of Crete
Department of Ophthalmology
Heraklion, Greece

Antonio Guirao, PhD
Laboratorio de Optica
Departamento de Física
Universidad de Murcia
Campus de Espinardo (Edificio C)
Murcia, Spain

Farhad Hafezi, MD
IROC AG, Institut für Refractive und Ophthalmo Chirurgie
Zürich, Switzerland

Gene Hilmantel, OD, MS
Food and Drug Administration
Center for Devices and Radiological Health
Office of Device Evaluation
Division of Ophthalmic and Ear, Nose, and Throat Devices
Rockville, Md

Arthur Ho, MOptom, PhD
Vision Cooperative Research Center
Sydney, Australia

Heidi Hofer, PhD
Center for Visual Science
University of Rochester
Rochester, NY

Howard C. Howland, MS, PhD
Department of Neurobiology and Behavior
Cornell University
Ithaca, NY

David Huang, MD, PhD
Cole Eye Institute
The Cleveland Clinic
Cleveland, Ohio

Hans Peter Iseli, MD
IROC AG, Institut für Refractive und Ophthalmo Chirurgie
Zurich, Switzerland

Mirko Jankov, MD
Departamento de Oftalmologia, Santa Casa de São Paulo, Brasil
Setor de Bioengenharia, Departamento de Oftalmologia,
Universidade Federal de São Paulo/EPM, Brasil

Joel A.D. Javier, MD
Cornea and Refractive Surgery Service
Department of Ophthalmology
Massachusetts Eye and Ear Infirmary
Boston, Mass

Vikentia J. Katsanevaki, MD, PhD
University of Crete Medical School
Vardinoyannion Eye Institute of Crete
Heraklion, Crete, Greece
University Hospital of Crete
Department of Ophthalmology
Heraklion, Greece

Douglas D. Koch, MD
Cullen Eye Institute
Baylor College of Medicine
Houston, Tex

Gilles Lafond, MD, FRCS(C)
Centre Hospitalier de l'Université Laval
Québec City, Canada

Michele Lagana, OD
Research Clinic
Bausch & Lomb
Rochester, NY

Junzhong Liang, PhD
VISX Incorporated
Santa Clara, Calif

Henia Lichter, MD
Emory Vision
Atlanta, Ga

Nick Mamalis, MD
John A. Moran Eye Center
University of Utah
Salt Lake City, Utah

Fabrice Manns, PhD
Department of Biomedical Engineering
University of Miami College of Engineering
Coral Gables, Fla

Susana Marcos, PhD
Instituto de Optica
Consejo Superior de Investigaciones Científicas
Madrid, Spain

Matthias Maus, MD
VisuMed AG
Cologne, Germany

Marguerite B. MacDonald, MD
Southern Vision Institute
New Orleans, La

James S. McLellan, PhD
Schepens Eye Research Institute
Boston, Mass

Ulrich Mester, MD
Department of Ophthalmology
Bundesknappschaft's Hospital
Sulzbach, Germany

Sergiy Molebny, MSc
National Technical University of Ukraine
Kiev, Ukraine
Tracey Technologies, LLC
Houston, Tex

Vasyl Molebny, PhD, DSc
Institute of Biomedical Engineering of the Academy of Technological Sciences of Ukraine
Kiev, Ukraine

Michael Mrochen, PhD
IROC AG, Institut für Refractive und Ophthalmo Chirurgie
Swiss Federal Institute of Technology, Institute of Biomedical Engineering
Zurich, Switzerland

Zoltan Z. Nagy, MD, PhD
1st Department of Ophthalmology
Semmelweis University
Budapest, Hungary

Daniel R. Neal, PhD
WaveFront Sciences
Albuquerque, NM

Ioannis Pallikaris, MD, PhD
University of Crete Medical School
Vardinoyannion Eye Institute of Crete
Heraklion, Crete, Greece
University Hospital of Crete
Department of Ophthalmology
Heraklion, Greece

Sophia I. Panagopoulou, PhD
University of Crete Medical School
Vardinoyannion Eye Institute of Crete
Heraklion, Crete, Greece

Seth Pantanelli, BS
Department of Biomedical Engineering
University of Rochester
Rochester, NY

George H. Pettit, MD, PhD
Alcon Orlando Technology Center
Orlando, Fla

Patricia Piers
Department of Applied Research
Pfizer Groningen BV
Groningen, Netherlands

Sotiris Plainis, PhD
Research Associate
Optometry and Neuroscience
Manchester, United Kingdom

Jason Porter, MS
Center for Visual Science
University of Rochester
Rochester, NY

Dan Z. Reinstein, MD, MA (Cantab), FRCSC
London Vision Clinic
St. Thomas' Hospital
Kings College London
University of London
London, United Kingdom
Weill Medical College of Cornell University
New York, NY
Centre Hospitalier National d'Ophtalmologie des Quinzes Vingts
Paris, France

Austin Roorda, PhD
University of Houston College of Optometry
Houston, Tex

Christian A. Sandstedt, PhD
Calhoun Vision, Inc
Pasadena, Calif

Leisa Schmid, PhD
The Laservision Centre
Southport Qld
Australia

Eckhard Schroeder, PhD
Carl Zeiss Meditec AG
Jena, Germany

Daniel M. Schwartz, MD
University of California
San Francisco Medical School
Department of Ophthalmology
San Francisco, Calif

Jim Schwiegerling, PhD
Department of Ophthalmology and Optical Sciences
University of Arizona
Tucson, Ariz

Theo Seiler, MD, PhD
IROC AG, Institut für Refractive und Ophthalmo Chirurgie
Zürich, Switzerland

Mario G. Serrano, MD
Scientific Director
Bogota Laser Refractive Institute
Bogota, Colombia

Steven Slade, MD
Private and Clinical Practice Faculty
University of Texas at Houston
Houston, Tex

Erin D. Stahl
Durrie Vision
University of Kansas Medical Center
Kansas City, Kan

P. Randall Staver, MS
Emory Vision
Atlanta, Ga

R. Doyle Stulting, MD, PhD
Emory Vision
Atlanta, Ga

N.E. Sverker Norrby, PhD
Department of Applied Research
Pfizer Groningen BV
Groningen, Netherlands

Gustavo E. Tamayo, MD
President
Bogota Laser Refractive Institute
Aruba Laser Refractive Institute
Bogota, Colombia

Natalie Taylor, PhD
SensoMotoric Instruments GmbH
Teltow, Germany

Winfried Teiwes, Dr Ing
SensoMotoric Instruments GmbH
Teltow, Germany

Larry N. Thibos, PhD
School of Optometry
Indiana University
Bloomington, Ind

Keith P. Thompson, MD
Emory Vision
Atlanta, Ga

Daniel Topa
WaveFront Sciences
Albuquerque, NM

Stefan Tuess, Dip Eng
VisuMed AG
Cologne, Germany

Hartmut Vogelsang, PhD
Carl Zeiss Meditec AG
Jena, Germany

Liliana Werner, MD, PhD
John A. Moran Eye Center
University of Utah
Salt Lake City, Utah

David R. Williams, PhD
Center for Visual Science
University of Rochester
Rochester, NY

Geunyoung Yoon, PhD
Department of Ophthalmology
University of Rochester
Rochester, NY

Foreword

Twenty years ago, a few groups across the world started to investigate the application of excimer lasers in ophthalmology.

There was a group in New York, which included Steve Trokel, Dobly Srinivasan, and a young student named Ron Krueger, that did basic research regarding photoablation of the cornea. (As a side note, the term photoablation was not yet coined.) Other groups sprung up in London (John Marshall) and in Berlin (Josef Wollensak and Theo Seiler). Very soon, we started using the excimer laser for therapeutic ablations in 1986 and we commenced pilot trials on photorefractive keratectomy in 1988.

The focus of this photorefractive approach was to correct myopic refractive errors. Based on the refractive experience with radial keratotomy, the expectations of doctors and patients regarding quality of vision were low. The typical criterion of success was that 60% of the operated eyes were within ±1 diopter (D) from emmetropia, and the criterion of safety was that less than 5% of the eyes lost two Snellen lines or more. Patients suffered severe pain during the first days after surgery and it took a month before normal visual acuity was obtained.

The next step in the evolution was to make the operation more tolerable for the patient. Laser in-situ keratomileusis (LASIK) came along, offering a much faster visual rehabilitation within days and significantly less pain after surgery. The early dreams of an extended refractive range of correction (up to -20 D), however, did not come true. Also, the quality of vision was still not a high priority; most of the scientific reports did not even mention glare and low contrast visual acuity.

Human vision has many dimensions, among others are form recognition, movement recognition, and color vision. In the standard ophthalmology practice, only a tiny part of this multidimensional network called vision is examined. High contrast visual acuity tested by means of Snellen charts is the most common method of examination, but it is descriptive only for a small portion of vision, even of form recognition. Patient complaints about deteriorated vision after ablative refractive surgery led us to other alternative examination methods—such as contrast sensitivity testing, low contrast visual acuity, glare testing, and aberrometry—to quantify these complaints. During these evaluations, we learned that we have to individualize the ablation profile in order to not deteriorate vision, especially mesopic vision.

This individualization of ablation is the next step in the evolution of refractive surgery and is the main topic of this book. We have entered a new era in refractive surgery and have to perform much basic research, not only in physiologic optics but also including neuronal processing of optical information. Such basic research involves natural scientists and, therefore, we should not be surprised to find many PhDs among the authors in this book.

A serious bottleneck of any new development in medicine is the education of medical practitioners who are handicapped by the conventional medical education that is based only marginally on natural science and more on a "medicine as an experience" science. This book is an excellent approach to overcoming this problem; it merges basic science and clinical experience.

I read this book with great pleasure (and learned a lot) and wish the reader the same pleasure in understanding the "new" refractive surgery to the benefit of our patients.

Theo Seiler, MD, PhD
Professor
Institut für Refraktive und Ophthalmo-Chirurgie (IROC)
Zurich, Switzerland

Introduction

In the span of 20 years, excimer refractive surgery has developed from a hotly debated hypothesis based on a handful of animal experiments into a widely accepted technology that has been successfully applied to millions of patients. This success has been due to the many people who devoted extraordinary efforts to understanding the nature of the interaction of far ultraviolet (UV) light with the cornea and to developing the complex technology that has been so successful in correcting human refractive errors. Ronald Krueger has been one of the few people who was and is present for this technical evolution and symbolizes the struggle of the early years and the movement toward maturation, success, and acceptance of the technology. At the outset, Ron, as a medical student, explored the tissue interactions of the high-powered pulsed UV lasers. He helped develop data measuring ablation thresholds and rates and explored the ultra-structure of both the acute lesions and the healed ablated areas in the corneas of rabbit and then monkey eyes.

These experiments gave increasing confidence that tissue could be removed from the cornea with a predictable pattern. The recognition of tissue removal of layers less thick than a quarter of the wavelength of light was strong evidence that this would be a potent technology for the reshaping of the cornea and the controlled modification of the optical properties of the eye. It was the successful ablation of a 3.5 mm series of circles in monkey corneas that drove the investment into commercial development of the instrumentation. However, the barriers to successful expression of the technology appeared formidable. It was evident from considerations of tissue ablation rates that exposure times of 15 seconds to almost 1 minute would be necessary for adequate tissue removal to achieve the bulk of optical corrections. It was also evident that, for this technology to succeed, it would have to be extremely safe with a biological and optical complication rate that was very, very low.

In spite of the difficulties that were immediately apparent, the limitations of existing technology for the correction of refractive errors were widely recognized and alternate solutions were avidly sought. The ametropic patient was frustrated by the technical limitations of his or her spectacles and contact lenses and the ophthalmic surgeon was inhibited by the complication rate, unpredictability, and optical imperfections of existing refractive surgical techniques. The energy generated by this desire by patients for alternate surgical technology and the surgeon's frustration with the status quo became the driving force behind the enormous investment of time, energy, and capital into the development of clinically practical excimer laser systems.

The first commercial prototype designed to reshape the cornea was shown at the academy exhibition floor in 1987 and generated interest, resistance, and disbelief. There was enthusiastic interest in an alternate technology to radial keratotomy, marked resistance to the idea that anyone would touch the center of a normal cornea, and general disbelief in the idea that it could ever be made safe enough to engender wide acceptance.

However, early success led to the development of increasingly accurate excimer laser systems that forced the development of increasingly accurate optical analyzers of the eye. First came marked improvements in corneal topography and a widely distributed clinical instrument evolved from what had been an esoteric laboratory tool present in only a handful of centers. The increasing necessity of precision alignment during the protracted ablation drove the development of precision trackers and alignment technologies. Finally, as the accuracy of the clinical results approached our ability to measure the manifest refraction, improvements in refractive technology were sought. This has resulted in the development of aberrometers using wavefront technology and has produced clinical devices that have become simple to use yet allow precision analysis of the optical details of the eye. This development has been the first major change in refractive technology since the manifest refraction evolved in the mid-19th century.

The importance of this development is reflected in this new book, which covers the optical theories underlying aberration analysis and the practical application of the technology. Raymond Applegate has been a pioneer in optical analysis of the eye and Scott MacRae an avid clinical investigator of the details of excimer laser refractive surgery. They explore in detail the basis of this new technology. The results show that when the sphere and cylinder and also the higher-order symmetrical and asymmetrical aberrations are corrected, not only has the resulting visual acuity improved but, equally important, the quality of vision has also improved. We have seen the virtual disappearance of unwanted optical effects as we have seen an overall improvement in visual acuity. We can anticipate that understanding aberration patterns will also allow development of patterns that will increase the depth of field of the final refraction and do much to ease the discomfort of the presbyopic eye.

Wavefront customized ablation is also a tool that allows us to handle complex and difficult problems that have had no ready surgical solutions in the past. Not only can aberrations be reduced in normal eyes, but the technology allows us to improve vision in injured or previously operated eyes that had been beyond our technical abilities.

Wavefront customized visual correction is one of those rare technical advances that not only makes the technique more effective in terms of quality of vision, but also has increased its safety. It is this latter perception that will drive acceptance of excimer laser surgery to become an alternative to the 1000-year-old technology of spectacles and the 65-year-old technology of contact lenses. The detailing of the refractive measurement of the eye as well as the maturation of the laser technology have gradually eroded the objections of ophthalmic surgeons and have made refractive surgery a legitimate alternative standard of care to spectacles and contact lenses. It is important to understand new technology as we use it clinically. This book brings together—from many diverse sources—all the elements needed to understand and apply this essential new technology.

Stephen Trokel, MD
Professor of Clinical Ophthalmology
Columbia University Medical Center
New York, NY
December 19, 2003

Preface

What is this book about? Is this book a second edition to *Customized Corneal Ablation: The Quest for Super Vision*, which was published 3 years ago, or the second volume in a series of wavefront customization books with new material and new ideas that are nonrepetitive, but additive to the previous volume? In some respects, it is a little of both—a second edition and a second volume. Although some of the chapters are of similar content, the bulk of the material in this book is newer and broader than the material in the first book. Even the title, *Wavefront Customized Visual Corrections: The Quest for Super Vision II*, talks about a more general overview of customization of vision rather than specific corneal ablation. Much of this broad coverage of the field of wavefront customization is well outlined by the various sections of the book, which expand upon the previous book. Yet in a similar way, it still covers the basic science as well as the clinical science of each section.

In Section I, the first five chapters of the book cover introductory concepts of wavefront customization. These introductory concepts begin with the introduction of customization in the first chapter, followed by a review of where we have been in Chapters 2 and 4. Finally, we outline the concepts of where we are going with customization in Chapters 3 and 5.

In Section II, we deal with the measurement and reporting of wavefront aberrometry. In the Basic Science subsection, a great deal of important information is presented regarding the assessment of optical quality and visual performance in Chapters 6 and 7, as well as new metrics for predicting wavefront aberration impact on vision and improvements in sampling and fitting in Chapter 8 and 9, respectively. The impact of chromatic aberration, aging changes, and other temporal aspects of aberrations are covered in Chapters 10, 11, and 12. Finally, the impact of accommodation dynamics and pupil size is covered in Chapters 13 and 14, respectively.

In the Clinical Science subsection, the commercially available aberrometers are conceptually described in terms of their diagnostic parameters and capabilities. Shack-Hartmann aberrometry, which is the most popular method of recording wavefront error, is covered in Chapters 15 and 16, while retinal imaging aberrometry using Tscherning and ray tracing principles are covered in Chapters 17 and 18, respectively. Finally, the unique methods of retinoscopic double pass aberrometry as well as spatially resolved refractometry are covered in Chapters 19 and 20, with a closing evaluation of the comparative reproducibility of multiple wavefront devices in Chapter 21.

Section III reviews similar concepts to the information in the previous book, however with modification and in-depth expansion based on new information over the past 3 years. The physics and technology requirements of customized corneal ablation, including eye tracking and alignment, are covered in Chapters 22, 23, and 24. Chapter 25 replaces the chapter on corneal biomechanics that appeared in the previous book and covers the important potential limitation of predictability in customized corneal ablation outcomes. Finally, in the Clinical Science subsection, data of the customized ablation platforms and outcomes are reported for each of the laser systems, including Alcon, VISX, Bausch & Lomb, Carl Zeiss Meditec, WaveLight, and Nidek in Chapters 26 through 31, respectively.

Beyond customized corneal ablation, new concepts of customization regarding ocular lenses are covered in Section IV. The four chapters in this section cover the following: biomaterials for wavefront customization in Chapter 32, customized contact lenses in Chapter 33, aspheric profile intraocular lenses in Chapter 34, and laser adjustable intraocular lenses in Chapter 35.

Finally, in Section V, customization extends beyond that which we measure with just an aberrometer. In the Basic Science subsection, corneal topography in customization and synchronizating corneal surface aberrations with total ocular aberrations are covered in Chapters 36 and 37, while vector compensation for wavefront and topographic astigmatism is covered in Chapter 38. In the last three clinically oriented chapters, customized topographic ablation using the VISX CAP method and a surgeon-guided retreatment of irregular astigmatism are addressed in Chapters 39 and 40, with Chapter 41 probing into customized presbyopia correction—a new and exciting development of clinical customization used for expanding the dynamic range of vision correction.

The final section and chapter of the book covers the future of customization, which is a forward look into where we are going in this field. In all, the concepts addressed in this book cover a broad view of the many aspects of customization and reveal a central theme and purpose for pursuing and expanding our knowledge in this area—the quest for super vision. We welcome the reader to participate in this journey with us, as the insights we cover in this book and new concepts revealed in future books are all part of a collective sharing and expansion of knowledge for which not only the authors, but also the readers play an important part.

Ronald R. Krueger, MD, MSE
Raymond A. Applegate, OD, PhD
Scott M. MacRae, MD

Section I

Introduction

Chapter 1

An Introduction to Wavefront-Guided Visual Correction

Scott M. MacRae, MD; Raymond A. Applegate, OD, PhD; and Ronald R. Krueger, MD, MSE

We live in a time of wondrous change. Customized correction of refractive errors using wavefront technology is revolutionizing the way we think of and treat refractive errors. There are two reasons for this paradigm shift. The first is that wavefront technology has allowed us to treat not only second-order aberrations, sphere and cylinder, but also higher-order aberrations such as coma and spherical aberrations which exist in normal individuals as well as postrefractive surgery patients. There is an important transformation occurring in ophthalmic optics.

> We have been correcting second-order aberrations such as myopia, hyperopia, and astigmatism for the past 200 years and are now on the verge of being able to detect and correct higher-order aberrations with laser refractive surgery, contact lenses, and intraocular lenses (IOLs).

The second major shift is perhaps even more fundamental. Until now, eye care practitioners have worked primarily to preserve vision in their patients but have not seen it as their role to enhance vision beyond what nature has designed. With the advent of adaptive optics, it seems possible to correct most of the eye's aberrations and improve contrast beyond what we viewed as normal previously. For some patients, this is a trivial improvement, but in some cases, visual performance can be improved considerably. Thus, there is a subtle but important shift in our view of ophthalmic optics and the potential of the human visual system. This book explores the intricate shift in thinking that wavefront technology and adaptive optics have introduced to this exciting field.

Wavefront Correction Strategy: Normalization vs Customization

Normalization

There are two major strategies taken in correcting higher-order aberration. The first is to take wavefront data from a population, such as the amount of positive spherical aberration in postmyopic laser in-situ keratomileusis (LASIK) eyes, and apply a correction factor that minimizes the positive corneal spherical aberration noted in subsequent treatments. This same strategy is used when one measures the spherical aberration in preoperative cataract surgery eyes and compensates for this by incorporating negative spherical aberration in the IOLs used to treat this population. This strategy uses information from an average (normalized) population and applies it to the population being treated using wavefront sensing to minimize higher-order aberration. It is not a "customized" correction but a "normalized" correction based on an average in a population of similar age. This strategy tends to be used with radially symmetric higher-order aberration, such as spherical aberration. It is not, however, a customized correction.

> Normalization is different from customization because it uses a normalized correction based on an average in the population rather than an individual customized wavefront to determine the treatment.

Customization

The second strategy is to use wavefront measurements to guide higher-order aberration correction for each eye on a "customized" basis. This strategy is being employed by most of the excimer laser companies and surgeons who are attempting to correct lower- and higher-order aberrations using customized ablation.

In reality, laser manufacturers use a combination of these two strategies even in customized ablation. Eyes are measured for spherical aberration preoperatively, but empirical "correction factors" are introduced by laser manufacturers to compensate for the increase in spherical aberration, which is introduced by the laser procedure itself. This combination strategy is employed to optimize the result for each eye.[1]

What is Customization?

Webster's Dictionary defines customize as "to build, fit, or alter according to individual specifications or needs."[2]

We all customize. In a sense, our lives are customized based on our genetics, background, and environment. In a similar way, customized corneal ablation is based on our patients' underlying genetics, which largely determine their anatomy and in turn their refractive error. Corneal customization is based on our ability to detect significant optical abnormalities or wavefront errors and correct them. This chapter will outline the various ways we as clinicians and surgeons can customize treatment to optimize our patients' vision while maximizing safety.

One Size Does Not Fit All

Customized ablation attempts to optimize the eye's optical system using a variety of spherical, cylindrical, aspherical, and asymmetrical treatments based on an individual eye's optics and anatomy, as well as the patient's needs and preferences. Customization can be used to improve optical quality in normal eyes, as well as eyes with atypical optical aberrations caused by corneal scarring, penetrating keratoplasty, central islands, decentered ablations, lenticular abnormalities, and spherical IOL implants.

> Customized correction involves three forms of customization: functional, anatomical, and optical. All three need to be utilized to optimize the patient's results.

Ways to Customize

Vision is a complex process and can be divided into at least two broad subsections: optics and neural processing. Customization of corneal laser treatment to correct the refractive errors of the eye falls under the optics section. Translating the retinal image into a neural precept is neural processing. The focus of this book is on new methods to create an optimal retinal image. Creating an optimal retinal image requires consideration of several interactive factors. These factors can be broken into three classes: 1) functional, 2) anatomical, and 3) optical (Table 1-1).

Functional Factors in Customization

Functional factors require an understanding of the patient's individual needs and circumstances, including the patient's age, refraction, occupation, and personal optical requirements (eg, monovision), as well as adaptability. Let us explore two of these areas in more detail.

Age Considerations

Experience has taught us that age is an important consideration when treating patients with laser refractive surgery. A number of studies have shown that myopic patients over the age of 40 to 45 are more susceptible to hyperopic overcorrection.[3-5] Further, in our experience, treating younger patients with myopia more aggressively and hyperopia less aggressively than recommended with current age adjusted nomograms results in higher patient satisfaction. The reason is that young eyes generally have a large range of accommodation, so a slight hyperopic overcorrection is not as devastating. Conversely, we tend to treat older patients more aggressively for hyperopia and less aggressively for myopia to leave them emmetropic or slightly myopic since they have limited accommodative amplitudes. On the other hand, older myopic eyes that are overcorrected would be blurred at both distance and near. Further, a slight undercorrection for the older myope can provide functional near vision for many near tasks.

Monovision and Mini-Monovision

In addition to appropriate age adjustments, presbyopic patients may also benefit from monovision, which renders one eye mildly myopic (typically the nondominant eye) by 1 to 1.5 diopters (D), or mini-monovision (0.25 to 0.75 D). There are many factors affecting whether or not monovision is appropriate for a particular patient, including his or her occupational and recreational needs, and perhaps most importantly, motivation. If he or she has never experienced monovision, fitting the patient with disposable contact lenses to simulate monovision is very helpful in guiding him or her in his or her decision for or against monovision.[6,7]

Anatomical Factors in Customization

Anatomical factors require the consideration of individual anatomical variations of each eye, including the patient's pupil size in bright and dim light conditions,[8-13] and the corneal diameter and thickness prior to surgery. LASIK flap considerations are dependent on ablation design, and corneal thickness limits the amount of refractive error that can be safely treated.

LASIK Flap Considerations

LASIK flaps are often customized depending on ablation design,[14-16] thickness,[13] and diameter,[14] and whether one is treating myopia, hyperopia, or astigmatism. One of the authors prefers a flap size 0.5 to 1 millimeter (mm) larger than the total diameter of the ablation. Since most surgeons prefer to avoid recutting a flap on retreatment, it is preferable to create a larger diameter flap (9.5 mm) when possible (even in myopes) to allow for room to perform a hyperopic retreatment if overcorrection occurs. Studies done on flap thickness and diameter indicate there is considerable variation in flap thickness as well as diameter with commonly used microkeratomes.[17-19] For instance, patients with thin corneas and high refractive error require special consideration. These eyes may require the surgeon to use a thinner flap (120 to 160 as opposed to 180 microns [μm]) and may require reducing the ablation optical zone based on the patient's mesopic pupil size, age, and functional needs. Intraoperative pachymetry may also be more accurate in defining the amount of residual bed after the flap is created with the microkeratome.[20] One study evaluated the Chiron 160 microkeratome (Chiron Vision Corp, Claremont, Calif) fixed plate and found that the mean corneal cap thickness measured 124.8 ± 18.5 μm, indicating the corneal flaps were thinner than predicted by the manufacturers' plate depth measurements.[17] Another study showed progressive thinning/thickening of the flap in the direction toward the hinge, as well as variation in flap diameter, depending on the microkeratome used.[18]

Ablation Diameter Considerations

Hyperopic ablations require larger total diameter ablations (8.5 to 10 mm) compared to myopic ablations (6 to 9.5 mm).[15,21] Individuals with higher astigmatism (> 1.5 D) require larger flaps if they are to have round ablation optical zones with minimal aberrations. Ablation optical zones and their transition to normal corneas that encompass the entire pupil under scotopic conditions are preferable to ablation optical zones that do not encompass the pupil under all physiological pupil diameters.[8-12,22] Larger astigmatic errors require larger transition zones to ensure a smooth transition and avoid regression.[23] Individuals with large amounts of myopic or mixed astigmatism may also benefit from crosscylin-

Table 1-1
Interactive Factors to Consider for Customized Correction

Functional Customization Factors Based on the Needs of the Patient

- Age
- Presbyopia
- Patient's occupational and recreational needs
- Refraction
- Psychological tolerance

Anatomical Factors to Consider for Customized Correction

- Corneal diameter and thickness
- Pupil size (also important for optical customization)
- Anterior chamber depth
- Anterior and posterior lens shape
- Axial length

Optical Factors to Consider for Customized Correction

- Customization based on corneal topography
- Customization based on wavefront measurements
  - Shack-Hartmann wavefront sensor
  - Crosscylinder aberrometer (developed by Howland and Howland)
  - Tscherning aberrometer
  - Tracey system
  - Slit-light bundle
  - Spatially resolved refractometer
  - Others

der ablation that reduces the amount of cylinder to be corrected in each meridian by 50%. This is because one can reduce tissue removal by 20% to 30%, minimize coupling effects, and perhaps improve the optics of the ablation.[24,25] In short, one should consider the ablation design before determining the optimal flap design.

Corneal Thickness Considerations

In corneas that are too thin to safely leave at least a 250-µm bed after LASIK, some surgeons recommend photorefractive keratectomy (PRK), laser epithelial keratomileusis (LASEK), the use of a phakic IOLs, or a combined refractive surgery-IOL procedure.

> We anticipate that the ocular anatomy (eg, posterior cornea shape, anterior chamber depth, the anterior and posterior lens shape as well as thickness) will be interactive and relevant factors when determining which optical designs are optimal for each patient.

For instance, a 18 D myope may be a better candidate for a bioptics procedure, which combines a phakic IOL with LASIK, rather than having LASIK alone.[26,27] The advent of customized contact lenses opens the possibility that thinner kerataconic corneas may be treated with a customized contact lens, as discussed in Chapter 33. Tamayo and coworkers have attempted to correct some kerataconics with customized ablation using the CAP method described in Chapter 39. It remains to be seen which methods are preferable for this patient group.

Optical Customization

Corneal Topographic-Guided Ablation

Corneal first surface aberrations and/or shape can be calculated from corneal elevation data derived from corneal topography measurements[12,28-38] and used along with a standard refraction to design ablative corrections. Using such an approach should reduce aberrations in highly aberrated corneas, but may be detrimental (ie, induce more aberrations) in normal eyes. That is, the potential for visual enhancement beyond the 20/20 level is unknown because formulating the ideal shape for the cornea is not dependent on corneal first surface aberrations alone. Instead, an optimal compensating optic (one that reduces the aberrations of the normal eye) must be designed to negate the aberrations of the whole eye. Corneal topographic-guided ablation has the greatest potential in patients with visual loss known to be related to large corneal topographic abnormalities.

Corneal topography-guided ablation has been attempted on patients with regular and irregular astigmatism, decentered ablations, and central islands.[39-41] The results have been encouraging with regular astigmatism and decentered ablations but require refinement with irregular astigmatism.[38] The irregular astigmatism group is more challenging but may ultimately benefit more from corneal topographic-guided ablation as the systems become more refined.

In a large study on quality of life,[42] it was noted that the second strongest indicator (after visual acuity) of improved quality of life after penetrating keratoplasty was the amount of postoperative astigmatism. Many patients after corneal transplantation complain of not being able to see despite 20/25 to 20/40 vision with a spectacle correction. On closer scrutiny, many of these patients are found to have higher-order aberrations (irregular astigmatism) that produce poor vision. These patients could benefit greatly if we could predictably treat patients with post-trauma or surgical astigmatism who have large amounts of corneal surface irregularity. As one of the remaining frontiers in corneal surgery, correcting very irregular corneal surfaces is explored in detail in Section III of this book. These eyes are particularly challenging because they may have regular and irregular astigmatism amounts that exceed the astigmatic dynamic range of the current wavefront sensors, which is typically around 6 to 8 D. This corneal topography-driven customization may be a helpful first stage treatment to reduce regular and irregular astigmatism, making the cornea symmetric. In the second stage, the more subtle aberrations could be treated with Shack-Hartmann driven customized ablation, which treats the aberrations of the whole eye and removes the more subtle aberrations.

> It is important to stress that corneal topographic-guided ablations will probably be helpful in individuals with topographic abnormalities, but they yet to demonstrate their usefulness in patients with relatively normal corneas with regular astigmatism.

Most experienced refractive surgeons use corneal topography to confirm that the astigmatism is regular and that there is reasonable consistency between the refraction astigmatism and that noted on corneal topography, but their astigmatic treatment is based on the refraction, not the corneal topography. The refraction accounts for the entire optics of the eye, not just the cornea. Algorithms that utilize both refraction and corneal topography are worthy of exploration, and this topic is explored in Chapter 38.

Wavefront-Guided Corneal Ablation

Wavefront-guided corneal ablation is designed to correct the traditional sphere and cylindrical error of the eye and reduce the eye's higher-order optical aberration. Ablative corrections that reduce the optical aberrations of the eye will increase retinal image resolution (eg, acuity) and contrast, which in turn should allow one to see the world with finer detail and higher contrast (see Chapters 2, 6, and 7). When perfected, such corrections could well lead to providing our patients with better than normal vision and an era in which the expected outcome is "super vision."

> The greatest gain in correcting higher-order aberrations is in improving contrast, not visual acuity, which has added an extra margin of safety for refractive surgeons.

Measurement of the ocular aberrations can be accomplished in several ways, including using an objective aberroscope,[43] a Shack-Hartmann (sometimes known as Hartmann-Shack) wavefront sensor,[44] a Tscherning wavefront sensor,[45] a spatially resolved refractometer,[46] or one of many other new approaches beginning to appear on the market. These techniques measure the eye's wavefront aberrations including second (sphere and cylindrical), asymmetric or coma-like (third, fifth, ... order), symmetric or spherical-like aberrations (fourth, sixth,... order). While the systems all utilize ray tracing in one form or another, each system has a unique way of measuring the displacement of a ray of light from its ideal position, which in turn defines the slope of the wavefront and then by integration, the actual wavefront. The difference between the actual wavefront and an ideal wavefront defines the aberrations of the eye. In turn, the aberrations of the eye define the form of an ideal or customized laser treatment. Such technology is already improving refractive surgery outcomes[42] as is documented in Chapters 26 to 31.

Adaptive Optics

Laboratory studies by Liang and Williams[44], which use adaptive optics on humans, indicate that polychromatic vision may improve two-fold, especially in low light conditions when the pupil is more dilated. Such an improvement would aid a wavefront enhanced normal driver on a wet, rainy night in seeing a cyclist at a much greater distance and with more confidence. In real world terms, objects would have sharper borders and higher contrast (see Chapter 6).

Quantifying the optical aberrations of the eye will not only allow us to design corrections for subtle aberrations but also look into the eye to see retinal detail in vivo with unprecedented resolution and contrast (see Chapter 5). One can measure the optical aberrations of the eye with a wavefront sensor and correct for the wavefront error with a technique called *adaptive optics*, typically a deformable mirror. Such a combination has been built and can be thought of as an adaptive optic ophthalmoscope. The adaptive optic ophthalmoscope has already resulted in our ability to observe live human photoreceptors as small as 2 to 3 µm in diameter and human capillaries as small as 6 µm in diameter. This technology has allowed investigators to further characterize the three types of photoreceptors (short, medium, and long wavelength) in living subjects.[47] As the technology matures and becomes clinically viable, such devices will help us to detect subtle abnormalities of the retina, better understand their pathophysiology, allow for earlier intervention, and monitor therapeutic interventions (see Chapter 5).

New Forms of Wavefront Sensing and Customization

> It is likely that future wavefront systems will combine both corneal topographic and whole eye (ie, Shack-Hartmann) wavefront sensors to separate the corneal wavefront from the whole eye wavefront.

These systems would be useful diagnostic tools to distinguish corneal from whole eye aberrations. For instance, clinicians are sometimes interested in distinguishing whether a corneal scar or an IOL is causing a visual loss. This could be determined using a combined corneal and whole eye wavefront sensing system. If the IOL was causing the aberrations, the corneal wavefront would be normal but the whole eye wavefront sensing would be abnormal. There has been more recent interest in a preoperative corneal wavefront demonstration that may be helpful to design a wavefront-guided IOL implant. This exciting area is covered in

Chapter 34, which raises interesting possibilities to improve pseudophakic IOL correction. Newer wavefront sensors with better sensitivity and higher dynamic range can be developed and these challenges are discussed in Chapter 16.

Summary

As we review the many new and evolving techniques for treating our patients with customized ablation, it is obvious that there is a rapid evolution of technology and thought. Newly refined diagnostic technology such as wavefront sensing and more sophisticated spot laser delivery systems with eye tracking give the refractive surgical team much greater flexibility to tackle the often challenging optical abnormalities we encounter. Wavefront technologies are now expanding to influence the design of IOLs and contact lenses. The next decade in refractive surgery has the promise of providing tremendous gains in visual function by increasing retinal image contrast and, to a more limited extent, resolution. In this book, we explore the concepts and methods on which the promise of improved, unaided vision are based. This next decade promises even more remarkable gains in the quest for the Holy Grail of "super vision."

References

1. Porter J, MacRae S, Yoon G, Roberts C, Cox IG, Williams DR. Separate effects of the microkeratome incision and laser ablation on the eye's wave aberration. *Am J Ophthalmol*. 2003;136(2):327-337.
2. *Webster's Ninth New Collegiate Dictionary*. Springfield, Mass: Merriam Webster, Inc Publishers; 1983:318.
3. Seiler T, Wollensak J. Myopic photorefractive keratectomy with the excimer laser: one-year follow-up. *Ophthalmology*. 1991;98:1156-1163.
4. Tengroth B, Epstein D, Fagerholm P, et al. Excimer laser photorefractive keratectomy for myopia: clinical results in sighted eye. *Ophthalmology*. 1993;100:739-745.
5. Chatterjee A, Shah S, Doyle SJ. Effect of age on final refractive outcome for 2342 patients following photorefractive keratectomy. *Invest Ophthalmol Vis Sci*. 1996;37(suppl):S57.
6. DePaolis M, Aquavella J. Refractive surgery update: how to respond to common questions. *Contact Lens Spectrum*. 1993;8(12):48.
7. Aquavella J, Shovlin J, Pascucci S, DePaolis M. How contact lenses fit into refractive surgery. *Review of Ophthalmology*. 1994;1(12):36.
8. Applegate RA, Gansel KA. The importance of pupil size in optical quality measurements following radial keratotomy. *Corneal and Refractive Surgery*. 1990;6:47-54.
9. Maloney RK. Corneal topography and optical zone location in PRK. *Corneal and Refractive Surgery*. 1990;6:363-371.
10. Applegate RA. Acuities through annular and central pupils following radial keratotomy. *Optom Vis Sci*. 1991;68:584-590.
11. Roberts CW, Koester CJ. Optical zone diameters for photorefractive corneal surgery. *Invest Ophthalmol Vis Sci*. 1993;34:2275-2281.
12. Diamond S. Excimer laser photorefractive keratectomy (PRK) for myopia present status: aerospace considerations. *Aviat Space Environ Med*. 1995;66:690-693.
13. Martínez CE, Applegate RA, Klyce SD, McDonald MB, Medina JP, Howland HC. Effect of pupil dilation on corneal optical aberrations after photorefractive keratectomy. *Arch Ophthalmol*. 1998;116:1053-1062.
14. Machat JJ, Slade SG, Probst LE, et al. *The Art of LASIK*. 2nd ed. Thorofare, NJ: SLACK Incorporated; 1998:50-53.
15. Gimbel HV, Anderson Penno EE. *Lasik Complications: Prevention and Management*. 2nd ed. Thorofare, NJ: SLACK Incorporated; 1998:60-61.
16. MacRae SM. Excimer ablation design and elliptical transition zones. *J Cataract Refract Surg*. 1999;25:1191-1197.
17. Sutton HF, Reinstein DZ, Holland S, Silverman RH. Anatomy of the flap in LASIK by very high frequency ultrasound scanning. *Invest Ophthalmol Vis Sci*. 1998;39(4):S244.
18. Maldonado MJ, Ruiz-Oblitas L, Mununera JM, Aliseda D, Garcia-Layana A, Moreno-Montanes J. Optical coherence tomography evaluation of the corneal cap and stromal bed features after laser in situ keratomileusis for high myopia and astigmatism. *Ophthalmology*. 2000;107(1):81-78.
19. Behrens A, Langenbucher A, Kus MM, Rummelt C, Seitz B. Experimental evaluation of two current-generation automated microkeratomes: the Hansatome and the Supratome. *Am J Ophthalmol*. 2000;29(1):59-67.
20. Flanagan GW, Binder, PS. Precision of flap measurements for laser in situ keratomileusis in 4428 eyes. *J Refract Surg*. 2003;19(2):113-123.
21. Dierick HG, Missotten L. Corneal ablation profiles for correction of hyperopia with the excimer laser. *J Refract Surg*. 1996;12:767-773.
22. Applegate RA, Gansel KA. The importance of pupil size in optical quality measurements following radial keratotomy. *Corneal and Refractive Surgery*. 1990;6:47-54.
23. Machat JJ. *Excimer Laser Refractive Surgery: Practice and Principles*. Thorofare, NJ: SLACK Incorporated; 1996:248-249.
24. Chayet AS, Montes M, Gomez L, Rodriguez X, Robledo N, MacRae S. Bitoric laser in situ keratomileusis for the correction of simply myopic and mixed astigmatism. *Ophthalmology*. 2001;108(2):303-308.
25. Vinceguerra P, Sborgia M, Epstein D, Azzolini M, MacRae S. Photorefractive keratectomy to correct myopic or hyperopic astigmatism with a crosscylinder ablation. *J Refract Surg*. 1999;15(2 Suppl):S183-185.
26. Zaldivar R, Davidorf JM, Oscherow S, Ricur G, Piezzi V. Combined posterior chamber phakic intraocular lens and laser in situ keratomileusis: bioptics for extreme myopia. *J Refract Surg*. 1999; 15(3):299-308.
27. Moser C, Kampmeier J, McDonnell P, Psaltis D. Feasibility of intraoperative corneal topography monitoring during photorefractive keratectomy. *J Refract Surg*. 2000;16:148-154.
28. Hemenger P, Tomlinson A, Caroline PJ. Role of spherical aberration in contrast sensitivity loss with radial keratotomy. *Invest Ophthalmol Vis Sci*. 1989;30:1997-2001.
29. Howland HC, Glasser A, Applegate RA. Polynomial approximations of corneal surfaces and corneal curvature topography. In: *Noninvasive Assessment of the Visual System Technical Digest*. Washington, DC: Optical Society of America; 1992;3:34-37.
30. Applegate RA, Howland HC, Buettner J, Yee RW, Cottingham Jr AJ, Sharp RP. Corneal aberrations before and after radial keratotomy (RK) calculated from videokeratometric measurements. In: *Vision Science and Its Applications, 1994 Technical Digest Series*. Vol 2. Washington, DC: Optical Society of America; 1994:58-61.
31. Howland HC, Buettner J, Applegate RA. Computation of the shapes of normal corneas and their monochromatic aberrations from videokeratometric measurements. In: *Vision Science and Its Applications, 1994 Technical Digest Series*. Vol 2. Washington, DC: Optical Society of America; 1994:54-57.
32. Hemenger P, Tomlinson A, Oliver K. Corneal optics from videokeratographs. *Ophthalmic Physiol Opt*. 1995;1:63-68.
33. Applegate RA, Howland HC, Hilmantel G. Corneal aberrations increase with the magnitude of the RK refractive correction. *Optom Vis Sci*. 1996;73:585-589.
34. Applegate RA, Howland HC. Refractive surgery, optical aberrations, and visual performance. *J Refract Surg*. 1997;13:295-299.

35. Applegate RA, Howland HC, Sharp RP, Cottingham AJ, Yee RW. Corneal aberrations, visual performance and refractive keratectomy. *J Refract Surg*. 1998;14:397-407.

36. Oshika T, Klyce SD, Applegate RA, Howland HC, El Danasoury MA. Comparison of corneal wavefront aberrations after photorefractive keratectomy and laser in situ keratomileusis. *Am J Ophthalmol*. 1999;127:1-7.

37. Oshika T, Klyce SD, Applegate RA, Howland HC. Changes in corneal wavefront aberrations with aging. *Invest Ophthalmol Vis Sci*. 1999;40:1351-1355.

38. Applegate RA, Hilmantel G, Howland HC, Tu EY, Starck T, Zayac EJ. Corneal first surface optical aberrations and visual performance. *J Refract Surg*. 2000;16:507-514.

39. Lafond G, Solomon L. Retreatment of central islands after photorefractive keratectomy. *J Cataract Refract Surg*. 1999;25:188-196.

40. Manche EE, Maloney RK, Smith RJ. Treatment of topographic central islands following refractive surgery. *J Cataract Refract Surg*. 1998;24:464-470.

41. Buzard KA, Fundingsland BR. Treatment of irregular astigmatism with a broad beam excimer laser. *J Refract Surg*. 1997;13:624-636.

42. Musch DC, Farjo AA, Meyer RF, et al. Assessment of health-related quality of life after corneal transplantation. *Am J Ophthalmol*. 1997;124:1-8.

43. Howland HC, Howland B. A subjective method for the measurement of monochromatic aberrations of the eye. *J Opt Soc Am*. 1977;67:1508-1518.

44. Liang J, Williams DR. Aberrations and retinal image quality of the normal human eye. *J Opt Soc Am A*. 1997;14(11):2873-2883.

45. Mrochen M, Kaemmerer M, Seiler T. Wavefront-guided laser in situ keratomileusis: early results in three eyes. *J Refract Surg*. 2000;16:116-121.

46. Webb RH, Penney CM, Thompson KP. Measurement of ocular wavefront distortion with a spatially resolved refractometer. *Appl Opt*. 1992;31:3678-3686.

47. Roorda A, Williams DR. Objective identification of M and L cones in the living human eye. *Invest Ophthalmol Vis Sci*. 1998;39(4):957.

Chapter 2

A Review of Basic Wavefront Optics

Austin Roorda, PhD

Introduction

In the last decade, technological advances in wavefront sensing and adaptive optics have made it possible to measure, correct, or alter the aberration structure of the eye. These advances have already reached the clinic, where wavefront-guided ablations are quickly becoming standard practice. Furthermore, new applications of wavefront sensing, as they apply to contact lenses or intraocular lenses (IOLs) for example, are on the horizon. As a result, it is becoming a necessity for the practicing optometrist or ophthalmologist to have a working understanding of a barrage of new concepts, terms, definitions, and theory related to wavefront optics. The old belief that wave aberrations, function fitting, and point spread functions (PSFs) should be relegated to the didactic portion of the eye doctor's professional training no longer applies.

> It is becoming a necessity for the practicing optometrist or ophthalmologist to have a working understanding of a barrage of new concepts, terms, definitions, and theory related to wavefront optics.

The goal of this chapter is to define and describe the aspects of optics and image formation that are important for this rapidly growing field. This is only an overview. For the most part, it should provide a sufficient working understanding of the concepts and methods that are commonly used. This chapter is not intended to be a thorough treatment of the field. For that, the reader should refer to the literature that is available. Some good reference books are listed in the Bibliography at the end of this chapter.

Geometrical Optics: Relationships Between Pupil Size, Refractive Error, and Blur

We begin with the most basic and most important properties of the optical system: the relationship between refractive error and pupil size. Both refractive error and pupil size are equally important in governing the size of the blur in an out of focus image. This is illustrated in Figures 2-1A and 2-1B where the same refractive error gives rise to a blur on the retina that changes linearly with pupil size. This is the reason why when the lights are turned down, students in the back of the room who normally can tolerate some myopia begin to squint or have to put on glasses. It is also the reason why some people only have to wear glasses when they are driving at night. The myopia does not change with light condition, but the pupil size does, and so does the blur on the retina.

> Pinhole glasses limit vision by decreasing available light and increasing the adverse effects of diffraction.

This phenomenon relates directly to depth of focus. Being able to tolerate your refractive error indicates that you have a long depth of focus. Increasing the depth of focus can be achieved directly through pupil size, which is why people squint. Squinting is a voluntary way of changing your pupil size, by effectively making your eyelids the pupil. The improvement is not uniform, however, since the pupil is only reduced in the vertical direction. Try looking at a simple cross sketched on a piece of paper. Hold it about 5 centimeters (cm) from your eye and try to resolve it. If you squint, you will see the horizontal bar come into focus. The reason the horizontal bar is in focus is because only the vertical spread of the blur has been reduced.

So why don't we simply prescribe pinhole glasses, and forget about the refractive error altogether? The answer is light and resolution. When the eye gets more light to form the image, it processes the information faster and more reliably. The loss of resolution induced by diffraction effects with small pupils will be discussed in later sections.

Physical Optics

Light as a Wave

The phenomena described in the previous section can be explained entirely by geometrical optics. However, the rules of geometrical optics (eg, light travels in straight lines) are not really true. Phenomena are often observed that violate these rules. This is where the area of physical optics comes in. Even the physical optical model of light is not entirely true, but it is sufficient to explain all of the remaining optics of image formation that will be covered in this chapter.

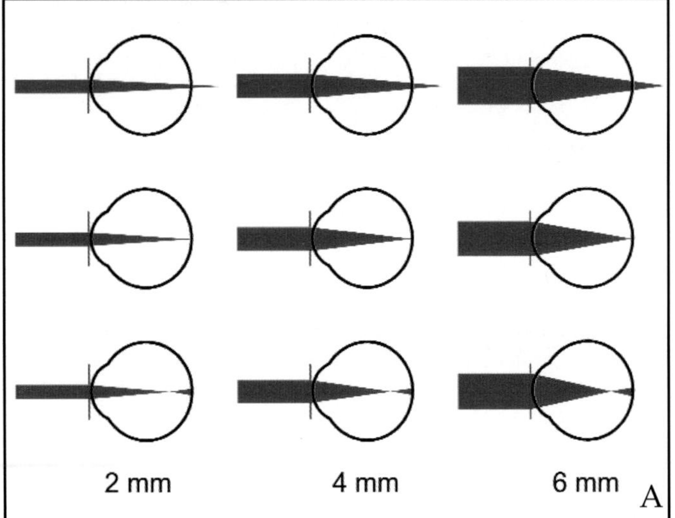

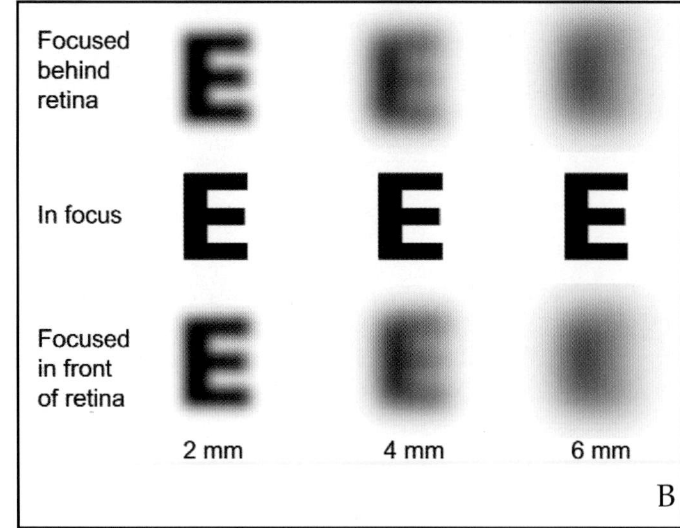

Figure 2-1. (A) The three rows show hyperopic, emmetropic, and myopic eyes, respectively. The eyes are shown for 2, 4, and 6 millimeter (mm) pupils. The retinal blur depends equally on pupil size and refractive error, with the larger pupils experiencing the most image degradation from a defocus error. (B) Simulations of the letter E for the conditions illustrated in A.

> The rules of geometrical optics (eg, light travels in straight lines) are not really true.

In physical optics, we describe light as a wave. The basic properties of this wave are the wavelength, frequency, and velocity; three terms that are intimately related. Since all light travels at the same speed (in a vacuum, approximately in air), then the shorter wavelengths of light have to oscillate faster to cover the same distance. This gives rise to the basic equation:

$$f = \frac{c}{\lambda} \qquad (1)$$

where c, the speed of light in vacuum, is constant at 3.0×10^8 meters per second (m/s). This leaves the frequency, f, inversely related to the wavelength, λ. When light travels through a different media, like glass or water, it slows down, but the frequency remains the same. Hence, the more general relationship:

$$f = \frac{V_n}{\lambda} \qquad (2)$$

where n is the index of refraction of the medium and V is the velocity of light, which is always equal to or less than c.

The reason equation 2 is important to discuss is because phase delays or advancements, or aberrations, are often brought about by altering the index of refraction that the light is passing through (eg, replacing cornea with air). This will be discussed further later, as we define the wavefront and wave aberrations.

> A *phase delay* or *advancement* is when any portion of a wavefront is behind (delayed or retarded) or advanced from its ideal location.

The wave model can be used to explain phenomena like the interference of light. The interference of light occurs similarly to interference of waves of water in a pond. When the crest of one light wave meets the crest of a second light wave, the crests add and undergo constructive interference. Conversely, when the crest of one light wave meets the trough of another, then the light waves cancel and undergo destructive interference. When two traveling light waves have their crests lined up, they are said to be *in phase*. Whenever the crest of one wave does not line up with the crest of a second light wave, the two waves are said to be *out of phase*. The relative phase of light and its associated interference is the basis for the formation of the PSF discussed below.

The Wavefront

A light is a source of energy that generates radiating waves of light, much like the waves that appear when you drop a pebble into a water tank. The crest of the wave continues to move outward in a circular pattern. The curved line that follows the crest of the wave at any instant in time is called the *wavefront*. Said differently, for light, the wavefront joins the emerging light waves at a single point in time. When light emerges from a point source, this wavefront takes on a spherical shape. As the wavefront moves further and further from the source, a segment of the surface of the wavefront will get flatter and flatter, until the wavefront finally takes the shape of a plane.

> The wavefront joins the emerging light waves at a single point in time.

From a geometrical perspective, one treats the emerging light as rays, which by law will always travel perpendicular to the direction of the wavefront. Rays are an inefficient representation, since it takes many rays to describe how light emerges from a source. It takes only one wavefront to efficiently describe how light is traveling as it emerges from a source. Nonetheless, the rays are included in the figures to provide an alternate and more intuitive representation of the light.

As discussed above, you can slow light down by passing it through a media of higher refractive index (eg, glass). In doing so, the wavefront of the light will necessarily change. Figure 2-2

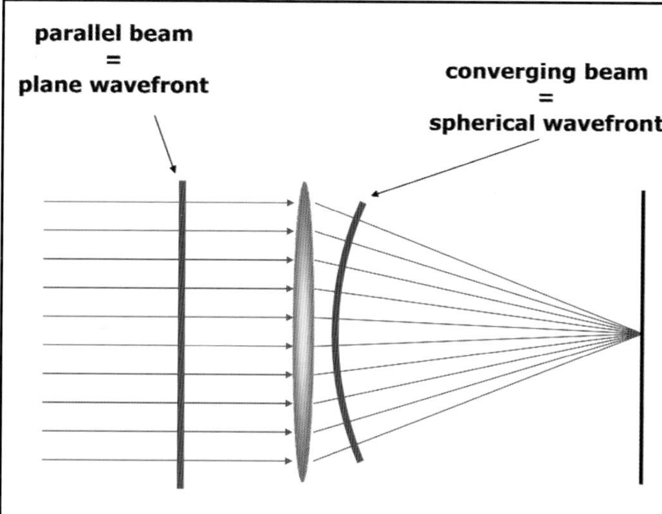

Figure 2-2. The relationship between the wavefront and light rays. The light rays travel perpendicular to the wavefront at all points.

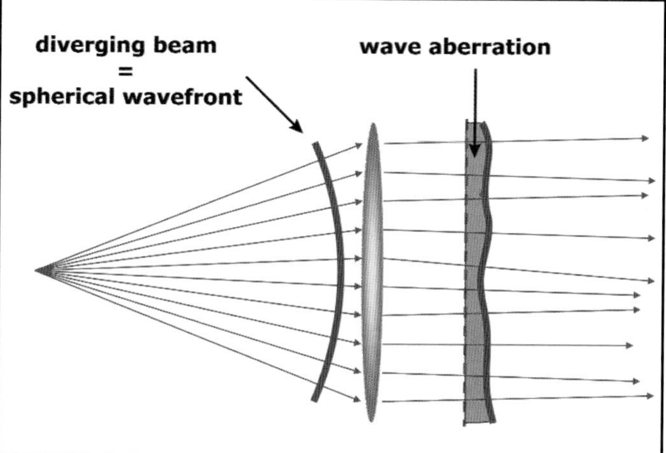

Figure 2-4. The wave aberration, illustrated in gray, is the difference between the ideal wavefront and the aberrated wavefront.

shows the effect that a lens has on a parallel incident wavefront. The light passing through the thicker portion of the lens is delayed more than on the edges, making the wavefront curve inward. Since light travels perpendicular to the direction of the wavefront, this curved wavefront shape describes light that is focusing to a point. The same lens can be used for incident light that is diverging. When the diverging light passing through the lens emerges as a plane wavefront (parallel beam), that light is said to be originating from the primary focal point of the lens.

Wave Aberration

When the wavefront is interrupted by media of a different index, then the emerging wavefront shape is often one that is not planar, nor does it converge to a point or diverge as though it is coming from a point. This will occur if the surface of the interrupting media is not smooth or if the index of refraction of the media is not constant. A wavefront that deviates from its intended shape is called an *aberrated wavefront*. Aberrated wavefronts even arise from centered lenses with spherical refracting surfaces (Seidel aberrations).

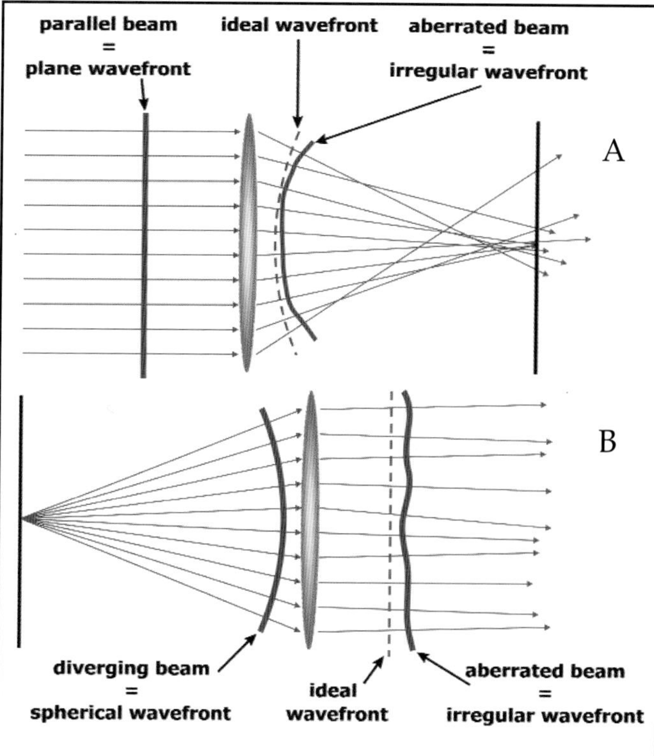

Figure 2-3. The aberrated wavefront for (A) light coming from a distant object and (B) light emerging from the approximate primary focal point of the lens. The emerging light neither converges to a point nor does it form a parallel beam, resulting in an irregular-shaped wavefront.

> A wavefront that deviates from its intended shape is called an *aberrated wavefront.*

The wave aberration is defined as the difference between the actual aberrated wavefront and the ideal or intended wavefront (Figure 2-3). Since the wavefront defines a surface, the wave aberration also defines a surface, since it is simply a map of the separation between two surfaces (Figure 2-4).

> Spherical refracting surfaces are not ideal because they do not refract light to a perfect spherical wavefront.

As stated earlier, light, which is often represented by rays, always travels perpendicular to the wavefront. Therefore, once the wavefront with all its aberrations is known, one can also determine how well that wavefront can produce an image.

> *Wave aberration* is defined as the difference between the actual aberrated wavefront and the ideal or intended wavefront.

For convenience, the wave aberration is often fit with a mathematical equation. This is analogous to fitting a line or a quadratic function to some data points, except in this case, the data are in two dimensions (over the pupil aperture) and the shapes are very complex. The Zernike polynomial is a set of basis functions (or shapes) that are fitted to the data. Each basis function has a coefficient, the value of which indicates the amount of that particular aberration that composes the wave aberration. The convenience of the Zernike polynomial is that it contains shapes that have some functional meaning, like defocus, astigmatism, coma, and spherical aberration. In addition, the Zernike polynomial has other complex shapes, with equally complex names, like quadrafoil or secondary astigmatism. These aberrations are present in the eye, however, and also need to be considered in the fit.

> The favorite choice for fitting wave aberration data is the Zernike polynomial equation.

Diffraction

Simply put, *diffraction* is defined as "...any deviation of light rays from a rectilinear path which cannot be interpreted as reflection or refraction."[1] It is a tendency for light to bend around edges. To explain diffraction, we employ Huygens principle, which states that any wavefront can be considered as being composed of an infinite array of point sources propagating light in the forward direction. When the wavefront is propagating undisturbed, the array of point sources combines and interferes to produce a a new wavefront that follows the previous one. The reason this is important is to explain diffraction. When the wavefront is interrupted by an aperture, the only point sources that are allowed to interfere are restricted to those that pass through the aperture. The resultant intensity pattern in the image plane (after superimposing the waves from the array of point sources) takes on a different shape. In the limit, when the aperture becomes very small, the parallel beam will be reduced to a wave that propagates in all directions. The less the original wavefront is disrupted by the aperture (ie, larger aperture), the less diffraction will take place.

> *Diffraction* is defined as "...any deviation of light rays from a rectilinear path which cannot be interpreted as reflection or refraction."[1]

> The less the original wavefront is disrupted by the aperture (ie, larger aperture), the less diffraction will take place.

Diffraction and Interference

Diffraction and wavefront phase variations combine in the simple lens. The physical size of the lens defines an aperture, and the shape of the lens alters the phase or changes the shape of the wavefront. Likewise, in the eye, the pupil acts as an aperture and suffers from diffraction, and the optics alter the wavefront of the light. Using Huygens principle again, one must simply reduce the emerging light to an array of point sources, along the altered wavefront over a size that is limited by the aperture. The point sources combine and interfere to form an intensity distribution across the retina.

Metrics to Define Image Quality

How image quality is defined, particularly for the human eye, is not well known. Although we have made much progress in our ability to measure accurately the wave aberrations of the eye, our ability to use that information to predict how well the eye "sees" is just now beginning to advance quickly (see Chapter 8). It is currently an area that is being investigated widely. Common textbook definitions of image quality often fail to predict visual quality in the human eye because of the large degree of aberration and a failure to appreciate how the human visual system translates the retinal image into a visual percept. Nonetheless, the common optical metrics are still used in vision science and have beneficial uses.

The Point Spread Function

When the wavefront that enters the eye comes from a point source (ie, forming a perfect diverging, converging, or parallel wavefront), then the intensity distribution that lands on the retina is called the PSF. In other words, the PSF is the image that an optical system forms of a point source. The point source is very important for defining optical systems, since the point source is the most fundamental object. Under most circumstances, any object can be considered as an array of independent point sources, each producing its own PSF. These all overlap to form an image of that object. The operation of overlapping the PSF from the array of points that make up the object is called a *convolution* (see p. 13).

> The PSF is the image that an optical system forms of a point source.

If the PSF is itself a point, then you have a perfect imaging system. But no such system exists. Even if wave aberrations are corrected, diffraction will broaden the PSF.

In the best possible imaging system, the image formation will be limited only by diffraction (hence the term *diffraction-limited*). Under these conditions, the light heading toward the retina will have a spherical shape. The PSF of the eye can be calculated as long as one knows the wave aberration, the transmission of the optical system, and the shape and size of the aperture (pupil). The equation that is used generally takes the following form:

$$PSF\,(r_i,\,\theta_i) = K * \left| FT \left\{ P\,(r,\,\theta) * e^{\frac{-i\,2\pi\,W\,(r,\,\theta)}{\lambda}} \right\} \right|^2 \qquad (3)$$

where FT represents the Fourier transform operator and K is a constant. The function inside the curly brackets is the complex (or generalized) pupil function The pupil function has two components, an amplitude component, $P\ (r,\ \theta)$, and a phase component that contains the wave aberration, $W\ (r,\ \theta)$. The amplitude component, $P\ (r,\ \theta)$, defines the shape, size, and transmission of the optical system. The most common shape for the aperture function is a circular aperture. The size is simply the size of the pupil that the pupil function defines. A clear optical system would have a value of unity at all points across the pupil function. To model variable transmission, one would represent pupil function as the fraction of transmitted light as a function of pupil location. Variable transmission may arise because of absorption in the lens. Variable transmission can also be used to model how the eye "sees" by incorporating phenomena like the Stiles-

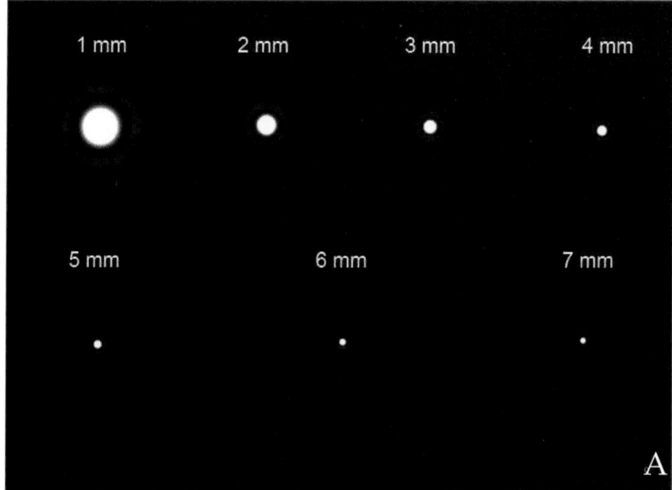

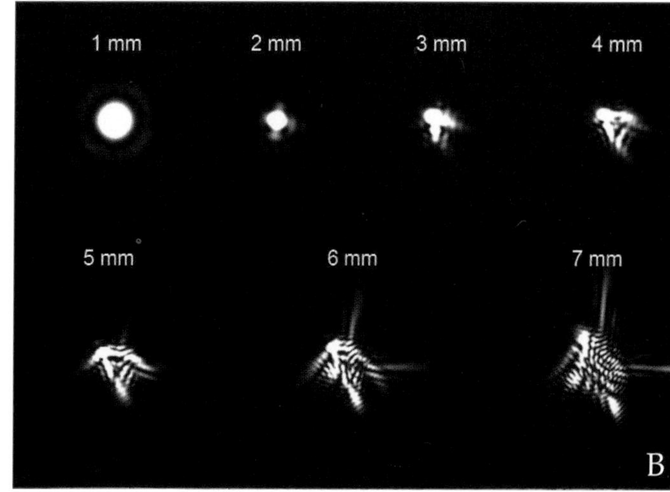

Figure 2-5. (A) The PSF for increasing pupil sizes in a perfect eye. Each PSF has the shape of the Airy disk, but the size decreases as the pupil size increases. (B) The PSF for increasing pupil sizes in a typical human eye. For small pupils, the PSF approximates an Airy disk, but as the pupil size increases, aberrations take over and the PSF broadens and takes an irregular shape.

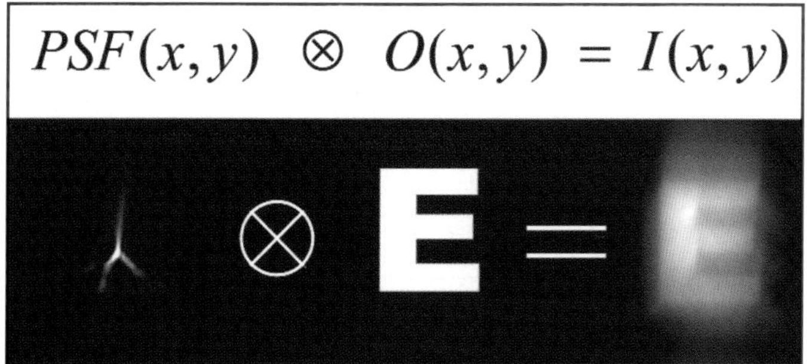

Figure 2-6. Pictorial explanation of the convolution operation. A perfect version of a letter E is blurred, point by point by the PSF, to produce a simulation of the blurred image.

Crawford effect. In this case, the amplitude component of the pupil function would take the form of a Gaussian function. Another reason to use a nonuniform aperture function would be to model the effect of a nonuniform beam entering or exiting the eye. The actual calculation of the Fourier transform will not be discussed in this chapter. Once the concepts are understood, computations like the Fourier transform can be done numerically using one of many common software packages like Matlab (The MathWorks, Natick, Mass).

> We will never be able to achieve a diffraction-limited correction over a large aperture with refractive surgery, contact lenses, or an IOL. The reasons are many and include the fact that the needed correction varies with object distance, the wavelength of light, and the fact that the eye's aberration structure varies with time. The goal is to minimize the eye's aberration over all physiologic pupil sizes.

> *Stiles-Crawford effect:* Light entering the pupil at various locations is not equally efficient at eliciting a visual response. Typically, light near the center of the pupil is more efficient at eliciting a visual response than light near the edge.

When the optical system has a circular aperture and no aberrations ($W[r, \theta] = 0$), the PSF takes the shape of the Airy disk. The angular size of the Airy disk depends on pupil size and on the wavelength of light, according to the following equation:

$$\theta = \frac{1.22 \times \lambda}{a} \qquad (4)$$

where θ is the angle subtended at the nodal point of the optical system between the peak and the first minimum of the disk, λ is the wavelength of light, and a is the diameter of the pupil. When wavelength and pupil diameter are expressed in common units (say, meters) the angle has units of radians. To convert radian to degrees, the value must be multiplied by $180/\pi$.

> Radians and degrees are two different ways to break up an angle into units. In a circle, there are 2π radians, or 360 degrees. In a half circle, there are π radians, or 180 degrees.

Figures 2-5A and 2-5B show the PSF calculated for a diffraction-limited eye as a function of pupil size and also for a typical eye whose aberrations were known. The image quality in the typical human eye degrades quickly as the pupil size increases.

Convolution

The convolution is an operation used to generate a simulation of a blurred image. It is useful because it provides a physical sense of the appearance of objects other than points. One can consider that any diffuse object is composed of an infinite array of point sources, each with its respective intensity, position, and color. The convolution operation gives each one of those points the shape of the PSF. The actual mathematics involved are more complex, but the concept is very simple.

When performing the convolution, it is important to maintain the appropriate sizes of the object with respect to the PSF. The PSF has a fixed size, spanning typically up to 0.5 degree visual angle in a normal 5 mm pupil. The convolved image will appear different depending on the angular size of the object. Figure 2-6 illustrates the convolution operation. Figure 2-7 shows how dif-

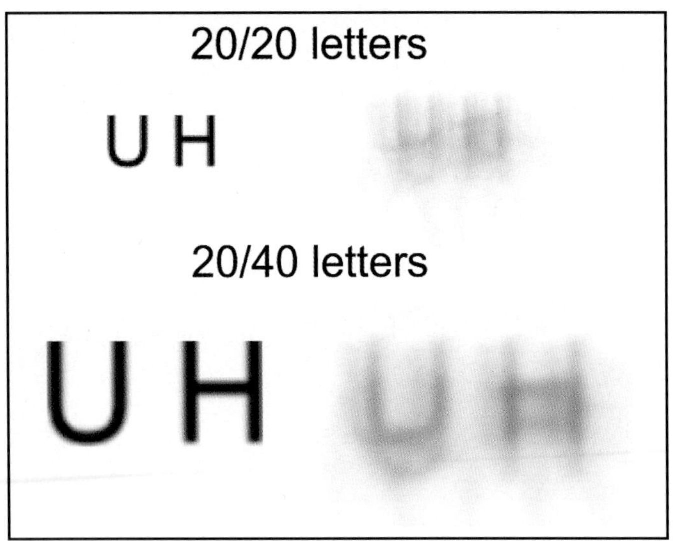

Figure 2-7. Two letters sizes convolved with the same PSF. Under most circumstances, smaller features and letters are degraded more than larger letters when they are convolved with the same PSF.

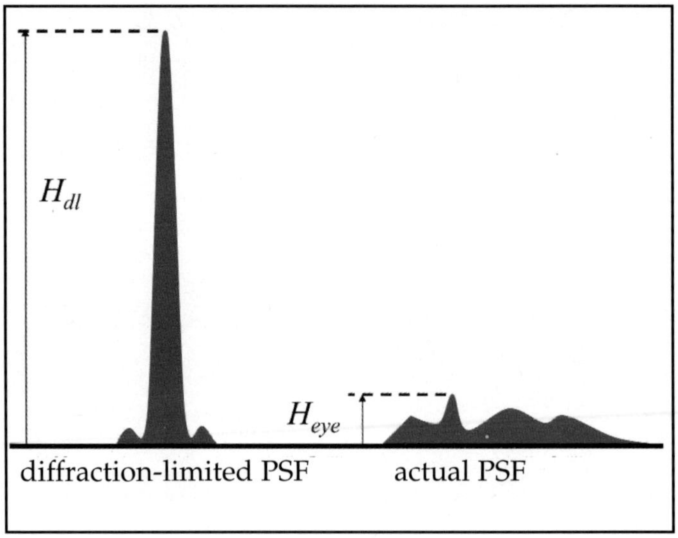

Figure 2-8. Pictorial definition of the Strehl ratio. The maximum value of the Strehl ratio is 1, which occurs when the optical system is diffraction-limited.

ferent letter sizes appear when they are convolved by the same PSF. As expected, the 20/20 letters are less legible than the 20/40.

Strehl Ratio

The Strehl ratio is a measure of the peak height of the PSF. It is expressed as a ratio between the peak height of the PSF over the peak height for the same optical system if it were diffraction-limited (Figure 2-8). Thus, the Strehl ratio ranges from 0 to 1, where a value of 1 indicates a diffraction-limited optical system. An optical system that has a Strehl ratio of 0.8 or greater is commonly considered to be diffraction-limited. A typical eye has a Strehl ratio for a 5 mm pupil of about 0.05 as long as defocus and astigmatism are corrected. However, for a 1 mm pupil, the Strehl ratio can be quite high, approaching 1. This does not imply that the 1 mm pupil has better image quality than the 5 mm pupil, it only means that the smaller aperture is closer to being diffraction-limited. As pupil sizes get smaller, the Strehl ratio will increase, but increased diffraction makes the image quality worse.

> The Strehl ratio is expressed as a ratio between the peak height of the PSF over the peak height for the same optical system if it were diffraction-limited.

An alternative method to calculate the Strehl ratio is to compute the ratio of the volume under the modulation transfer function (MTF) between the diffraction-limited and the aberrated conditions. Again, the best possible value for the Strehl ratio is 1.

Root Mean Square Aberration

The root mean square (RMS) is a measure of the magnitude of the wave aberration. As the name implies, the RMS is the square root of the mean of the square of all the wave aberration values across the pupil aperture. This can be calculated directly once the wave aberration is known. However, the RMS is more simply calculated if the Zernike polynomials are used to fit the wave aberration. As long as the Zernikes are normalized (see Appendix 1), the RMS is calculated as the square root of the sum of the squares (or the vector summation) of the Zernike coefficients. The following equation shows such a calculation:

$$\text{RMS} = \sqrt{Z^{-2}_2 + Z^{0}_2 + Z^{2}_2 + Z^{-3}_3 + \ldots} \qquad (5)$$

where each Z represents the coefficient for its corresponding Zernike term. This simple calculation is possible because the Zernike polynomials are an orthogonal set of functions. That is, there is no similarity or correlation in the shape between any two polynomials when compared over the extent of a circle with a radius of 1. The use of Zernike polynomials allows one to assess the contribution to the total aberration of any set of terms. For example, the RMS of the defocus and astigmatism is calculated as the vector sum of Zernike coefficients 3 through 5 (in the OSA standard notation [see Appendix 1]). The RMS of higher-order aberrations is calculated as the vector sum of the coefficient for all terms above second order. The RMS is limited, however, since it is a single number that indicates the magnitude of the aberration, but not its shape.

> In statistical terms, the RMS error is simply the standard deviation of the wavefront error.

> RMS error has limited utility as an ideal single metric for visual performance because it does not show how a given aberration affects visual performance.[2,3]

Modulation Transfer Function

Objects in space can be represented as an array of point sources, hence the PSF is an important image quality metric. Likewise, objects in space can also be represented as a superposition of sinusoidal gratings of various spatial frequencies, orien-

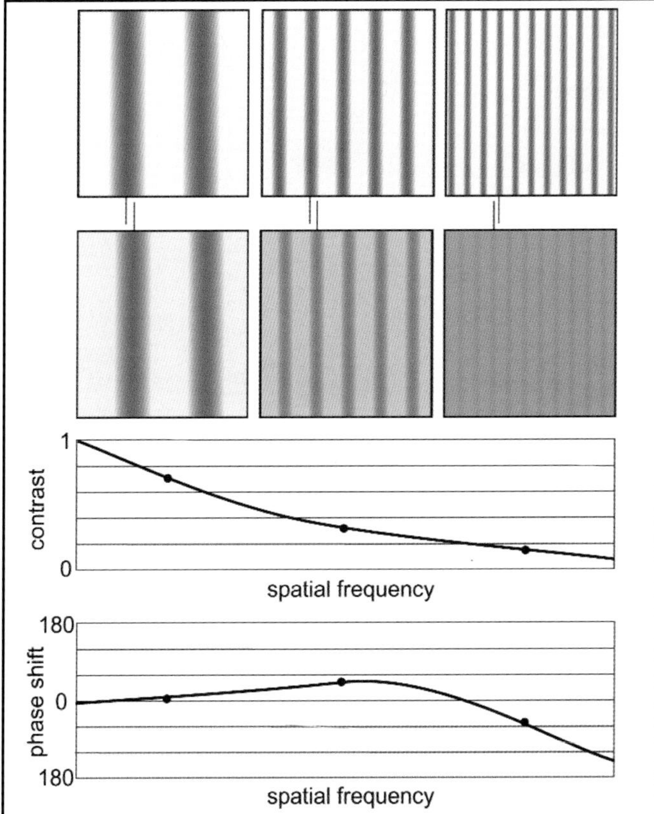

Figure 2-9. Pictorial demonstration of the calculation of the MTF and the PTF. The first row shows the objects, which are 100% contrast vertical sinusoidal gratings with low, medium, and high spatial frequencies. After passing through the imaging system, the gratings have less contrast and the peak locations (phase) are shifted. The MTF plots the change in contrast relative to the original object. The PTF plots the change in the phase of the same grating. This procedure may be different for each orientation of the gratings. The OTF is the combination of the MTF and the PTF for all grating orientations.

tations, and phases. This is called *Fourier*, or *frequency, space*. It is an equally adequate way to represent objects. Representing objects in this way is convenient since it allows us to consider objects in terms of their spatial frequency content. A person, for example, is composed of many spatial frequencies, from low (torso, arms, legs) to high (facial features, hair, etc). We all know that fine detail, or high spatial frequencies, are the first to get lost when you degrade an image. When you are out of focus, you can still make out a person (low spatial frequencies), but you may not identify his or her fine facial features (high spatial frequencies). This is what the MTF measures. The MTF indicates the ability of an optical system to reproduce (transfer) various levels of detail (spatial frequencies) from the object to the image. Its units are the ratio of image contrast over the object contrast as a function of spatial frequency. It is the optical contribution to the contrast sensitivity function (CSF).

> Objects in space can also be represented as a superposition of sinusoidal gratings of various spatial frequencies, orientations, and phases. This is called *Fourier*, or *frequency, space*.

The MTF can be calculated directly by imaging simple sinusoidal objects with different spatial frequencies and measuring their contrast. The more common way to produce the MTF, however, is by taking the Fourier transform of the PSF or calculating it directly from the pupil function (see p. 12). A point source (commonly called a *delta function* in physics) is comprised of all spatial frequencies. It follows that its Fourier transform (which is an operation that decomposes an object into its spatial frequencies components) produces a frequency spectrum that is equal to one for all spatial frequencies in all directions. The PSF, having been filtered by the optical system, has lost much of the spatial frequencies that originally composed the object, particularly the high spatial frequencies. The Fourier transform of the PSF shows what spatial frequencies remain and at what contrast. Therefore, the Fourier transform of the PSF produces directly the MTF.

Phase Transfer Function

When spatial frequencies get transferred to the image plane, the location of the bright and dark bars, called the *phase*, of the reduced-contrast grating may also be shifted. For example, if the peak of the sinusoid in the image is displaced by one quarter of a wave cycle, then the phase transfer at that spatial frequency is given a value of 90 degrees, or $\pi/4$. The shift in the sinusoid arises from asymmetry in the PSF. For example, if one took a PSF with coma and convolved it with a sinusoidal grating, the peak positions of the grating pattern would shift in the image plane from that of the diffraction-limited system.

Optical Transfer Function

The MTF and the phase transfer function (PTF) combine to form the optical transfer function (OTF). Like the PSF, the OTF is an entirely adequate and complete way to present how an image is formed by the optical system. Figure 2-9 shows pictorially how the MTF and PTF are calculated.

Relationships Between Wave Aberration, PSF, and OTF

To summarize, the wave aberration, the PSF, and the OTF are all intimately related. Once the wave aberration is known, the PSF and OTF can be calculated. The relationships between the three are typically through the Fourier transform. From wave aberration to PSF, one takes the Fourier transform of the complex pupil function. The OTF is the Fourier transform of the PSF.

Figure 2-10 shows a few examples going from wave aberration to the MTF. When the wave aberration is flat, the PSF is compact. A compact PSF gives rise to a broad MTF, since more frequencies can be transferred to images with a small PSF. When the wave aberration is high, the PSF is broad, which gives rise to a narrow MTF.

Chromatic Aberration

Chromatic aberration in the eye describes differences in image formation as a function of wavelength. Chromatic aberration arises entirely because the index of refraction of media is not the same for all wavelengths. Typically, the index of refraction is higher as the wavelength decreases. This is commonly called *chromatic dispersion*. If a refracting media (eg, the cornea) has a higher index of refraction, then it follows that its focusing power will be higher. This is why human eyes remain myopic for blue

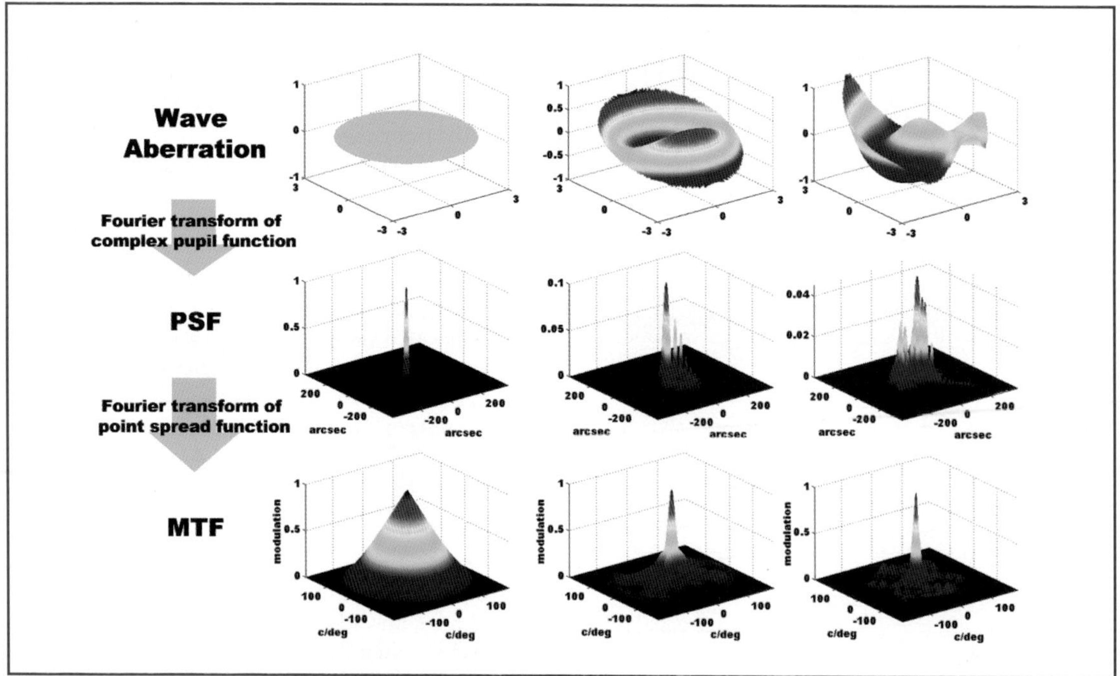

Figure 2-10. Wave aberration, PSF, and MTF for three different wave aberrations. The first row shows wave aberrations where the z-axis is in microns and the x-y axis is in millimeters. The second row shows the PSF with relative intensity on the z-axis and distance in seconds of arc in the x-y directions. The third row shows modulation in the z-direction and spatial frequency in cycles/degree in the x-y directions. The first column is for a flat wavefront (no aberration). The PSF is the Airy disk and the MTF drops nearly linearly from 1 to 0 at the cutoff frequency, which for 550 nanometer (nm) light and a 6 mm pupil size is 190 c/deg. The aberration in the second column is pure coma, and the aberration in the third column is for the aberrations from a typical human eye. When aberrations are present, the PSF broadens and becomes more irregular. The MTF shows that with aberrations, contrast drops quickly and in a nonuniform manner for all high spatial frequencies.

light after they are corrected for green or yellow light. The changing power and its corresponding change in focal length of the eye as a function of wavelength is defined as the longitudinal chromatic aberration. Chromatic aberration in a typical eye results in a chromatic difference of refraction that spans 2 diopters (D) between 400 and 700 nm.[4] That might seem surprising, especially considering that a refractive error of 0.25 D is noticeably blurry to a patient. The eye can tolerate this amount of chromatic aberration because it has reduced sensitivity at the extent of the visible spectrum. Most of the brightness in a broad spectral (white light) target comes from wavelengths near the peak of the spectral luminosity function (555 nm), over which the chromatic difference of refraction is within ± 0.25 D.[5]

> Chromatic aberration arises entirely because the index of refraction of media is not the same for all wavelengths.

Chromatic aberrations also cause a lateral shift in the retinal image as a function of wavelength. The shift is called *transverse chromatic aberration* and occurs whenever the pupil is displaced from the best optical axis of the eye, which is not an uncommon occurrence.[5]

Under everyday viewing conditions, the eye is exposed to the entire visible spectrum of wavelengths, with most objects having broad spectral components. Therefore, it is very important to consider chromatic aberration when computing retinal image quality. The white light PSF, for example, has to be computed as the sum of a range of PSFs across the spectrum. For each wavelength, the PSF will be different because of longitudinal and transverse chromatic aberration, as well as differences in diffraction with wavelength.

It should be noted that custom corneal ablation cannot correct chromatic aberration of the eye. In fact, recent reports suggest that the presence of a small amount of monochromatic aberration can mask the deleterious effects of chromatic aberration.[6] Once monochromatic aberrations are corrected, chromatic aberrations may pose more of a problem.

Retinal Sampling and the Nyquist Sampling Limit

The image that lands on the retina is sampled by a set of discrete photoreceptors that tile the retinal surface. The sampling imposes an upper boundary on what the eye can resolve. This upper boundary is called the *Nyquist sampling limit*. Nyquist sampling limit states that spatial frequencies are only properly detected when they are less than one half of the sampling frequency. For example, in order to detect a spatial frequency of 100 c/deg, the sampling frequency has to be at least 200 c/deg. The basic concept is shown pictorially in Figure 2-11 and more schematically in Figure 2-12.

In the human eye, the highest density of cone photoreceptors is in the central fovea. This high density offers a sampling rate of

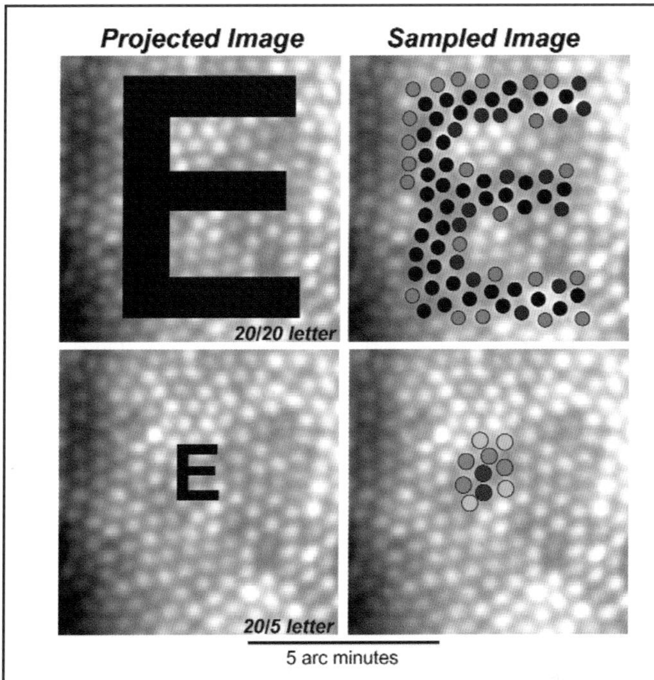

Figure 2-11. Limits imposed by the discrete photoreceptor array. An ideal image landing on the retina is sampled by the mosaic. If there are insufficient numbers to sample the image, as is illustrated for a 20/5 letter on foveal cones, then the letter is unreadable. As long as there are sufficient cones to sample the image, the images are legible and sampling is not a concern.

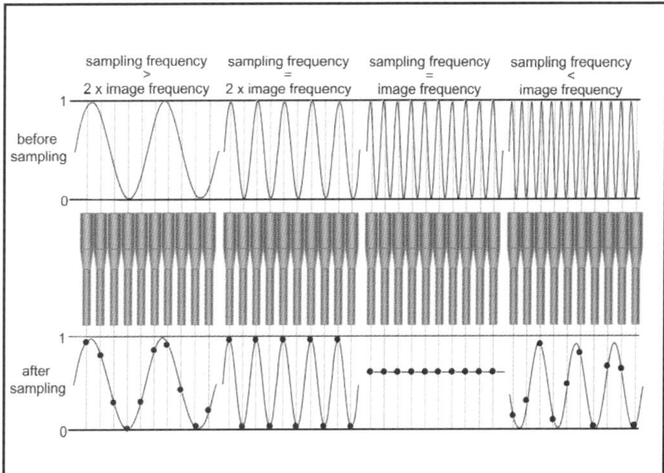

Figure 2-12. Illustration of the sampling limit. The figure shows sinusoidal gratings of increasing spatial frequency landing on a photoreceptor array. The lower row shows the sampled image. Sampling frequencies of at least two times the image frequency are adequate to produce a faithful representation of the image. When the image frequency is the same as the sampling frequency, nothing is transmitted. For other subsampled frequencies, the sampled image is misinterpreted as one with a lower spatial frequency. Such erroneous sampled images are called *aliases*. In the human eye, these aliases take on irregular shapes because of the nonuniform packing of the cones.[13] This illustration also overestimates the modulation of the sampled images because it ignores the fact that the cones sample the light over an area, not over a single point.[14]

about 120 c/deg,[7,8] which means that a typical eye cannot properly detect frequencies that are higher than about 60 c/deg. These frequencies are comparable to those that compose a 20/10 line on a letter acuity chart. When the frequency that lands on the retina is higher than the Nyquist limit, then the potential for aliasing occurs.

> When an image is undersampled, it is misinterpreted and referred to as an *aliased image* because it misrepresents the original image.

Another factor affecting image quality that is imposed by the retina is through the tuning properties of the cone photoreceptors, called the *Stiles-Crawford effect*.[9] Light entering the cones at an oblique angle are perceived as being less bright than light entering on the axis. The effect is strong enough to make light entering the margins of a 6 mm pupil half as bright as light entering the center of the pupil (assuming that the cones are pointing toward the center of the pupil of the eye).[10] The consequence of the Stiles-Crawford effect is that light from the margins of the pupil, where aberrations are worse, will contribute less to overall image quality than light from the center of the pupil. The effect is small and may be more important for out-of-focus images than for governing best image quality in the eye.[11,12] Nonetheless, these effects should not be ignored when considering perceived image quality in the eye.

Conclusion

This chapter provides some basic optics related to image formation that should help the reader as he or she goes through this book. For more thorough study, the reader is encouraged to read the books listed in the Bibliography.

Acknowledgments

Preparation of this chapter was supported in part by the National Science Foundation's "Center for Adaptive Optics," a Science and Technology Center managed by the University of California at Santa Cruz under cooperative agreement No. AST-9876783.

References

1. Sommerfeld A. Zur mathematischen theorie der Beugunserscheinenungen. *Nachr Kgl Acad Wiss Gottingen*. 1894;4:338-342.
2. Applegate RA, Sarver EJ, Khemsara V. Are all aberrations equal? *J Refract Surg*. 2002;18:S556-S562.
3. Applegate RA, Marsack J, Ramos R. Interaction between aberrations can improve or reduce visual performance. *J Cataract Refract Surg*. 2003;29(8):1487-1495.
4. Bennett AG, Rabbetts RB. *Clinical Visual Optics*. 2nd ed. London: Butterworths; 1989.

5. Thibos LN, Bradley A, Still DL, Zhang XX, Howarth PA. Theory and measurement of ocular chromatic aberration. *Vision Res.* 1990;30:33-49.
6. McLellan JS, Marcos S, Prieto PM, Burns SA. Imperfect optics may be the eye's defense against chromatic blur. *Nature.* 2002;417:174-176.
7. Curcio CA, Sloan KR, Kalina RE, Hendrickson AE. Human photoreceptor topography. *J Comp Neurol.* 1990;292:497-523.
8. Williams DR. Topography of the foveal cone mosaic in the living human eye. *Vision Res.* 1988;28:433-454.
9. Stiles WS, Crawford BH. The luminous efficiency of rays entering the eye pupil at different points. *Proc R Soc Lond B Biol Sci.* 1933;112:428-450.
10. Applegate RA, Lakshminarayanan V. Parametric representation of Stiles-Crawford functions: normal variation of peak location and directionality. *J Opt Soc Am A.* 1993;10:1611-1623.
11. Atchison DA, Scott DH, Strang NC, Artal P. Influence of Stiles-Crawford apodization on visual acuity. *J Opt Soc Am A.* 2002;19:1073-1083.
12. Roorda A. Human visual system: image formation. In: Hornack JP, ed. *Encyclopedia of Imaging Science and Technology.* New York: Wiley & Sons; 2002:539-557.
13. Williams DR. Aliasing in human foveal vision. *Vision Res.* 1985;25:195-205.
14. Chen B, Makous W. Light capture by human cones. *J Physiol.* 1989;414:89-109.

Bibliography

Fourier Optics

Bracewell R. *The Fourier Transform and Its Applications.* New York: McGraw-Hill; 1965.

Goodman JW. *Introduction to Fourier Optics.* New York: McGraw-Hill; 1968.

Wavefront Fitting and Image Quality Metrics

Cubalchini R. Modal wavefront estimation from phase derivative measurements. *J Opt Soc Am.* 1979;69:972-977.

Malacara D, DeVore SL. Interferogram evaluation and wavefront fitting. In: Malacara D, ed. *Optical Shop Testing.* 2nd ed. New York: Wiley-Interscience; 1996:455-499.

Smith WJ. *Modern Optical Engineering.* 2nd ed. New York: McGraw Hill, Inc; 1990.

Optics of the Eye

Atchison DA, Smith G. *Optics of the Human Eye.* Oxford: Butterworth-Heinemann; 2000.

Bennett AG, Rabbetts RB. *Clinical Visual Optics.* 2nd ed. London: Butterworths; 1989.

Charman WN. Optics of the human eye. In: Cronly-Dillon J, ed. *Visual Optics and Instrumentation.* Boca Raton, Fla: CRC Press Inc; 1991:1-26.

Roorda A. Human visual system: image formation. In: Hornack JP, ed. *Encyclopedia of Imaging Science and Technology.* New York: Wiley & Sons; 2002:539-557.

Vision

Rodieck RW. *The First Steps in Seeing.* Sunderland, Mass: Sinauer Associates; 1998.

Wandell BA. *Foundations of Vision.* Sunderland, Mass: Sinauer Associates; 1995.

Chapter 3

How Far Can We Extend the Limits of Human Vision?

David R. Williams, PhD; Jason Porter, MS; Geunyoung Yoon, PhD; Antonio Guirao, PhD; Heidi Hofer, PhD; Li Chen, PhD; Ian Cox, PhD; and Scott M. MacRae, MD

Introduction

Methods to correct the optics of the human eye are at least 700 years old. Spectacles have been used to correct defocus at least as early as the 13th century[1,2] and to correct astigmatism since the 19th century.[3] Though it is well established that the eye suffers from many more monochromatic aberrations than defocus and astigmatism-aberrations we will refer to as higher-order aberrations—there has been relatively little work on correcting them until recently. In 1961, Smirnov, an early pioneer in the characterization of the eye's higher-order aberrations, suggested that it would be possible to manufacture customized lenses to compensate for them in individual eyes.[4] Recent developments increase the probability that Smirnov's suggestion may soon be realized. More rapid and accurate instruments for measuring the ocular aberrations are available, most notably the Shack-Hartmann wavefront sensor, first applied to the eye by Liang et al.[5] Moreover, there are new techniques to correct higher-order aberrations. Liang et al showed that a deformable mirror in an adaptive optics system can correct the eye's higher-order aberrations.[6] This study was the first to demonstrate that the correction of higher-order aberrations can lead to supernormal visual performance in normal eyes. Presently, the visual benefits of adaptive optics can only be obtained in the laboratory due to the relatively large size and high cost of conventional deformable mirrors. Alternative wavefront correctors that are less expensive and more compact, such as Microelectromechanical Systems (MEMS) technology and liquid crystal spatial light modulators, offer the exciting possibility of developing new diagnostic tools incorporating adaptive optics that every clinician would ultimately be able to afford. Nevertheless, the success of adaptive optics encourages the implementation of higher-order correction in everyday vision through customized contact lenses, intraocular lenses (IOLs), or laser refractive surgery. Lathing and laser ablative technologies now exist that can create arbitrary surfaces on contact lenses, offering the possibility of truly customized contact lenses. It has also been shown that conventional IOLs do not produce optimal retinal image quality after cataract surgery, and an IOL that is designed to compensate for the corneal aberrations of the eye would yield better visual outcomes.[7] Finally, there is a major ongoing effort to refine laser refractive surgery to correct other defects besides conventional refractive errors.[8-11]

Ultimately, the visual benefit of attempts to correct higher-order aberrations depends on two things. First, it depends on the relative importance of these aberrations in limiting human vision, and second, on the finesse with which these aberrations can be corrected in everyday vision. The emphasis of this chapter is on the first of these issues: How large are the visual benefits that will accrue from correcting higher-order aberrations and under what conditions will they be realized? We review what is known about the fundamental limits on visual acuity and provide theoretical and empirical evidence concerning the visual significance of higher-order aberrations. There are optical, cone mosaic, and neural factors that limit the finest detail we can see, and an understanding of all three is required to appreciate how much vision can be improved by correcting higher-order aberrations in addition to defocus and astigmatism. For example, as we will see later, improving the eye's optics is not always a good thing. Due to the nature of the limits on visual resolution set by the cone mosaic, improving the optical quality of the eye too much can actually lead to a decline in visual performance on some tasks. Before tackling this apparent paradox, however, we need to review some fundamental aspects of the optical quality of the retinal image.

Optical Limits on Vision

An understanding of the limits the eye's optics place on vision requires a succinct description of the optical quality of the eye, independent of neural factors. In this chapter, we will use the modulation transfer function (MTF) to characterize the ability of the eye's optics to create a sharp image on the retina. The MTF characterizes the quality of an optical system, whether it is a camera, a telescope, or the human eye. The curves of Figure 3-1 show the MTFs for eyes at two pupil sizes, 3 and 7.3 millimeters (mm). These curves reveal how faithfully the eye's optics can form an image of sine waves of different spatial frequency. Sine waves describe the variation in intensity across simple patterns of alternating light and dark bars used as visual stimuli. The x-axis of the MTF represents sine waves with spatial frequency varying from low, corresponding to a large angular spacing between adjacent white bars, to high spatial frequency (ie, fine gratings). Though not as familiar to the clinician as Snellen letters, sine wave gratings also produce a response not only from the optics, but also from the photoreceptor mosaic and the neural visual system, and can provide a richer characterization of how well each stage in the visual system performs. Sine waves

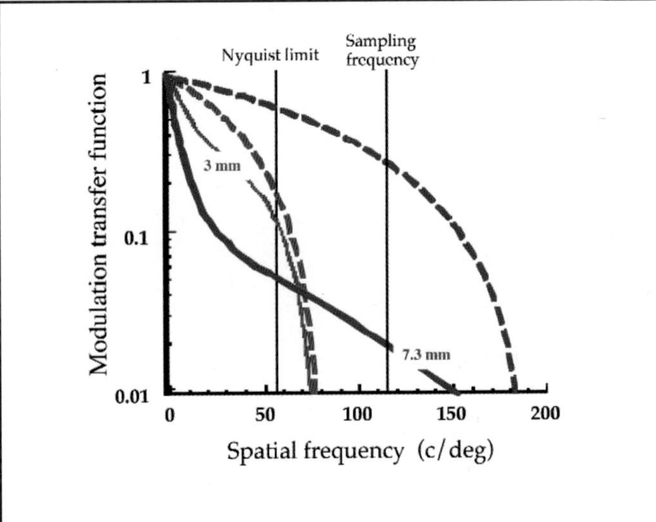

Figure 3-1. Solid curves show MTFs of the eye (averaged across 14 subjects) for two pupil sizes (3 and 7.3 mm diameter) with the correction of astigmatism and defocus, calculated from wavefront sensor measurements of the eye's wave aberration.[12] Dotted curves show the MTF for the same pupil sizes in hypothetical eyes that are free from aberrations and scatter so that the only source of image blur is diffraction. The wavelength was 670 nanometers (nm). The vertical line at 57 cycles/degree (c/deg) corresponds to the Nyquist sampling limit for the average human foveal cone mosaic. The vertical line at 114 c/deg indicates the mosaic sampling frequency.

can be added together to create any visual scene the eye might care to look at. The crucial implication of this fact is that if you know how well the eye images sine waves of different spatial frequency, it is possible to predict the retinal image for any visual scene. Intuitively, the eye's MTF at low spatial frequencies reveals how well the eye images large features in visual scenes, whereas the response to high frequencies tells us how well the eye images fine detail, closer to the limits of visual acuity. The y-axis of the MTF is the modulation transferred by the eye's optics and corresponds to the ratio of the contrast of the sine wave image on the retina to that of the original sine wave pattern viewed by the eye. The more blurring by the eye's optics, the more the modulation transfer departs from a perfect value of 1 and approaches 0.

There are three sources of image blur in the human eye: scatter, diffraction, and aberrations. Even though scatter can degrade vision in older and/or pathological eyes, we will not discuss scatter here because it is generally a minor source of image blur in younger, normal eyes. Diffraction at the eye's pupil is an important source of image blur when the pupil is small, becoming less important with increasing pupil size. The dashed lines in Figure 3-1 show the MTF of eyes that suffer only from diffraction and are free of aberrations. The MTF extends to much higher spatial frequencies (ie, there is less blur from diffraction) for the 7.3 mm pupil than the 3 mm pupil. The highest spatial frequency (expressed in c/deg) that can be imaged on the retina of an aberration-free eye is $\pi p/180\lambda$, where p is the diameter of the pupil and λ the wavelength. Thus, for a 3 mm pupil and a wavelength of 670 nm, the highest spatial frequency that could be viewed in an aberration-free eye is 78 c/deg (190 c/deg for a dilated pupil of 7.3 mm). Blurring by diffraction is unavoidable, quite unlike aberrations, which can be corrected.

The solid curves show the MTFs of normal human eyes for the same 3 and 7.3 mm pupil sizes, but including the blurring effects of the eye's higher-order aberrations as well as diffraction. We have not included blur due to defocus and astigmatism, which conventional spectacles can correct. At low spatial frequencies, the 7.3 mm curve lies below the 3 mm curve because the blurring from aberrations increases strongly with increasing pupil diameter. The central area in the dilated pupil typically has better optical performance than the pupil margin. The aberration-free MTFs lie above the MTFs that include higher-order aberrations, especially for the larger pupil. These results suggest that a rather large increase in retinal image contrast could be achieved by correcting higher-order aberrations when the pupil is large. However, this analysis overestimates the benefit of correcting higher-order aberrations for at least two reasons. First, it does not take account of the limitations on visual acuity imposed by the photoreceptor mosaic and subsequent neural processing, a topic we will address next. Second, this analysis is valid only in monochromatic light, whereas vision normally involves broad band, polychromatic light. As we will see later, in addition to suffering from higher-order monochromatic aberrations, the eye suffers from chromatic aberration that also blurs the retinal image in polychromatic (white light) illumination. Chromatic aberration in an optical system such as the eye causes light rays of different wavelengths to be focused at different positions.

Limits Imposed by the Photoreceptor Mosaic on Vision

The image formed on the retina (or retinal image) is a spatially continuous distribution of light intensity, but the cone mosaic is made of photoreceptors that discretely sample the image. This sampling process results in the loss of information about the retinal image because the brain can never know about the behavior of the retinal image between the sample locations defined by the cone mosaic. The information loss caused by sampling superficially resembles that by optical blurring in that it is high spatial frequencies (ie, fine details in the retinal image) that are affected most. However, there the similarity ends. Optical blurring is a reduction in contrast in the retinal image, whereas sampling does not generally reduce contrast but rather causes errors in the brain's interpretation of the retinal image.

The term used to describe errors due to sampling is *aliasing*. This is because sampling causes high spatial frequencies in the image to masquerade or alias as low spatial frequencies. Figure 3-2A shows this effect for a one-dimensional array of photoreceptors that is sampling two sinusoidal gratings with different spatial frequencies. Notice that the light intensity is identical at each of the sample locations. The cone mosaic is blind to the fact that the retinal images differ between the sample locations defined by the photoreceptors. Since the photoreceptor mosaic does not retain any information that these two images are in fact different, the brain cannot hope to distinguish them. The brain interprets the pattern as the low frequency alternative whether the low or high spatial frequency is in fact present. Figure 3-2B shows aliasing for an array of sample locations taken from an image of the human cone mosaic. When the fundamental spatial frequency of a grating is low, such as for a 30 c/deg grating, the mosaic has an adequate number of samples to represent it and aliasing does not occur.

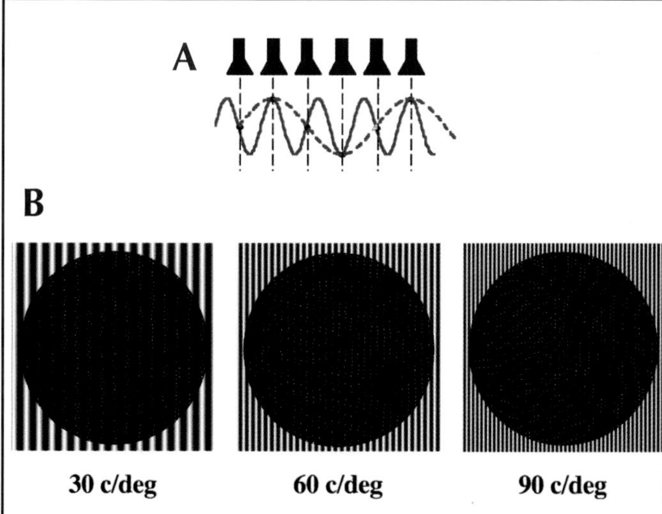

Figure 3-2. (A) Two sinusoidal stimuli sampled by an array of cones. The spatial frequency of one stimulus (solid line) is three times the frequency of the other (dashed line). The cone response is identical for the two patterns, illustrating aliasing, the ambiguity introduced by sampling. (B) Three sinusoidal patterns seen through the same sampling resembling the cone mosaic. After sampling, the high-frequency pattern (90 c/deg) appears as a distorted, low-frequency pattern, though the sampling rate is adequate for the low frequency pattern (30 c/deg). The finest grating pattern that this mosaic can distinctly resolve is set at the Nyquist sampling limit of approximately 60 c/deg.

> The 60 c/deg grating represents the highest spatial frequency that can be adequately sampled and represented by this typical photoreceptor mosaic.

However, when the spatial frequency becomes higher, as for the 90 c/deg grating, a low frequency pattern emerges. The irregularity of the low frequency alias is a result of the disorder in the cone mosaic. A 30 c/deg grating has the same spacing between bright bars as the spacing between the horizontal strokes in a 20/20 Snellen letter E. A 60 c/deg grating has a bar spacing corresponding to that of a 20/10 Snellen letter E, and so on.

How can we quantify the limits imposed by the spacing of cones on vision?

> Helmholtz knew that the finest grating that the eye could resolve required at least one sample for each light and each dark bar of the grating.[3] This simple intuition is captured in modern terms by the sampling theorem, which states that the highest frequency that can be recovered without aliasing from a sampling array is one half the sampling frequency of the array.[13]

The sampling frequency of the array is the reciprocal of the spacing between samples, which in this case is the spacing between rows of cones at the fovea.

> Half the sampling frequency is the so-called Nyquist sampling limit. Anatomical and psychophysical estimates of the spacing between rows of foveal cones indicate an average of about 0.51 minutes of arc, which makes the average sampling rate 118 c/deg and the average Nyquist sampling limit half that, or about 59 c/deg.

Table 3-1 compares the results of several studies. The conversion between columns in Table 3-1 has been made assuming triangular packing of cones.[14] The Nyquist limit indicates the finest grating patterns that human foveal vision can reasonably expect to resolve in the sense of being able to see the regular stripes of the grating imaged on the retina. Indeed, estimates of the foveal visual acuity for gratings generally agree with the Nyquist sampling limit. In some circumstances, subjects can obtain correct information about, for example, the orientation of a grating at spatial frequencies slightly higher than the Nyquist sampling limit,[15] but the perception of a distinct grating pattern ends at spatial frequencies near the Nyquist sampling limit.

At spatial frequencies above the Nyquist sampling limit, gratings appear more like wavy zebra stripes and appear coarser than the actual gratings on the retina, as shown in Figure 3-3. Williams[14,16] studied these perceptual effects with a laser interferometer, extending earlier reports by Bergmann,[17] Byram,[18] and Campbell and Green,[19] showing conclusively that they result from aliasing by the cone mosaic. Laser interferometry is a method to project gratings, in the form of interference fringes, on the retina that are not blurred by the eye's optics. Gratings with spatial frequencies over 200 c/deg can be imaged on the retina without any appreciable loss of contrast. In the range between 0 and 45 c/deg, interference fringes can be seen as regular stripes across the central foveal region. As the spatial frequency increases toward 60 c/deg, the bars of the fringes can be seen only in a progressively smaller region of the fovea. At about 60 c/deg, the fine, regular bars are lost, and most subjects report the appearance of an annulus of fine wavy lines as shown in Figure 3-3. The annulus corresponds to aliasing by cones just outside the foveal center, which are more widely spaced, and alias at a lower spatial frequency than in the foveal center. As spatial frequency increases, this annulus of wavy lines collapses to a circular patch at a frequency of 90 to 100 c/deg. Subjects describe this patch as resembling a fingerprint or a pattern of zebra stripes. Between 150 and 160 c/deg, the zebra stripe pattern disappears. Due to the sampling limits imposed by the cone mosaic, no matter how much one could improve the eye's optics, one would not expect an increase in visual acuity beyond about 60 c/deg in the average human eye.

Aliasing can potentially distort the appearance of not only grating stimuli but of any visual scene that contains spatial frequencies above the Nyquist sampling limit. For example, sharp edges would be expected to take on a jagged appearance. There are also errors in the color appearance of fine details, referred to as *chromatic aliasing*, caused by the fact that the retina contains three cone submosaics for color vision, each sampling the visual scene even more coarsely than the combined mosaic.[20] Aliasing errors are not generally visible in everyday viewing conditions, partly because the blurring of the retinal image by the eye's optics plays a protective role. This is illustrated in Figure 3-1 which shows that the optical MTF does not allow much contrast in the retinal image at spatial frequencies that exceed the foveal cone Nyquist sampling limit. At the Nyquist sampling limit, the retinal image contrast never exceeds about 10% for any pupil

Table 3-1
Estimates of Human Foveal Cone Sampling

Source	Density (cones/mm²)	Spacing (microns)	Spacing (min of arc)	Nyquist (c/deg)	Acuity (min)
Østerberg (1935)[21]	147 x 10^3	2.43	0.50	60	1
Miller (1979)[22]	128 x 10^3	2.6	0.54	55.9	1.07
Yuodelis and Hendrikson (1986)[23]	208 x 10^3	2.04	0.42	71.4	0.84
Curcio et al (1987)[24]	162 x 10^3	2.57 ± 0.71	0.53 ± 0.15	56.6	1.06
Curcio et al (1990)[25]	197 x 10^3	2.55 ± 0.52	0.53 ± 0.11	56.6	1.06
Williams (1985)[16]	126 x 10^3	2.62 ± 0.17	0.54 ± 0.04	55.6	1.08
Williams (1988)[14]	129 x 10^3	2.59 ± 0.12	0.54 ± 0.02	55.6	1.08
Average	157 x 10^3	2.49	0.51	58.8	1.03

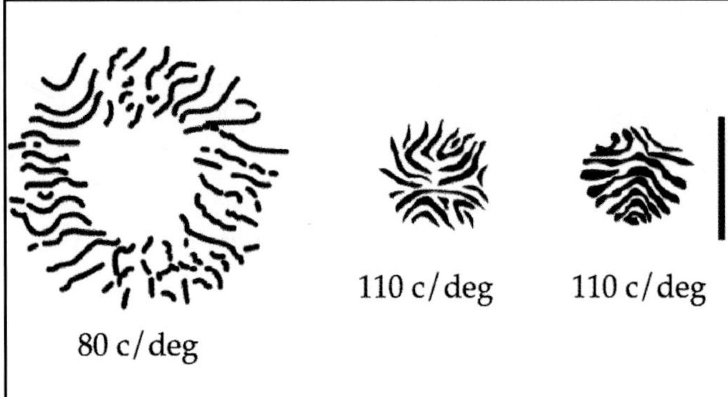

Figure 3-3. Drawing of the appearance of an 80 c/deg and a 110 c/deg (two subjects) interference fringe. Scale bar corresponds to 1 deg of visual angle.[16] The zebra stripe appearance results from aliasing by the cone mosaic.

size, and it is usually far less than this since the contrast in the original scene is usually much less than 100%.

For aliasing to disrupt vision in ordinary scenes, the optical quality of the eye would have to be considerably better than it is.

An indication that this is the case comes from the observation that aliasing errors are not seen in ordinary vision outside the fovea. At an eccentricity of about 4 degrees, the optical quality of the eye is essentially the same as that at the foveal center, yet the Nyquist sampling limit has declined by a factor of about 3. The fact that aliasing is not visible at this eccentricity suggests that the MTF of the eye could be extended by at least a factor of 3 at the fovea without running the risk of incurring aliasing errors there. This realization runs counter to the prevailing view that evolution has matched the optics of the eye and the spacing of foveal cones. Instead, it appears that the optics could afford to be substantially better in the average eye without introducing an important loss of image fidelity due to foveal aliasing. Even in controlled laboratory conditions, it is difficult to produce aliasing effects without the use of interference fringe stimuli. This is true even in extrafoveal vision, which is less protected from aliasing by the eye's optics. Increasing the optical quality of the eye runs a greater risk of causing aliasing outside the fovea. But even outside the fovea, unusually high contrast stimuli are required to cause aliasing and careful attention must be paid to the eye's refractive state.

This is good news for attempts to correct higher-order aberrations in the eye because it suggests that the deleterious effects of sampling and aliasing will not interfere with vision and will not reduce the visual benefit of improving retinal image contrast.

Neural Limits on Vision

Are the postreceptoral retina and the brain equipped to take advantage of the improved optical quality that customized correction can provide? There would be little point in improving the eye's optics if the brain were incapable of resolving the high spatial frequencies restored by a customized correction. Experimentally, this question has been explored by measuring the *contrast sensitivity function* (CSF) with laser interference fringe stimuli.

The CSF is a measure of how sensitive subjects are to gratings of different spatial frequencies. The CSF is determined by finding the threshold contrast at which the subject can detect a sinusoidal grating at each of a number of spatial frequencies. The reciprocal of the threshold is the contrast sensitivity.

At high spatial frequencies, the CSF steadily decreases with spatial frequency, which means that the subject needs higher contrast to detect finer details. This is true even when interference fringes are used to eliminate optical blurring in the eye, as shown in Figure 3-4. This shows that, just as the optics blur the retinal image, the postreceptoral visual system blurs the neural image. The important point is that, despite the neural blur, the nervous system is equipped with the machinery to resolve spatial frequencies as high as the foveal cone Nyquist sampling limit. This makes it quite likely that it can take advantage of improvements in retinal image contrast for spatial frequencies up to the limits set by the photoreceptor mosaic. Indeed, we will show direct empirical evidence for this later.

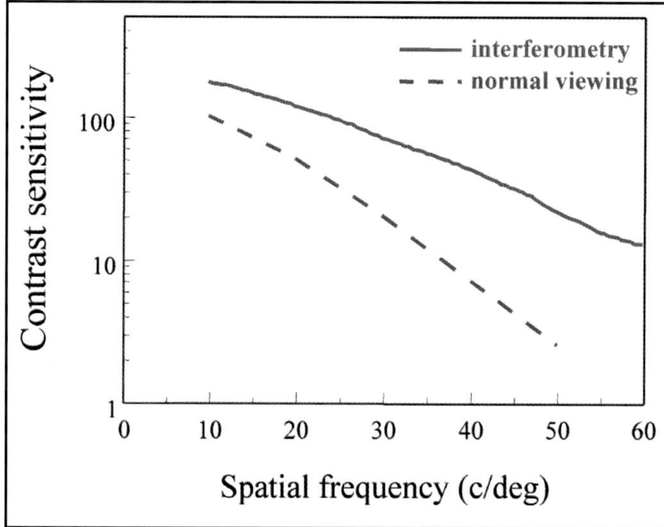

Figure 3-4. CSF measured with interferometry (neural CSF) and CSF for normal viewing conditions for a pupil of 3 mm.[26]

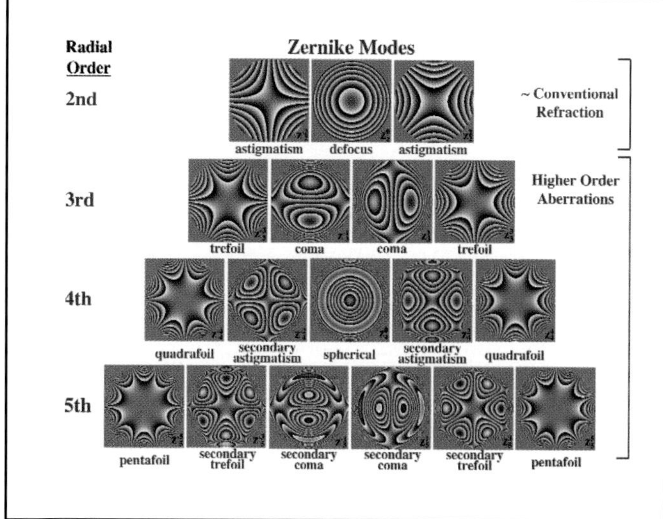

Figure 3-5. Zernike Pyramid. An arbitrary wave aberration can be decomposed into individual Zernike modes. The second-order Zernike modes, which are defocus and two astigmatism terms, can be corrected with a conventional refraction. Higher-order aberrations correspond to Zernike modes of third order and higher.

Visual Benefit of Higher-Order Correction Based on Wave Aberration Measurements

This section describes an analysis of the visual benefit of correcting higher-order aberrations based on measurements of the aberrations found in a large population of eyes. Based on subjective observations of a point source of light, Helmholtz argued that the eye suffered from a host of aberrations that are not found in conventional, man-made optical systems.[27] There have been a number of methods developed to quantify these aberrations.[4,28-33] Liang et al[5] developed a technique based on the Shack-Hartmann principle[34] that provides a rapid, automated, and objective measure of the wave aberration simultaneously at a large number of sample points across the eye's pupil. Using this technique, Liang and Williams provided what is arguably the most complete description to date of the wave aberration of the eye.[12] They measured the eye's aberrations up to 10 radial orders, quantifying the irregular aberrations predicted by Helmholtz and subsequent investigators.[28,29,35]

The wave aberration can be described as the sum of a number of component aberrations such as defocus, astigmatism, coma, spherical aberration, as well as other higher-order aberrations. The wave aberration can be decomposed into these constituent aberrations in much the same way that Fourier analysis can decompose an image into spatial frequency components. For an optical system such as the eye, it is convenient to use Zernike polynomials as the basis functions because of their desirable mathematical properties for circular pupils. In addition, it has been shown using principal components analysis that Zernike polynomials are robust basis functions that adequately capture the majority of aberration variance typically found in human eyes.[36,37] Figure 3-5 shows in two dimensions the first five radial orders (18 Zernike modes) in the Zernike Pyramid of aberrations (excluding piston, tip, and tilt) that are used to compose the eye's wave aberration. Each mode has a value that indicates its magnitude of wavefront error, usually expressed in microns, corresponding to its root mean square (RMS) or standard deviation across the pupil (see Appendix 1).

> Defocus is one of the simplest Zernike modes and is the mode that is most closely associated with the spherical refractive error. (Sometimes Zernike defocus does not correspond to the spherical refractive error because higher-order aberrations can also influence the spherical refractive error.)

Clinicians are familiar with defocus in myopia and hyperopia, expressed in diopters (D), which corresponds to the reciprocal of the focal length in meters. In an eye that suffers from defocus alone, the relationship between diopters and the RMS wavefront error is:

$$\text{Diopters (D)} = -\frac{4\sqrt{3}Z^0_2}{(\text{pupil radius})^2}$$

where Z^0_2 is the magnitude of the Zernike defocus mode in microns and the pupil radius is in mm. In a normal eye that suffers from defocus and additional aberrations, this equation is only approximately correct, as higher-order aberrations can influence estimates of a patient's best subjective refraction.[38]

From the wave aberration, we can calculate the eye's MTF and phase transfer functions (PTFs), which provide a complete description of retinal image quality. The MTF and PTF can be obtained from the complex autocorrelation of the pupil function, where the pupil function includes the pupil aperture and the wave aberration.[13] Alternately, the point spread function (PSF) captures the same information as the MTF and PTF. The PSF is the Fourier transform of the MTF and PTF. Intuitively, it is the image on the retina of a single point of light, such as the image on the retina when the eye is looking at a star. Figure 3-6 illustrates the PSFs produced by each individual Zernike mode on the retina. We can also calculate any retinal image by the convolution of the object with the PSF. An example of this is shown in Figure 3-7, which illustrates how the retinal image of a visual stimulus sometimes used in psychophysical experiments, called a *binary noise stimulus*, is blurred due to the PSF corresponding to each Zernike term.

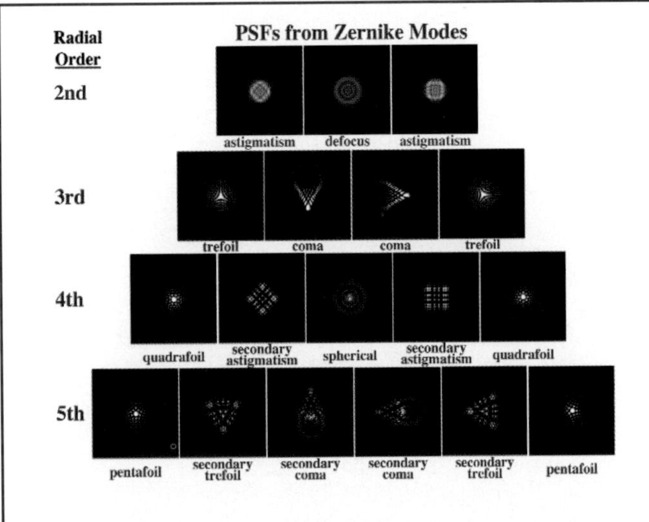

Figure 3-6. Pyramid of PSFs (add-point spread function) obtained from each individual Zernike mode in monochromatic light (550 nm). A PSF is what one would see if looking at a point source of light.

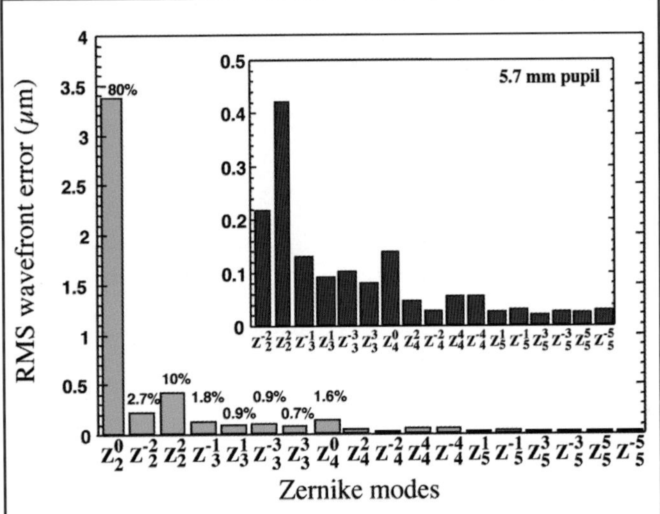

Figure 3-8. Mean absolute RMS values for 18 Zernike modes as measured from a population of 109 normal human subjects for a 5.7 mm pupil. The inset excludes the first Zernike mode corresponding to defocus (Z^0_2) and has an expanded ordinate to illustrate the magnitudes of the higher-order aberrations. Percentages labeled above the first eight modes designate the percent of the variance accounted for by each mode.

The beauty of this is that we can compute from the aberrations, which are defined in the eye's pupil, the impact they will have on the quality of the image formed on the retina. Both diffraction and aberrations are taken into account and it is only light scatter that is ignored, as it is usually small in younger, normal eyes. This computational link between pupil and retina is very valuable because we can use it to deduce the relative importance of different aberrations on image quality. This is critical for deciding which aberrations are worth correcting and which are less important.

An important feature of the eye's wave aberration is that it is a single function that captures all optical defects in both the cornea and the lens. The final retinal image quality depends on the combined effects of the cornea and the lens rather than on the

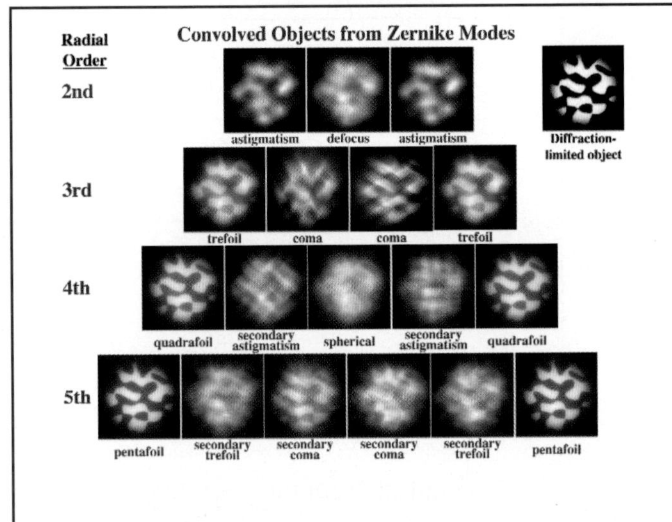

Figure 3-7. Pyramid of retinal images obtained by convolving the PSF produced by each individual Zernike mode (see Figure 3-6) with a binary noise stimulus (the object) in monochromatic light (550 nm). The original object, blurred only by the effect of diffraction, is shown in the top right corner. Aberrations near the center of the pyramid tend to blur the object more than aberrations at the edge.

optical quality of each isolated component. For example, in young eyes, the spherical aberration introduced by the cornea is usually reduced by the lens.[39] Other corneal aberrations may also be compensated by the lens in younger subjects.[40,41] These results have important implications for customized correction because they emphasize the necessity to capture the total wave aberration. For example, if the ablation profile in customized laser refractive surgery were computed solely from corneal topography, the final aberrations of the eye could be larger in some cases than before ablation.

For the same amount of RMS wavefront error of each aberration, it is clear from Figure 3-7 that aberrations at the edges of the Zernike pyramid have less subjective blur than those closer to the center of the pyramid.

Population Statistics of the Wave Aberration

A conventional refraction (sphere, cylinder, and axis) typically corrects for only three components of the wave aberration (one defocus and two astigmatic modes). However, if one hopes to achieve a diffraction-limited correction of the eye's optics, a complete description of the wave aberration of normal eyes would require at least 42 individual Zernike modes (corresponding to eighth order) for a large pupil diameter of 7.3 mm.[12] The average magnitudes of the lowest 18 monochromatic aberrations (up to and including fifth order) are presented in Figure 3-8 for 109 normal subjects between the ages of 21 and 65 years (mean age of 41 years) with natural accommodation. Each adult had a spherical refraction between 6 D and -12 D and a refractive astigmatism no larger than -3 D, and no pathological eyes were included in this study.[36] Verifying earlier results reported by Howland and Howland[30] from a smaller subset of eyes, there is a general tendency for the magnitude of the aberrations to decrease with increasing order. The aberration with the largest magnitude is

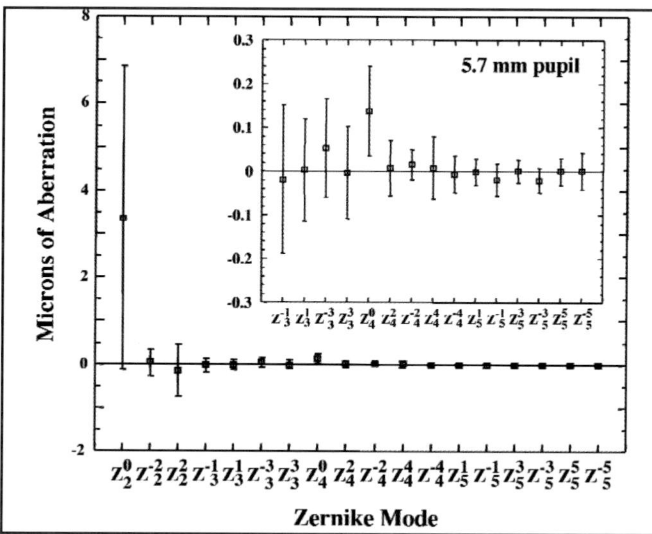

Figure 3-9. Mean values of the first 18 Zernike modes in the population of 109 human subjects for a 5.7 mm pupil. The error bars indicate plus and minus one standard deviation. The inset excludes the first three Zernike modes corresponding to defocus and astigmatism (Z^0_2, Z^{-2}_2, and Z^2_2) and has an expanded ordinate to illustrate the variability of the higher-order aberrations.

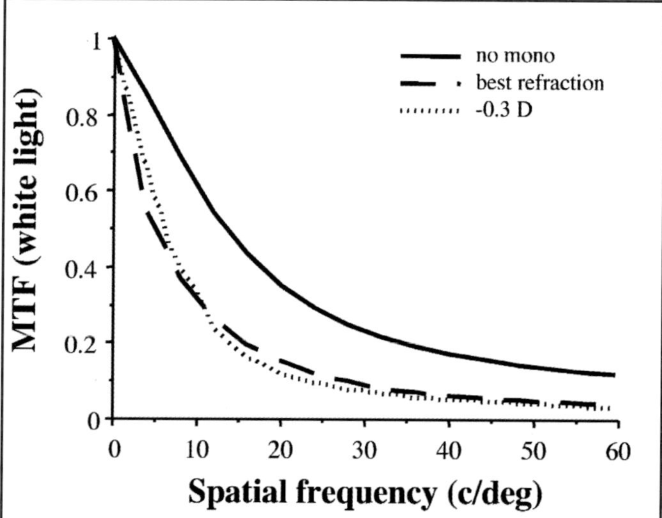

Figure 3-10. White light MTFs (5.7 mm pupil) when correcting all of the eye's monochromatic aberrations (solid line) and when only -0.3 D of defocus are present in the eye (dotted line). The average MTF showing the best correction of defocus and astigmatism from the normal population with higher-order aberrations still present (dashed line) is very similar to the MTF of an eye with only -0.3 D of sphere.

defocus, Z^0_2, followed by the two Zernike modes representing astigmatism, Z^{-2}_2 and Z^2_2. Defocus is expected to be the largest aberration, but it is especially large in this population because the majority of the subjects were patients at a local clinic and tended to be myopic. Higher-order aberrations in this figure correspond to all those beyond the first three. The 15 higher- order aberrations shown here in aggregate account for about two-thirds as much of the variance of the wave aberration as the two modes associated with astigmatism.

In addition to examining the magnitude of each mode, we can also look at the distribution of each Zernike coefficient in the same population. These results, displayed in Figure 3-9, show that each Zernike coefficient, with the exception of spherical aberration, has a mean value that is approximately zero. The mean RMS wavefront error for spherical aberration in this population was 0.138 ± 0.103 µm (5.7 mm pupil).

> This indicates that the normal population typically has a tendency toward a slight positive spherical aberration, where the peripheral light rays are focused in front of the central light rays.

Population Statistics of the Visual Benefit of Higher-Order Correction

The magnitude and distribution of monochromatic aberrations in the population of human eyes shown above does not directly provide information on the degree to which higher-order aberrations constructively or destructively interact with each other to improve or degrade retinal image quality. Figure 3-10 compares the white light MTF produced by the eye's higher-order aberrations with that of an eye containing defocus alone. As illustrated in the figure, the average MTF from the normal population for the best correction of defocus and astigmatism (with higher-order aberrations left uncorrected) is nearly identical to the MTF of a hypothetical eye suffering from only -0.3 D of pure defocus, or sphere. The average RMS wavefront error of the higher-order aberrations in the population is equivalent to that produced by -0.3 D of defocus alone, approximately 0.35 microns (µm) (5.7 mm pupil). Of course, these values can be highly variable from patient to patient depending on the amount of higher-order aberration present in each individual eye.

One measure we have developed to inform us directly about the visual improvement resulting from a perfect, theoretical correction of the eye's higher-order aberrations is a quantity we call the *visual benefit*. It is the increase in retinal image contrast at each spatial frequency that would occur if one were to correct all monochromatic aberrations instead of just correcting defocus and astigmatism as one does with a conventional refraction. More specifically, the visual benefit is the ratio of the eye's polychromatic (white light) MTF when all the monochromatic aberrations are corrected to that when only defocus and astigmatism are corrected, as shown in Figure 3-11.

Because customized correction with contact lenses, IOLs, and laser refractive surgery would involve everyday viewing conditions in which the spectra of objects are broad band or polychromatic, we chose to calculate the visual benefit for white light instead of monochromatic light of a single wavelength. The eye suffers from chromatic aberration of two kinds, *axial* and *transverse*. The axial chromatic aberration is the chromatic difference of focus on the optical axis of the eye. Short wavelength (blue) light is brought to a focus nearer to the cornea and lens than the long wavelength (red) light so that only one wavelength in a broad band stimulus can be in focus on the retina at any one time. Wald and Griffin[42] and many other researchers have measured the axial chromatic aberration of the eye. There is almost no variation from observer to observer because all eyes are made of essentially the same materials with the same chromatic dispersion. The total chromatic difference of focus is approximately 2 D over the entire visible spectrum of wavelengths the eye can detect. We have included axial chromatic aberration in the calcu-

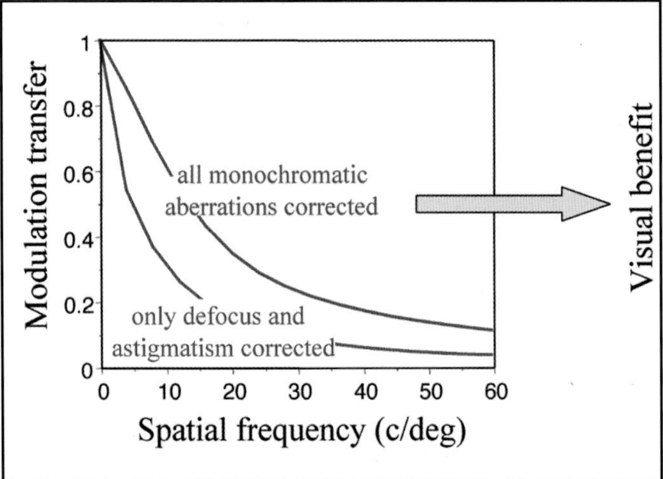

Figure 3-11. The visual benefit is obtained as the ratio between the MTF in white light with no monochromatic aberrations and the eye's MTF in white light with only astigmatism and defocus corrected. The MTF in white light was calculated from the polychromatic PSF determined by integrating the monochromatic PSF affected by the eye's chromatic aberration across the spectrum and weighted with the ocular spectral sensitivity. The baseline MTF corresponding to a conventional correction was calculated by finding the amount of defocus and astigmatism required to maximize the volume of the CSF obtained as the product of the MTF and the neural CSF.

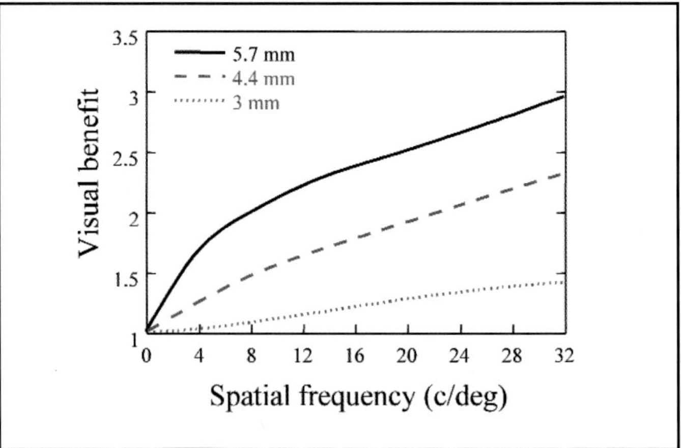

Figure 3-12. Visual benefit at each spatial frequency for three pupil diameters, averaged across a normal population of 109 subjects.

lation of the MTF because, as we will see later, it can have large effects on retinal image quality when one is trying to eliminate all of the aberrations in the eye.

The transverse chromatic aberration (TCA) is the wavelength-dependent displacement of the image position on the retina. In our experience, foveal TCA does not typically reduce retinal image quality very much.

The white light MTF is computed from the polychromatic PSF, which is calculated by first summing the monochromatic PSFs defocused by axial chromatic aberration, shifted by TCA, and weighted by the spectral sensitivity of the eye at each wavelength. The modulus of the Fourier transform of the white light PSF is the white light, or polychromatic, MTF. A visual benefit of 1 corresponds to no benefit of correcting higher-order aberrations. A value of 2 would indicate a two-fold increase in retinal image contrast provided by correcting higher- order aberrations (in addition to defocus and astigmatism). Though the visual benefit is calculated from retinal image quality, the visual benefit is directly applicable to visual performance as assessed with contrast sensitivity measurements. That is, a visual benefit of 2 will lead to a two-fold increase in contrast sensitivity as well as a two-fold increase in retinal image contrast.

Figure 3-12 shows the mean values of the visual benefit across a population of 109 normal subjects, for three different pupil sizes, as a function of the spatial frequency.[43] For a pupil of 3 mm, the visual benefit is modest. For small pupils, diffraction dominates and aberrations beyond defocus and astigmatism are relatively unimportant. A small visual improvement might be realized for the 3 mm pupil at high spatial frequencies (about 1.5 at 32 c/deg). In bright daylight conditions, the natural pupil of most normal eyes is so sufficiently small (~3 mm) that the retinal image would not be greatly affected by aberrations. However, for mid and large pupils, because of the well-known fact that the aberrations grow with increasing pupil size,[12,44] an important visual benefit can be obtained across all spatial frequencies by correcting the monochromatic higher-order aberrations. For example, with a 5.7 mm pupil, the average visual benefit across the population is about 2.5 at 16 c/deg and about 3 at 32 c/deg. This would correspond to a distinct improvement in the sharpness of the retinal image. Thus, for the normal population, the visual benefit of a customized ablation would be greatest in younger patients or individuals who tend to have large pupils, and in situations such as night driving.

> Visual benefit is directly applicable to visual performance as assessed with contrast sensitivity measurements. That is, a visual benefit of 2 will lead to a two-fold increase in contrast sensitivity as well as a two-fold increase in retinal image contrast.

What fraction of the population could benefit by correcting the higher-order aberrations? Just as there is large variability in the population in the amount of astigmatism present, so there is variability in the amount of higher-order aberrations. Patients with larger amounts of higher-order aberrations will derive much more visual benefit from higher-order correction than others. The frequency histograms in Figure 3-13 show how much the visual benefit, for a 5.7 mm pupil, varies among eyes in the normal population of 109 normal subjects and in a small cohort of four kerataconic patients. The distributions of visual benefit at spatial frequencies of 16 c/deg and 32 c/deg are shown because they correspond roughly to the highest frequencies that are detectable by normal subjects viewing natural scenes.

> Some normal eyes have a visual benefit close to 1 (ie, show almost no benefit of correcting higher-order aberrations). At the other extreme, some normal eyes show a benefit of more than a factor of 5.

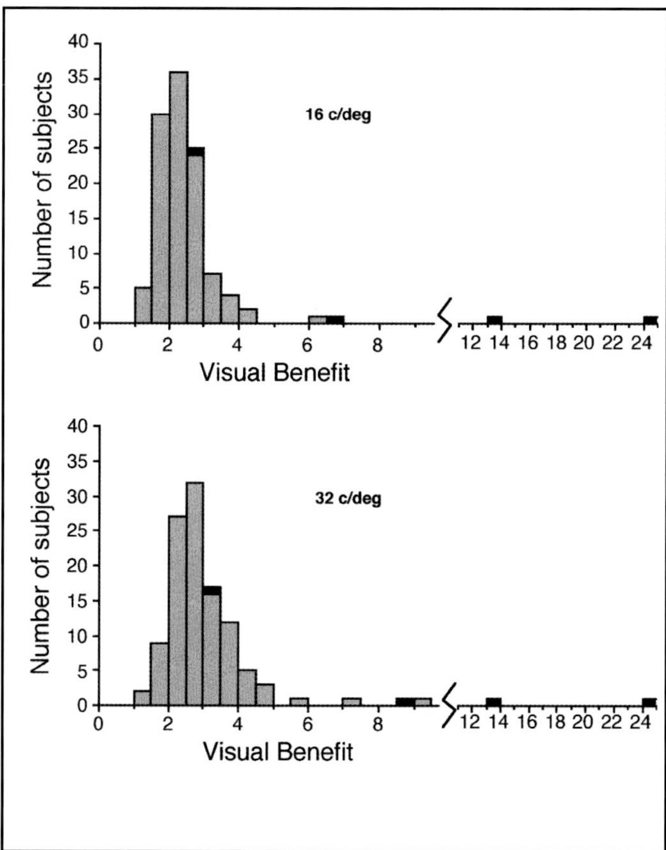

Figure 3-13. Histogram of the visual benefit, at 16 c/deg and 32 c/deg, of correcting higher-order aberrations in white light for a population of 109 normal subjects (green) and a sample of four kerataconic patients (black). Pupil size is 5.7 mm.

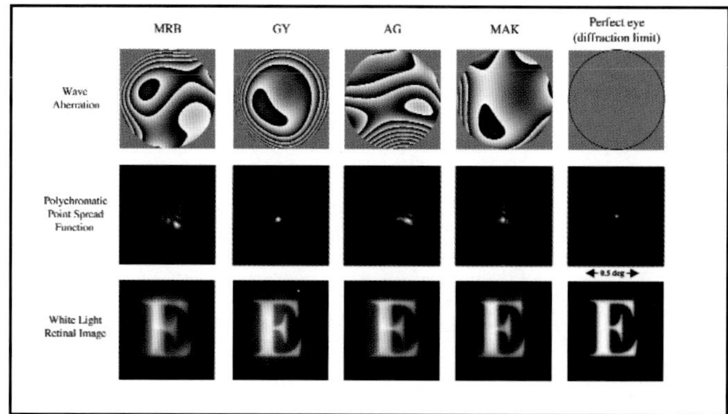

Figure 3-14. The wave aberrations of four typical eyes and a perfect diffraction-limited eye for 5.7 mm pupils are shown at the top. Their corresponding PSFs, computed from the wave aberrations, are shown in the middle row. The bottom row shows the convolution of the PSF with a Snellen letter E, subtending 30 minutes of arc. This shows the retinal image of the letter given the wave aberration measured in each eye. Note the increased blurring in the real eyes compared with the diffraction-limited eye. The calculations were performed assuming white light, axial chromatic aberration in the eye, and that a wavelength of 555 nm was in best focus on the retina.

Editor's note:

The normal population studies by Porter et al[36] demonstrate that some people would have a higher visual benefit from higher-order aberration correction and others would not.[43] We have found this to be true in the clinical excimer laser studies noted later in this book on wavefront-guided customized ablation (Chapters 26 to 31, specifically Chapter 28, Figure 28-7).

S. MacRae, MD

To provide a better indication of the typical visual benefits that subjects would incur with customized correction, Figure 3-14 shows the effect of correcting higher-order aberrations on the retinal image in white light for four subjects over a 5.7 mm pupil. In each case, the PSF computed from the wave aberration is convolved with a letter E subtending 30 minutes of arc, roughly corresponding to the 20/100 line on the Snellen chart. The letters are substantially more blurred than that in the diffraction-limited case, in which there is little or no influence of aberrations. We emphasize that these are the retinal images expected from these eyes and do not necessarily represent the perceptual experience these subjects would have of the retinal images, which is also determined by neural processing.

The visual benefit in the kerataconic patients is typically much larger than that of the normal eyes. One of the subjects of the sample, who is in the early stages of keratoconus, would have a visual benefit similar to the normal population. But the other three show larger benefits than any subject does in the normal population (one of them as high as a factor of 25). Figure 3-15 shows the average visual benefit in the sample of four kerataconics for the three pupil sizes. These patients can expect a large benefit at all pupil sizes. Based on this information, the development of technologies to correct the idiosyncratic higher-order aberrations of such patients would be an especially valuable outcome of wavefront sensing. The wavefront sensor coupled with calculations such as these can efficiently screen those patients who stand to gain the largest benefit from customized correction.

The Visual Benefit of Higher-Order Correction Measured With Adaptive Optics

The analysis so far has been based on calculation and theory. It would be helpful if a reliable, noninvasive method existed that allowed higher-order aberrations to be quickly corrected in normal eyes, so that the actual visual benefit could be assessed. Fortunately, adaptive optics provide just such a method. Figure 3-16 shows a simplified drawing of an adaptive optics system for the eye that is in use in our lab at the University of Rochester.[12,45] The complete system requires a wavefront sensor to measure the wave aberration of the eye and a wavefront corrector to compensate for the aberrations.

The correcting element in our system is a deformable mirror with 97 actuators (or small mechanical pistons) mounted behind it that can reshape the mirror in such a way as to temporarily correct most of the particular aberrations found in each patient's eye.

In addition to the wavefront sensor and corrector, the adaptive optics system has an optical path that allows the subject to view visual stimuli, such as sine wave gratings or Snellen letters, through the deformable mirror.

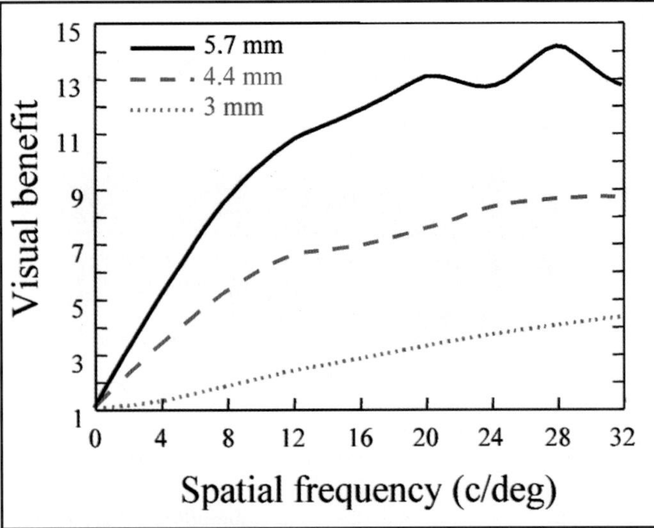

Figure 3-15. Average visual benefit in a sample of four keratoconic patients, for three pupil diameters.

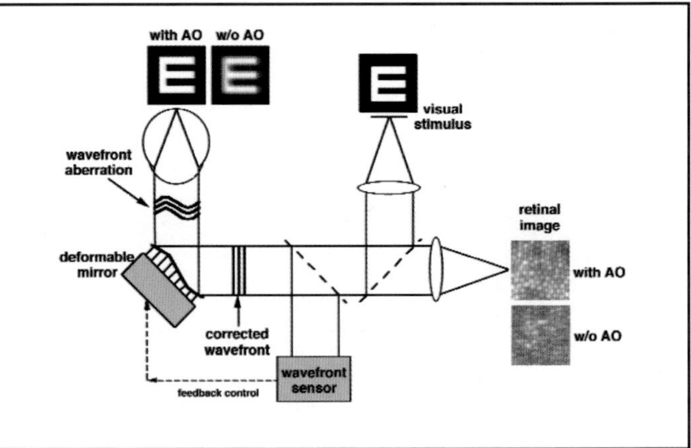

Figure 3-16. Schematic of the University of Rochester adaptive optics system for the human eye.

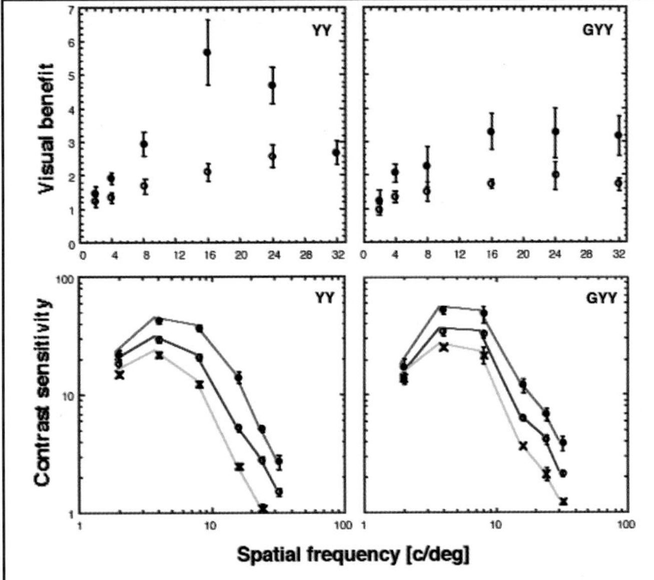

Figure 3-17. The measured contrast sensitivity (lower panels) and visual benefit (upper panels) for two subjects when correcting various aberrations across a 6 mm pupil: both monochromatic and chromatic aberrations (filled circles), monochromatic aberrations only (open circles), and defocus and astigmatism only (x symbols).

> Subjects viewing the world through adaptive optics can have a sharper image of it than they have ever had before. Adaptive optics can also correct the aberrations for light leaving the eye, which makes it possible to obtain very high resolution images of the living retina[46] as well as to improve vision.

Contrast Sensitivity With and Without Higher-Order Correction

To assess the benefit of correcting higher-order aberrations, we measured the contrast sensitivity of the eye following correction with adaptive optics compared with the contrast sensitivity following a conventional refraction to correct defocus and astigmatism only. Figure 3-17 shows the CSF (lower panels) and visual benefit (upper panels) for two subjects with only defocus and astigmatism corrected (x symbols), after correcting the higher-order monochromatic aberrations as well as defocus and astigmatism (open circles), and after correcting both monochromatic aberrations and chromatic aberration (filled circles). In this case, visual benefit is calculated from the ratio of the CSFs instead of the ratio of MTFs, but its meaning is otherwise identical. Chromatic aberrations, both axial and transverse, were eliminated by placing a narrow band interference filter between the eye and the stimulus.

The results are similar for both subjects. The contrast sensitivity when correcting most monochromatic aberrations with a deformable mirror is higher than when defocus and astigmatism alone are corrected. This illustrates that higher-order aberrations in normal eyes reduce visual performance. Moreover, correcting both chromatic and monochromatic aberrations provides an even larger increase in contrast sensitivity.

Figure 3-17 also shows the visual benefit of correcting various aberrations, defined as the ratio of contrast sensitivity when correcting monochromatic and chromatic aberrations (filled circles) and when correcting monochromatic aberrations only (open circles) to that when correcting defocus and astigmatism only. Contrast sensitivity when correcting monochromatic aberrations only is improved by a factor of 2 on average at 16 and 24 c/deg. The maximum visual benefits for the two subjects are approximately a factor of 5 (YY) and 3.2 (GYY) at 16 c/deg when both monochromatic aberrations and chromatic aberration were corrected.

The Role of Chromatic Aberration

These results illustrate that the maximum increase in retinal image contrast that could be achieved requires correcting the chromatic aberrations as well as the monochromatic aberrations. Figure 3-18 shows the average maximum theoretical visual benefit computed from the wave aberrations of 17 subjects for a 6 mm pupil. Correcting monochromatic aberrations alone provides a large benefit of a factor of about 5 at middle and higher spatial frequencies.

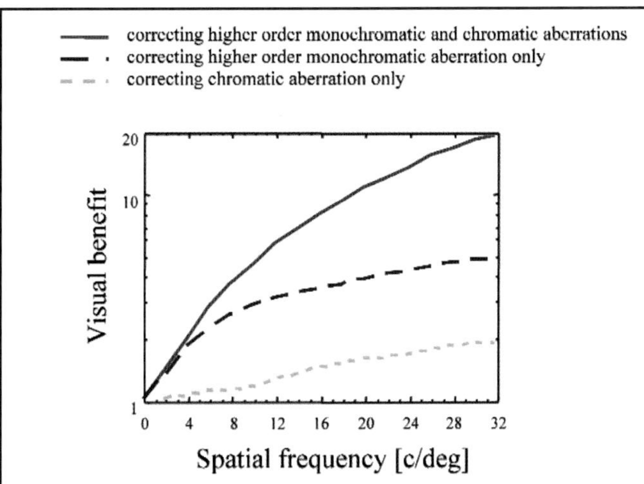

Figure 3-18. The maximum visual benefit of correcting higher-order monochromatic aberrations and/or chromatic aberration for a 6 mm pupil. A perfect correction method was assumed. The monochromatic MTFs were computed every 10 nm from 405 to 695 nm assuming an equally distributed energy spectrum. The reference wavelength assumed to generate no chromatic aberration was 555 nm where the photopic spectral sensitivity is maximal. The axial chromatic aberration data of Wald and Griffin[42] was used after rescaling it to the reference wavelength of 555 nm. Estimates of foveal transverse chromatic aberration from Thibos et al[47] were also considered in the calculation. For both monochromatic and white light conditions, the amounts of defocus were chosen to maximize the MTF at 16 c/deg.

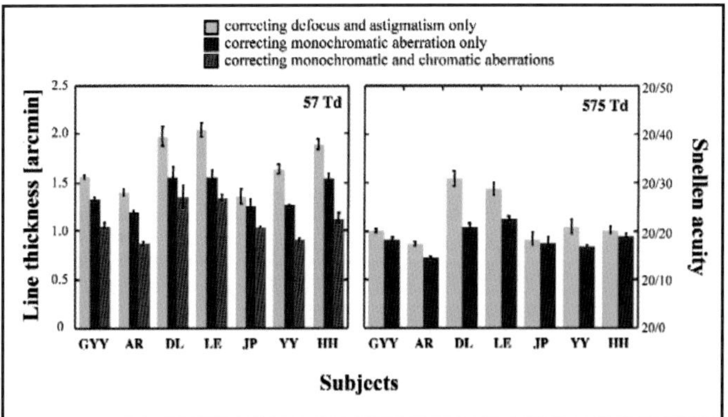

Figure 3-19. Measured visual acuity for seven subjects when correcting various aberrations for a 6 mm pupil. Two retinal illuminance levels, 57 (left) and 575 Td (right), were used. A color cathode ray tube (CRT) was used to display the acuity target, a single letter E. The spectrum of the CRT was a reasonable example of the broadband spectrum considered in natural scenes. The letter E with one of four different orientations was displayed at 100% contrast. From trial to trial, the orientation of the letter was varied randomly among four orientations: the normal orientation and rotations of 90, 180, and 270 degrees. Subjects indicated the orientation of the letter by pressing one of four keys. The psychometric function based on 40 trials was derived using the QUEST procedure[50] and acuity was taken as the line thickness of the letter for which 82% of responses were correct. Chromatic aberration was removed using a 10 nm bandwidth interference filter.

> The theoretical benefit of correcting both chromatic and monochromatic aberrations is substantially larger than that when correcting higher-order monochromatic aberrations only.

In theory for these subjects, correcting both could increase contrast sensitivity by a factor of almost 20 at 32 c/deg. These theoretical benefits are larger than we measured empirically (see Figure 3-17) because the adaptive optics system is incapable of perfect correction.

Campbell and Gubisch found that contrast sensitivity for monochromatic yellow light, which cannot produce chromatic aberration, was only slightly greater than contrast sensitivity for white light.[48] One of the reasons that axial chromatic aberration is not as deleterious under normal viewing conditions as one might expect is that it is overwhelmed by the numerous monochromatic aberrations.[49] This is shown in Figure 3-18. The visual benefit when only chromatic aberration is corrected is relatively small since the effect of higher-order aberrations on retinal image quality dilutes the benefit of correcting chromatic aberration. There is a larger gain when monochromatic aberrations are corrected without correcting chromatic aberration. Correcting both at the same time produces even larger benefits. The challenge is to devise a method to correct the chromatic aberrations of the eye along with the monochromatic aberrations. This cannot be achieved with laser refractive surgery. Multilayer contact lenses that could correct chromatic aberration with conventional methods would be too bulky, and decentration would obliterate any benefit. Reducing the bandwidth of illumination is simple to implement and is effective, but it also eliminates color vision and greatly reduces luminance. No practical solution to this problem currently exists. Even if it did exist, as we will see later, perfect correction of all aberrations does come at the expense of depth of field.

Snellen Acuity With and Without Higher-Order Correction

Due to the ubiquitous use of Snellen acuity in the clinic, we have also measured the increase in Snellen visual acuity provided by correcting higher-order aberrations as well as defocus and astigmatism. Figure 3-19 shows visual acuity at a low (mesopic, 57 Td, left) and a high (photopic, 575 Td, right) retinal illuminance. Before the measurement, defocus and astigmatism were subjectively corrected with a trial lens, if necessary. Correcting monochromatic aberrations provides an average increase for the seven subjects of a factor of 1.2 at 575 Td and 1.4 at 57 Td. All subjects reported an obvious subjective increase in image sharpness when higher-order aberrations were corrected compared with the conventional refraction. Correcting both monochromatic and chromatic aberrations improves visual acuity by a factor of 1.6. Therefore, visual acuity reveals a small benefit of correcting higher-order monochromatic aberrations.

> Though reliable improvements in letter acuity can be measured when higher-order aberrations are corrected with adaptive optics, visual acuity is a far less sensitive measure of the benefits of correcting higher-order aberrations than contrast sensitivity.

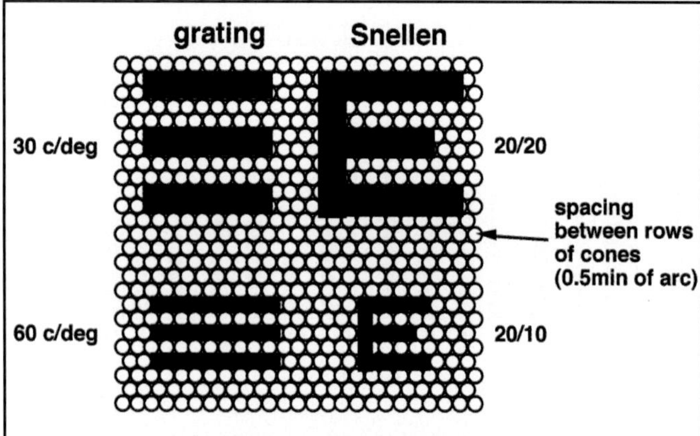

Figure 3-20. The grating and the Snellen letter E sampled by the foveal cone mosaic with a triangular arrangement. 20/20 vision (5 minutes of visual angle) and 20/10 vision (2.5 minutes) roughly correspond to 30 c/deg and 60 c/deg, respectively. The spacing between cones is about 0.5 minutes.

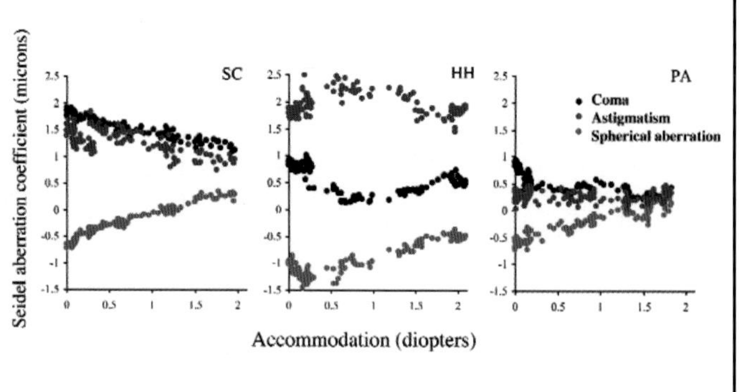

Figure 3-21. Changes in some of the eye's aberrations with accommodation. Pupil size is 4.7 mm. The Seidel aberrations were calculated from wave aberration measurements made with a real-time Shack-Hartmann wavefront sensor at a rate of 25 Hz while the subjects smoothly changed accommodation from the far point to a vergence of about 2 D.

This is because the contrast sensitivity curve is steep at the acuity limit and a large increase in contrast sensitivity slides the intersection of the curve with the x-axis only a short distance. Another reason why visual acuity may underestimate the benefit of correcting higher-order aberrations is that cone sampling considerations will ultimately limit acuity even when improvements in retinal image contrast can continue to provide improved contrast sensitivity at lower spatial frequencies. How does Snellen acuity compare with grating acuity? (see Chapter 7) Figure 3-20 shows a mosaic of foveal cones assuming a triangular arrangement, the 20/20 and the 20/10 letters E, and gratings of 30 and 60 cycles/deg. Approximately an array of 10 x 10 cones samples the 20/20 letter. Clinical visual acuity is usually defined as letter acuity using a standard letter chart observed at a set distance. The size of the smallest letter that can be recognized is taken as the clinical visual acuity of the subject. The most widely used system of acuity notation is the Snellen fraction: V = d/D, where d is distance at which a given letter can just be discriminated and D is distance at which the same letter subtends 5 minutes of arc of visual angle. The reading distance is usually 6 meters (m) (20 feet [ft]). At that distance, the letter size corresponding to 20/20 vision (6/6 in m) is 5 minutes of arc in height. Acuity of 20/200 means that the subject can read at 20 ft a letter that subtends 5 minutes at 200 ft (ie, the smallest letter that this subject can read at 6 m would subtend 50 minutes). A subject subtends 2.5 with 20/10 vision could read at 6 m a letter that subtends 2.5 minutes of arc. The 20/20 letter E may be regarded as being composed of three black horizontal lines and two interdigitated white lines, which have the same spacing as a grating with a spatial frequency of 0.5 c/min, or 30 c/deg. A 20/10 letter has the same stroke periodicity as a 60 c/deg grating. If human grating acuity approaches 60 c/deg, one may well wonder why the average Snellen acuity is not 20/10. For one thing, the detection of gratings is a very different task than the recognition of Snellen letters. In Snellen acuity, the subject can be influenced by literacy and past experience. Letters present low spatial frequency cues due to the symmetry or asymmetry in the form that can help recognize them. Grating targets usually extend over a larger visual angle than their equivalent Snellen letters, which increases their visibility. All these factors make the comparison between Snellen and grating acuity problematic. As mentioned above, increasing retinal image quality with higher-order correction generally is expected to have a smaller effect on high contrast visual acuity than contrast sensitivity, whether measured with gratings or letters. We suggest that visual benefit, as we have defined it based on retinal image contrast, is a more robust and useful measure of the outcome of correcting higher-order aberrations. If an acuity measure is to be used, an alternative is low contrast visual acuity, which should be more sensitive than high contrast visual acuity.

Additional Considerations in Higher-Order Correction

We have already discussed the role that pupil diameter and chromatic aberration play in the visual benefit of higher-order correction. This section discusses additional factors that need to be considered to evaluate the ultimate benefits that customized correction will be able to produce.

Accommodation

Any attempt to improve the eye's optics with a customized correction will only be beneficial if the values of the eye's aberrations are relatively fixed. If, for any reason, the eye's optics are not stable, the ability to improve vision will be limited. The eye's higher-order aberrations change substantially with accommodation. What implications will this have for the visual benefit that could be obtained with a customized correction? Figure 3-21 shows how a few of the eye's aberrations—coma, astigmatism, and spherical aberration—varied for a 4.7 mm pupil in three subjects as they smoothly changed their accommodation from distant (far point) to near accommodation (a change of about 2 D or 0.5 m).[51] Although the nature of the change in the eye's higher-order aberrations generally varies for different subjects, it is clear that for each subject there are substantial, systematic changes in the aberrations that depend on accommodative state. This means that a higher-order correction tailored for distance vision would not be appropriate for near viewing and vice versa.

For the same three subjects, the effect of accommodative state on the monochromatic visual benefit that could be attained with a higher-order correction is illustrated in Figure 3-22. The blue

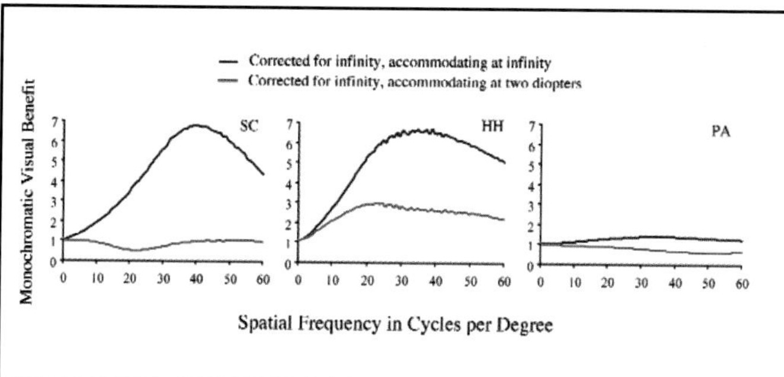

Figure 3-22. The effect of accommodative state on visual benefit. For the same three subjects as in Figure 3-21, the visual benefit in monochromatic light was computed for different accommodative states from wave aberrations measured with a Shack-Hartmann wavefront sensor. Pupil size is 4.7 mm.

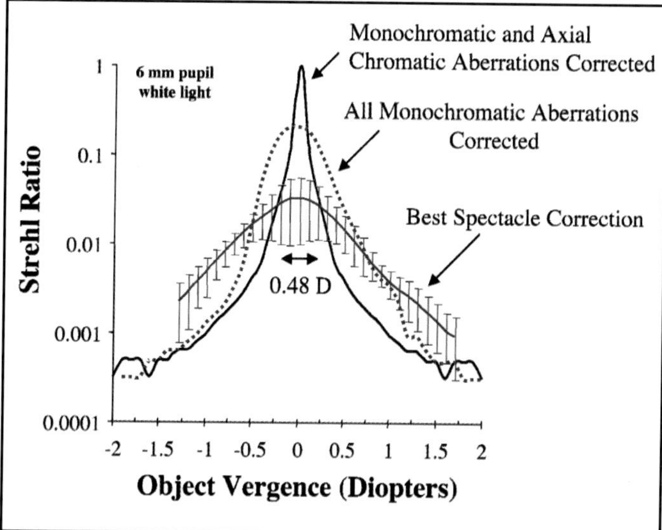

Figure 3-23. Average changes in the Strehl ratio as a function of light vergence in white light when correcting defocus and astigmatism alone (solid red curve), when correcting all monochromatic aberrations (dotted blue curve), and when correcting both monochromatic and axial chromatic aberrations (solid black curve). These data were calculated based on wave aberration measurements obtained from 13 eyes and incorporated axial chromatic aberration (6 mm pupil). Correcting higher-order aberrations increases image quality over a 1.25 D range, but results in worse image quality outside of this range when compared with a spectacle correction. Correcting both monochromatic and chromatic aberrations can optimize image quality at the expense of a further reduction in the depth of focus.

curve for each subject shows the visual benefit that would be obtained with the ideal corneal ablation profile designed to eliminate the eye's higher-order aberrations when the subject is accommodating at infinity. This is the maximum obtainable visual benefit for each subject. The pink curve shows the subject's visual benefit obtained with this same ablation profile, but now when the subject is actually accommodating at 2 D instead of infinity. It is important to keep in mind that defocus is not responsible for the drop in visual benefit. In fact, it has been assumed that the subject has perfect accommodation. This was implemented by zeroing the residual Zernike defocus. (*Note*: although the focal plane for best image quality does not necessarily correspond to the plane where Zernike defocus is equal to 0, for relatively small pupil sizes and mild wave aberrations, zeroing the Zernike defocus is usually a good approximation to the best focal plane.) This shows that a customized corneal ablation profile tailored to perfectly correct all higher-order aberrations at one accommodative state will be less effective when the accommodative state is substantially changed. In this situation, the custom correction is little better, and maybe even somewhat worse, than a traditional spherocylindrical correction. Though the changes of the wave aberration with accommodation limit the conditions under which a customized static correction of the eye's aberrations would provide a benefit in young people who can still accommodate, it does not imply that such a correction would have no use. This limitation is not particularly severe because it does not apply to presbyopes. Even in younger people, there would be value in designing a lens to correct for distance vision.

The failure to focus correctly on the target, or accommodative lag, will also diminish the visual benefit of higher-order correction. Accommodative lag typically increases as the luminance of the stimulus is reduced and can yield an error in defocus of 0.3 D or more in low luminance conditions.[52] We showed in Figure 3-10 that the image blur produced by 0.3 D of defocus is nearly identical to that produced by the higher-order aberrations alone. This implies that one needs to maintain accurate accommodation in order to reap the full benefit of a customized higher-order correction. An error as slight as 0.3 D in a patient's ability to focus in dim lighting conditions will greatly reduce the visual benefit obtained by correcting the eye's higher-order aberrations, which are highest for large pupil diameters. Despite these limitations, we believe that it is advantageous to correct for higher-order aberrations generally for distance corrections because the pupil constricts with accommodation, making higher-order aberrations less problematic.

Depth of Focus

A customized correction of higher-order aberrations may also reduce the eye's depth of focus. We can see this effect in Figure 3-23, which illustrates how the eye's Strehl ratio changes as a function of light vergence for three separate conditions in white light (6 mm pupil). The Strehl ratio is an image quality metric defined as the ratio of the peak value of the eye's PSF with aberrations to that of a diffraction-limited system. A perfect, diffraction-limited system has a Strehl ratio of 1, with image quality typically becoming worse as the Strehl ratio approaches 0. As shown in Figure 3-23, correcting all of the eye's monochromatic aberrations improves image quality over a range of nearly 1.25 D, outside of which image quality is actually better with a conventional spectacle correction. Correcting all of the eye's monochromatic and axial chromatic aberrations can yield the highest Strehl ratio and best image quality at the expense of an additional reduction in the depth of focus (0.48 D range). An analysis of the real impact of a reduction in the eye's depth of field with higher-order correction has yet to be performed.

Slow Changes in the Wave Aberration Over Time

Another issue that is important to consider in evaluating the feasibility of a customized corneal ablation procedure is whether, for a fixed accommodative state, the wave aberration is stable over long periods of time. If higher-order aberrations were not

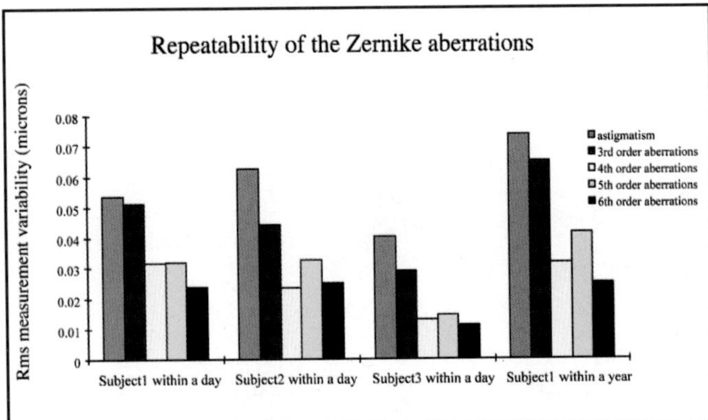

Figure 3-24. Repeatability of the Zernike aberration measurement for Zernike coefficients of different radial orders. This figure shows the average RMS variability of different orders of Zernike coefficients measured several times throughout a single day for three subjects. Pupil size was approximately 6 mm. The RMS measurement variability of the different Zernike orders over the course of 1 year is also shown for one of the subjects. The Zernike coefficients were measured with a Shack-Hartmann wavefront sensor. Since the measurement variability includes experimental errors specific to the particular Shack-Hartmann wavefront sensor, measurement noise, and errors due to pupil centration, it represents an upper boundary to the actual instability in the wave aberration.

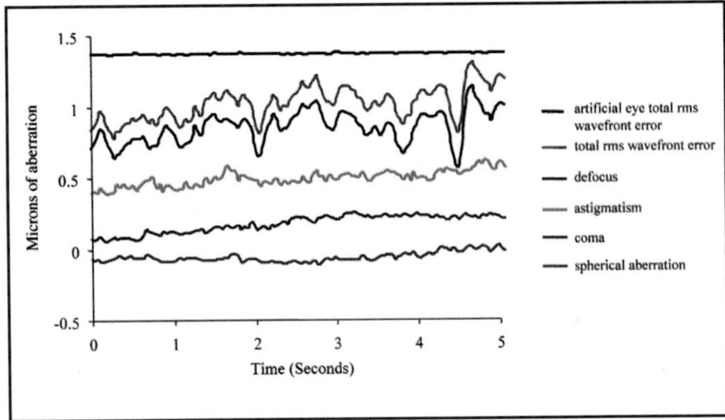

Figure 3-25. Short-term temporal instability in the eye's wave aberration. Aberrations were measured with a real-time Shack-Hartmann wavefront sensor while the subject attempted to fixate steadily on a high contrast target at 2 D. Pupil size is 4.7 mm.

stable, there would be little point in performing a customized corneal ablation. This issue can be addressed by examining the repeatability with which the wave aberration can be measured within a single day and within an entire year. Figure 3-24 shows the RMS between-measurement variability in the wave aberration, expressed in microns, for three subjects with 6 mm pupils. Each measurement was made with a long integration time to minimize the influence of short-term instability in the wave aberration, to be discussed later. Within-a-day variability depends on the Zernike order considered, but generally ranges between 0.01 and 0.06 µm. This RMS within-a-day variability is about nine times smaller than the average magnitude of aberration for the second-order aberrations and about three times smaller than the average magnitude of aberration for the third- and fourth-order modes. It is likely that the actual variability in the wave aberration is smaller than this since much of the variability is probably due to changes in pupil position and other sources of measurement error rather than actual changes in the wave aberration that would affect vision.

Figure 3-24 also shows repeatability data for one eye over a much longer time scale. The wave aberration for this eye was measured on three occasions spanning more than an 8-month period, and showed a RMS between-measurement variability of less than 0.08 µm in every case, only slightly worse than the within-a-day variability, both of which are minimal. These results imply that, for a fixed accommodative state, the wave aberration of the eye is stable both within a day and probably over a period of many months as well. Although similar data for more subjects would be required to make a definitive statement about longer periods, the evidence that is available indicates that a custom surgical procedure to correct higher-order aberrations would be of value to the patient for an extended period of time.

The evidence that is available indicates that a custom surgical procedure to correct higher-order aberrations would be of value to the patient for an extended period of time.

Although we believe the wave aberration to be fairly stable over relatively long time periods, it is known that spatial vision does deteriorate with age.[53] In addition to neural factors, a significant steady increment in ocular aberrations with age has been found,[54,55] which produces a degraded retinal image in the older eye. Both changes in the crystalline lens[56,57] and changes in the cornea[58,59] are responsible. However, the cause of the degradation of the eye's optical quality is the loss of the aberration balance between cornea and lens that seems to be present in the younger eye.[60] These factors may ultimately limit the longevity of an effective customized correction and suggest that an adjustable customized correction would be optimal.

Rapid Changes in the Wave Aberration Over Time

The experiments described above address the issue of the long-term stability of the wave aberration, but they do not consider the possibility that the short-term stability of the eye might be poor. Rapid temporal fluctuations in the wave aberration might also reduce the value of a static correcting procedure such as a customized corneal ablation. All the calculations described thus far have assumed that the eye's aberrations are perfectly static in time, and the contrast sensitivity measurements described earlier are usually conducted with paralyzed accommodation so that at least some of the dynamics would have been suppressed compared with normal viewing.

Microfluctuations in accommodation, even during attempted steady-state accommodation, have been documented and studied since 1951;[61,62] however, measurement of the short-term instability of the eye's higher-order aberrations has not been possible until recently. Figure 3-25 shows the short-term temporal variability of the eye's total RMS wavefront error and of some of the Zernike aberrations for one subject measured over 5 seconds. For comparison, the total RMS wavefront error measured for a static artificial eye is also shown.[63] It can be seen from this figure that the eye's higher-order aberrations do exhibit temporal instability.

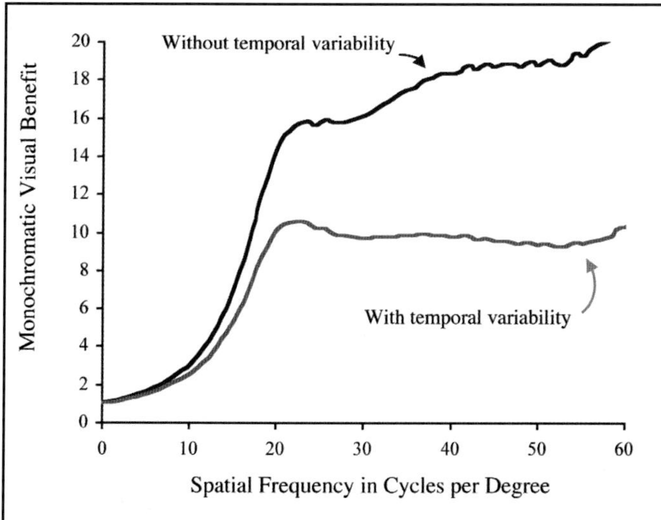

Figure 3-26. The effect of short-term temporal instability in the eye's wave aberration on the visual benefit of a perfect custom correction. The time-averaged monochromatic visual benefit for different conditions was calculated from wave aberration measurements made with a real-time Shack-Hartmann wavefront sensor. Pupil size is 5.8 mm. The blue curve is the benefit that could be obtained in the absence of temporal instability; this is the benefit that would be achieved with a perfect customized correction. The pink curve is the visual benefit obtained with a perfect customized correction of the static component of the eye's wave aberration when the effects of temporal instability are included; it is the best optical quality that can be achieved with any static correction method.

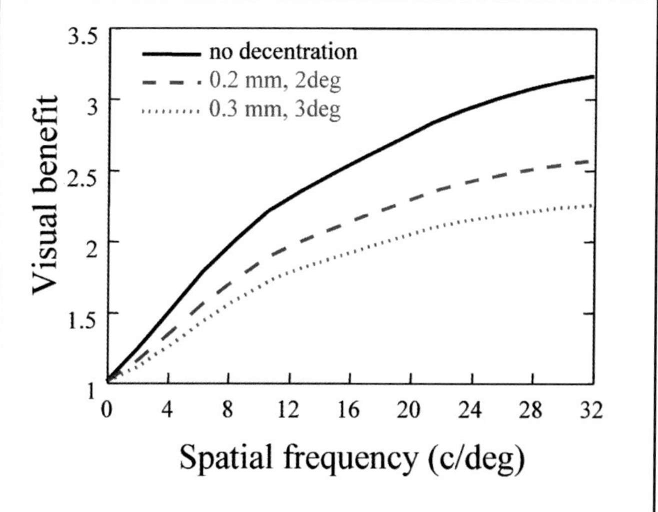

Figure 3-27. Mean visual benefit in white light across 10 eyes with 7 mm pupils, calculated when an ideal correcting method is perfectly centered and for decentrations within an interval of translation and rotation characterized with a standard deviation of 0.2 mm, 2 deg, and 0.3 mm, 3 deg, respectively. The visual benefit was obtained as the ratio between the MTF in white light when the monochromatic aberrations are corrected and the MTF achieved with an optimum correction of defocus and astigmatism.

> By far the largest source of short-term instability in the eye's wave aberration is due to the microfluctuations in accommodation (or defocus).

Figure 3-26 shows the theoretical effect of this short-term variability in the eye's aberrations on the maximum visual benefit that can be obtained in one subject with a perfect customized corneal ablation procedure for a 5.8 mm pupil. The calculations were performed assuming a perfect correction of the static component of the eye's wave aberration and also perfect correction of the eye's chromatic aberration, implying that a perfect corneal ablation procedure, in the absence of temporal instability, would result in diffraction-limited performance. The effect of temporal instability is similar to the effect of chromatic aberration in that it only fully reveals itself when higher-order aberrations are very small. The blue curve indicates the monochromatic visual benefit of a perfect correction, for this subject, if the aberrations were perfectly static. The pink curve shows how the visual benefit is decreased when the effect of the temporal instability in the wave aberration is taken into account. Temporal instability causes very little reduction in visual benefit for the low spatial frequencies and a reduction of about a factor of 2 at higher spatial frequencies. Even so, the visual benefit for the perfect custom correction of the eye's static aberrations (pink curve) is still quite substantial, indicating that a perfect customized correction would still be of benefit to this subject.

Decentration Errors

The benefit from the correction of the higher-order aberrations will be reduced by decentrations of the correcting method. A customized contact lens will translate and rotate to some extent with respect to the cornea. Also, the eye is not completely static during a laser refractive surgery procedure. Calculations for an ideal correcting phase-plate model suggest, contrary to what one might expect, that reasonable decentrations do not detract greatly from the potential benefit of correcting higher-order aberrations.[64,65] Even with fixed translations or rotations of up to 0.6 mm and 30 degrees, a correction of the higher-order aberrations would still yield an improvement over a typical spherocylindrical refraction.

> Even with fixed translations or rotations of up to 0.6 mm and 30 degrees, a correction of the higher-order aberrations would still yield an improvement over a typical spherocylindrical refraction.

Maximum translations and rotations reported for soft contact lenses[66] and measurements of the motion of the eye during the laser surgery treatment[67] allow us to estimate the typical decentration of an ideal correcting method. Figure 3-27 shows the impact of movements within a reasonable interval (characterized by a standard deviation of 0.2 to 0.3 mm for translation, and 2 to 3 degrees for rotation) on the visual benefit in white light. The eye's chromatic aberration overwhelms the effect of residual aberrations caused by decentrations. The visual benefit is as high as 2.50 at 32 c/deg, only somewhat less than the ideal case with no decentration.

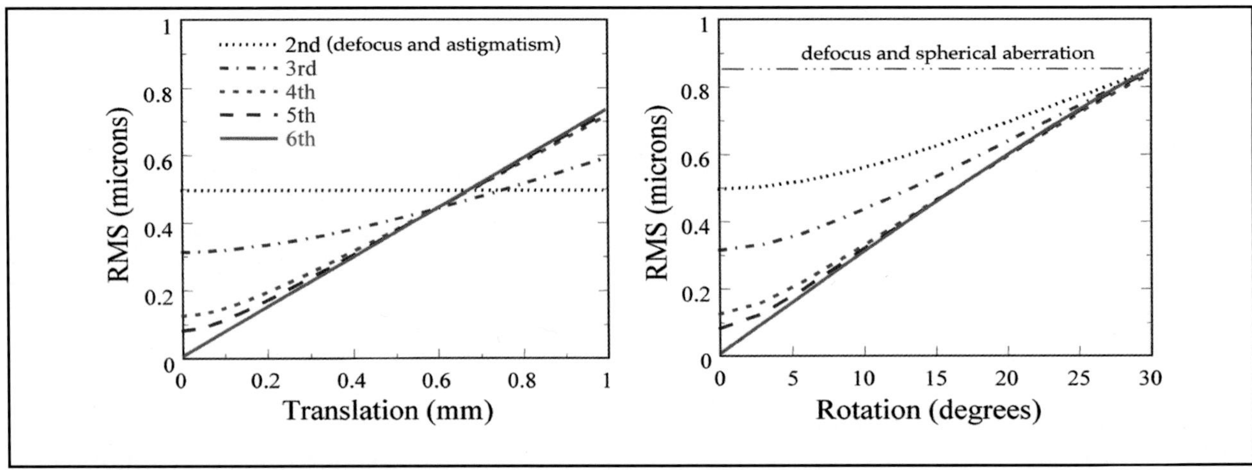

Figure 3-28. RMS of the residual wave aberration (mean value across 10 eyes, 7 mm pupils) as a function of fixed translations and rotations, when the ideal correcting method corrects the higher-order aberrations up to second, third, fourth, fifth, and sixth order. For example, a method designed to compensate for the aberrations up to fourth order leaves uncorrected the aberrations higher than fourth order and there is a residual RMS even with perfect centration due to the incomplete correction. The RMS is a measure of the total amount of aberration.

Correcting progressively higher orders of aberration will result in progressively lower tolerances to decentration. Figure 3-28 shows the impact of translation and rotation on a correction that includes different orders of aberration (up to second, third, fourth, fifth, and sixth order). The ordinate is a measure of the amount of residual aberrations remaining in the eye. While a perfectly centered correcting method continues to provide improvement in image quality when it is designed to correct more orders, the benefit of correcting additional orders decreases when decentration increases. This fact indicates that the higher-order corrections are more sensitive to translation and rotation. If the expected decentration of the correction is too large, then it is not worth correcting all the higher-order aberrations that one can measure.

However, as a general statement, nearly 50% of the eye's higher-order aberrations would still be eliminated in a customized correction that was statically translated by 0.3 to 0.4 mm and rotated by 8 to 10 degrees.

Of course, the types of decentrations that typically occur during laser in-situ keratomileusis (LASIK) are not necessarily as simplistic as the previously considered model in which the entire higher-order correction has been statically displaced and/or rotated on the eye. Dynamic eye movements in a conventional or customized procedure can also introduce additional aberrations in laser refractive surgery. Finally, another important caveat is that the process of removing corneal tissue in refractive surgery could also induce other aberrations not accounted for in the phase-plate model.

Effect of Beam Size on Customized Refractive Surgery

The success of customized laser refractive surgery depends on using a laser beam that is small enough in diameter to produce the fine ablation profiles needed to correct the eye's higher-order aberrations. Just as an artist requires a finer paintbrush for more detailed work, the laser refractive surgeon requires a smaller diameter laser beam to achieve a successful customized ablation. Based on wave aberration data from real eyes, we theoretically calculated the effect of changing the laser beam size on the expected benefit of a customized refractive surgery procedure.[68] We calculated the residual aberrations that would remain in the eye for beam diameters ranging from 0.5 to 2 mm, estimated retinal image quality, and conducted a Fourier analysis to study the spatial filtering properties of each beam size. The laser beam acts like a spatial filter, smoothing the finest features in the ablation profile. The quality of the customized correction declines steadily when the beam size increases, as large diameter laser beams decrease the ability to correct finer, higher-order aberrations in the eye.

A beam diameter of 2 mm is capable of correcting defocus and astigmatism while beam diameters of 1 mm or less may effectively correct aberrations up to fifth order. A top-hat laser beam of 1 mm (or an equivalent Gaussian profile with a full width at half maximum [FWHM] of 0.76 mm) is small enough to achieve a customized ablation for typical human eyes.

For more information on the requirements for a customized correction of the eye's aberrations, refer to Chapter 22.

The Rationale for Pursuing Higher-Order Correction

Even though we must consider the implications of the aforementioned hurdles in the path to effective customized correction, it is clear from the population statistics that substantial benefits can be had for some eyes in the normal population. As previously shown in Figure 3-13, there are some subjects who have a visual benefit of nearly 1, indicating that they have excellent optics and would not benefit from a customized correction. However, there are also many normal subjects who possess inferior optical quality and would experience large visual benefits from a customized correction, particularly for large pupil sizes (such as in nighttime con-

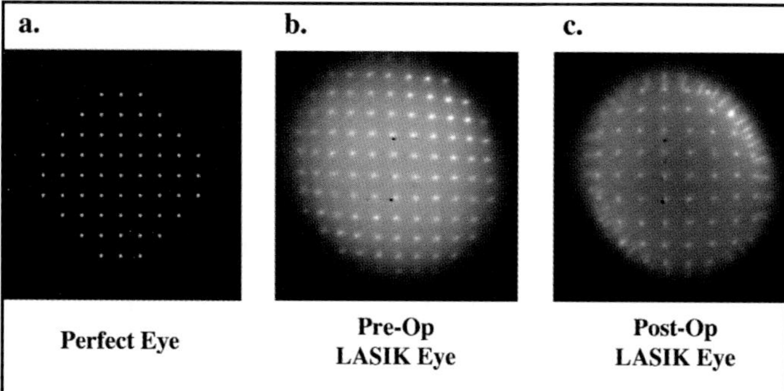

Figure 3-29. The Shack-Hartmann spot array pattern for a perfect eye (A), a normal aberrated eye (B), and the same eye following LASIK surgery (C).

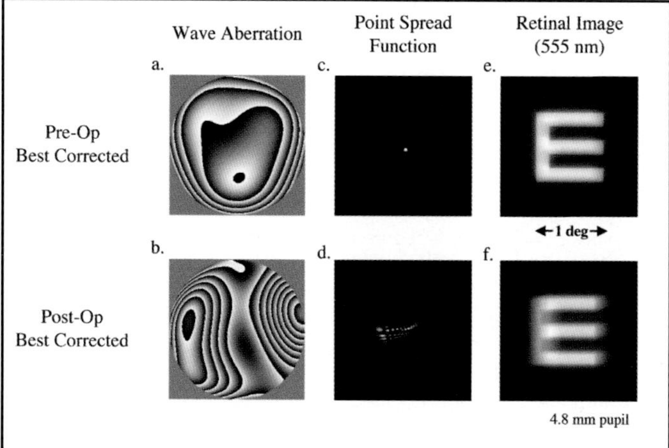

Figure 3-31. The wave aberrations across a 4.8 mm pupil for the same LASIK patient's left eye before surgery with his best correction (A) and after surgery with his best correction (B), and his corresponding PSFs (C and D). The aberrations have become more severe for the patient over this moderately larger pupil diameter. For the wave aberrations shown in (A) and (B), the subject's best refraction was again determined by adjusting the amount of defocus and astigmatism needed to maximize the Strehl ratio in their corresponding PSF. The patient's best corrected PSF before and after surgery was convolved with the letter E in monochromatic light (555 nm) to produce the retinal image shown in (E) and (F). After surgery, higher-order aberrations become the dominant source of degradation in the quality of the letter E.

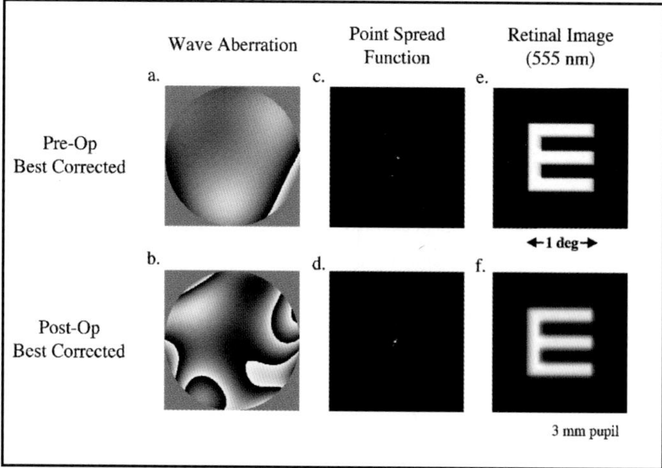

Figure 3-30. The wave aberrations across a 3 mm pupil for the LASIK patient's left eye before surgery with his best correction (A) and after surgery with his best correction (B), and his corresponding PSFs (C and D). For the wave aberrations shown in (A) and (B), the subject's best refraction was determined by adjusting the amount of defocus and astigmatism (or all three second-order Zernike modes) needed to maximize the Strehl ratio in their corresponding PSF. (E) and (F) show the result of convolving the letter E in monochromatic light (555 nm) with the patient's best corrected PSF before and after surgery. After surgery, higher-order aberrations become the dominant source of degradation in the quality of the letter E.

ditions). Of course, pathological patients, such as kerataconics, would experience the greatest gains in visual performance.

In addition to correcting higher-order aberrations in these populations, it is important to examine and attempt to correct for the higher-order aberrations that are being introduced by current refractive surgical procedures. Figure 3-29 shows three images obtained from a Shack-Hartmann wavefront sensor. The details of its operation will be explained in Chapter 7. A perfect eye, shown in Figure 3-29A, produces a spot pattern that is regular and possesses uniform spots that are equally spaced. An aberrated eye produces a Shack-Hartmann array containing spots that are displaced from their ideal, perfect locations. The larger the displacements of these spots, the greater the amount of aberration that is present in an image. Adjacent to the perfect eye is the Shack-Hartmann array for the patient before LASIK surgery. The preoperative spherocylindrical refraction of this unoperated eye was -7.75 -2.00 x 57. The third picture in this sequence shows the Shack-Hartmann array for the same subject 4 months following LASIK surgery. The postoperative refraction for this LASIK eye was +0.25 -0.50 x 172. As seen in the figure, the spots in the center of the pupil are fairly uniform and evenly spaced while the spots in the periphery become distorted and elongated as the spacing between the spots becomes dramatically compressed. This indicates that the aberrations are becoming more severe as we move away from the center of the pupil, which is characteristic of the pin cushion appearance of spherical aberration.

We can more easily determine how the aberration structure of the patient has changed following surgery by analyzing the pre- and postoperative Shack-Hartmann arrays to determine the corresponding wave aberrations. These results are shown in Figure 3-30 for a 3 mm pupil diameter and in Figure 3-31 for a 4.8 mm pupil diameter. The step size of an individual contour line in the wave aberration is 0.56 μm. Due to the large compression and overlapping of the spots in the periphery of the postoperative eye, we were unable to accurately determine the wave aberration for pupil diameters larger than 5 mm. The eye's PSF for any pupil size up to 5 mm may then be determined from the wave aberration, yielding a complete description of the imaging properties of the entire eye.

For the smaller pupil size of 3 mm, we see that there is not a dramatic difference between the wave aberration before and after surgery. This is to be expected since the eye's aberrations are mainly limited by diffraction for small pupil diameters. By convolving the letter E with the eye's PSF, we can directly observe how the eye's wave aberration degrades the retinal image. Even for this small pupil size, the letter E shows a reduction in image quality

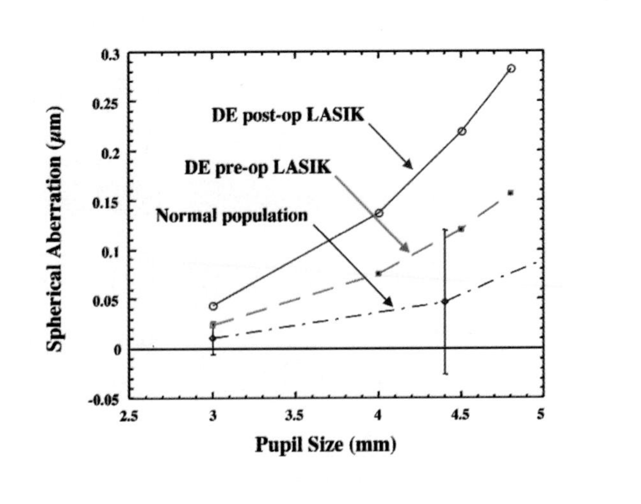

Figure 3-32. Spherical aberration (in microns) for the normal population of 109 subjects (dash-dotted blue line), the patient before LASIK surgery (dashed green line), and the patient after LASIK surgery (solid red line) as a function of pupil size. The error bars for the normal population represent plus and minus 2 standard deviations from the mean value, encompassing approximately 95% of the normal population. The patient's preoperative values for spherical aberration fit in with the normal population. However, after LASIK surgery, the patient's spherical aberration doubles in magnitude as a result of the procedure.

after surgery when compared with the preoperative E, indicating that the surgery has produced higher-order aberrations.

The same trends occur to a larger degree in Figure 3-31 for the 4.8 mm pupil. The best-corrected postoperative LASIK eye produces a retinal image of the letter E whose quality is inferior to that formed by the best-corrected preoperative eye. As the pupil size increases from 3 to 4.8 mm, the postoperative LASIK patient has noticeably poorer retinal image quality than his or her typical, unoperated eye and would see even worse for larger pupil diameters. The wave aberration after surgery for the postoperative LASIK eye is fairly smooth in the center of the pupil, as evidenced by the low density of contour lines. However, the density of the contour lines increases at the edge of the pupil, indicating the presence of more severe aberrations in the periphery of the pupil. This increase in aberration structure at the pupil edge is primarily due to a steepening of the cornea near the transition zone of the ablation.[69]

The predominant higher-order aberration exhibited by this LASIK patient and several other LASIK patients[69-71] after surgery is spherical aberration, which often increased two- to four-fold with conventional LASIK.

See Chapter 7 for similar evidence obtained from corneal topographic measurements. Corneal topography correlates with wavefront variance.[72]

Figure 3-32 shows the increase in spherical aberration for this LASIK patient as a function of pupil diameter. Before surgery, the preoperative values of spherical aberration for the patient are comparable to those expected from the normal population data. After surgery, the magnitude of spherical aberration in the post-LASIK eye becomes twice as large as the unoperated values. This postoperative value will become even larger as the pupil diameter increases from a moderate size of 4.8 mm to a fully dilated size of 6 or 7 mm, severely degrading nighttime vision.

The results from this LASIK patient and the population data suggest that there is a need to refine corrective techniques that can eliminate the eye's higher-order aberrations. Abnormal eyes, such as kerataconics, and eyes containing large amounts of higher-order aberrations, such as the patient discussed here, will obviously benefit the most from a customized correction. Normal eyes, particularly in low illumination conditions with large pupil diameters, can also substantially benefit from a customized correction. Wavefront sensing is a key technology that will be instrumental in optimizing these techniques to maximize the potential benefit each individual patient will be able to receive from a customized correction.

References

1. Willoughby Cashell GT. A short history of spectacles. *Proc Roy Soc Med.* 1971;64:1063-1064.
2. Rubin ML. Spectacles: past, present and future. *Surv Ophthalmol.* 1986;30:321-327.
3. Helmholtz H. *Helmholtz's Treatise on Physiological Optics.* New York: Optical Society of America; 1924.
4. Smirnov MS. Measurement of the wave aberration of the human eye. *Biophysics.* 1961;687-703.
5. Liang J, Grimm B, Goelz S, Bille J. Objective measurement of the wave aberrations of the human eye using a Shack-Hartmann wavefront sensor. *J Opt Soc Am A.* 1994;11:1949-1957.
6. Liang J, Williams DR, Miller DT. Supernormal vision and high-resolution retinal imaging through adaptive optics. *J Opt Soc Am A.* 1997;14:2884-2892.
7. Guirao A, Redondo M, Geraghty E, Piers P, Norrby S, Artal P. Corneal optical aberrations and retinal image quality in patients in whom monofocal intraocular lenses were implanted. *Arch Ophthalmol.* 2002;120(9):1143-1151.
8. MacRae SM, Schwiegerling J, Snyder R. Customized corneal ablation and super vision. *J Refract Surg.* 2000;16:S230-S235.
9. Mrochen M, Kaemmerer M, Seiler T. Wavefront–guided laser in situ keratomileusis: early results in three eyes. *J Refract Surg.* 2000;16:116-121.
10. Mrochen M, Kaemmerer M, Seiler T. Clinical results of wavefront-guided laser in situ keratomileusis 3 months after surgery. *J Cataract Refract Surg.* 2001;27:201-207.
11. Panagopoulou SI, Pallikaris IG. Wavefront customized ablations with the WASCA Asclepion workstation. *J Refract Surg.* 2001;17:S608-S612.
12. Liang J, Williams DR. Aberrations and retinal image quality of the normal human eye. *J Opt Soc Am A.* 1997;14:2873-2883.
13. Goodman JW. *Introduction to Fourier Optics.* 2nd ed. New York: McGraw-Hill; 1996
14. Williams DR. Topography of the foveal cone mosaic in the living human eye. *Vision Res.* 1988;28:433-454.
15. Williams DR, Coletta NJ. Cone spacing and the visual resolution limit. *J Opt Soc Am.* 1987;14:1514-1523.
16. Williams DR. Aliasing in human foveal vision. *Vision Res.* 1985;25:195-205.
17. Bergmann C. Anatomical and physiological findings on the retina. *Zeitschrift für rationelle Medicin II.* 1857;83-108.
18. Byram GM. The physical and photochemical basis of visual resolving power. Part II. Visual acuity and the photochemistry of the retina. *J Opt Soc Am.* 1944;34:718-738.
19. Campbell FW, Green DG. Optical and retinal factors affecting visual resolution. *J Physiol.* 1965;181:576-593.
20. Williams DR, Sekiguchi N, Haake W, Brainard D, Packer O. The cost of trichromaticity for spatial vision. In: Valberg A, Lee BB, eds. *From Pigments to Perception: Advances in Understanding Visual Processes.* Series A/Vol 203. New York: Plenum Press; 1991:11-22.

21. Østerberg GA. Topography of the layer of rods and ones in the human retina. *Acta Ophthalmol.* 1935;13:1-97.
22. Miller WH. Ocular optical filtering. In: Autrum H, ed. *Handbook of Sensory Physiology.* Vol VII/6A. Berlin: Springer-Verlag; 1979:70-143.
23. Yuodelis C, Hendrikson A. A qualitative analysis of the human fovea during development. *Vision Res.* 1986;26:847-856.
24. Curcio CA, Sloan KR, Packer O, Hendrickson AE, Kalina RR. Distribution of cones in human and monkey retina: individual variability and radial asymmetry. *Science.* 1987;236:579-582.
25. Curcio CA, Sloan KR, Kalina RR, Hendrickson AE. Human photoreceptor topography. *J Comp Neurol.* 1990;292:497-523.
26. Williams DR. Visibility of interference fringes near the resolution limit. *J Opt Soc Am A.* 1985;2:1087-1093.
27. Helmholtz H. *Popular Scientific Lectures.* New York: Dover Publications, Inc; 1962.
28. Van den Brink G. Measurements of the geometrical aberrations of the eye. *Vision Res.* 1962;2:233-244.
29. Berny F, Slansky S. Wavefront determination resulting from Foucault test as applied to the human eye and visual instruments. In: Dickenson JH, ed. *Optical Instruments and Techniques.* Newcastle, Del: Oriel Press; 1969:375-386.
30. Howland HC, Howland B. A subjective method for the measurement of monochromatic aberrations of the eye. *J Opt Soc Am.* 1977;67:1508-1518.
31 Walsh G, Charman WN, Howland HC. Objective technique for the determination of monochromatic aberrations of the human eye. *J Opt Soc Am A.* 1984;1:987-992.
32. Campbell MCW, Harrison EM, Simonet P. Psychophysical measurement of the blur on the retina due to optical aberrations of the eye. *Vision Res.* 1990;30:1587-1602.
33. Webb RH, Penney CM, Thompson KP. Measurement of ocular wavefront distortion with a spatially resolved refractometer. *Appl Opt.* 1992;31:3678-3686.
34. Platt B, Shack RV. Lenticular Hartmann screen. *Opt Sci Center Newsl.* 1971;5:15-16.
35. Howland HC, Buettner J. Computing high order wave aberration coefficients from variations of best focus for small artificial pupils. *Vision Res.* 1989;29:979-983.
36. Porter J, Guirao A, Cox IG, Williams DR. Monochromatic aberrations of the human eye in a large population. *J Opt Soc Am A.* 2001;18:1793-1803.
37. Thibos LN, Hong X, Bradley A, Cheng X. Statistical variation of aberration structure and image quality in a normal population of healthy eyes. *J Opt Soc Am A.* 2002;2329-2348.
38. Guirao A, Williams DR. A method to predict refractive errors from wavefront aberration data. *Optom Vis Sci.* In press.
39. El Hage SG, Berny F. Contribution of crystalline lens to the spherical aberration of the eye. *J Opt Soc Am.* 1973;63:205-211.
40. Artal P, Guirao A. Contribution of cornea and lens to the aberrations of the human eye. *Optics Letters.* 1998;23:1713-1715.
41. Artal P, Guirao A, Berrio E, Williams DR. Compensation of corneal aberrations by the internal optics in the human eye. *J Vision.* 2001;1:1-8.
42. Wald G, Griffin DR. The change in refractive power of the human eye in dim and bright light. *J Opt Soc Am A.* 1947;321-336.
43. Guirao A, Porter J, Williams DR, Cox IG. Calculated impact of higher order monochromatic aberrations on retinal image quality in a population of human eyes. *J Opt Soc Am A.* 2002;19:620-628.
44. Artal P, Navarro R. Monochromatic modulation transfer function for different pupil diameters: an analytical expression. *J Opt Soc Am A.* 1994;11:246-249.
45. Hofer H, Chen L, Yoon GY, Singer B, Yamauchi Y, Williams DR. Improvement in retinal image quality with dynamic correction of the eye's aberrations [abstract]. *Optics Express* [serial online]. 2001;8,:631-643. Available at: http://www.opticsexpress.org/oearchive/source/31887.htm. Accessed October 22, 2003.
46. Roorda A, Williams DR. The arrangement of the three cone classes in the living human eye. *Nature.* 1999;397:520-522.
47. Thibos LN, Bradley A, Still DL, Zhang X, Howarth PA. Theory and measurement of ocular chromatic aberration. *Vision Res.* 1990;30:33-49.
48. Campbell FW, Gubisch RW. The effect of chromatic aberration on visual acuity. *J Physiol.* 1967;192:345-358.
49. Yoon GY, Cox I, Williams DR. The visual benefit of the static correction of the monochromatic wave aberration. *Invest Ophthalmol Vis Sci.* 1999;40(Suppl):40.
50. Watson AB, Pelli DG. QUEST: A Bayesian adaptive psychometric method. *Perception & Psychophysics.* 1983;33:113-120.
51. Artal P, Hofer H, Williams DR, Aragon JL. Dynamics of ocular aberrations during accommodation. Paper presented at: Optical Society of America Annual Meeting; 1999.
52. Johnson CA. Effects of luminance and stimulus distance on accommodation and visual resolution. *J Opt Soc Am.* 1976;66:138-142.
53. Owsley C, Sekuler R, Siemsen D. Contrast sensitivity throughout adulthood. *Vision Res.* 1983;23:689-699.
54. Artal P, Ferro M, Miranda I, Navarro R. Effects of aging in retinal image quality. *J Opt Soc Am A.* 1993;10:1656-1662.
55. Guirao A, Gonzalez C, Redondo M, Geraghty E, Norrby S, Artal P. Average optical performance of the human eye as a function of age in a normal population. *Invest Optom Vis Sci.* 1999;40:203-213.
56. Cook CA, Koretz JF, Pfahnl A, Hyun J, Kaufman PL. Aging of the human crystalline lens and anterior segment. *Vision Res.* 1994;34:2945-2954.
57. Glasser A, Campbell MCW. Presbyopia and the optical changes in the human crystalline lens with age. *Vision Res.* 1998;38:209-229.
58. Oshika T, Klyce SD, Applegate RA, Howland HC. Changes in corneal wavefront aberrations with aging. *Invest Ophthalmol Vis Sci.* 1999;40:1351-1355.
59. Guirao A, Redondo M, Artal P. Optical aberrations of the human cornea as a function of age. *J Opt Soc Am A.* 2000;17:1697-1702.
60. Artal P, Berrio E, Guirao A, Piers P. Contribution of the cornea and internal surfaces to the change of ocular aberrations with age. *J Opt Soc Am A.* 2002;19:137-143.
61. Arnulf A, Dupuy O, Flamant F. Les microfluctuations d'accommodation de l'oiel et l'acuite visuelle pur les diametres pupillaires naturels. *CR Hebd Seanc Acad Sci Paris.* 1951;232:349-350.
62. Arnulf A, Dupuy O, Flamant F. Les microfluctuations de l'oiel et leur influence sur l'image retinienne. *CR Hebd Seanc Acad Sci Paris.* 1951;232:438-450.
63. Hofer H, Artal P, Singer B, Aragon JL, Williams DR. Dynamics of the eye's wave aberration. *J Opt Soc Am A.* 2001;18:497-506.
64. Guirao A, Williams DR, Cox IG. Effect of rotation and translation on the expected benefit of an ideal method to correct the eye's higher-order aberrations. *J Opt Soc Am A.* 2001;18:1003-1015.
65. Guirao A, Williams DR, Cox IG. Method for optimizing the benefit of correcting the eye´s higher order aberrations in the presence of decentrations. *J Opt Soc Am A.* 2002;19:126-128.
66. Tomlinson A, Ridder III WH, Watanabe R. Blink-induced variations in visual performance with toric soft contact lenses. *Optom Vis Sci.* 1994;71:545-549.
67. Schwiegerling J, Snyder RW. Eye movement during laser in situ keratomileusis. *J Cataract Refract Surg.* 2000;26:345-351.
68. Guirao A, Williams DR, MacRae SM. Effect of beam size on the expected benefit of customized laser refractive surgery. *J Refract Surg.* 2003;19(1):15-23.
69. Oshika T, Klyce SD, Applegate RA, Howland HC, El Danasoury MA. Comparisons of corneal wavefront aberrations after photorefractive keratectomy and laser in situ keratomileusis. *Arch Ophthalmol.* 1999;127:1-7.
70. Thibos LN, Hong X. Clinical applications of the Shack-Hartmann aberrometer. *Optom Vis Sci.* 1999;76:817-825.

71. Williams DR, Yoon GY, Porter J, Guirao A, Hofer H, Cox I. Visual benefit of correcting higher order aberrations of the eye. *J Refract Surg*. 2000;16:S554-S559.

72. Applegate RA, Hilmantel G, Howland HC, Tu EY, Starck T, Zayac EJ. Corneal first surface optical aberrations and visual performance. *J Refract Surg*. 2000;16:507-514.

Chapter 4

Ophthalmic Wavefront Sensing: History and Methods

Howard C. Howland, MS, PhD

Introduction

> Prior to the introduction of refractive surgery, the wavefront aberration of the eye played a very small role in anyone's thinking about the optics of the eye.

This is because in normal eyes, even at relatively large apertures, the wavefront aberration generally does not degrade the image quality below 20/20 vision.

However, with the advent of refractive surgery, very large amounts of spherical aberration and coma were induced in eyes treated with radial keratotomy, photorefractive keratectomy, or laser in situ keratomileusis.[1,2] While generally not significant at small pupil sizes, these induced aberrations became important at low light levels and large pupil apertures. This spurred an increased interest both in the measurement of higher-order monochromatic aberrations and techniques for eliminating them.

> Induced aberrations are important at low light levels and large pupil apertures.

Methods of Detection of Wavefront Aberration

The primary methods of wavefront aberration detection and reconstruction have been based either on interferometry or ray tracing.

> *Interferometer:* Any of several optical, acoustical, or radio-frequency instruments that use interference phenomena between a reference wave and an experimental wave, or between two parts of an experimental wave, to determine wavelengths, wave velocities, distances, and directions.

The Twymann-Green interferometer (Figure 4-1), described in almost every book on physical optics, works by first dividing and then recombining a collimated beam of light after its divided beams have been reflected from a test and a reference surface. Only if the surfaces are identical and correctly aligned will no interference fringes be visible in the final, recombined beam. Otherwise, the resulting interference fringe pattern will provide a topographic map (in steps of one wavelength) of the wavefront aberration difference surface.

> All ocular wavefront sensors that have been reduced to viable clinical devices have been based on ray tracing and reconstruction of the wavefront aberration surface.

> Interferometric methods have not found much application in physiological optics, primarily due to difficulties in stabilizing the eye and constructing appropriate reference surfaces with which to compare (eg, corneal shape).

All of the other methods have been based on ray tracing and reconstruction of the wavefront aberration surface by integrating the slopes of an array of beams intersecting the eye's entrance pupil. In physical optics, these methods were first realized by Hartmann[3] at the turn of the last century. About 5 years earlier, Tscherning[4] had constructed and described an apparatus, which he named an "aberroscope" (Figure 4-2), from a grid superimposed on a 5 diopter (D) spherical lens. Viewing a distant point source of light through the aberroscope, a subject could see a shadow image of the grid on his or her retina. From the distortions of the grid, one could infer the aberrations of the eye.

> Tscherning's aberroscope was attacked and dismissed by Gullstrand, and possibly due to this, its use was temporarily abandoned.

Sixty years later, Bradford Howland invented the crossed cylinder aberroscope[5] (Figure 4-3) to investigate the aberrations of camera lenses. Instead of using a spherical lens to shadow the grid on the retina, he used a crossed cylinder lens of 5 D with the negative cylinder axis at 45 degrees. The advantages of this over the Tscherning aberroscope are 1) diffraction blurs the grid lines along their axes, producing a sharper grid, 2) the point of zero

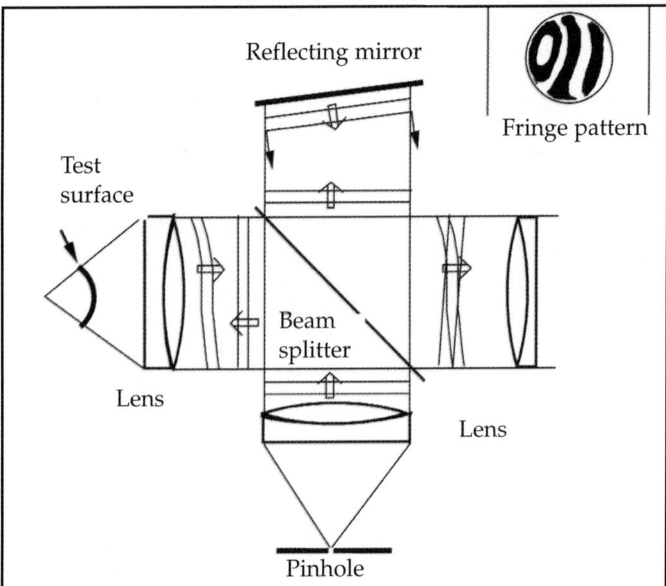

Figure 4-1. Twymann-Green interferometer. A collimated light source enters a beam splitter where light in one path is focused onto a curved surface (arrow [eg, a cornea]) and reflected back through the beam splitter. This beam is then combined with (and interferes with) the second beam, which has passed through the beam splitter and is reflected from a reference reflecting mirror. If the test spherical surface was perfectly centered with its center at the focal point of the lens and the reference mirror tilted, a set of perfectly parallel fringes would be seen by the observer.

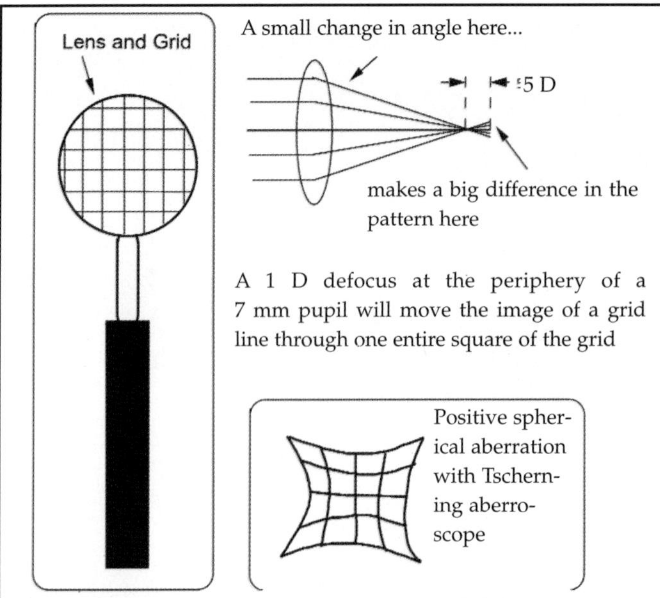

Figure 4-2. The Tscherning aberroscope. The aberroscope is shown at the left and consists of a +5 D lens with a grid consisting of about 1 millimeter (mm) squares. To use it, the subject views a distant point source of light that is focused in front of his or her retina by the aberroscope's lens. The grid is then shadowed on the subject's retina and the distortions of the grid are noted and drawn by the subject. A grid corresponding to positive spherical aberration is depicted.

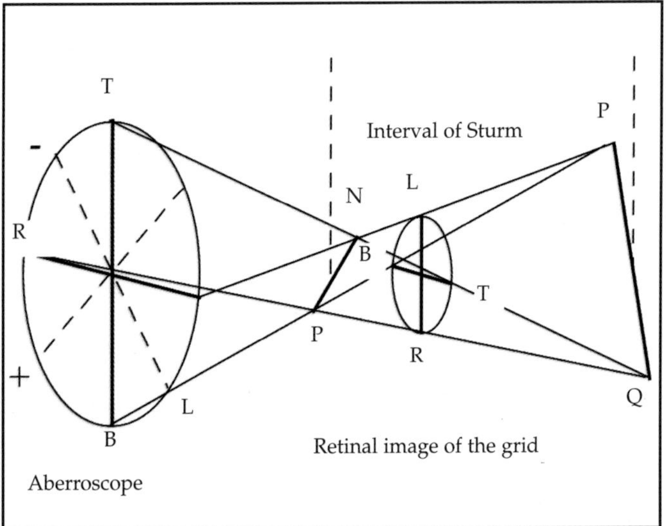

Figure 4-3. The optics of the crossed cylinder aberroscope. The construction and use is similar to that of the Tscherning aberroscope. However, in place of a +5 D spherical lens, a ±5 D crossed cylinder lens is employed. This causes the grid to be shadowed in the interval of Sturm. In this arrangement, diffraction smears the images of the lines along their lengths, making the image sharper than that of the Tscherning aberroscope.

defocus of the eye is clearly indicated by the horizontal and vertical orientation of the central grid lines, and 3) the distorted grid lines represent the ray intercept plots of classical optics.

Another 20 years passed before a subjective aberroscope was used to investigate and characterize the monochromatic aberrations of 55 eyes.[6] The principal results of that study were that 1) third-order coma-like aberrations dominate the aberration structure of the normal eye at all physiological pupil sizes and 2) there was about one order of magnitude difference in root mean square (RMS) wavefront aberration between the best and the worst eye in the study. This was the first time that comatic aberrations had been measured, as opposed to estimated, in any eye. This study also introduced the use of Zernike polynomials to describe the wavefront aberration of the human eye.

> Howland and Howland were the first to introduce Zernike polynomials to describe the wavefront aberration of the human eye.

The crossed cylinder aberroscope was improved by introducing an ophthalmoscopic track and photographing grid patterns on the retina,[7] making it an objective technique. More recently, an objective Tscherning aberroscope method has been adapted for clinical use.[8]

Another subjective method to find the wavefront aberration of the human eye was that of Smirnov,[9] wherein a grid is viewed by the entire aperture of the eye, minus a single central intersection viewed through a small aperture, which is made to scan the entire pupil sequentially. Smirnov measured the topographies of seven eyes and commented on them.

Since then, Webb and colleagues[10] (Figure 4-4) have made a modern implementation of Smirnov's method called the *spatially resolved refractometer* that computes the wavefront aberration and reduces it to Zernike polynomials in a matter of minutes. It shows remarkable repeatability.

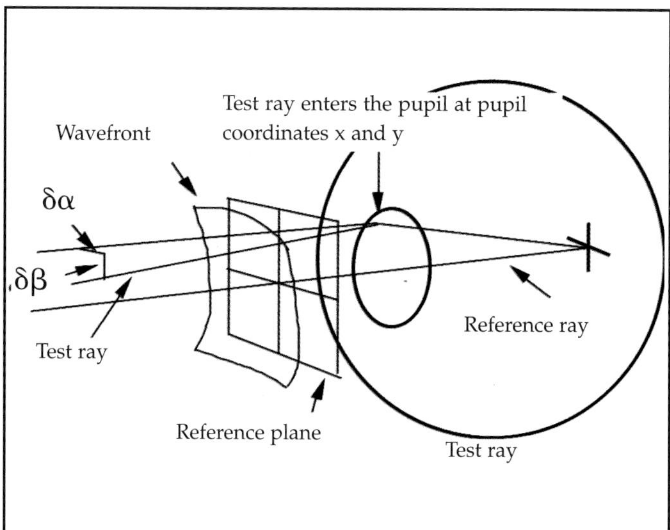

Figure 4-4. Optics of a spatially resolved refractometer. A reference beam enters the center of the pupil (or alternatively the entire pupil) and forms a reference mark at the fovea. A second beam that can scan the pupil enters a small portion of the pupil and its entrance angles are adjusted by the subject so that it intersects the reference mark at the fovea. From a knowledge of the entrance angles of the test ray at multiple positions on the pupil, the wavefront can be reconstructed.

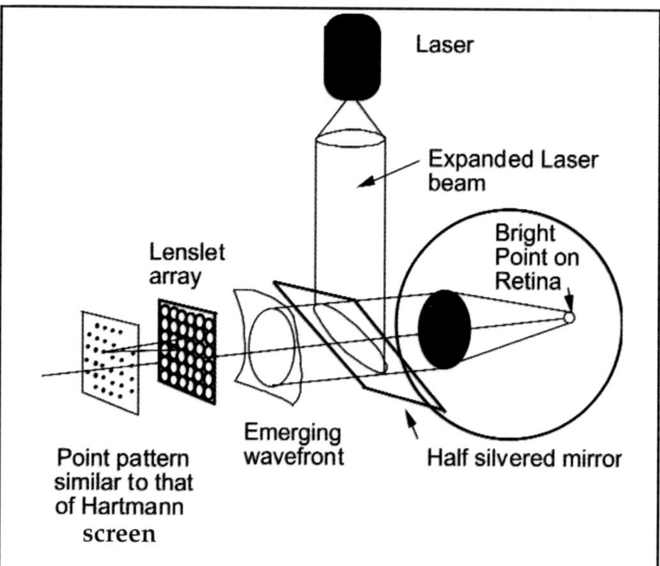

Figure 4-5. Optics of a Shack-Hartmann device. A laser beam is expanded, collimated, and focused to a point on the retina. The emerging beam from this point source is focused onto a lenslet array that forms a point pattern that is captured by a video camera. The pattern obtained is compared with that of an aberration-free beam, and again the wavefront is computed from the displacements of the points from their unaberrated pattern.

Lastly, the Shack-Hartmann wavefront sensor (Figure 4-5), a method initiated in astronomy to analyze the aberrations of the atmosphere above a telescope in real time, was adapted by J. Bille and J. Liang in Heidelberg and developed by Liang, Williams, and colleagues in Rochester to image the human fundus by removing the aberrations of the eye with a deformable mirror.[11] The measurement is made by focusing a bright spot of light on the retina and projecting the quasi-planar wavefront onto a lenslet array that focuses spots of light on a charged-coupled device (CCD) video array. Just as in the Tscherning aberroscope, the displacement of the spots from their unaberrated positions yields the average slopes of the wavefront at each lenslet's position.

Wavefront Aberration of the Cornea

With the advent of modern corneal topographers that used targets of many mires, together with a digital camera and computer processing, it became possible to compute the shape of the cornea and, hence, its wavefront aberration from the mire images. This was first done to assay the aberrations of corneas that had undergone refractive surgery.[12] However, the technique is of general utility in determining the internal aberrations of the eye by subtracting the corneal Zernike coefficients from the corresponding coefficients describing the wavefront aberration of the whole eye.

One issue that has not been totally resolved in computing the corneal wavefront aberration is what shaped surface should be used as a reference shape for the nonaberrated cornea? The most commonly used reference surface has been the best fitting sphere, followed by an ellipsoid of revolution.

Commercial Machines for Wavefront Measurement

Recently, due to the popularity of refractive surgery, a number of commercial wavefront measuring machines have come on the market. One such product is depicted in Figure 4-6. This machine includes an infrared refractor, a corneal topographer, and a Shack-Hartmann device for measuring total ocular aberrations. Both corneal and total Zernike coefficients are calculated. By subtracting the corneal Zernike coefficients from their corresponding total ocular Zernike coefficients, one may obtain the wavefront aberration of the internal optics. Such machines are finding clinical applications in disease conditions that influence the aberrations of the eye, such as studies of tear film breakup[13] or cataracts,[14] as first suggested by Applegate and Thibos.[15]

An Emerging Picture of "Normal" Wavefront Aberration of the Eye

Now that the wavefront aberrations of many eyes are being measured by many machines, we are rapidly gaining a picture of what the normal wavefront aberration may be. The RMS deviation of the wavefront aberration surface from a plane (outside the eye) or perfect sphere (inside the eye) has become the most common single metric used to characterize the aberrations of the eye. However, RMS wavefront aberration is not well correlated with visual performance.[16] On a log-log correlation over three orders of magnitude, wavefront RMS deviation accounts for approximately half of the variance in high and low contrast acuity.[17]

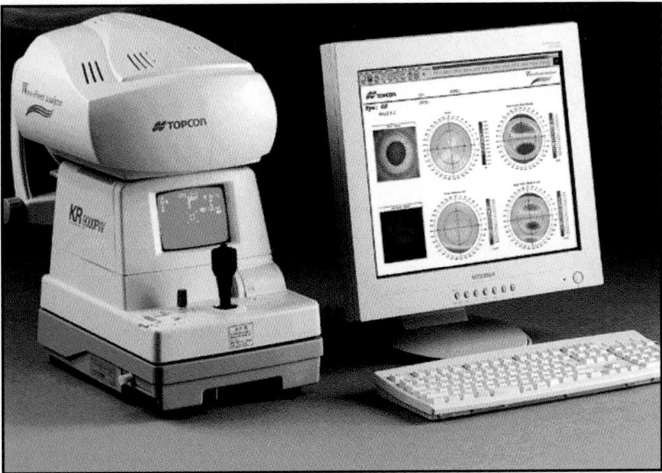

Figure 4-6. A commercially available Shack-Hartmann wavefront sensor. In this machine (Topcon KR 9000 PW [Topcon America Corp, Paramus, NJ]), a Shack-Hartmann wavefront sensor is combined with a corneal topographer and a conventional infrared refractometer. The monitor displays a corneal topographic map and a corresponding topographic map of the aberrations of the entire eye.

Metrics of optical quality that are more predictive of visual performance are discussed in Chapter 8. RMS wavefront error generally increases with about the third power of the pupil radius.[18]

> RMS wavefront aberration is not well correlated with visual performance.[16]

There is evidence that RMS wavefront aberration increases with increasing age above 20 years or so.[18]

However, for young adults, a rule of thumb derived from several studies shows that the RMS wavefront aberration in micrometers may be approximated by the equation: RMS = $r^3/100$, where r is the pupil radius in millimeters.[19] Furthermore, 95% of all RMS values at that pupil radius should lie within a factor of 3 of this value.

Conclusion

There exists today a variety of subjective and objective methods for assaying the wavefront aberration of human eyes, which span a wide range in cost, complexity, and accuracy. Many of these methods have now been realized in commercial machines, which have found a variety of applications, not only in refractive surgery, but also in the study of disease and the characterization of the wavefront aberration of normal eyes. Due to the unique advantages of each method, we may expect to see their continued use in the future.

References

1. Martinez CE, Applegate RA, Klyce SD, McDonald, MB, Medina JP, Howland HC. Effect of pupillary dilation on corneal optical aberrations after photorefractive keratectomy. *Arch Ophthalmol.* 1998;116: 1053-1062.
2. Oshika T, Klyce SD, Applegate RA, Howland HC, el Danasoury MA. Comparison of corneal wavefront aberrations after photorefractive keratectomy and laser in situ keratomileusis. *Am J Ophthalmol.* 1999;127(1):1-7.
3. Hartmann J. Bemerkungen ueber den Bau und die Justierung von Spektrographen. *Zeitschrift fuer Instrumentenkunde.* 1900;20:47.
4. Tscherning M. Die monochromatischen aberrationen des menschlichen. *Auges Z Psychol Physiol Sinn.* 1894;6:456-471.
5. Howland B. Use of crossed cylinder lens in photographic lens evaluation. *Appl Opt.* 1960;7:1587-1588.
6. Howland HC, Howland B. A subjective method for the measurement of monochromatic aberrations of the eye. *J Opt Soc Am.* 1977; 67:1508-1518.
7. Walsh G, Charman WN, Howland HC. Objective technique for the determination of monochromatic aberrations of the human eye. *J Opt Soc Am A.* 1984;1:987-992.
8. Mierdel P, Krinke HE, Wiegand W, Kaemmerer M, Seiler T. A measuring device for the assessment of monochromatic aberrations in human eyes. *Ophthalmologe.* 1997;94(6):441-445.
9. Smirnov HS. Measurement of the wave aberration in the human eye. *Biophys.* 1961;6:52-66.
10. Webb RH, Burns SA, Penney M. Coaxial spatially resolved refractometer. United States Patent 6,000,800. 1999.
11. Miller-Donald T, Williams DR, Morris GM, Liang M. Images of cone photoreceptors in the living human eye. *Vision Res.* 1996;36(8):1067-1079.
12. Applegate RA, Johnson CA, Howland HC, Yee RW. Monochromatic wavefront aberrations following radial keratotomy. In: *Technical Digest, Noninvasive Assessment of the Visual System.* Washington, DC: Optical Society of America; 1989:98-102.
13. Koh S, Maeda N, Kuroda T, et al. Effect of tear film break-up on higher-order aberrations measured with wavefront sensor. *Am J Ophthalmol.* 2002;134(1):115-117.
14. Kuroda T, Fujikado T, Maeda N, Oshika T, Hirohara Y, Mihashi T. Wavefront analysis in eyes with nuclear or cortical cataract. *Am J Ophthalmol.* 2002;134(1):1-9.
15. Applegate RA, Thibos LN. Localized measurement of scatter due to cataract. *Invest Ophthalmol Vis Sci.* 2000;41(Suppl):S3.
16. Applegate RA, Sarver EJ, Khemsara V. Are all aberrations equal? *J Refract Surg.* 2002;18:S556-S562.
17. Applegate RA, Hilmantel G, Howland HC, Tu EY, Starck T, Zayac EJ. Corneal first surface optical aberrations and visual performance. *J Refract Surg.* 2000;16:507-514.
18. Howland HC. High order wave aberration of eyes. *Ophthalmol Physiol Opt.* 2002;22(5):434-439.
19. McLellan JS, Marcos S, Burns SA. Age-related changes in monochromatic aberrations of the human eye. *Invest Ophthalmol Vis Sci.* 2001;42(6):1390-1395.

Chapter 5

Retinal Imaging Using Adaptive Optics

Austin Roorda, PhD and David R. Williams, PhD

Introduction

The optical system of the human eye is fraught with aberrations. This fact was documented as early as 1801 by Thomas Young,[1] but perhaps Helmholtz stated it best when he wrote "Now, it is not too much to say that if an optician wanted to sell me an instrument [the eye] which had all these defects, I should think myself quite justified in blaming his carelessness in the strongest terms and giving him back his instrument."[2] These ocular aberrations blur the retinal image and limit our ability to see, but they also impose a limit on one's ability to look into the eye since, for ophthalmoscopy, the optics of the eye serve as the objective lens. For years, these aberrations were considered to impose fundamental limits on what can be imaged[3] in the retina, but recent developments have demonstrated that these limits can be overcome. The most notable recent developments include the first application of the Shack-Hartmann wavefront sensing technique to accurately measure the aberrations of the human eye,[4,5] which was soon followed by the successful application of adaptive optics (AO) to compensate for these optical aberrations.[6]

> Helmholtz: "Now, it is not too much to say that if an optician wanted to sell me an instrument [the eye] which had all these defects, I should think myself quite justified in blaming his carelessness in the strongest terms and giving him back his instrument."[2]

History of Adaptive Optics

The original problem that AO was proposed to solve was that of image degradation arising in ground-based telescopes due to turbulence in the earth's atmosphere. Babcock, in 1953, wrote a paper in which the basic concepts of an AO system were described.[7] Due to the technological difficulties associated with AO, it was not until 1977 that the first successful application was demonstrated.[8] The technological development was largely due to an infusion of funds from the military, who appreciated the potential benefits of AO, largely for imaging (and targeting) foreign satellites from ground-based installations.[9] Much of the military's information was declassified in 1992, a move that accelerated progress for all applications, including astronomy and vision science. At the present time, AO technology is still maturing and developing and there is much scope for improvement. Today, virtually every major telescope has or is planning to establish an AO program. By comparison, the history of AO for ophthalmic imaging is just over 10 years old. AO was first used in a scanning laser ophthalmoscope in 1989 by Dreher et al.[10,11] Their wavefront corrector was a 13-element segmented mirror, and the correction was limited to the astigmatism of the eye. The information used to control the mirror was the patient's prescription since they had not yet developed the wavefront sensing technology required to close the loop on the AO system. The images they obtained were only slightly better than without correction; not surprising given the low-order of the correction. Nonetheless, they clearly appreciated the potential optical benefits of correcting the ocular aberrations with AO. It wasn't until 1997 that the first closed loop AO system for the eye was demonstrated that could correct higher-order aberrations other than defocus and astigmatism.[6] This device provided the highest transverse resolution to date of images of the human retina, allowing single cells to be clearly resolved. It also was used to demonstrate that vision could be improved by correcting higher-order aberrations as well as the defocus and astigmatism corrected by ordinary spectacles.

Methods

Mathematics of Imaging

In order to image the retina, we must consider the optics of the eye as an integral part of the ophthalmoscope. The pupil of the eye plays a major role in how much light and image quality we ultimately receive back from the retina. Imaging systems, such as the eye, transmit spatial frequencies at various contrasts that ultimately compose an image. The curve that defines the transmitted contrast as a function of changing spatial frequency is called the *modulation transfer function*, or MTF. High contrast transmission of higher spatial frequencies leads to higher image detail and resolution. In any optical system, the maximum spatial frequency that can be transmitted is defined by the following equation:

$$f_{\text{cutoff}} = \frac{d}{57.3\lambda}$$

where d is the diameter of the pupil and λ is the wavelength of the light. The cutoff frequency, f_{cutoff}, is the maximum spatial

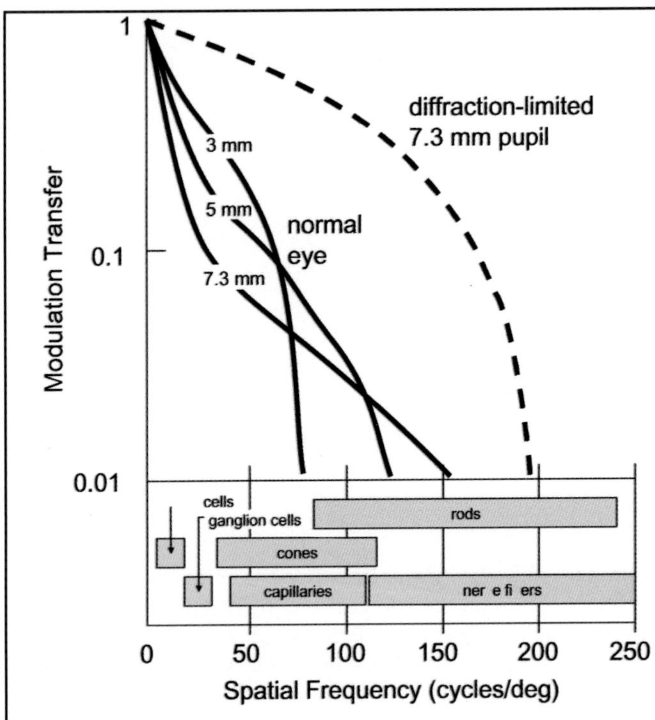

Figure 5-1. MTFs and retinal features as a function of spatial frequency. The solid lines show the average MTFs for three pupil sizes: 3 mm (12 eyes), 5 mm (14 eyes), and 7.3 mm (14 eyes).[5] The diffraction-limited MTF for a 7.3 pupil is also shown (dashed line) to illustrate the improvements in contrast offered by correcting the aberrations of a 7.3 mm pupil. The lower part of the plot shows the typical sizes of photoreceptors,[39] ganglion cells,[40] retinal pigmented epithelium (RPE) cells,[41] and capillaries[42] in the retina. Their spatial frequencies are based on their sizes. Because the sizes of the retinal cells change with location in the retina, they span a range of spatial frequencies. For example, cone photoreceptors are about 2.50 micrometers (μm) in the fovea but increase to about 10.00 μm in the far periphery.[28] (Adapted from Miller D. Retinal imaging and vision at the frontiers of adaptive optics. *Physics Today.* 2000;53:31-36.)

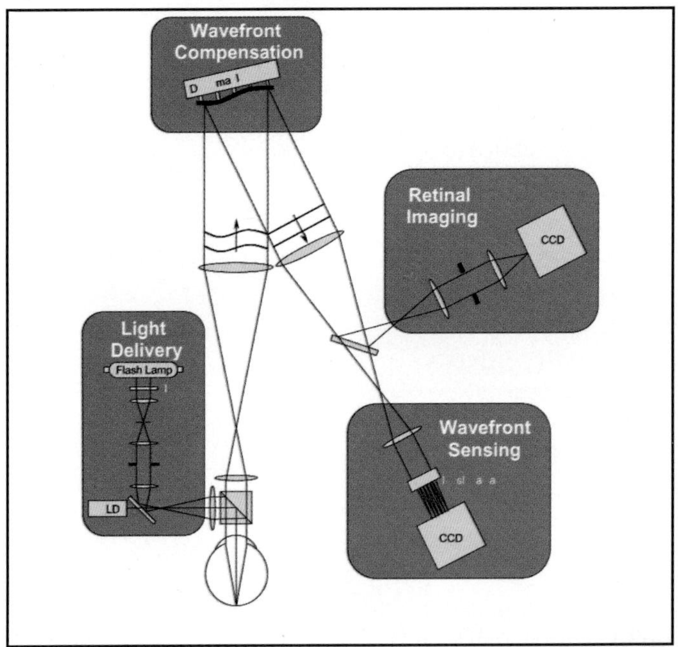

Figure 5-2. Optical system for wavefront sensing and correction. The eye focuses a collimated beam from a laser onto the retina. The light reflected from the retina forms an aberrated wavefront at the pupil, which is measured by the Shack-Hartmann wavefront sensor. A deformable mirror, conjugate with the pupil, is used to compensate for the eye's wave aberration. After compensation is achieved, the retina is imaged by sliding a mirror into place to open the retinal imaging arm. For imaging the retina, a krypton flash lamp delivered a 4-millisecond (ms) flash, illuminating a 1 degree diameter retinal patch.

frequency (in cycles per degree [c/deg]) that is transmitted through the optical system. For a diffraction-limited eye, spatial frequencies that are lower than f_{cutoff} are imaged with increasing contrast to a maximum contrast of 100% at 0 c/deg. This formula sets a minimum on the pupil size that is required to image the smallest structures in the retina. For example, the foveal cones have a spatial frequency that peaks at about 120 c/deg.

Transverse means in the plane of the retina, as opposed to *axial*, which is depth into the retina.

According to the formula, the pupil size required to image these cones would have to be greater than 4.30 millimeters (mm) (for 632 nanometers [nm] of light). Practically, the size has to be greater because the transmitted contrast at the cutoff is, by definition, zero. But the human eye is not diffraction-limited for pupil sizes greater than 1 mm[12] and even though information up to the cutoff frequency is still transmitted, it is transmitted with such low contrast that the effective cutoff frequency is much lower. Aberrations increase with pupil size to such an extent that the blur they cause more than offsets the gains in image quality that diffraction predicts. The overall best pupil size for transverse imaging over spatial frequencies from 0 to 30 c/deg is usually between 2 and 3 mm.[12] Figure 5-1 shows MTFs for the average human eye compared with the MTFs for the same eyes if they had diffraction-limited optics. So, in order to benefit from the larger pupils that the eye offers (up to ~8 mm), one must compensate for the aberrations.

Conventional Ophthalmoscopy With Adaptive Optics

A schematic layout of a typical flood-illumination AO ophthalmoscope is shown in Figure 5-2. Like all AO systems, two main components, a wavefront sensor and a wavefront corrector, are required. The wavefront sensor is used to measure the aberrations of the optical system that are to be corrected. Different wavefront sensing techniques might be used, but the technique that is integrated into the Rochester AO ophthalmoscope is the Shack-Hartmann wavefront sensor.[6,13] The wavefront corrector in the Rochester ophthalmoscope is a deformable mirror or DM (Xinetics Inc, Devens, Mass). The DM consists of a 2 mm thin facesheet attached to 97 lead magnesium niobate (PMN) actuators bonded to a base. Each actuator can locally push or pull the mirror over a range spanning ±2 microns (μm), allowing for compensation of wave aberrations with peak-to-valley magnitudes of up to 8 μm. Alternative techniques to compensate the wave aberrations are being explored because the high cost and large size of these DMs prohibit commercialization of the technology.

> The mirror shape required to compensate the aberrations is simply one-half the magnitude of the actual wavefront aberration.

In the AO ophthalmoscope, the wavefront sensor and the DM are integrated into the same system. The patient sits in the instrument and his or her eye is brought into alignment with the instrument axis. The first aberration measurement of the eye is made with the DM in an initially flattened state. The wavefront sensor measures the slope of the wavefront at a discrete number of points and the appropriate DM actuator voltages that are required to compensate the aberrations are calculated and sent to the mirror. The mirror shape required to compensate the aberrations is simply one-half the magnitude of the actual wavefront aberration. Rather than attempting to correct the aberrations all in one step, an iterative procedure is used in which a small number of measurement and correction cycles converge smoothly on the best correction. The present system can reach 0.8 hertz (Hz) closed loop bandwidth when running at a 30 Hz sampling rate.

> Since there are a limited number of actuators in the DM and the eye has a small fraction of very high-order aberrations, a perfect correction is not possible.

One usually continues the iterations until the wavefront aberration asymptotes to a minimum value. With a 97 actuator DM, the system can reduce the eye's residual root mean square wavefront error over a 6.8 mm pupil to values lower than 0.05 μm. Once the wavefront is flattened, a dichroic mirror that is placed in the path directs the corrected beam of light from the eye into the retinal camera, which looks at the retina through the compensating mirror.

> Dichroic mirrors reflect one band of wavelengths of light while simultaneously transmitting another. They are commonly used in instruments that use two different wavelengths in the optical system to perform two tasks (eg, wavefront sensing and retinal imaging).

The human retina is not a source of light so, to take an image, the retina is flood-illuminated over a 1 degree circular patch with light from a krypton flash lamp. Narrow-bandwidth interference filters are placed in the illumination path to control the wavelength of the imaging light.

Scanning Laser Ophthalmoscopy With Adaptive Optics

> A scanning laser ophthalmoscope (SLO) differs from conventional imaging in that the SLO captures an image over time by detecting the scattered light from a focused point as it scans across the retina in a raster pattern.[14]

This imaging modality offers several noted advantages over conventional ophthalmoscopes. First, one can use more sensitive detectors, such as a photomultiplier tube or an avalanche photodiode, to detect the light rather than using an inherently noisier and less sensitive charged coupled device (CCD) camera.

> A CCD is an integrated circuit comprised of an array of light sensitive pixels that build up a charge proportional to the amount of incident light and convert the charge for each pixel into a digital gray scale value. These devices are most commonly used to obtain digital images in camera systems.

More importantly, SLOs are relatively insensitive to image degradation due to scatter in the optics. SLOs also have the ability to do optical sectioning in the retina. These two advantages are facilitated by passing the scattered light through a small aperture conjugate to the retina, called the *confocal pinhole*, prior to detection.

SLOs are similar to conventional ophthalmoscopes in that they rely on the optical system of the eye as the objective lens for imaging. Hence, an SLO suffers from the same image quality losses due to aberrations. It follows that the AO technique can offer the same benefits to this imaging technique. Roorda and colleagues at the University of Houston have recently incorporated AO into an SLO (AOSLO).[15] A schematic layout of the instrument is shown in Figure 5-3. There are two main differences in the AO system of the AOSLO compared to a flood illuminated system. First, the AOSLO wavefront sensor measures aberrations from the entire raster-scanned area of the retina. This is possible because the light from the raster is "descanned" on its return path in the SLO.

> *Descanned* means light scattered from the eye reverses its ingoing path and reflects from the scanning mirror again, thereby "undoing" the scanning motion and leaving the beam stationary, or nonscanning, which allows it to pass through a small pinhole prior to detection.

The second difference is that the wave aberrations are corrected on the way into the eye (to get a small focused spot) and on the way out of the eye (to get a small focused spot at the confocal pinhole).

Both the Rochester flood-illuminated camera and the Houston AOSLO achieve about a three-fold benefit in lateral resolution with adaptive optics. In the AOSLO, however, a further benefit is that it has axial resolution, or the ability to do optical slicing, and it can image the retina in real-time.

Results

Conventional Adaptive Optics Ophthalmoscopy

Photoreceptor Images

Human cone photoreceptors comprise the earliest stage in receiving the retinal image. Images of the photoreceptors are

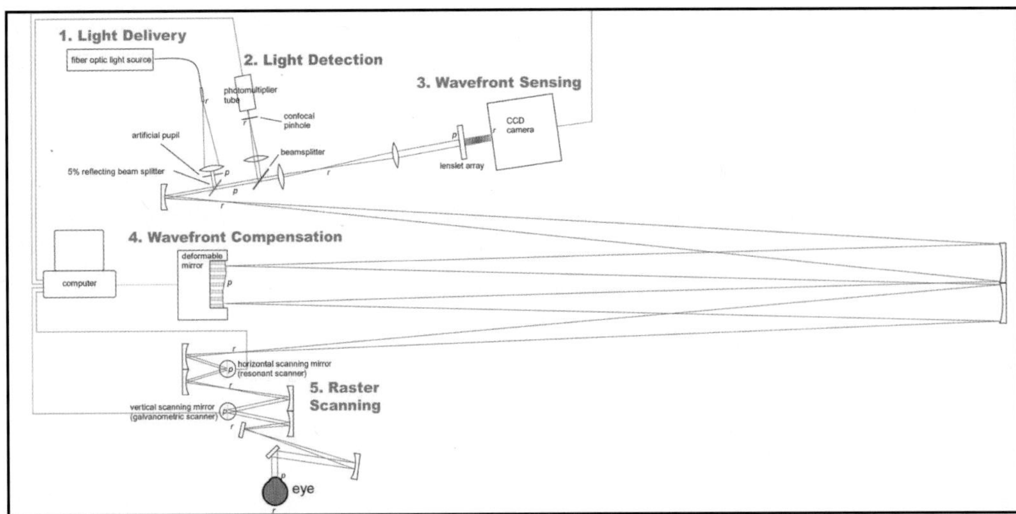

Figure 5-3. Schematic of the Houston Adaptive Optics Scanning Laser Ophthalmoscope (AOSLO). The AOSLO optics are comprised of five major components: 1) Light delivery: The source is a single mode fiber optic that can be coupled to any type of laser. We currently use a 660 nm laser diode. 2) Light detection: The scattered light is focused with a collector lens to the confocal pinhole (100 mm fl collector lens; 3.5 mm exit beam; 80 mm pinhole in these examples). A GaAs PMT module (Hamamatsu Corp, Japan) is used to detect the scattered light. 3) Wavefront sensing: A Shack-Hartmann wavefront sensor is used to measure the wave aberrations. The lens array samples the wavefront at 241 points over a 6.3 mm pupil (0.4 mm lenslet spacing in a square grid). 4) Wavefront compensation: Aberrations are compensated for both ingoing and outgoing light with a XinEtics 37-channel deformable mirror. 5) Raster scanning: The beam is scanned on the retina with a resonant (16 kilahertz [kHz] sinusoidal scan)/galvanometric (30 Hz sawtooth scan) scan mirror combination. Pupil and retinal conjugate points are labeled *p* and *r*, respectively, throughout the optical path.

important for learning about the fundamental properties of vision as well as for diagnosing retinal disease. Most effort on the Rochester AO ophthalmoscope to date has been concentrated on imaging cone photoreceptors, and that effort has produced the best pictures ever of the cone mosaic in the living human eye.

> AO noninvasive imaging has produced the best images of the cone mosaic in the living human eye.

> *Signal-to-noise* is the ratio of the signal (what you want to see—the cone mosaic) to the noise (information that degrades the signal).

Examples of the types of images that can be obtained are shown in the three panels on Figure 5-4. The image on the left is a single snapshot taken after only defocus and astigmatism have been corrected in the eye.[6,16] Prior to the implementation of AO, sphere and cylinder were the only corrections that were applied to improve image quality. In the case shown here, the aberrations for the subject were sufficiently low so that some photoreceptor structure could be seen in the uncompensated images. This ability to resolve photoreceptors without using AO had already been documented by other groups who showed similar results.[17-20] Nonetheless, the improvement in image quality obtained after AO compensation (see the middle panel in Figure 5-4) is striking. In the compensated image, the fine structures are better resolved and have higher contrast than in the uncompensated image. The bright spots in the image are cone photoreceptors, which at this retinal location are about 5 µm in diameter. Nearly all photoreceptors are resolved in a single image. Registration of multiple images, as shown on the rightmost image, improves the signal-to-noise ratio in the image to an extent where all photoreceptors are resolved. Even the smallest cones across the very center of the fovea have been resolved, as shown in Figure 5-5, which is a composite of many frames taken around the central 2.2 degrees of one subject.

Arrangement of S, M, and L Cones

Over 200 years ago, Thomas Young proposed that the human retina was comprised of three cone types,[21] but it was not possible to determine the spatial arrangement of those cones prior to the development of high-resolution imaging with AO. While retinal densitometry has been used for years to measure the pigment concentration in cone photoreceptors,[22] the advantage of using AO is that it allows one to perform the same measurements on individual photoreceptors. Full details of this experiment are described elsewhere[16] but a brief description follows. All photoreceptor images were taken with 550 nm light; a wavelength chosen to maximize the absorptance by L and M cone photopigments. Individual cones were classified by comparing images when the photopigment was fully bleached with those taken when it was either dark-adapted or exposed to a light that selectively bleached one photopigment. Images of fully bleached retinas were obtained following exposure to 550 nm light. Images of dark-adapted retina were taken following 5 minutes of dark adaptation. The S cones were distinguished from M and L cones by comparing fully bleached and dark-adapted images. Since the S cones absorb negligibly while the M and L cones absorb strong-

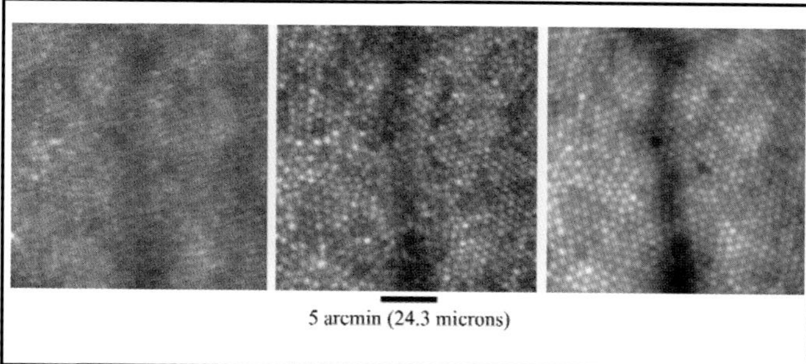

Figure 5-4. Images before and after adaptive compensation for the right eye of a living human subject. All three images are of the same retinal area located 1 degree from the central fovea. Images were taken with 550 nm light (25 nm bandwidth) through a 6 mm pupil. The dark, vertical band down the center of each image is an out-of-focus shadow of a blood vessel. The image to the far left shows a single snapshot taken after defocus and astigmatism have been corrected. The middle image is a snapshot after additional aberrations have been corrected with adaptive optics. The image to the far right shows the benefits in image quality obtained by registering and averaging multiple frames, 61 in this example.

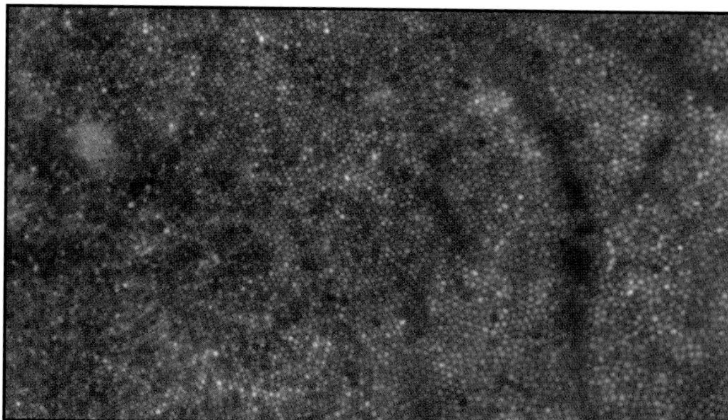

Figure 5-5. Image of the center of the living human fovea obtained with the Rochester Adaptive Optics Ophthalmoscope. Because of the 1 degree field of view of the instrument, this larger image was constructed by merging a number of overlapping images centered at different locations. The height of the image is 0.98 degrees high and its width is 2.2 degrees wide, extending from 0.7 degrees temporal to 1.5 degrees nasal retina. Note the increase in cone spacing with increasing distance from the foveal center.

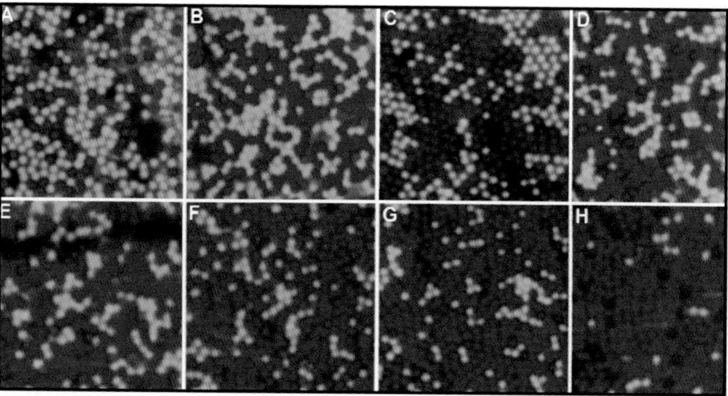

Figure 5-6. Images of the cone mosaics of eight subjects with normal color vision, obtained with the combined methods of adaptive optics imaging and retinal densitometry developed by Roorda and Williams.[16] The images are false colored so that blue, green, and red are used to represent the S, M, and L cones, respectively. (The true colors of these cones are yellow, purple, and bluish-purple). The mosaics illustrate the enormous variability in L/M cone fractions. The L:M cone ratios are A, 0.33; B, 1.04; C, 1.12; D, 1.5; E, 2.00; F, 2.33; G, 4.00; and H, 19.00. Images were taken either 1 or 1.25 degree from the foveal center.

ly at the imaging wavelength of 550 nm, the S cones reflect relatively more light than the M and L cones, which absorb the light and appear dimmer. Once the sparse population of S cones was identified, they were removed from analysis so that the M and L cones could be distinguished. To distinguish L from M cones, images were taken immediately following either of two bleaching conditions. In the first bleaching condition, dark-adapted retina was exposed to a 650 nm light that selectively bleached the L pigment. In the second, a 470 nm light selectively bleached the M pigment. The image following the 650 nm bleach revealed relatively brighter, low absorptance L cones that had been heavily bleached and darker, high absorbing M cones spared from bleaching. The absorptance images for the 470 nm bleach showed the opposite. Densitometric measurements were repeated in this way until the signal-to-noise in the data was sufficiently high to confidently identify the individual cones. Pseudocolor images of the arrangement of the cones near the fovea for eight human retinas are shown in Figure 5-6. The figure shows L:M ratios ranging from 0.33:1 to 19:1.

> S, M, and L cones: S is short wavelength sensitive cones, M is medium wavelength sensitive cones, and L is long wavelength sensitive cones.

Angular Tuning

> The angular tuning of the cones is often referred to as the *Stiles-Crawford effect* after the individuals who discovered the fact that in most eyes light entering the edge of the pupil is less effective in eliciting a visual response than light entering more centrally in the pupil.

It is well known that human photoreceptors act as waveguides. High resolution AO imaging can be brought to bear on some remaining questions about these waveguiding properties by looking at how each individual photoreceptor contributes to the overall directional properties. For example, it is suggested, based on psychophysics[23] and reflectometric measurements from an ensemble of cones,[24] that all the cones are narrowly tuned. This question can be answered directly now that individual cones can be resolved in living eyes. In the AO ophthalmoscope, the directional properties of individual cones were measured by determining how efficiently light is coupled into the cones as a function of illumination angle.

If less light gets into a cone because it is illuminated away from the cone's optical axis, then the reflected light from that cone will also be less.[25,26] Images were taken of the same cone mosaic under identical conditions except that the illumination angle was controlled by translating a 2 mm entrance pupil beam to different locations in the pupil. The images in Figure 5-7 are of

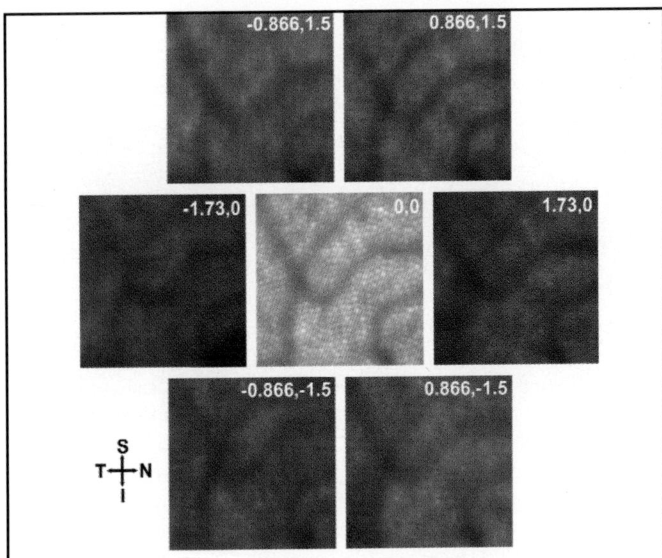

Figure 5-7. Composite of seven images of the same patch of retina taken with different entrance beam locations. Each image is a registered sum of 10 images. The number in the upper right corner of each image shows the position of the entrance beam relative to the central illumination beam location. The central location was centered with the best estimation of the Stiles-Crawford peak. The symbols S, I, N, and T indicate the superior, inferior, nasal, and temporal directions in retinal space. The reflectance of each cone changes as the illumination angle moves off the axis of the photoreceptor.

the same retinal patch taken with seven different entrance pupil positions. An angular tuning function was fit to over 200 contiguous cones in the images. The main result was that some disarray can be seen in the individual cones, but it is very small, accounting for less than 1% of the breadth of the overall tuning of an ensemble of cones.[27] Thus, the angular tuning of ensembles of cones is a good measure of the angular tuning of a single cone photoreceptor.

> The angular tuning of ensembles of cones is a good measure of the angular tuning of a single cone photoreceptor.

Adaptive Optics Scanning Laser Ophthalmoscopy

Optical Sectioning

The retina is a thin, mostly transparent, multilayered tissue. Its thickness is typically 300 µm from the nerve fibers on the surface to the retinal pigment epithelium. Beneath the retina is the choroid, which is primarily composed of blood vessels that nourish the retinal pigment epithelium and the back of the eye. Because of its complex structure, it is desirable to be able to image the retina in three dimensions. The improvement in optical sectioning in the AOSLO is important because current instruments report a maximum axial resolution (full width at half maximum [FWHM] of the axial point spread function [PSF]) of greater than 300 µm, which is about the thickness of the neural retina.

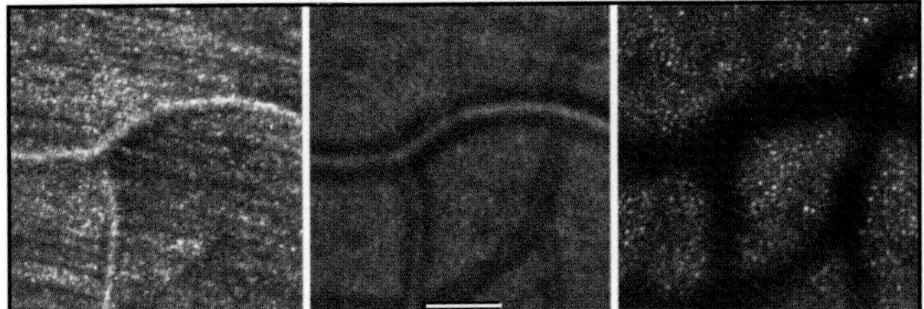

Figure 5-8. The three images are of a retinal location that is about 1.5 mm from the fovea. Each panel shows a different optical section of the retina, starting with the nerve fiber layer, and a blood vessel that runs across the retinal surface. The second panel reveals a second blood vessel and other capillaries that run beneath the nerve fibers. The final panel shows the mosaic of cone photoreceptors, which lie about 300 µm below the retinal surface. The scale bar on the middle figure represents about 100 µm.

> AOSLO allows noninvasive optical sectioning in real time of the microscopic structure of the living human retina.

Improved axial sectioning has allowed for direct imaging of specific layers in the retina, such as nerve fibers, capillary layers, and photoreceptors. Figure 5-8 shows a series of optical sections of an area in a living human retina located about 4 degrees (1.2 mm) from the fovea. The sequence of images reveals the three dimensional structure of the retina.

Blood Flow

The AOSLO images at 30 frames per second. This allows us to track dynamic changes in the retina, such as blood flow. The movement of single white blood cells has been observed in the smallest capillaries. Moreover, this blood flow can be observed directly without the use of fluorescein. The movement is impossible to observe in static frames, but digital videos can be found at www.opt.uh.edu/research/aroorda/aoslo.htm.

The Future of Adaptive Optics Ophthalmoscopy

Clinical Applications

Early diagnosis and treatment of retinal disorders have been hampered by the inability to resolve microscopic structures in the living human eye. In many cases, the retinal disease is detected only after significant and irreversible retinal damage has occurred. Since early detection and appropriate treatment is the best way to maintain good vision, it is important that we develop instruments that are sensitive to the specific changes, like photoreceptor loss, that are known to occur with these disorders.

> Rods are difficult to see because they are barely inside the resolution limits of the eye and because of low contrast due to the fact that, unlike cones, they do not direct their reflected light toward the pupil.

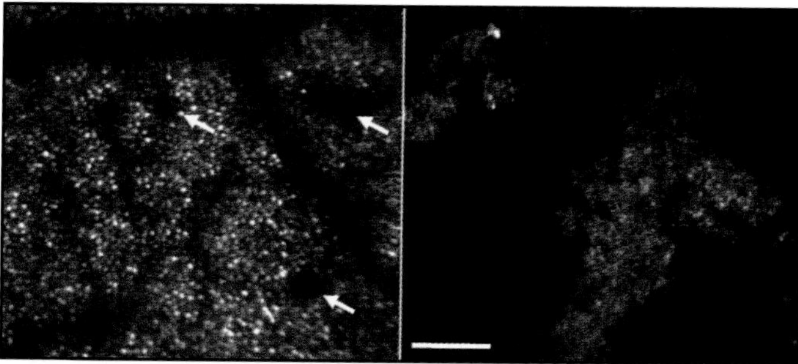

Figure 5-9. The two images are taken from different locations of the retina of a diabetic patient. The left image is focused on the photoreceptor layer, and shows shadows of small microaneurysms in the capillaries just nasal to the fovea. The right image shows a detail of a hard exudate that is about 2.5 degrees temporal to the fovea. The area outside the hard exudate appears dark because the photoreceptor layer is beyond the focal plane. The scale bar on the figure represents about 100 μm.

The increased contrast and resolving power offered with AO imaging will provide this sensitivity. More importantly, this increased sensitivity will open the possibility of testing the effectiveness of treatment interventions and also learning more about the mechanisms of the retinal disease.

To date, little AO imaging effort has been spent on the study of features other than the cone photoreceptors. To develop the instrument for clinical applications, it is desirable to expand the range of features that can be imaged (eg, rods, nerve fibers, and retinal pigment epithelium cells). Rods outnumber the cones by 20:1 in the human eye.[28] They are not important for central vision, but they have important roles in peripheral and night vision and rods are also the first photoreceptors to be affected in common retinal diseases like retinitis pigmentosa. Rods have never been resolved with the AO ophthalmoscope, but it remains a real possibility and a future challenge. Nerve fibers have diameters of about 3 μm and the striated patterns they produce are readily seen in conventional fundus images. With AO, we should be able to resolve individual nerve fibers and even measure their diameters.

> AO imaging will soon allow individual nerve fibers to be resolved, providing a powerful new tool for cutting edge research in glaucoma, as well as the monitoring and evaluation of therapy designed to alter the natural history of glaucoma.

Figure 5-9 shows two AOSLO pictures from preliminary investigations of the retina of a diabetic patient. The two images show microaneurysms and a detailed view of hard exudates.

Resolution, however, is not the only challenge to overcome for microscopic retinal imaging. Contrast is also a major limiting factor. Figure 5-1 illustrates that the contrast of features are improved in an image by improving the MTF, but successful imaging still relies on the object having its own intrinsic contrast. For example, RPE cells, whose health is implicated in several important retinal diseases, are difficult to see. The problem is not that they are too small, but rather because they have such low contrast. The low contrast is mainly due to the fact that to see the RPE, one must look through the strong reflection from the photoreceptor layer. Likewise, ganglion cells have low contrast, but in this case it is because they are transparent, a necessary requirement for tissue that lies anterior to the photoreceptors. Successful imaging of the broad range of structures in the retina will likely demand the marriage of AO ophthalmoscopy (either conventional or SLO) with other imaging and detection modalities, such as optical coherence tomography, differential interference contrast microscopy, or fluorescein angiography.

Alternate Technologies

> Developing and expanding the scope of the use of AO for basic and clinical investigations will require that AO technology become simpler to use, more compact, and less expensive.

The DM is the most effective technology for AO, but these devices are large and expensive and an economical, smaller version of DM technology is not likely. However, alternate technologies are on the horizon. For more details on these alternate technologies, the reader is referred to some recent publications.[29-31] For vision science, the best choice for an alternate wavefront corrector may depend on the particular imaging application. For example, the requirement of using polarized light for liquid crystal wavefront correcting devices might be a drawback for some applications but an advantage for others. Economical wavefront correctors such as phase plates[32] or membrane mirrors,[33] which have limitations, might be sufficient for many applications. On the other hand, for the best imaging possible, high temporal bandwidth to compensate for small eye movements, tear film changes, and accommodative fluctuations will be necessary.[34]

The most promising new technologies are in Micro Electrical Mechanical Systems, or MEMS. The manufacturing process, similar to that used for computer chips, can be done inexpensively and in mass quantities once a suitable system has been designed. The first MEMS DM for ophthalmic applications was demonstrated in 2002 by Doble et al,[35] where they corrected an eye over a 6 mm pupil down to 0.12 μm. Although the level of improvement did not reach performance of the Xinetics DM, the results were promising and efforts to make MEMS mirrors that are suitable for vision applications are continuing in several laboratories.

Beyond Imaging

Since AO can be used to image the retina with high spatial resolution, it follows that AO can be used to deliver light to the retina with the same precision. This opens a number of possibilities that range from studying the perception of aberration-free retinal images to realizing the potential for pinpoint laser treatment of the retina.

Prior to the development of AO for vision applications, studies of the perception of high spatial frequency retinal images could only be done by producing interference fringes on the retina.[36,37] This was and remains a very useful and productive technique, but the complexity of the retinal image is limited to sinusoidal gratings. Using AO, any complex near aberration-free image can be projected on the retina. Projection of such images is already being used to test the potential benefits of aberration-correcting refractive surgical techniques.[38] While there are some obvious benefits to vision, such as an improvement in contrast sensitivity, it remains to be seen whether or not hyperacuity tasks might be compromised by improving retinal image quality. Delivering small spots of color to the single photoreceptor cells might also be used to learn about the early stages of color processing in the human retina.

For clinical applications, laser systems can be equipped with AO to potentially pinpoint the treatment of features as small as individual capillaries or single cells. Using this technology, laser treatments like photocoagulation or photodynamic therapy can be restricted to a localized region, thereby preserving neighboring functional tissue in the retina. Finally, a real-time high resolution image offers the opportunity to do eye tracking measurements with unprecedented resolution.

Conclusion

With new technologies on the horizon and a host of new scientists and companies developing their own AO programs, the future promises to be exciting and productive for years to come.

AO in ophthalmoscopy is still a young field. Both the technology and the ideas of how to apply it are still developing. With new technologies on the horizon and a host of new scientists and companies developing their own AO programs, the future promises to be exciting and productive for years to come.

Acknowledgments

Preparation of this chapter was supported by the following grants: NSF "Center for Adaptive Optics" a Science and Technology Center managed by the University of California at Santa Cruz under cooperative agreement number AST-9876783 to AR and DRW, NIH/NEI grant RO1 EY13299 to AR and NIH/NEI grant RO1 EY04367.

References

1. Young T. On the mechanism of the eye. *Phil Trans Roy Soc London.* 1801;91:23-88.
2. Helmholtz H. *Helmholtz's Treatise on Physiological Optics.* Washington, DC: Optical Society of America; 1924.
3. Snyder AW, Miller WH. Photoreceptor diameter and spacing for highest resolving power. *J Opt Soc Am.* 1977;67:696-698.
4. Liang J, Grimm B, Goelz S, Bille JF. Objective measurement of wave aberrations of the human eye with use of a Hartmann-Shack wavefront sensor. *J Opt Soc Am A.* 1994;11:1949-1957.
5. Liang J, Williams DR. Aberrations and retinal image quality of the normal human eye. *J Opt Soc Am A.* 1997;14:2873-2883.
6. Liang J, Williams DR, Miller D. Supernormal vision and high-resolution retinal imaging through adaptive optics. *J Opt Soc Am A.* 1997;14:2884-2892.
7. Babcock HW. The possibility of compensating astronomical seeing. *Pub Astr Soc Pac.* 1953;65:229-236.
8. Hardy JW, Lefebvre JE, Koliopoulis CL. Real-time atmospheric compensation. *J Opt Soc Am.* 1977;67:360-369.
9. Benedict R, Breckinridge JB, Fried DL. Atmospheric-compensation technology: introduction. *J Opt Soc Am A.* 1994;11:257-262.
10. Dreher AW, Bille JF, Weinreb RN. Active optical depth resolution improvement of the laser tomographic scanner. *Appl Opt.* 1989;28: 804-808.
11. Bille JF, Dreher AW, Zinser G. Scanning laser tomography of the living human eye. In: Masters BR, ed. *Noninvasive Diagnostic Techniques in Ophthalmology.* New York: Springer-Verlag; 1990:528-547.
12. Campbell FW, Gubisch RW. Optical quality of the human eye. *J Physiol.* 1966;186:558-578.
13. Hofer H, Chen L, Yoon G, Singer B, Yamauchi Y, Williams DR. Improvement in retinal image quality with dynamic correction of the eye's aberrations. *Optics Express.* 2001;8:631-643.
14. Webb RH, Hughes GW, Pomerantzeff O. Flying spot TV ophthalmoscope. *Appl Opt.* 1980;19:2991-2997.
15. Roorda A, Romero-Borja F, Donnelly WJ, Queener H, Hebert TJ, Campbell MCW. Adaptive optics scanning laser ophthalmoscopy. *Optics Express.* 2002;10:405-412.
16. Roorda A, Williams DR. The arrangement of the three cone classes in the living human eye. *Nature.* 1999;397:520-522.
17. Miller D, Williams DR, Morris GM, Liang J. Images of cone photoreceptors in the living human eye. *Vision Res.* 1996;36:1067-1079.
18. Roorda A, Campbell MCW. Confocal scanning laser ophthalmoscope for real-time photoreceptor imaging in the human eye. *Vision Science and its Applications: Technical Digest.* 1997;1:90-93.
19. Wade AR, Fitzke FW. In vivo imaging of the human cone-photoreceptor mosaic using a confocal laser scanning ophthalmoscope. *Lasers and Light in Ophthalmology.* 1998;8:129-136.
20. Marcos S, Navarro R, Artal P. Coherent imaging of the cone mosaic in the living human eye. *J Opt Soc Am A.* 1996;13:897-905.
21. Young T. On the theory of light and colours. *Phil Trans Roy Soc London.* 1802;91:12-48.
22. Rushton WAH, Baker HD. Red/green sensitivity in normal vision. *Vision Res.* 1964;4:75-85.
23. MacLeod DIA. Directionally selective light adaptation: a visual consequence of receptor disarray? *Vision Res.* 1974;14:369-378.
24. Marcos S, Burns SA. Cone spacing and waveguide properties from cone directionality measurements. *J Opt Soc Am A.* 1999;16:995-1004.
25. van Blokland GJ. Directionality and alignment of the foveal receptors, assessed with light scattered from the human fundus in vivo. *Vision Res.* 1986;26:495-500.
26. Burns SA, Wu S, Chang He J, Elsner AE. Variations in photoreceptor directionality across the central retina. *J Opt Soc Am A.* 1996;14:2033-2040.
27. Roorda A, Williams DR. Optical fiber properties of individual human cones. *Journal of Vision.* 2002;2:404-412.
28. Curcio CA, Sloan KR, Kalina RE, Hendrickson AE. Human photoreceptor topography. *J Comp Neurol.* 1990;292:497-523.
29. Tyson RK. *Principle of Adaptive Optics.* 2nd ed. San Diego, Calif: Academic Press; 1998.
30. Tyson RK, ed. *Adaptive Optics Engineering Handbook.* New York: Marcel Dekker; 2000.
31. Séchaud M. Wave-front compensation devices. In: Roddier F, ed. *Adaptive Optics in Astronomy.* Cambridge: Cambridge University Press; 1999:57-91.
32. Burns SA, Marcos S, Elsner AE, Bará S. Contrast improvement for confocal retinal imaging using phase correcting plates. *Optics Letters.* 2002;27:400-402.
33. Fernández EJ, Iglesias I, Artal P. Closed-loop adaptive optics in the human eye. *Optics Letters.* 2001;26:746-748.
34. Hofer H, Artal P, Aragon JL, Williams DR. Dynamics of the eye's wave aberration. *J Opt Soc Am A.* 2001;18:497-506.

35. Doble N, Yoon G, Bierden P, Chen L, Olivier S, Williams DR. Use of a microelectromechanical mirror for adaptive optics in the human eye. *Optics Letters.* 2002;27:1537-1539.
36. Westheimer G. Modulation thresholds for sinusoidal light distributions on the retina. *J Physiol.* 1960;152:67-74.
37. Arnulf MA, Dupuy MO. La transmission des contrastes par le système optique de l'oeil et les seuils de contrastes retinines. *C R Acad Sci (Paris).* 1960;250:2757-2759.
38. Yoon G, Cox I, Williams DR. The visual benefit of static correction of the monochromatic wave aberration. *Invest Ophthalmol Vis Sci.* 1999;40(Suppl):40-40.
39. Curcio CA, Hendrickson A. Organization and development of the primate photoreceptor mosaic. In: Osborne NN, Chader GJ, eds. *Progress in Retinal Research.* Oxford: Pergamon; 1991:89-120.
40. Kolb H, Linberg KA, Fisher SK. Neurons of the human retina: a Golgi study. *J Comp Neurol.* 1992;318:147-187.
41. Zinn KM, Benjamin-Henkind JV. Anatomy of the human retinal pigment epithelium. In: Zinn KM, Marmor MF, eds. *The Retinal Pigment Epithelium.* Cambridge: Harvard University Press; 1979:3-31.
42. Snodderly DM, Weinhaus RS, Choi JC. Neural-vascular relationships in central retina of Macaque monkeys (Macaca fascicularis). *J Neuroscience.* 1992;12:1169-1193.

Section II

Wavefront Diagnostics and Standards

Basic Science Section

Chapter 6

Assessment of Optical Quality

Larry N. Thibos, PhD and Raymond A. Applegate, OD, PhD

Contemporary visual optics research is changing our mindset, our way of thinking about the optical system of the eye, and in the process is redefining the field of visual optics. In the past, optical imperfections of the eye were conceived as simple refractive errors—defocus, astigmatism, and perhaps a bit of prism. Although clinical students learned about other kinds of optical imperfections, such as spherical aberration, coma, oblique astigmatism, and the other Seidel aberrations, those concepts were confined to courses in optical theory, not to clinical practice. This is for good reason: these higher-order aberrations of the eye could not be measured routinely in the clinic, and even if they could, we did not have the means to correct them optically at a reasonable cost to patients. Furthermore, since the effects of such aberrations on visual function were largely unknown, there was little reason to suppose that correcting them would do any good for the patient's vision. However, the introduction of laser refractive surgery, with its potential for removing as well as introducing unwanted optical aberrations into the eye, demands changes in established ways of thinking and answers to these unresolved issues.

Today, optical imperfections of the eye are being re-examined within a comprehensive theoretical framework that expresses the combined effect of all the eye's aberrations in a two-dimensional aberration map of the pupil plane. An aberration map is similar in concept to corneal topographic maps used to describe the corneal surface. The major difference is that a corneal map describes the curvature of a physical surface, whereas an aberration map describes the difference between a wavefront of light and a reference wavefront. By concentrating our attention on light instead of the refracting surface, we gain an ability to compute image quality on the retina for simple points of light, for clinical test targets, or for any complex object in the real world. For example, Figure 6-1 shows a wavefront aberration map for a defocused eye from which the retinal image of an acuity chart may be computed. Such computations are poised to become routine clinical tools of the future for predicting the visual benefit of aberration correction to the patient, and for explaining the risks and visual consequences of unintended increases in optical aberrations following refractive surgery or other forms of treatment.

> An aberration map is similar in concept to corneal topographic maps used to describe the corneal surface.

Customized corneal ablation is a surgical procedure designed to improve the optical quality of the eye, thereby improving vision. To assess the outcome of this procedure requires measures of the direct effect on retinal image quality and secondary effects on visual performance and the quality of visual experience. A variety of methods for specifying optical quality are well established in the field of optics and may be readily applied to the optical image on the retina. Similarly, a variety of visual performance measures are sensitive to the optical quality of the retinal image and therefore may be used to assess the effect of refractive surgery on vision. However, optical limits normally imposed by the eye's optical aberrations may recede in the near future if refractive surgery, contact lenses, or intraocular lenses (IOLs) improve retinal image quality beyond limits imposed by the neural component of the visual system. If this occurs, then common measures of visual performance such as letter acuity, which are traditionally regarded as good measures of optical quality of the retinal image, may no longer be optically limited. When this happens, visual performance will be limited instead by the neural architecture and physiology of the retina and visual brain, thereby generating a demand for new measures of vision that are sensitive to even the smallest departures from perfect retinal image quality.

Measures of Optical Quality

The quality of an optical system may be specified in three different, but related, ways. The first method is to describe the detailed shape of the image for a simple geometrical object such as a point of light, or a line. The distribution of light in the image plane is called a point spread function (PSF) for a point object or a line spread function (LSF) for a line object. Simple measurements derived from these functions, such as the width (blur circle diameter) or height (Strehl ratio) of the intensity distribution, are taken as figures of merit that capture the blurring effects of optical imperfections.

The second method is a description of the loss of contrast suffered when an image of a sinusoidal grating object is cast. The sinusoidal grating is a very special object in optics because it has the unique property of producing images of the same form. In other words, a sinusoidal grating object forms sinusoidal images with the same spatial frequency (expressed in cycles/degree [c/deg]) and the same orientation.

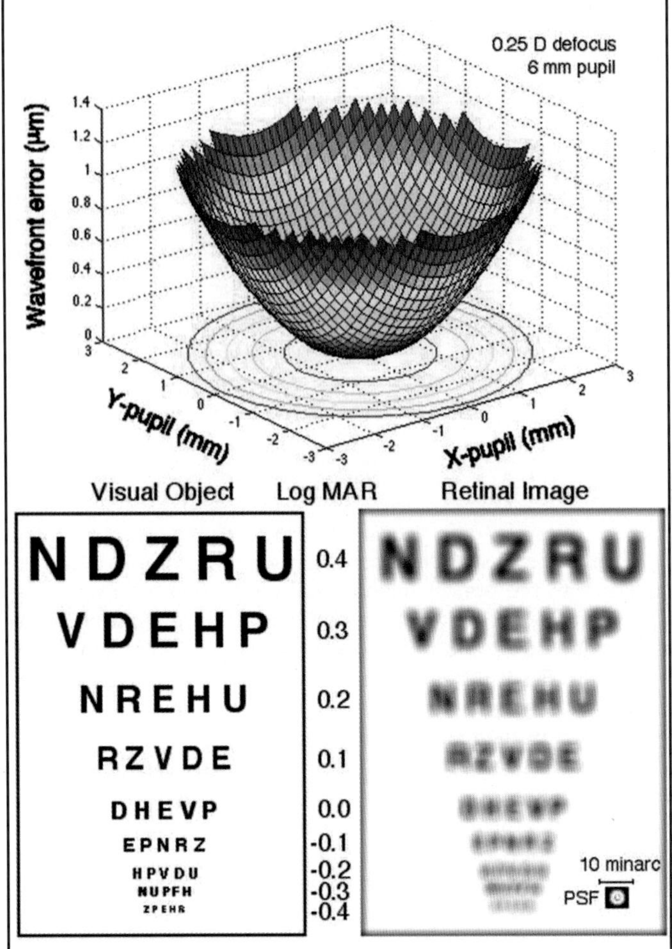

Figure 6-1. Effect of optical defocus (0.25 diopters [D], 6 millimeter [mm] pupil diameter) on the aberration map (top) and simulated retinal image of an eye chart (bottom). Method of calculation is to first determine the PSF, which is then convolved with the eye chart to yield the retinal image.

This property of sinusoidal grating objects, known as *preservation of form,* is strictly true only if the aberrations of the imaging system remain the same over the full extent of the object.

In visual science, a grating is usually described in polar form in terms of its spatial frequency and orientation. An alternative—rectangular form in terms of spatial frequency in two orthogonal x- and y-directions—is usually preferred in mathematical treatments.

Thus, gratings make it easy to specify the optical effect of the imaging system in terms of just two parameters: spatial contrast and spatial phase. The ratio of image contrast to object contrast captures the blurring effects of optical imperfections, and the variation of this ratio with spatial frequency and orientation of the grating object is called the modulation transfer function (MTF). The difference between the spatial phase of the image and the phase of the object captures the prismatic displacements induced by optical imperfections. The variation of this phase difference with spatial frequency and orientation of the grating object is called the phase transfer function (PTF). Taken together, the MTF and PTF define the optical transfer function (OTF) of an imaging system. One of the most important results of optical theory in the 20th century is the linking of the PSF, LSF, MTF, PTF, and OTF by means of a mathematical operation known as the Fourier transform.[1,2] Furthermore, given these characterizations of an imaging system, one may use optical theory to compute the expected retinal image for any visual object, thus overcoming the great handicap imposed on clinicians and visual scientists by the natural inaccessibility of the retinal image.

This chapter examines a third method for specifying optical quality in terms of underlying optical aberrations rather than the secondary effect of those aberrations on image quality. Such a description may be couched in terms of the deviation of light rays from perfect reference rays (ray aberrations) or in terms of the deviation of optical wavefronts from the ideal reference wavefront (wavefront aberrations). This aberration method is a more fundamental approach to the description of optical imperfections of eyes, from which all of the secondary measures of optical quality described above (PSF, LSF, MTF, PTF, and OTF) may be derived. It is also the most useful approach for customized corneal ablation since the aberration function of an eye is a prescription for optical perfection.

Definition and Interpretation of Aberration Maps

From a clinical perspective, perhaps the most useful interpretation of optical aberration maps is in terms of errors of optical path length (OPL). The OPL concept specifies the number of times a light wave must oscillate in traveling from one point to another. Since the propagation velocity of light is slower in the watery refractive media of the eye than in air, more oscillations will occur in the eye compared to the same physical distance in air. Thus, by defining OPL as the product of physical path length with refractive index, OPL becomes a measure of the number of oscillations executed by a propagating ray of light. This is an important concept because light rays emitted by a point source will propagate in many directions, but if all the rays have the same OPL, then every ray represents the same number of oscillations. Consequently, light at the end of each ray will have the same temporal phase and this locus of points with a common phase represents a wavefront of light. A propagating wavefront of light is defined by the locus of points in space lying at the same OPL from a common point source of light. To define the aberrations of an optical system, we compare the OPL for a ray passing through any point (x,y) in the plane of the exit pupil with the chief ray passing through the pupil center (0,0). The result is called the *optical path difference* (OPD). The aberration structure of the eye's optical system is summarized by a two-dimensional map showing how OPD varies across the eye's pupil.

For a perfect imaging system, the OPL is the same for all light rays traveling from the object point to the image point; therefore, OPD = 0 for all (x,y) locations in the pupil. In the case of an eye, this means that rays of light from a single point object that pass through different points in the pupil will arrive at the retinal image point having oscillated the same number of times. Such rays will have the same temporal phase and will, therefore, add constructively to produce a perfect image. If, on the other hand,

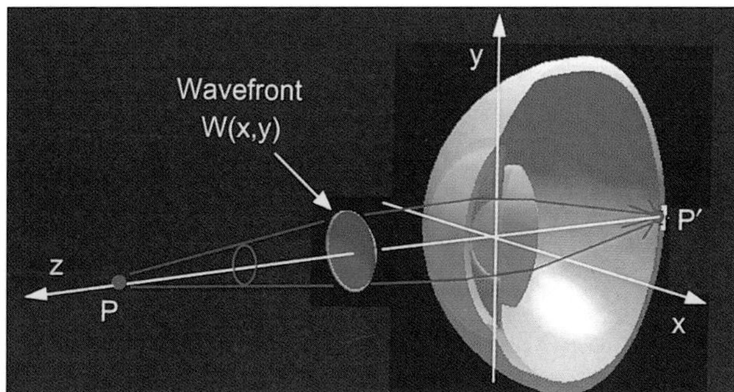

Figure 6-2. Example of a diverging wavefront from source P being focused to retinal point P′ by a myopic eye. Reversing the direction of light propagation, light reflected from retinal point P′ emerges from the eye as a wavefront converging on point P. When referenced to the x-y plane of the pupil, the wavefront shape W(x,y) is also an aberration map of the eye.

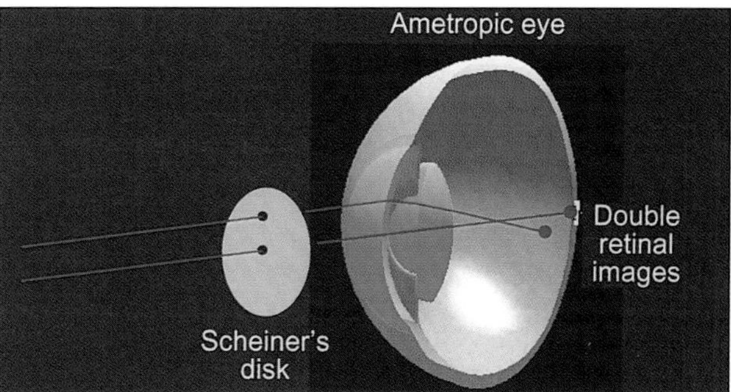

Figure 6-3. Scheiner's disk isolates rays, allowing their aberrated direction of propagation to be traced. An ametropic eye will form two retinal images for each object point when viewing through a Scheiner disk with two apertures.

light passing through different points in the pupil arrives with different phases because they traveled along paths of different OPLs, then the system is aberrated and the quality of the image will suffer. Thus, by conceiving of optical aberrations as differences in OPL it is easy to see how aberrations might arise due to:

1. Thickness anomalies of the tear film, cornea, lens, anterior chamber, posterior chamber, etc
2. Refractive index anomalies of the ocular media that might accompany inflammation, disease, aging, etc
3. Decentering or tilting of the various optical components of the eye with respect to each other

A concrete example of the OPL concept is illustrated in Figure 6-2. For a myopic eye with no other aberrations, the optical path is shorter for rays passing near the pupil margin compared to rays passing through the pupil center. Consequently, the best retinal image of a point object will be formed if we compensate for this variation in OPL by placing the point source at the eye's far point. Now the wavefront of light enters the eye as a concave wavefront such that the central rays arrive at the eye before the marginal rays, giving them a head start so that when they follow a longer optical path through the eye, they arrive in-phase with the marginal rays. In short, to obtain the optimum retinal image requires the optical distance from each object point to its image be the same for every path through the pupil. The wavefront aberration map indicates the extent to which this ideal condition is violated.

By reversing the direction of light propagation in Figure 6-2, we achieve a more practical definition of an aberration map for the eye. It follows from the preceding discussion that if the retinal point P′ is a source of light reflected out of the eye, then the shape of the emerging wavefront is determined by the variation of OPL across the eye's pupil. If the eye is optically perfect and emmetropic, this reflected wavefront would be a plane wave propagating in the positive z-direction. Thus, for distance vision, any departure of the emerging wavefront from the x-y plane is an optical aberration. On the other hand, for near vision, the reflected wavefront emerging from the eye must be compared with a spherical wavefront centered on the fixation point. In practice, the distance W(x,y) between the reflected wavefront emerging from the eye and the corresponding reference sphere is taken as a measure of the wavefront aberration function of the eye for the given viewing distance. By convention, positive aberrations occur when the marginal ray travels a shorter OPL than does the central (chief) ray, as in the case of a myopic eye shown in Figure 6-2. Therefore, by this sign convention, W(x,y) = -OPD(x,y).

In summary, the shape of a wavefront of light reflected out of the eye from a point source on the retina is determined by the OPD for rays passing through each point in the eye's pupil. Therefore, a map of OPD across the pupil plane is equivalent to a mathematical description, W(x,y), of the shape of the aberrated wavefront that emerges from the eye. Either may be used as an aberration map of the eye. Such maps are fundamental characterizations of the optical quality of the eye that may be used to compute other common metrics of image quality (eg, the PSF or OTF) from which we may compute the expected retinal image of any visual target.

Methods for Measuring Aberration Maps of Eyes

The current explosion of interest in optical aberrations of eyes has been spawned by new technology resting on an ancient principle. Nearly 400 years ago, the celebrated Jesuit philosopher and astronomer Christopher Scheiner, professor at the University of Ingolstadt and a contemporary of Kepler and Galileo, published his 1619 treatise *Optical Foundations of the Eye* some 75 years prior to the invention of the wave theory of light by Huygens. This pioneering book[3] described a simple device (illustrated in Figure 6-3) that is widely known in ophthalmology as Scheiner's disk.

> Scheiner reasoned that if an optically imperfect eye views through an opaque disk containing two pinholes, a single distant point of light such as a star will form two retinal images.

If the eye's imperfection is a simple case of defocus, then the double retinal images can be brought into register by viewing through a spectacle lens of the appropriate power. This design idea for an optometer for measuring refractive errors of eyes was first proposed by Porterfield in 1747 and was afterward improved by Thomas Young in 1845.

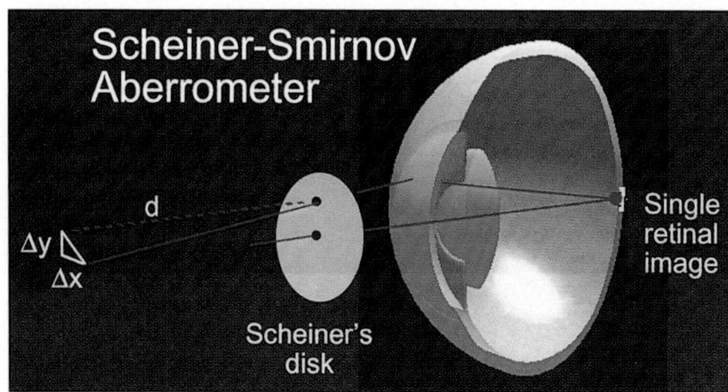

Figure 6-4. Smirnov's aberrometer used the principle of Scheiner's disk to measure the eye's optical imperfections separately at every location in the eye's entrance pupil.

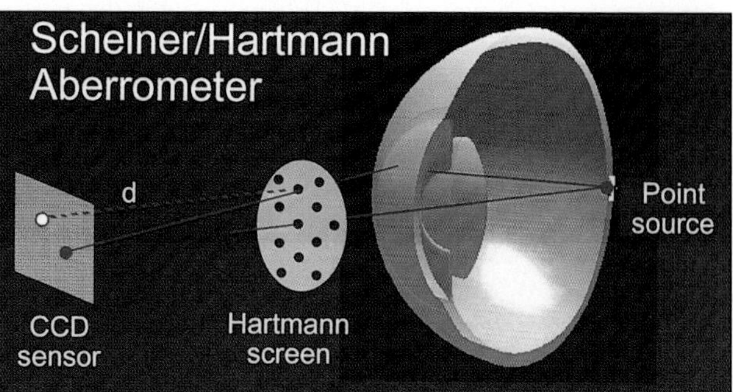

Figure 6-5. The Hartmann screen used to measure aberrations objectively is a Scheiner disk with numerous apertures.

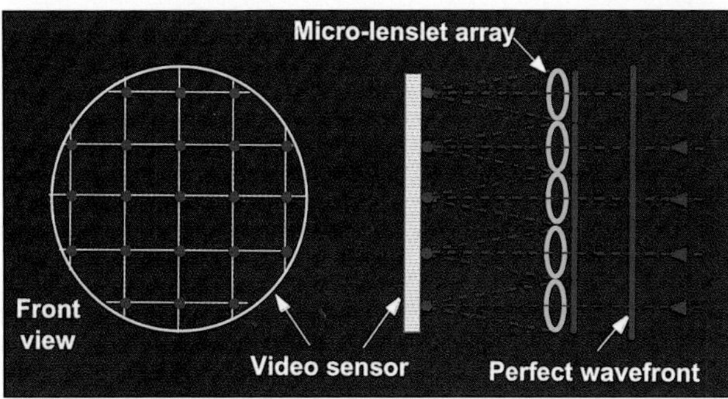

Figure 6-6. The Shack-Hartmann wavefront sensor forms a regular lattice of image points for a perfect plane wave of light.

A simple lens will not always bring the two retinal images into coincidence, however, so a more general method is needed for quantifying the refractive imperfection of the eye at each pupil location. Smirnov[4] was first to extend Scheiner's method by using a fixed light source for the central reference pinhole and a moveable light source for the outer pinhole, as illustrated in Figure 6-4. By adjusting the moveable source horizontally and vertically, the isolated ray of light is redirected until it intersects the fixed ray at the retina and the patient now reports seeing a single point of light. Having made this adjustment, the displacement distances Δx and Δy are measures of the ray aberration of the eye at the given pupil point.

Independent of these developments in ophthalmology, Scheiner's simple idea was reinvented by Hartmann for measuring the ray aberrations of mirrors and lenses.[5] Hartmann's method was to perforate an opaque screen with numerous holes, as shown in Figure 6-5. Each hole acts as an aperture to isolate a narrow bundle of light rays so they could be traced to determine any errors in their direction of propagation. Since rays are perpendicular to the propagating wavefront, any error in ray direction is also an error in wavefront slope. Thus, Hartmann's method is commonly referred to a *wavefront sensor.*

Seventy years later, Shack and Platt invented a better Hartmann screen using an array of tiny lenses that focus the light into an array of small spots, one spot for each lenslet.[5]

Their technique came to be known as Shack's modified Hartmann screen, or Shack-Hartmann for short. To see how the array of spot images can be used to determine the shape of the wavefront, we need to look at the wavefront in cross section, as shown in Figure 6-6. For a perfect eye, the reflected plane wave will be focused into a perfect lattice of point images, each image falling on the optical axis of the corresponding lenslet. By contrast, the aberrated eye reflects a distorted wavefront (Figure 6-7). The local slope of the wavefront is now different for each lenslet; therefore, the wavefront will be focused into a disordered collection of spot images. By measuring the displacement of each spot from its corresponding lenslet axis, we can deduce the slope of the aberrated wavefront as it entered the corresponding lenslet. Mathematical integration of slope yields the shape of the aberrated wavefront, which can then be displayed as an aberration map.

The first use of a Shack-Hartmann wavefront sensor to measure aberrations of human eyes was in 1994 by Liang and colleagues,[6] thus completing this historically meandering path to discover a fast, objective, reliable method for assessing the aberration structure of human eyes. Liang's concept of a Scheiner-Hartmann-Shack aberrometer is shown schematically in Figure 6-8. Because the shape of an aberrated wavefront changes as the light propagates, it is important to analyze the reflected wavefront as soon as it passes through the eye's pupil. To do this, a pair of relay lenses focuses the lenslet array onto the entrance pupil of the eye. Optically, then, the lenslet array appears to reside in the plane of the eye's entrance pupil where it can subdivide the reflected wavefront immediately as it emerges from the eye. The array of spot images formed by the lenslet array is captured by a video sensor and then analyzed by computer to estimate the eye's aberration map.

Normal and Clinical Examples

Four examples of aberration maps for normal healthy eyes are shown in Figure 6-9. By using a grayscale to encode wavefront height, we capitalize on the human visual system's natural abili-

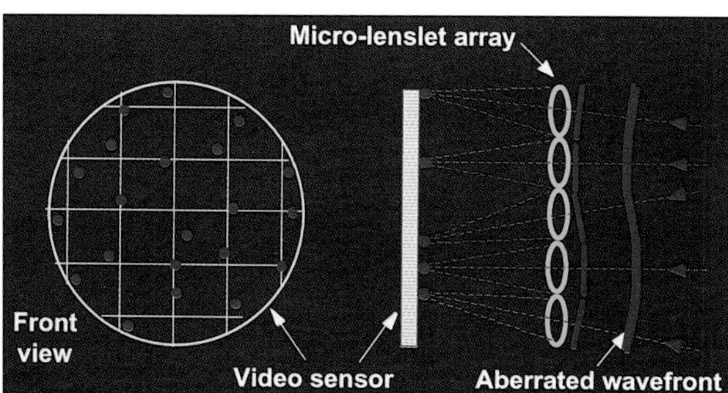

Figure 6-7. The Shack-Hartmann wavefront sensor forms an irregular lattice of image points for an aberrated wavefront of light.

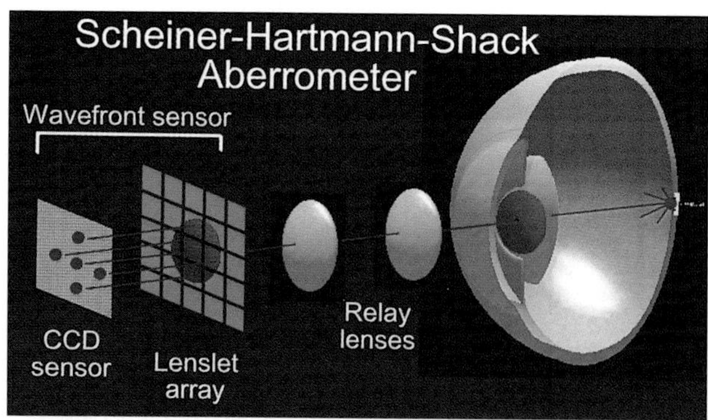

Figure 6-8. The modern aberrometer built on the Scheiner-Hartmann-Shack principle uses relay lenses to image the lenslet array into the eye's pupil plane. A video sensor (CCD) captures an image of the array of spots for computer analysis.

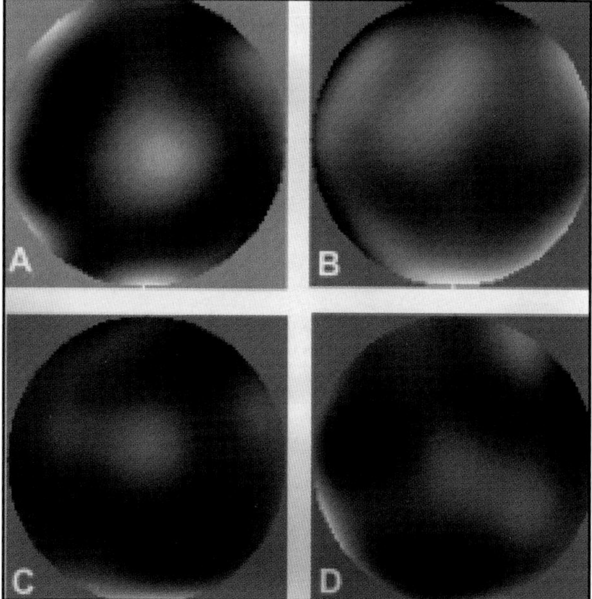

Figure 6-9. Examples of higher-order aberration maps for four normal, healthy individuals reconstructed from measurements taken with a Scheiner-Hartmann-Shack aberrometer, similar to that shown in Figure 6-8. Light areas in the map indicate the reflected wavefront is phase-advanced; dark areas indicate phase-retardance. The maximum difference between high and low points on each map is about 1 μm (Zernike orders 0 to 2 omitted for clarity).

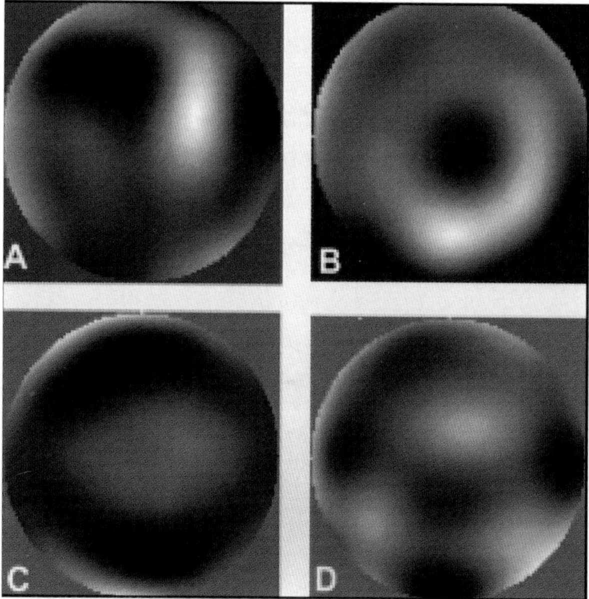

Figure 6-10. Examples of higher-order aberration maps from eyes with four different clinical conditions. (A) Dry eye. (B) Keratoconus. (C) Laser in-situ keratomileusis (LASIK) surgery. (D) Cataract. The maximum difference between high and low points on each map is about 10 μm except D, which is closer to 1 μm (Zernike orders 0 to 2 omitted for clarity).

ty to infer depth and structure from shading. The maximum difference between the highest and lowest points on each of these maps is about 1 micron (μm), which is a bit more than one wavelength of the light used to measure the eyes' aberrations (0.633 μm). Perhaps the most distinctive feature of these maps is the irregular shape of their smoothly varying shapes. Another important feature of aberration maps from normal eyes is the tendency to be relatively flat in the center of the pupil with aberrations growing stronger near the pupil margin. This is consistent with the literature showing that image quality is relatively good for medium-sized pupils but deteriorates as pupil diameter increases.[7,8]

For comparison, Figure 6-10 shows four examples of clinically abnormal eyes. Qualitatively, these maps have the same irregular, smoothly varying shapes as in normal eyes. The main difference is that the magnitude of the aberrations is about ten-fold larger; therefore, image quality is about ten-fold worse than normal. Another important abnormality of the kerataconic patient (B) in this figure and, to a lesser extent, the dry-eye patient (A) is the tendency to have large aberrations in the middle of the pupil. The implication of this result is that image quality will be subnormal for small pupils as well as for large pupils.

Limitations

Classical analysis of data from a Shack-Hartmann wavefront sensor takes no account of the quality of individual spots formed

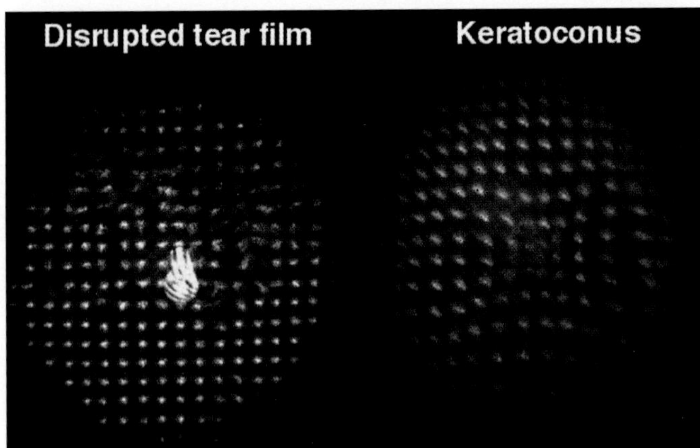

Figure 6-11. Examples of selective loss of image quality in individual spots for eyes with two different clinical conditions.

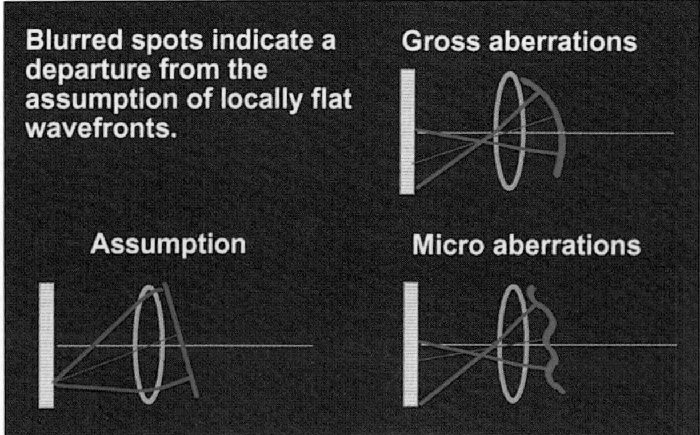

Figure 6-12. Blurring of individual spots detected by a Shack-Hartmann wavefront sensor may indicate the presence of gross aberrations of large magnitude or microaberrations. In either case, the blur is due to violation of the underlying assumption that the wavefront is locally flat over the lenslet aperture.

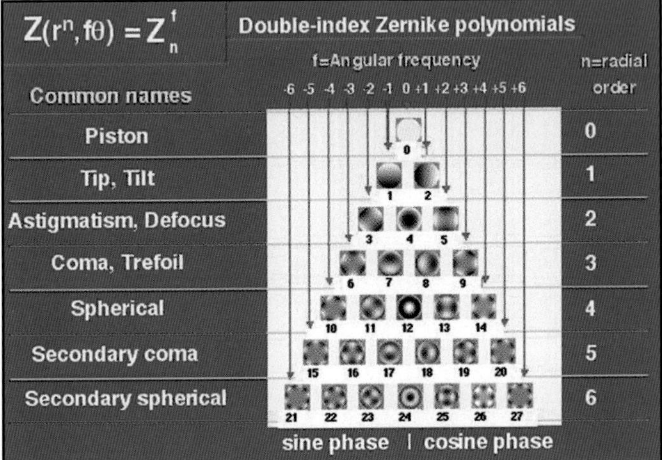

Figure 6-13A. Pictorial directory of Zernike modes used to systematically represent the aberration structure of the eye.

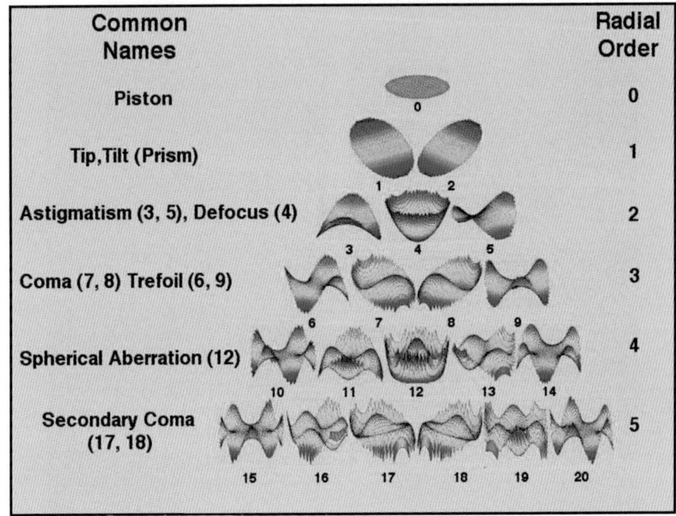

Figure 6-13B. Three-dimensional pictorial directory of Zernike modes 0 to 20.

by the lenslet array. Only the displacement of spots is needed for computing local slope of the wavefront over each lenslet aperture. However, experience has shown that the quality of dot images can vary dramatically over the pupil of a human eye as illustrated in Figure 6-11. The presence of blurred spots indicates a violation of the underlying assumption that the wavefront is locally flat over the face of the lenslet. Two possible reasons are illustrated in Figure 6-12.

The first possibility is that the gross aberrations of the eye are so large that the wavefront is significantly curved over the area of the lenslet. The result is a blurry spot that is difficult to localize. If the aberrations are large enough, neighboring spots can even overlap, which considerably complicates the analysis. The second possible limitation involves irregular aberrations on a very fine spatial scale. Perturbations of the wavefront within the lenslet aperture are too fine to be resolved by the wavefront sensor using classical methods. Rather than displacing the spots laterally, these "microaberrations" scatter light and blur the spots formed by the aberrometer. Although these blurry spots are problematic, they nevertheless contain useful information about the degree and location of scattering sources inside the eye, which may prove useful in clinical applications.[9]

Taxonomy of Optical Aberrations

One systematic method for classifying the shapes of aberration maps is to conceive of each map as the weighted sum of fundamental shapes or basis functions. One popular set of basis functions are the Zernike polynomials. This set of mathematical functions is formed as the product of two other functions, one of which depends only on the radius r of a point in the pupil plane, and the other depends only on the meridian θ of a point in the pupil plane. The former is a simple polynomial of the nth degree and the latter function is a harmonic of a sinusoid or co-sinusoid. A pictorial dictionary of the first 28 Zernike polynomials is arranged in the form of a pyramid of basis functions in Figures 6-13A and 6-13B. Every aberration map can be represented uniquely by a weighted sum of these functions. The process of determining the weighting coefficient required to describe a given aberration map is a least-squares curve-fitting process called *Zernike decomposition,* which results in a vector of Zernike

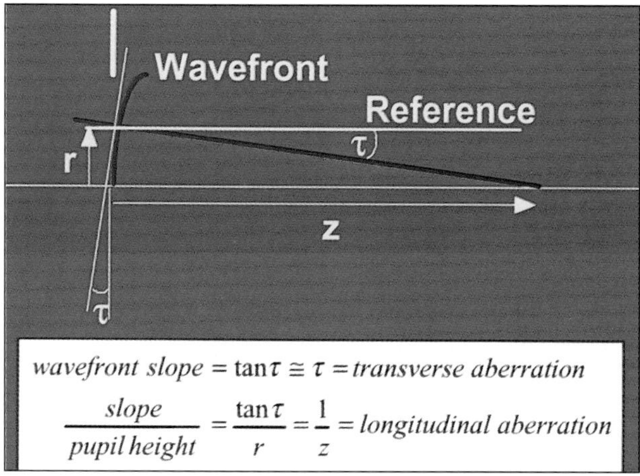

Figure 6-14. Relationship between wavefront, its first and second derivatives, and measures of transverse aberration (τ) and longitudinal aberration (1/z).

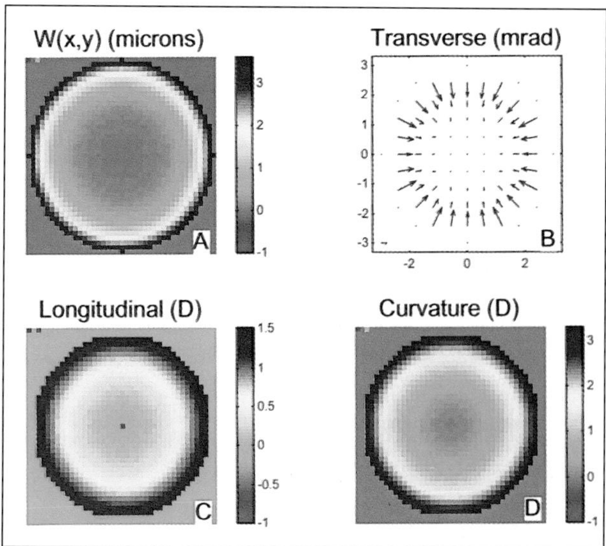

Figure 6-15. Four methods for displaying an aberration map. (A) Height of reflected wavefront from the (x,y) plane perpendicular to the path of the chief ray (line-of-sight for foveal vision). (B) Vector field map showing the displacement of each spot image from the optical axis of the corresponding lenslet. (C) Axial power map obtained by dividing average wavefront slope at each pupil location by the radial distance of the point from the pupil center. (D) Local curvature in the wavefront obtained by applying the Laplacian operator to the wavefront. Maps in C and D are calibrated in diopters.

coefficients. Mathematical details may be found in several standard reference works.[10,11]

Recently, the Optical Society of America sponsored a task force of visual optics researchers to develop standards for reporting optical aberrations of eyes. Recommendations of this task force were presented at the 2000 Topical Meeting on Vision Science and Its Applications and will be published in full in a future issue of *Trends in Optics and Photonics*, published by the Optical Society of America.[12]

Derivatives of the Aberration Map

Klein and colleagues have suggested[13] using the slopes (first partial derivatives in x and y directions) and curvature (average of second partial derivatives in x and y) of the aberration map to supplement the interpretation of the wavefront aberration function W(x,y). As illustrated in Figure 6-14, the slope of the wavefront aberration map may be interpreted as the transverse ray aberration, which is defined by angle τ between the aberrated ray and the nonaberrated reference ray. The associated focusing error is called the *longitudinal ray aberration* and is equal to 1/z D, which may be computed as the ratio of transverse aberration to ray height in the pupil plane.

To illustrate the derivatives of the aberration map, we evaluated the wavefront error for the Indiana eye model, a simple, reduced eye model with an aspheric refracting surface that has proved useful on previous occasions for studying the aberrations of the human eye.[14] In the specific example illustrated in Figure 6-15, the pupil diameter was 6 mm and the conic constant of the surface was set to 0.6, a value that generates a degree of spherical aberration that is typical of human eyes.[15] The wavefront aberration map W(x,y) for this model at the wavelength 589 nanometers (nm) (see Figure 6-15A) is nearly flat in the middle of the pupil but becomes increasingly curved near the pupil margin.

Slope (Transverse Aberration)

In a symmetrical optical system, the transverse aberration τ may be measured in any meridian, but for nonsymmetrical systems it is typically computed as the partial derivative of the aberration function in the vertical as well as horizontal directions. One way to simultaneously visualize the variation of the vertical and horizontal components of transverse aberration is with a vector field (see Figure 6-15B). Each arrow represents the transverse ray aberration for the pupil location marked by the tail of the arrow. The lengths of the horizontal and vertical components of each arrow give the horizontal and vertical components of angle τ, respectively. The calibration arrow in the lower left corner is 1 milliradian in length. The arrows all point toward the center of the pupil for this model eye, indicating that the light reflected out of the eye forms a converging wavefront. The arrows are longer near the pupil margin, indicating the steeper slope expected of spherical aberration.

In a perfect optical system, every ray from a point object will intersect the retina at the same location, but in an aberrated system, the intersection will be displaced by an amount and direction indicated by the arrows in Figure 6-15B. We can then visualize where each ray strikes the retina by collapsing all of the arrows so that their tails coincide (the ideal image point) with the head of each arrow, showing where the ray from the corresponding pupil location intersects the retina. In optical engineering, such visualization would be called a *spot diagram* and would be taken as a discrete approximation to the continuous PSF.

Slope Per Unit of Pupil Radius (Longitudinal Aberration)

From the geometry of Figure 6-14, we noted that the ratio of wavefront slope to r, the distance from the pupil center to the given point on the wavefront, is the inverse of the distance between pupil center and the point where the aberrated ray crosses the optical axis. This latter quantity is the traditional definition of longitudinal ray aberration (also known as *axial power*). In general, the longitudinal aberration has horizontal and verti-

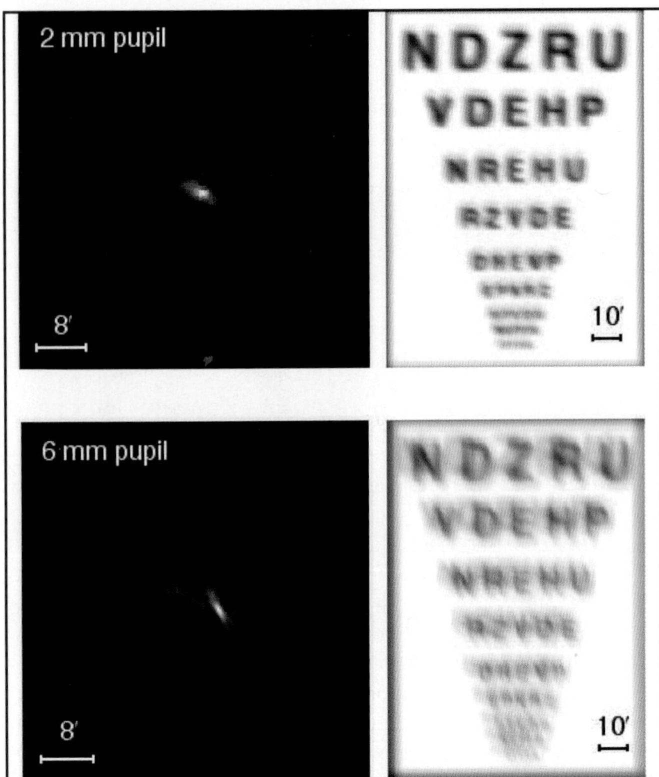

Figure 6-16. PSFs (left panels) and simulated retinal images of an eye chart (right panels) for the eye in Figure 6-10C analyzed for two pupil diameters (2 mm, 6 mm).

cal components just like the transverse aberration, which reflects the fact that the refracted ray may be skew to the optical axis. In practice, we simplify the situation by resolving the transverse ray arrow into radial and tangential components and then use the radial component to compute the longitudinal aberration. This allows us to reduce a vector plot, as in Figure 6-15B, into a scalar plot (see Figure 6-15C).

If the eye suffers only from defocus, then the longitudinal aberration is constant and equal to the spherical refractive error of the eye. For other aberrations, such as coma or spherical aberration, the longitudinal aberration varies with pupil location and may be depicted with a longitudinal aberration map like that shown in Figure 6-15C. The scale of this map is calibrated in diopters to enhance its clinical interpretation. For this particular example, the increased power near the margin represents 1.70 D of spherical aberration, which is the same result obtained by finite ray tracing.[15]

Curvature (Local Power)

The second derivative of the aberration function measures the rate of change of slope of the wavefront (ie, local curvature). The average curvature in the horizontal and vertical directions is called the *Laplacian* of the aberration map. An example of the Laplacian curvature map for the Indiana eye model is shown in Figure 6-15D. The scale of this map is also calibrated in diopters to enhance its clinical interpretation. Notice that the longitudinal aberration underestimates local curvature, which means that local segments of the wavefront come to focus before the rays intersect the optical axis. Some difference is to be expected because the traditional measure of longitudinal aberration is proportional to wavefront slope, whereas curvature is a measure of the rate of change of slope.

Related Measures of Optical Quality

PSF and Strehl's Ratio

The PSF is computed as the squared magnitude of the Fourier transform of a complex-valued pupil function built from the aberration map. Since the PSF represents the intensity distribution of light in the image of a point source, it should be a highly localized, bright spot. Diffraction sets a lower limit to the diameter of the spot and an upper limit to the intensity in the center of the spot. A common metric of image quality, called *Strehl's ratio*, is computed as the ratio of the actual intensity in the center of the spot to the maximum intensity of a diffraction-limited spot. As pupil diameter increases, the intensity of a diffraction-limited spot increases faster than the intensity of an aberrated spot, which tends to reduce Strehl's ratio. It is not uncommon for the PSF of human eyes to have multiple peaks, which complicates the simple notion of Strehl's ratio. More importantly, it signals the formation of two or more point images for a single point object. This condition of diplopia or polyplopia has great clinical significance because of its implications for visual performance and the quality of visual experience.[16,17]

Examples of PSFs computed from the wavefront aberration function displayed in Figure 6-10C are shown for small and large pupils in Figure 6-16. In the dark, this patient's natural pupil diameter was 6 mm, which was large enough to expose significant amounts of aberration introduced by refractive surgery. The effect of these aberrations was to blur the central spot while simultaneously spreading some of the light into a long, secondary, wispy tail. Since each point of light in an object will produce this same type of pattern, the retinal image of an eye chart will be blurred and contain a second, lower-contrast ghost image that hampers legibility. This situation may be contrasted with the much improved image quality for daylight viewing through a 2 mm pupil, which is small enough to exclude most of the aberrations of this patient's eye. Under these conditions, the PSF is more compact, which results in a clearer, more focused retinal image.

> The reader should be aware that to meet publication standards, PSFs are usually scaled arbitrarily to use the full range of gray levels available for reproduction. The results are potentially misleading. In reality, the total amount of light in the PSF is determined by the intensity of the point source, the eye's pupil diameter, and absorption losses in the ocular media.

MTF, PTF, and OTF

The OTF, comprised of the MTF and PTF, is computed as the inverse Fourier transform of the PSF. The MTF component represents the contrast of the retinal image for a sinusoidal grating target of 100% contrast. Diffraction sets an upper limit to the contrast of the retinal image and therefore the ratio of MTFs for a real eye to a diffraction-limited optical system is a measure of the losses of contrast due to aberrations. One implication of the Fourier transform relationship between the OTF and the PSF is that Strehl's ratio, defined as the ratio of intensities at the center

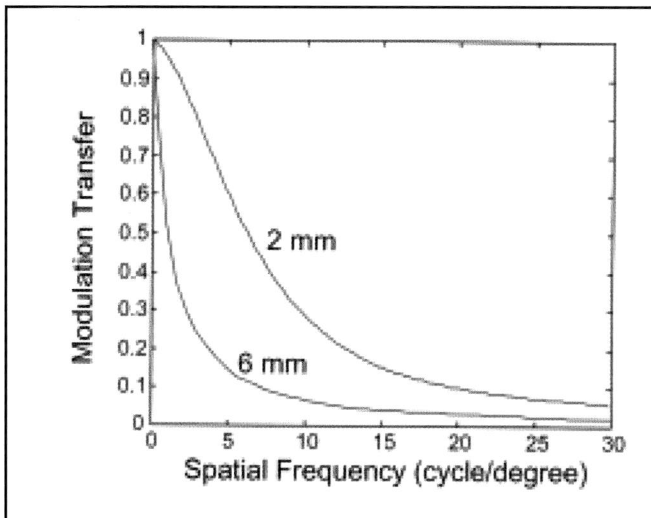

Figure 6-17. Radially averaged MTFs for the eye in Figure 6-10C analyzed for two pupil diameters (2 mm, 6 mm).

of the test PSF and a diffraction-limited PSF, is equal to the volume under the OTF of an aberrated system divided by the volume under the OTF for the same system without aberrations. In general, the OTF, PSF, and MTF are two-dimensional functions of spatial frequency and orientation, or equivalently, of spatial frequency in the x and y directions. Such functions may be reduced to one-dimensional graphs by averaging across orientation, a process called *radial averaging*.

Radially averaged MTFs for the LASIK patient in Figure 6-16 are shown in Figure 6-17 for small and large pupils. The transfer of contrast from object to image is from three to five times lower for the 6 mm pupil condition compared to the 2 mm condition over most of the visible range of spatial frequencies. It is to be expected that these optical losses would be reflected directly in visual performance measurements of contrast sensitivity for grating targets.

Acknowledgments

Preparation of this chapter was supported by National Institutes of Health (National Eye Institute) grants R01-EY-05109 to Dr. Thibos and R01-EY-08520 to Dr. Applegate and an unrestricted grant to the Department of Ophthalmology from Research to Prevent Blindness, New York, NY.

References

1. Gaskill JD. *Linear Systems, Fourier Transforms, and Optics*. New York, NY: John Wiley & Sons; 1978.
2. Goodman JW. *Introduction to Fourier Optics*. New York, NY: McGraw-Hill; 1968.
3. Scheiner C. Oculus, sive fundamentum opticum. *Innspruk*. 1619.
4. Smirnov MS. Measurement of the wave aberration of the human eye. *Biofizika*. 1961;6:687-703.
5. Shack RV, Platt BC. Production and use of a lenticular Hartmann screen. *J Opt Soc Am A*. 1971;61:656.
6. Liang J, Grimm B, Goelz S, Bille J. Objective measurement of the wave aberrations of the human eye using a Hartmann-Shack wavefront sensor. *J Opt Soc Am A*. 1994;11:1949-1957.
7. Campbell FW, Gubisch RW. Optical quality of the human eye. *J Physiol*. 1966;186:558-578.
8. Liang J, Williams DR. Aberrations and retinal image quality of the normal human eye. *J Opt Soc Am A*. 1997;14:2873-2883.
9. Thibos LN, Hong X. Clinical applications of the Shack-Hartmann aberrometer. *Optom Vis Sci*. 1999;76:817-825.
10. Born M, Wolf E. *Principles of Optics*. 7th ed. Cambridge, England: Cambridge University Press; 1999.
11. Malacara D. *Optical Shop Testing*. 2nd ed. New York, NY: John Wiley & Sons, Inc; 1992.
12. Thibos LN, Applegate RA, Schwiegerling JT, Webb R. Standards for reporting the optical aberrations of eyes. In: Lakshminarayanan V, ed. Vision Science and Its Applications. Vol TOPS-35. Washington, DC: Optical Society of America; 2000:232-244.
13. Klein SA, Garcia DD. Alternative representations of aberrations of the eye. *Vision Science and Its Applications*. Washington, DC: Optical Society of America; 2000:115-118.
14. Thibos LN, Ye M, Zhang X, Bradley A. The chromatic eye: a new reduced-eye model of ocular chromatic aberration in humans. *Appl Opt*. 1992;31:3594-3600.
15. Thibos LN, Ye M, Zhang X, Bradley A. Spherical aberration of the reduced schematic eye with elliptical refracting surface. *Optom Vis Sci*. 1997;74:548-556.
16. Woods RL, Bradley A, Atchison DA. Consequences of monocular diplopia for the contrast sensitivity function. *Vision Res*. 1996;36:3587-3596.
17. Woods RL, Bradley A, Atchison DA. Monocular diplopia caused by ocular aberrations and hyperopic defocus. *Vision Res*. 1996;36:3597-3606.

Chapter 7

Assessment of Visual Performance

Raymond A. Applegate, OD, PhD; Gene Hilmantel, OD, MS; and Larry N. Thibos, PhD

Introduction

For the first time in history, it is possible to clinically measure the optical defects of the eye beyond sphere and cylinder, quickly and efficiently in the clinical environment. By all indications, this technology will continue to work its way into clinical practice. There are several companies that are currently employing or planning to employ such technology to design refractive corrections intended to improve the optical quality of the retinal image beyond what is achievable with traditional spherocylindrical corrections. These "ideal" corrections may come in the form of customized corneal ablative corrections, contact lenses, intraocular lenses (IOLs), or in combination.[1]

> *Super vision* is vision that is significantly improved over that provided by more traditional forms of spherocylindrical corrections.

Currently, it is not clear that ideal corrections can be implemented routinely or that such corrections will routinely result in super vision. Super vision is vision that is significantly improved over that provided by more traditional forms of spherocylindrical corrections. Until just recently, surgeries generally increased corneal[2-5] and total eye aberrations.[6] Recent results with wavefront-guided surgery are encouraging (a decrease in the surgically induced aberrations) and increasing number of eyes where the higher-order aberrations are reduced from presurgical values, leading to an increasing number of eyes with 20/15 or better postsurgical acuity. However, despite the better outcomes, the majority of eyes are still seeing an increase in postsurgical higher-order aberrations. These results pose several questions with respect to the measurement of visual performance. What will the world look like with super vision?[7-10] Do we have tests of visual performance capable of quantifying the visual improvement in a clinically significant manner? When therapy induces new aberrations, do we have the tests necessary to quantify the visual complaints of our patients that have 20/20 vision but do not see as well as they used to, or whose vision changes with pupil size, or with time of day? To answer these questions, this chapter will:

1. Review the fundamental limits to visual performance imposed by optical imaging and photoreceptor sampling to determine the potential gains offered by ideal corrections
2. Examine the losses in vision induced by less than ideal refractive corrections and their implications for visual testing
3. Examine the nature of traditional and new clinical tests of visual performance in the context of fundamental limitations and the visual impact of less than ideal refractive corrections
4. Identify the characteristics of the ideal clinical test to measure subtle gains and losses in visual function

Fundamental Limits to Visual Performance

In the broadest sense, visual performance is limited by the quality of the retinal image and the ability of the neural system to translate the retinal image into a percept. A fundamental assumption in the design of an ideal correction is that our patients will see better with an ideal correction than with a conventional spherocylindrical correction. This assumption deserves careful examination. Specifically, what are the gains in visual performance that are expected with "ideal" refractive corrections?

The retinal image in the eye is principally affected by reflection, absorption, diffraction, aberration, and scatter. Reflection, absorption, and back scatter decrease the amount of light reaching the retinal plane. Diffraction, aberrations, and forward scatter reach the retinal plane and directly affect the quality of the retinal image. In an optically clear normal eye, forward scatter is relatively minor and will be ignored in this chapter. Diffraction and aberration effects on image quality directly impact the quality of the retinal image and are very pupil size dependent. It is therefore useful to start the discussion by exploring the possible gains in retinal image quality provided by aberration-free correction as a function of pupil size. These gains define the upper limit of retinal image quality for each pupil size. The gains in retinal image quality can be easily seen in the point spread function (PSF) and/or the optical transfer function (OTF). Both the PSF and OTF contain all the information necessary to fully describe image quality. Knowing one allows the calculation of the other. The benefit of understanding both is derived from the fact that sometimes the effects of diffraction and aberration are better illustrated and understood as changes in the PSF and sometimes they are better illustrated and understood as changes in the OTF. For the purposes of this chapter, we will use both to illustrate important points about optical quality.

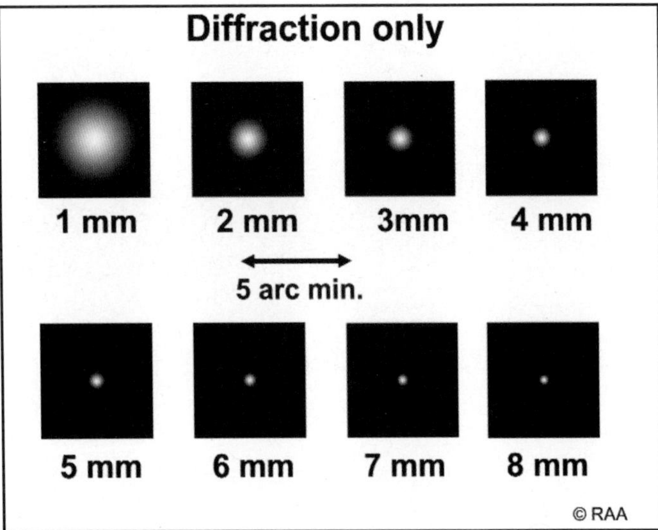

Figure 7-1. PSF as a function of pupil diameter for a diffraction-limited (aberration-free) eye.

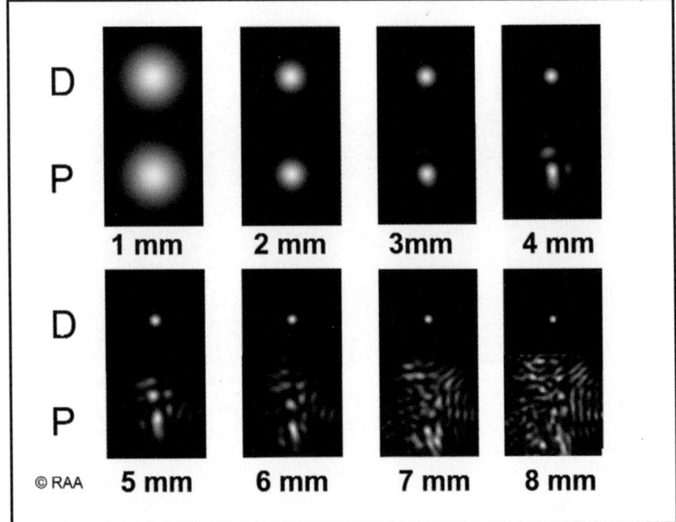

Figure 7-2. Top row of PSFs labeled D: PSFs as a function of pupil diameter for a diffraction-limited eye. Bottom row of PSFs: PSFs as a function of pupil diameter for a typical eye with best spectacle correction. Notice for the typical eye that for pupil diameters below 3 mm, diffraction is the major contributor to the PSF and above 3 mm, higher-order aberrations are the major contributor.

The PSF defines how a single object point is imaged by the optical system. Since any object can be broken down into an infinite number of points for imaging purposes, and given the PSF defines how each point is imaged, the PSF is a fundamental metric of optical quality. The more compact and symmetric the PSF, the higher will be the image fidelity. Likewise, improving the OTF by removing optical aberrations increases the contrast and spatial detail of the retinal image. The OTF has two parts: the modulation transfer function (MTF) and the phase transfer function (PTF). These will be discussed in more detail below. For now, suffice it to say that in a healthy visual system, increases in retinal image fidelity are reflected in percepts having higher contrast (increased modulation transfer) and sharper edges (decreased phase errors). These two components (MTF and PTF) of the OTF, like the PSF, are pupil size dependent and define the optical quality of the retinal image.

> The PSF defines how a single object point is imaged by the optical system.

Diffraction and Pupil Size

Diffraction occurs as light passes through a limiting aperture, such as the eye's pupil. The larger the pupil in an optical system, the less diffraction impacts image quality. Conversely, the smaller the pupil, the more diffraction degrades image quality. The effects of diffraction as a function of pupil size can easily be seen in the PSF of an aberration-free eye. Notice in Figure 7-1, that as the pupil size gets smaller, diffraction effects on the PSF increase. Diffraction effects are part of the explanation of why patients on pilocarpine (very small pupil) complain of poor quality vision. Small pupils degrade vision due to diffraction.

> The smaller the pupil, the more diffraction degrades image quality.

> In an eye that is free of optical aberrations, best image quality is obtained at the largest pupil size.

Of course, normal eyes are not aberration-free. In any typical normal eye best-corrected for spherocylindrical error, there are uncorrected higher-order aberrations. A direct consequence of these remaining optical aberrations is that there is a pupil size at which optical aberrations degrade image quality more than diffraction effects. As can be seen in Figure 7-2, in the normal eye with sphere and cylindrical error corrected, higher-order aberration effects start to degrade image quality more than diffraction at pupil diameters greater than 3 millimeters (mm). This is the principle reason patients do not like the quality of their vision when their pupils are dilated. That is, optical aberrations that are normally masked by a smaller pupil are now manifesting themselves.

> In the normal eye with sphere and cylindrical error corrected, higher-order aberration effects start to degrade image quality more than diffraction at pupil diameters greater than 3 mm.

The perfect optical correction would convert the typical eye's 8 mm PSF to a diffraction-limited image of a point (Figure 7-3). While this goal is unlikely to ever be reached, Figure 7-3 does pictorially define in a visually clear manner the maximum gain in image quality achievable by a perfect correction.

In these figures, notice that it is difficult to easily evaluate the image quality of anything other than a point by inspection of the PSF. That is, it is very difficult to predict how an extended object would appear by simply looking at any given PSF. The OTF helps to solve this problem by quantifying the MTF.

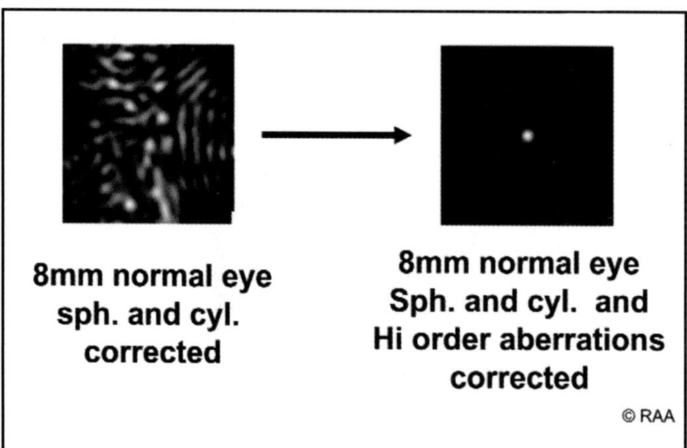

Figure 7-3. The goal of an ideal correction is to make the eye diffraction-limited over all pupil diameters. Correcting the optical defects of the typical normal eye will markedly improve the PSF for large pupil diameters.

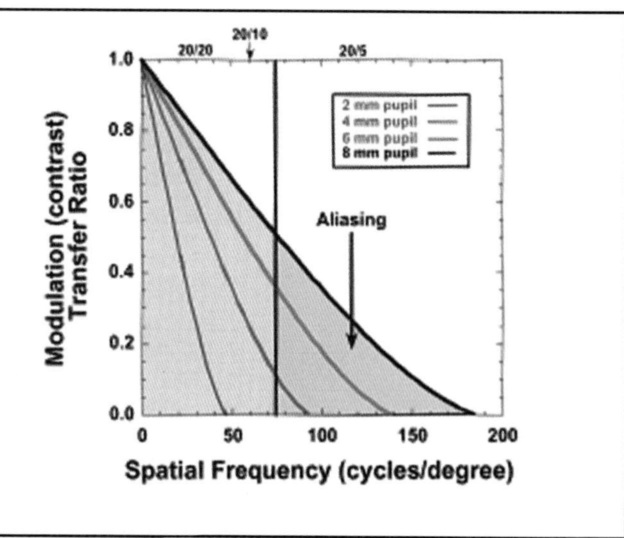

Figure 7-4. Diffraction-limited MTFs for four pupil sizes. If the object has 100% contrast, the stippled area identifies the spatial frequencies and contrast levels over which detection and recognition ("clear vision") are theoretically possible in the normal eye. The crosshatched area identifies the spatial frequencies and contrast levels over which detection of aliased images is possible. The area above the uppermost curve represents contrast that cannot be achieved in the retinal image. Calculations of the MTFs were made using 555 nanometers (nm) of light and methods detailed by Smith's equation.[29]

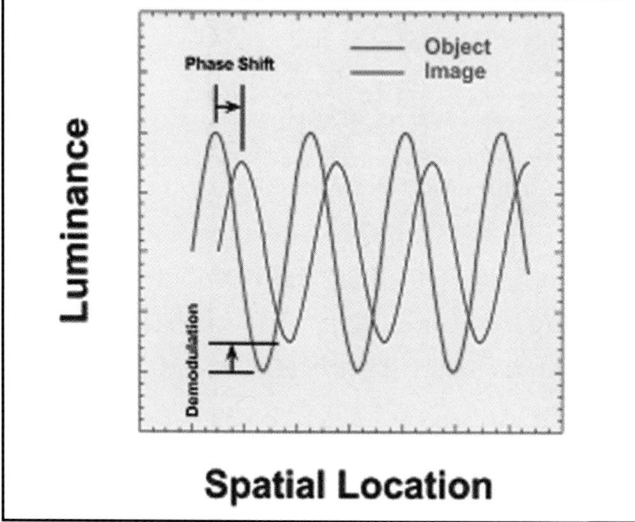

Figure 7-5. Luminance as a function of location for a sinusoidal object and image showing a 25% demodulation from object to image with a 100 degree phase shift, causing a change in image location.

Modulation Transfer Function and Pupil Size

The importance of pupil size to modulation transfer can be easily seen by viewing plots of the aberration-free (diffraction-limited) MTF of the eye for a variety of pupil sizes (Figure 7-4). The diffraction-limited MTF displays the ratio of image contrast to object contrast for perfect ocular optics as a function of the spatial frequency of a sinusoidal grating. The advantage of using sinusoidal gratings is two-fold. Sinusoidal objects are transferred to the image plane as demodulated (decreased contrast) sinusoidal images of the same frequency. Phase changes are reflected as a shift in the location of the grating image with respect to object location and do not alter the nature of the sinusoidal luminance pattern or its image modulation. In a diffraction-limited system (no optical aberration), there are no phase shifts. However, as aberrations increase, phase changes are very important and will be discussed later in this chapter. Second, through Fourier analysis, more complex patterns can be constructed as a summation of sinusoidal gratings of various frequencies, orientations, modulations, and phases. Conversely, objects can be decomposed into a series of sinusoidal gratings of various frequencies, orientations, modulations, and phases. Such decomposition allows the modulation of each frequency component to be reduced and phase shifted to reflect the impact of the eye's optics on any object. In turn, these demodulated and phase-shifted spatial frequencies permit the reconstruction of a retinal image as the photoreceptors would see it. For these reasons, the MTF and the PTF are standard and very powerful measures of optical quality in the optical industry.

Notice in Figure 7-4 that the eye's diffraction-limited MTF (no optical aberrations) reveals several interesting facts:

1. Only for a uniform field (0 spatial frequency) is the object modulation (contrast) transferred to the image plane with 100% efficiency (a modulation factor of 1). This efficiency is independent of pupil size
2. For all other frequencies, the modulation (contrast) transfer ratio is less than 1 and is pupil size dependent
3. For higher spatial frequencies, the modulation (contrast) transfer ratio increases as pupil size increases
4. The cut-off frequency (the spatial frequency at which the modulation goes to 0) increases as pupil size increases

Phase Transfer Function

The OTF is made up of two principle components: the MTF discussed above and the PTF. The PTF describes the phase shift of the image with respect to the object (Figure 7-5) as a function of spatial frequency. In a diffraction-limited optical system, object location and image location are identical and there are no phase shifts. In an aberrated optical system, phase shifts can become very important and can lead to what is commonly called *spurious*

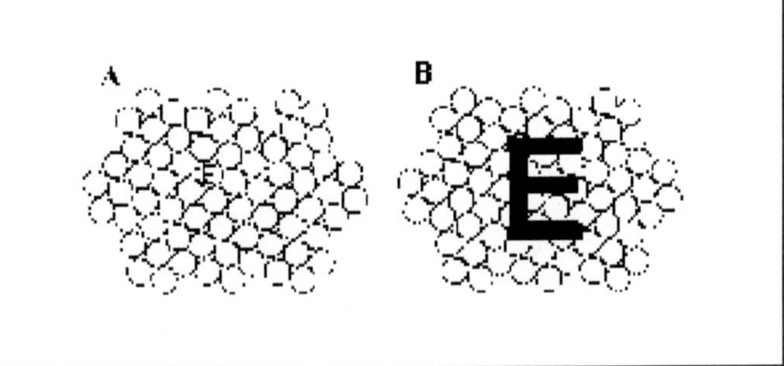

Figure 7-6. (A) If a letter E is imaged such that it falls within the borders of a single photoreceptor, then the letter E cannot be differentiated from a period. (B) To be seen as a letter, the E must be sampled by enough photoreceptors to differentiate the letter's component parts. (Reprinted with permission from Applegate RA. Limits to vision: can we do better than nature? *J Refract Surg.* 2000;16:S547-S551.)

resolution and *decreased visual performance*. These effects on vision are discussed later in this chapter.

Retinal Limitations

So far we have limited our discussion to optical considerations. There is also a fundamental retinal limitation to visual performance: the ability of the photoreceptors to sample the retinal image (see Chapter 3). Photoreceptors in the foveola are on the order of 2 micrometers (μm) in diameter. The response of the photoreceptor to an input signal is graded based on photon capture within the photoreceptor. That is, within a single photoreceptor, spatial (shape) information is lost. Consequently, to differentiate a letter E from a period, the components of the letter E must be distributed over an adequate number of receptors to allow the components of the letter to be detected (Figure 7-6). Thus, the coarseness of the foveola photoreceptor mosaic limits letter acuity independent of the quality of the optics to somewhere between 20/8 and 20/10 (depending on the biological variation in foveolar receptor diameters for the particular eye of interest). At spatial frequencies beyond 75 cycles/degree (c/deg) (20/8), visual percept will be distorted (aliased), limiting the ability of the nervous system to interpret a high quality retinal image (Figure 7-7). Therefore, in an optically aberrated eye capable of neural-limited acuity (20/8 to 20/10), improving the optics cannot improve acuity but will improve contrast for larger pupils.

> In an optically aberrated eye capable of neural-limited acuity (20/8 to 20/10), improving the optics cannot improve acuity but will improve contrast for larger pupils.

Receptor sampling limits should not be interpreted to mean that the visual system is incapable of seeing targets having finer detail. This simply is not true. The visual system can see targets having finer detail; however, they will not appear in their true form. Because of receptor undersampling, the appearance of the image is distorted, forming what is commonly called an *alias percept* of the actual object (see Figure 7-7). That is, the percept of the actual object takes on an appearance that can be quite different from the actual object. Consequently, photoreceptor sampling fundamentally limits acuity for larger pupils in the diffraction-limited eye.

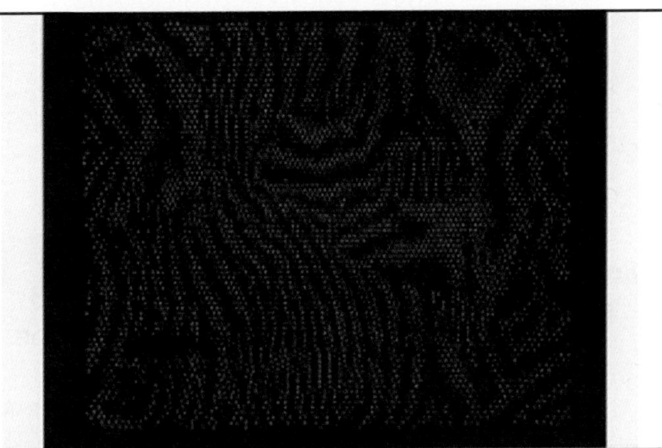

Figure 7-7. A simulated retinal view of an 80 c/deg grating (notice the edges of the pattern show the grating) being sampled by a primate foveolar retinal receptor mosaic. Undersampling creates an alias percept of the grating that appears as zebra stripes. (Photo courtesy of David Williams.) (Reprinted with permission from Applegate RA. Limits to vision: can we do better than nature? *J Refract Surg.* 2000;16:S547-S551.)

> Photoreceptor sampling fundamentally limits acuity for larger pupils in the diffraction-limited eye.

Losses in Vision Induced by Less Than Ideal Refractive Corrections and Their Implications for Visual Testing

In reality, we can only approach the diffraction limit as we minimize higher and higher orders of ocular aberration. The fact that we can only approach the ideal raises an interesting question: Do the same gains in contrast and cut-off frequency exist when aberrations remain in the system (ie, the system is not diffraction-limited)?

Modulation Transfer Function and Aberrations

Counter to the diffraction-limited case, in an optically aberrated system large pupils can be a disadvantage. First, the modulation transfer ratio can go negative, indicating a phase shift (light bars are now dark and dark bars are light). Second, in the diffraction-limited case (Figure 7-8), the modulation transfer ratio first goes to zero at the cut-off frequency and remains at zero. In the aberrated case, the function can cross zero several times before reaching the cut-off frequency. The extent of these effects is dependent on the magnitude and type of the residual optical aberration. To illustrate this point, in Figure 7-8 we plot MTFs for four pupil diameters in the presence (thinner lines) and absence (thicker lines) of 0.5 diopters (D) defocus.

These effects are better illustrated by looking at the change in the modulation transfer ratio and the first zero crossover of the MTF caused by moderate aberrations (Figure 7-9). Both of these figures show that with moderate defocus, increasing pupil diameter decreases optical performance. Consequently, to maximize the benefit of increasing the pupil diameter (decreased f#) the system needs to be essentially aberration free.

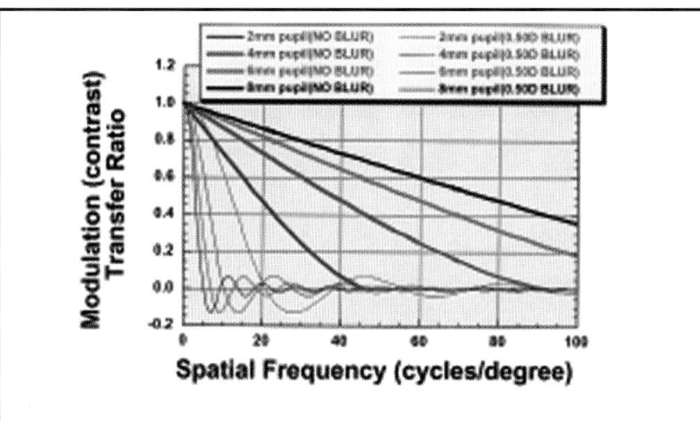

Figure 7-8. Diffraction-limited (no blur) MTFs (thick color-coded lines) and 0.5 D of defocus MTFs (color-coded thin lines) for four different pupil sizes. Calculations of the diffraction-limited MTFs were made using 555 nm light and methods detailed by Smith's equation.[29] Calculations of the defocus MTFs were made using a geometric approximation detailed by Smith's equation. Negative values reflect a phase shift and are discussed in the next section. (*Note*: A small error in the geometric approximation can be appreciated most clearly by the crossover of the 2 mm defocus MTF and the 2 mm diffraction MTF at low spatial frequencies. For larger pupil sizes in which the wavefront error is greater than 1 wavelength, the error in the geometric approximation of the defocus case is, for all practical purposes, inconsequential.)

> To maximize the benefit of increasing the pupil diameter, the system needs to be essentially aberration free.

Notice the following in Figures 7-8 and 7-9:

1. Counter to the diffraction-limited case, the larger the pupil, the larger the loss in image contrast and cut-off frequency
2. The defocus-induced losses in image contrast and cut-off frequency for the 2 mm pupil are less than for larger pupils, demonstrating why pinhole testing is effective clinically

Phase and Aberrations

So far, we have emphasized the effects of optical aberrations on retinal image contrast and the resulting visual perception. Equally important are shifts in spatial phase induced by optical aberrations. It is well known, for example, that defocus can introduce phase reversals into images so that dark bars become light and light bars become dark, an effect sometimes called *spurious resolution* (Figure 7-10). Similar effects occur for other aberrations besides defocus, which can lead to subtle notches and other anomalies in the contrast sensitivity function (CSF).[11,12] Therefore, one of the potential benefits of correcting ocular aberrations is that errors in spatial phase are corrected. This benefit is likely to be substantial for many aspects of visual function.

For example, the visual task of letter discrimination is strongly affected when optical defocus introduces phase reversals into some spatial frequency components of the target but not others (Figure 7-11). The upper row of images in Figure 7-11 demonstrates the devastating effect of phase reversals on letter legibility caused by optical blur. However, when these phase reversals

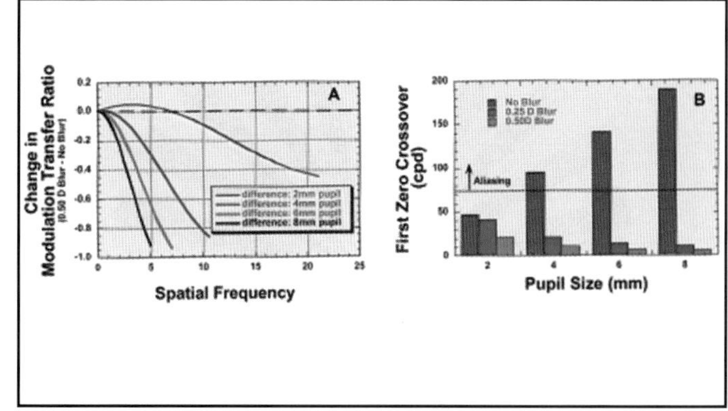

Figure 7-9. (A) The change in the MTF (0.5 D blur—no blur) as a function of spatial frequency up to the first zero crossover. Notice that the loss in MTF increases as pupil size increases. (The small gain in the MTF for the 2 mm pupil between 0 and approximately 7 c/deg is an error in the calculation due to ignoring the effects of diffraction in the calculation of the blur MTF.) For larger pupils, this error is essentially zero. (B) The MTF first zero crossover frequency as a function of pupil size for three levels of defocus.

are corrected, as shown in the bottom row of images, we see that the decrease in contrast induced by blur has relatively little impact. This simple demonstration shows that the phase shifts and phase reversals caused by optical aberrations can be more important than loss of contrast.

> The visual task of letter discrimination is strongly affected when optical defocus introduces phase reversals into some spatial frequency components of the target but not others.

Chromatic Aberration, Spherical Aberration, and the Neural Transfer Function

So far we have limited our discussion to monochromatic light, simple defocus, and phase. We have ignored the effects of chromatic aberration and have not shown the relationship between the neural threshold function and the optical MTF. In Figure 7-12, we model these interactions for a 6 mm pupil using the Indiana model eye. Introducing chromatic defocus (green line) into the model reduces the MTF significantly from the diffraction-limited case (black line). The MTF suffers more when spherical aberration is introduced, and performance is even worse when chromatic and spherical aberration are combined in the model.

The vertical separation between these curves tells us that by correcting the eye's chromatic aberration we could expect about five-fold improvement in image contrast at 30 c/deg. The improvement in image contrast would be approximately twelve-fold if we corrected the eye's spherical aberration, and we get approximately twenty-five-fold improvement in contrast at 30 c/deg by correcting both chromatic and spherical aberration.

Anticipated improvements in spatial resolution are not as dramatic as the improvements in contrast. The spatial frequency limit of detection without aliasing for the visual system is indicated graphically by the intersection of the optical MTF with the neural threshold function. This intersection occurs at approximately 30 c/deg (20/20) when both aberrations are included in the model. The intersection increases to 60 c/deg (20/10), a two-

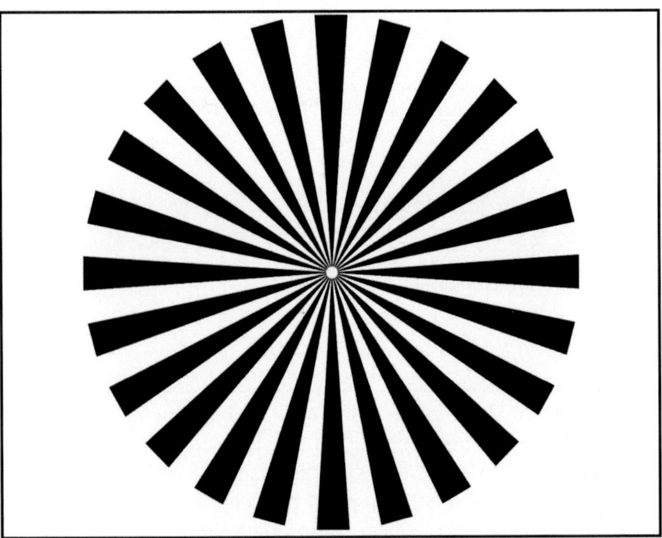

Figure 7-10. On the left is a focused image Seimen Star and on the right the same image blurred with 0.5 D defocus (6 mm pupil) showing phase reversal for higher frequencies (ie, notice how the higher frequency white part of the pattern just off center aligns with the dark part of the pattern in the periphery). Figure 7-8 shows the MTF for 0.5 D blur over a 6 mm pupil.

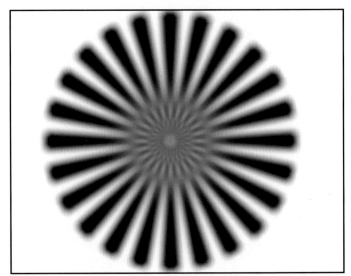

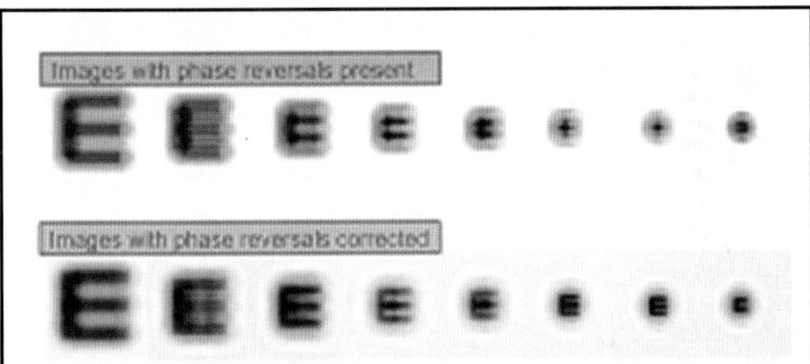

Figure 7-11. A blurred letter E with phase reversals at higher frequencies (top) and without phase reversal (bottom). Notice how phase reversal degrades the percept of the letter to the point in which the smaller letters (higher frequencies) are no longer legible. (Courtesy of Arthur Bradley.)[31]

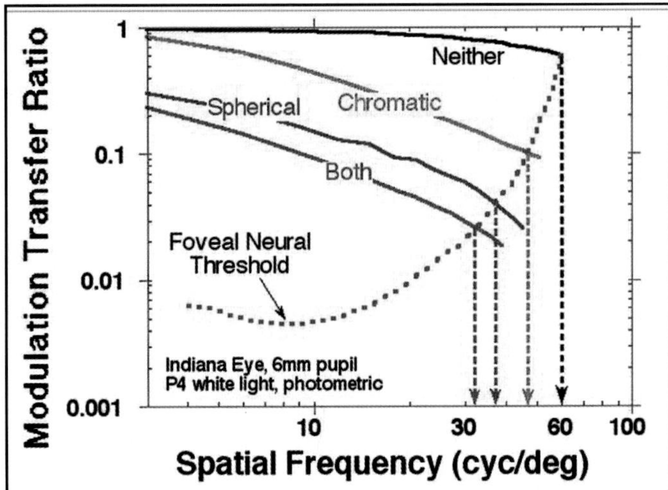

Figure 7-12. MTFs for a diffraction-limited case (black line), the chromatic aberration (green line), typical spherical aberration (blue line), both spherical and chromatic aberrations (red line), and the foveal neural threshold function. The foveal neural thresholds are measured by using gratings formed on the retina through interference, bypassing the optics of the eye. The points where each MTF crosses the foveal neural threshold function defines the limiting spatial frequency that the model can "see" (dashed arrows).

fold increase when both aberrations are removed. We may conclude from this analysis that the benefits of aberration correction are proportionally greater when measured in the contrast domain than when measured in the spatial domain.

Do clinical tests capitalize on these theoretical considerations to optimize sensitivity? In the next section, we will examine current methods to measure visual performance in the context of these theoretical considerations and the demands of the clinical environment.

Traditional Measures of Visual Performance

Clinically defining the quality of the visual percept is much more complex than defining the quality of the retinal image using objective measurement techniques. The retinal image defines the input to the visual system. The visual percept forms the basis for the final behavioral output after considerable cognitive processing. A proper treatment of the conversion of the retinal image to a visual percept is well beyond the scope of this chapter. Here we will try to give the reader a feel for the complexity and the issues involved in assessing visual performance, followed by a discussion of commonly used clinical measures of visual performance.

Clinically defining the quality of the visual percept is much more complex than defining the quality of the retinal image using objective measurement techniques.

Visual performance is multidimensional, with each dimension having its own set of tests. There are tests of color vision, temporal resolution (flicker fusion), variations in peripheral con-

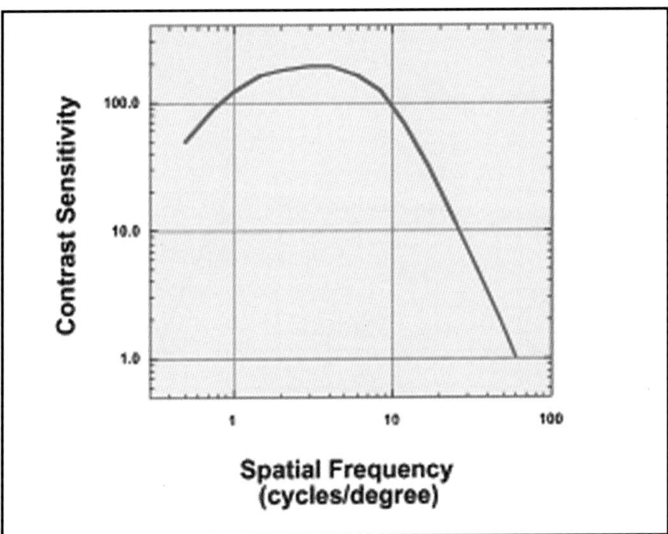

Figure 7-13. Typical log contrast sensitivity as a function of log spatial frequency for a normal eye.

trast sensitivity (perimetry), peripheral acuity, texture processing, motion processing, dynamic visual acuity (acuity while observing a moving target), visual attention (simultaneously identifying objects at two locations), localization (vernier) acuity, stereopsis, and many others. Although some of these may seem esoteric, some measure important aspects of visual function and are likely to work their way to prominence, particularly given the aging population. For example, a test of "useful field of vision" has been developed, which measures a subject's ability to identify the location of a car silhouette, eccentrically placed, while simultaneously performing a visual task at the point of fixation. Results from this test show a good correlation with incidence of automobile crashes in older drivers.[13]

Further, many aspects of human performance, though strongly dependent upon vision, do not require exceptional visual acuity and are not harmed by mildly reduced acuity. For example, driving a car[14] or shooting basketballs[15] is essentially unimpaired by having 20/40 rather than 20/20 or better acuity. On the other hand, some tasks are exquisitely sensitive to high levels of visual performance. In the Air Force, it is common wisdom that in a visual dogfight between two jet fighters, it is usually the pilot who first sees the enemy plane on the horizon who triumphs. For tasks such as these, improvements in the optics of the eye achieved through wavefront-guided laser surgery may mean the difference between success and failure. Superior vision does not necessarily mean exceptional performance; however, those who perform exceptionally generally have superior vision.

Measuring visual performance in a meaningful manner is not a simple matter, and principles of proper testing are often ignored in the clinical environment. The inherent variability of biological systems and the interpretive process dictate that reliable and sensitive tests must employ:

1. Small increments in task difficulty
2. Multiple trials at each level
3. A "forced-choice" methodology[16-18]
4. Scoring to the finest practical scale (eg, scoring by the number of letters read rather than by the number of lines read)

Acuity charts that have inconsistencies in letter size progression and number of letters per line (like the Snellen chart) make consistent scoring by the letter difficult. Further, and perhaps most importantly, clinicians and technicians are often satisfied if the patient can read the 20/20 line even though he or she may be able to read the 20/10 line. As a consequence, a patient who formerly had 20/10 vision can come in complaining of a vision loss that goes undetected. Such an experience leaves the patient thinking that he or she must be imagining things; or for the more confident patient, he or she may feel (more correctly) that you and your staff do not know what you are doing.

As a consequence of these and other factors (eg, quality of life measures), there is no one "silver bullet" test for measuring the quality of the visual percept and/or its impact on the quality of life. Despite this fact, every patient and clinician appropriately wants to know if refractive therapy improves vision. So what clinical tests best meet this need and why? Here we will focus on tests that are of particular relevance to refractive surgery and evaluating good but not perfect ocular optics. These tests center on tests of spatial processing (eg, acuity and contrast sensitivity).

> There is no one "silver bullet" test for measuring the quality of the visual percept and/or its impact on the quality of life.

Contrast Sensitivity

Although we would like to measure the MTF of the entire visual system (optics and neural pathways combined), such a MTF cannot be directly measured. To similarly characterize the visual system, one can measure the ability of the observer to detect sinusoidal gratings at threshold contrast as a function of spatial frequency. The resulting function is called the CSF. To carefully and accurately measure the CSF is too time-consuming for routine clinical use (generally 15 to 20 minutes per eye), particularly given current insurance reimbursement for such testing. Further, testing with sinusoidally varying luminance patterns is insensitive to changes in phase. Nonetheless, understanding how the visual system responds to contrast as a function of spatial frequency provides excellent insight into currently used clinical tests of spatial vision and those likely to meet clinical needs in refractive surgery.

In Figure 7-13, notice that with increasing spatial frequency, contrast sensitivity increases to a peak and then decreases. The decrease in contrast sensitivity at low spatial frequencies is attributable to neural processing.[19] The decrease in contrast sensitivity after the peak at moderate spatial frequencies is principally due to ocular optics.[19] In normal eyes that have excellent optics, the highest spatial frequency detected without aliasing will be neural limited. Functional human spatial vision is defined by space under the curve.

The CSF provides information about the visual system that is not given by high contrast acuity. For example, contrast sensitivity is more strongly related to certain visual tasks, such as face recognition, than is visual acuity.[20] Further, it is possible for high contrast acuity to remain normal or near normal, while contrast sensitivity in the midspatial frequencies is decreased. Such a midfrequency loss results in objects having a "washed out" appearance. Likewise, it is also possible for contrast sensitivity to be improved by custom ablation, while acuity remains constant. Consider a patient who has 20/15 or better best-corrected acuity before surgery. After refractive surgery that successfully eliminat-

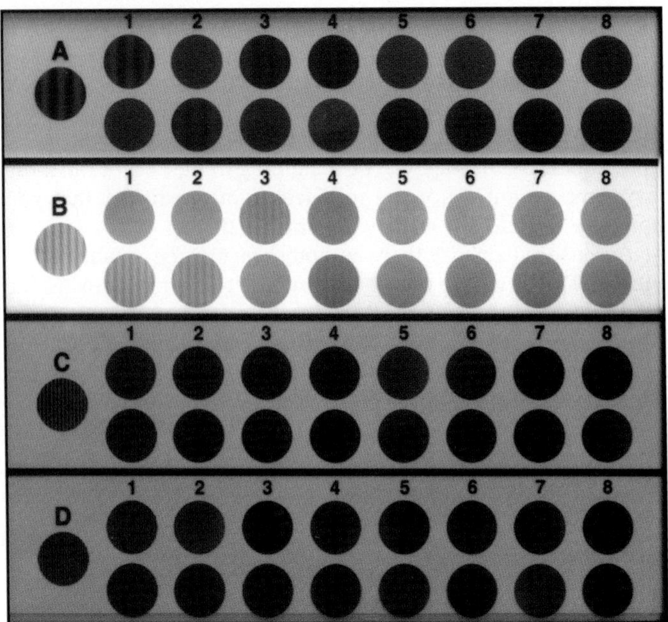

Figure 7-14. A clinical back illuminated chart from Vector Vision, Inc (Arcanum, Ohio) designed to test contrast sensitivity in the clinical environment. (Courtesy of Vector Vision Inc.)

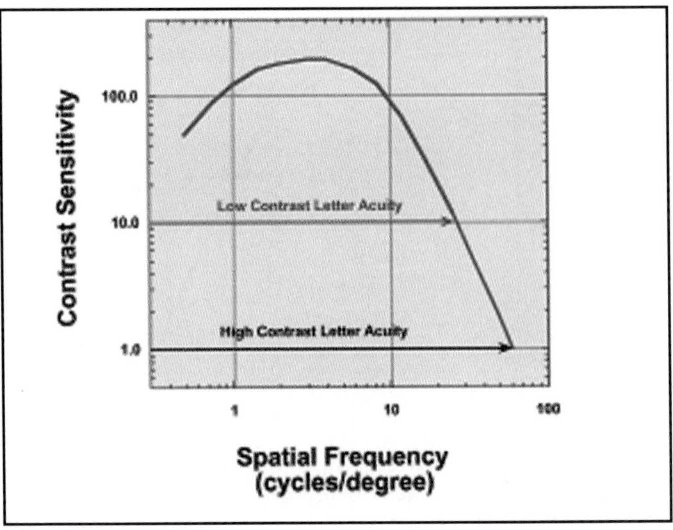

Figure 7-15. CSF showing that testing high or low contrast acuity samples spatial vision at a fixed contrast level and finds one point on the CSF curve. Acuity testing determines the highest spatial frequency (smallest letter) that can be seen at the fixed contrast level. Contrast is not varied in these tests.

ed the spherical and cylindrical error and reduced the higher-order optical aberration, photoreceptor spacing will quickly limit improvement in acuity. Nevertheless, such a surgical outcome will result in higher contrast images with crisper borders,[1,21] making it easier for the individual to drive or perform other tasks under foggy conditions or dim illumination. Such benefits are more likely to be reflected in measures of contrast sensitivity than they are in more traditional clinical measures like high contrast acuity.

Clinically, contrast sensitivity can be measured using patches of sinusoidal gratings. Figure 7-14 is a contrast sensitivity test developed by Vector Vision. Four spatial frequencies are presented (sections A to D). For each spatial frequency, the patient is to identify whether the disk containing the grating is on the top or on the bottom. At some point for each spatial frequency, the patient will be randomly guessing. The first missed identification is defined as the threshold.

High Contrast Visual Acuity

As the name implies, high contrast visual acuity employs high contrast letters of varying size to measure the smallest letters a patient can correctly identify. Letters are complex targets made up of a large number of frequencies having numerous orientations and modulations. Despite their complex nature, as letters get smaller and smaller, the spatial frequency content shifts to higher spatial frequencies. Consequently, in CSF space, high contrast acuity is a psychophysical measure that marches horizontally across the spatial frequency axis (toward smaller letters) near 100% contrast (CS of 1) until it hits the CSF curve (Figure 7-15). As a result, high contrast acuity is a surrogate measure of the highest spatial frequency that the visual system can process accurately (ie, the smallest high contrast letter that can be read).

An advantage of high contrast acuity tests is that they are relatively insensitive in the normal or near normal eye to minor changes in pupil size and minor variations in the higher-order aberrations. Consequently, high contrast visual acuity is not particularly sensitive to more subtle visual complaints commonly offered by refractive surgery patients (eg, the patient who reports, "I may see 20/20, but I do not see as well as I did, particularly at night").

Sensitivity can be increased by using state-of-the-art high contrast log minimum angle of resolution (MAR) acuity charts (Figure 7-16), forcing the patient to read until five letters are missed and defining the final acuity as the total number of letters read correctly up to the fifth miss. As a practical matter, when scoring acuity in this manner, one asks the patient to start reading the chart at the smallest line that he or she knows he or she can read. If he or she reads the entire line correctly, it is assumed that he or she can read all larger lines correctly and these larger unread letters are counted in the correct count as if they were read. If a patient misses a letter on the starting line, the patient is asked to read the next larger line before proceeding to smaller letters. Final log MAR acuity is defined as:

Final log MAR acuity = x – (LC x 0.02)

where x = the worst log MAR acuity for the test distance + 0.10 and LC = total number of letters read correctly.

Low Contrast Acuity

Using letters of constant low contrast shifts the acuity measurement line vertically in CSF space (see Figure 7-15). Notice that spatial frequencies requiring high contrasts will be below the detection threshold. A consequence of high spatial frequencies being below the threshold of detection and lower overall contrast for all frequencies is that the borders of visible letters are less distinct (letters are harder to read). Lowering letter contrast increases the test sensitivity, and more subtle changes in optical quality can be detected. Two prominent versions of the low contrast acuity test are the the low contrast log MAR chart and the Regan charts. The low contrast log MAR charts are constructed in an identical manner as the high contrast version except for the lower contrast, which with state-of-the-art computer programs (eg, CTView by Sarver and Associates, Inc, Celebration, Fla [www.sarverassociates.com]) can be set at any level and printed

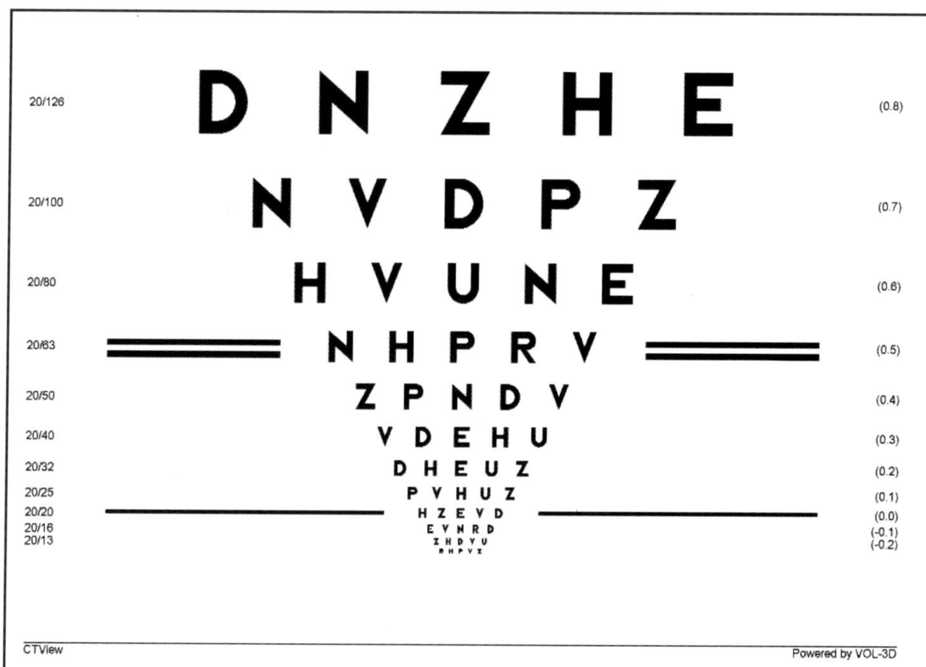

Figure 7-16. State-of-the-art log MAR chart generated using the CTView. (Courtesy of Ed Sarver.)

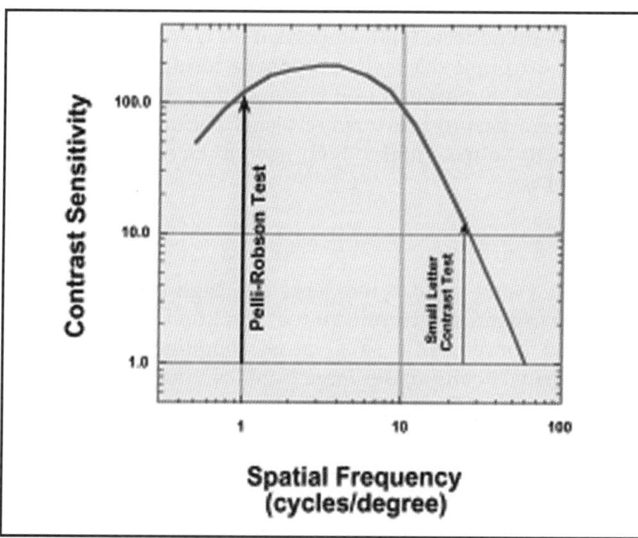

Figure 7-17. Letter contrast sensitivity tests use letters of a constant size (spatial frequency) and gradually decrease contrast of the letters.

out for use. The Regan charts[22] consist of four charts, each having a different contrast ranging from 4% to 96% (Weber contrast, ΔI/I). Both capitalize on state-of-the-art chart design by having a fixed number of letters in each line, a fixed scalar between lines, and separation between letters dependent on letter size.[20,22-24] At least three studies have found low contrast acuity to be a more sensitive measure of changes in visual function after refractive surgery than high contrast acuity.[6,25,26] Despite these findings, the correlation between high and low contrast acuity remains high (r^2 = 0.87), suggesting that the gains in test sensitivity are not as large as might be hoped.[27]

Pelli-Robson Large Letter Contrast Sensitivity

The Pelli-Robson test uses letters of equal legibility and a constant large size (20/640 or approximately 1 c/deg) and, unlike high or low contrast acuity, varies the contrast between letter presentations (Figure 7-17). Three letters are presented at each of 16 contrast levels. The letter contrast changes 0.15 log units for each level, starting at about 100% and decreasing to about 0.9%. The test has been shown to have good reliability[17] in measuring low frequency contrast sensitivity and has gained a fair amount of popularity among clinicians testing for neural problems. The choice of the large letter places the fundamental spatial frequency of the letter into the low frequency roll-off in the CSF due principally to neural processing. Using such a low spatial frequency makes the test more sensitive to neurologically induced changes in contrast sensitivity than optically induced changes. The reason is simple. Minor changes in optical properties have a greater effect on the higher spatial frequencies than they do on the low spatial frequencies, as seen in Figures 7-8, 7-9, and 7-12. Although it is wise to switch to the contrast domain to test for optical changes likely to be induced by refractive surgery, test sensitivity to improvements or degradations in the eye's optics will be increased by using smaller letters where the fundamental frequency is securely in the steep portion of the CSF and more sensitive to changes in the eye's optical properties.

Small Letter Contrast Test

Rabin's small letter contrast test[28] capitalizes on the steep slope of the CSF in the moderate to high spatial frequencies, which are more sensitive to changes in optical quality than lower frequencies (see Figure 7-17). As a consequence of the steep slope, small amounts of blur cause relatively large changes in contrast sensitivity and only small changes in spatial frequencies (Figure 7-18). The small letter contrast test is similar to the Pelli-Robson chart in that all letters are the same size, and successive rows have lower contrast. However, instead of using large letters, the letter size is approximately 20/25 (24 c/deg). There are 14 lines in the test with 10 letters in each line. Contrast decreases by 0.10 log unit on each successive line.[28] Unlike tests of contrast using sinusoidal gratings, this test should be sensitive to phase shifts as well as gains or losses in the MTF. Despite its excellent

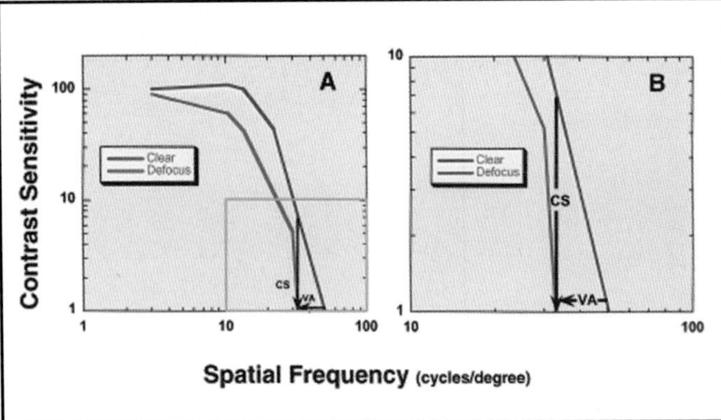

Figure 7-18. (A) A small amount of defocus causes the CSF to shift down, which causes a minor shift in cut-off frequency and a large change in contrast at high frequencies. (B) An enlargement of the light green square in panel A. (Adapted from Rabin J, Wicks J. Measuring resolution in the contrast domain: the small letter contrast test. *Optom Vis Sci.* 1996;73:398-403.)

design, the Rabin small letter contrast test has seen little clinical use to date.

The Ideal Clinical Test of Visual Function

In the normal visual system, we would like to believe that visual performance tests are a good surrogate measure for the optical quality of the retinal image. That is, as the retinal image improves, test performance improves and as the retinal image degrades, test performance degrades. Such an ideal test is fantasy. Visual systems vary in their capacity to interpret the retinal image and form a percept. It is unrealistic for such tests to perfectly mimic retinal image quality. Likewise, it is unrealistic to think that metrics of optical quality, even when they are modified to include neural processing, will perfectly reflect the final output of the visual system on any given task.

Fortunately, the reliance on visual performance tests to serve as a surrogate measure of retinal image quality will likely disappear over the next several years as sensitive new objective tests of retinal image quality make their way to the market. These new aberrometers will be able to quantify the aberration structure of the eye well beyond simple sphere and cylinder. Further, and perhaps more importantly, new metrics will be developed that reflect input from both the optical and neural stages of vision (see Chapter 8). In this new setting, visual performance tests will be used to define the relationship between retinal image quality, new metrics of visual quality based on our understanding the optics and visual system.[31-34] Differences between retinal image quality and new tests of visual performance will be used to explore the nature of refractive amblyopia and new causes of refractive amblyopia. For example, it may be the case that "ideal" refractive corrections improve the retinal image quality but that visual performance does not improve to the neural limit accordingly.[1]

What Design Characteristics Should Ideal Visual Performance Tests Have?

Key design characteristics include:

1. Ease of use for clinicians and technical support staff
2. Easy for the patient to understand
3. Fast—the test should be able to be administered and scored in less than 1 minute per eye
4. Variable contrast and spatial frequency
5. Small increments in task difficulty
6. Multiple trials at each test level
7. Use a "forced-choice" methodology
8. Computer generated, scored, and random generation of test targets
9. Allow the pupil to physiologically dilate
10. Infrared pupil size monitoring

The Rabin small letter contrast test meets many of these test requirements. However, it cannot be overemphasized that visual function following refractive surgery is highly dependent upon pupil size. Much of the interest in visual performance after refractive surgery is concerned with large pupil conditions. The reason is two-fold. First, aberrations induced by refractive surgery (as performed prior to the year 2000) increased dramatically under large pupil conditions. Consequently, visual performance decreased with increasing pupil size.[2,25,26] Second, the effects of diffraction increase with decreasing pupil size. Thus, the visual benefit (more contrast and sharper borders)[8,21] of correcting the eye's higher-order aberrations is increasingly masked by diffraction as pupil size decreases. Consequently, until ideal corrections are perfected, it is important for clinicians and scientists to report pupil sizes when reporting results of visual performance tests. Reporting pupil size is critical when correlating optical aberrations to measures of visual performance. For the correlation to be meaningful, both have to be measured at the same pupil size.

Tests Allowing Large Physiological Pupil Diameters

Current visual performance tests (eg, high or low contrast acuity) are generally performed under conditions of high illumination and consequently small pupil conditions. In order to measure visual acuity under large pupil conditions, it has been necessary to either artificially dilate the pupil with mydriatics or use low levels of lighting for the chart and for the surrounding environment.

As an alternative, Stanley Klein has suggested a new type of chart using single bright letters presented against a dark background (on a monitor) in a dark room and decreasing letter size to threshold (personal communication, S Klein, October 1999). Under these conditions the pupil would be physiologically dilated. This innovative concept may be considered a new twist on what may be one of the oldest methods of testing visual acuity. One can imagine shepherds in ancient Greece sitting in a field at night comparing their abilities to resolve two closely positioned stars. Klein's suggestion lends itself to modern methods of computer display with all its advantages. However, as currently suggested, Klein's test does not capitalize on the sensitivity of the contrast domain to subtle changes in optical quality. The test could be easily altered to test in the contrast domain similar to the Rabin small letter contrast test.

Summary

New refractive therapy, whether it increases or reduces ocular higher-order aberrations (beyond sphere and cylinder), is changing how we view and test visual performance. Key points are:

1. New, more sensitive tests of visual performance need to be developed that capitalize on the visual system's sensitivity to contrast and phase
2. With the advent of clinically practical wavefront sensing and new metrics that reflect optical and neural processing, the need to use measures of visual performance as a surrogate measure of retinal image quality will diminish
3. Differences between retinal image quality and visual performance measures will be used to explore amblyopia
4. Improvements in retinal image quality of the normal eye will not be reflected by large gains in traditional acuity tests
5. New tests should allow full physiological pupil dilation
6. Both retinal image quality and visual performance measures need to be reported as a function of pupil diameter

Acknowledgments

Preparation of this chapter was supported by National Institutes of Health (National Eye Institute) grants R01-EY08520 to Dr. Applegate, R01-EY05109 to Dr. Thibos, HEAF funds from the University of Houston, CORE Grant R43 EY014754 to the College of Optometry, University of Houston, and the Visual Optics Institute of the College of Optometry, University of Houston. We thank Arthur Bradley for permission to reproduce Figure 7-11.

References

1. Applegate RA. Limits to vision: can we do better than nature? *J Refract Surg*. 2000;16:5547-5551.
2. Applegate RA, Howland HC, Sharp RP, Cottingham AJ, Yee RW. Corneal aberrations and visual performance after radial keratotomy. *J Refract Surg*. 1998;14:397-407.
3. Martinez CE, Applegate RA, Klyce SD, McDonald MB, Medina JP, Howland HC. Effect of pupil dilation on corneal optical aberrations after photorefractive keratectomy. *Arch Ophthalmol*. 1998;116:1053-1062.
4. Oliver KM, Hemenger RP, Corbett MC, et al. Corneal optical aberrations induced by photorefractive keratectomy. *J Refract Surg*. 1997;13:246-254.
5. Oshika T, Klyce SD, Applegate RA, Howland HC. Comparison of corneal wavefront aberrations after photorefractive keratectomy and laser in situ keratomileusis. *Am J Ophthalmol*. 1999;127:1-7.
6. Seiler T, Kaemmerer M, Mierdel P, Krinke HE. Ocular optical aberrations after photorefractive keratectomy for myopia and myopic astigmatism. *Arch Ophthalmol*. 2000;118:17-21.
7. Liang J, Williams DR. Effect of higher order aberrations on image quality of the human eye. *Vis Sci Appl Tech Digest* (OSA). 1995;1:70-73.
8. Liang J, Williams DR, Miller DT. Supernormal vision and high resolution retinal imaging through adaptive optics. *J Opt Soc Am A*. 1997;14:2884-2892.
9. MacRae SM, Schwiegerling J, Snyder R. Customized corneal ablation and supervision. *J Refract Surg*. 2000;16:S230-S235.
10. Yoon GY, Williams DR. Visual benefits of correcting the higher order monochromatic aberrations and the longitudinal chromatic aberration in the eye. Paper presented at: The 2000 Vision Science and its Applications Annual Meeting; February 11-14, 2000; Sante Fe, NM.
11. Woods RL, Bradley A, Atchison DA. Monocular diplopia caused by ocular aberrations and hyperopic defocus. *Vision Res*. 1996;36:3597-3606.
12. Woods RL, Bradley A, Atchison DA. Consequences of monocular diplopia for the contrast sensitivity function. *Vision Res*. 1996;36:3587-3596.
13. Owsley C, Ball K, McGwin G, et al. Visual processing impairment and risk of motor vehicle crash among older adults. *JAMA*. 1998;279:1083-1088.
14. Owsley C. Vision and driving in the elderly. *Optom Vis Sci*. 1994;71:727-735.
15. Applegate RA. Set shot shooting performance and visual acuity in basketball. *Optom Vis Sci*. 1992;69:765-768.
16. Bailey IL, Bullimore MA, Raasch TW, Taylor HR. Clinical grading and the effects of scaling. *Invest Ophthalmol Vis Sci*. 1991;32:422-432.
17. Elliott DB, Bullimore MA. Assessing the reliability, discriminative ability, and validity of disability glare tests. *Invest Ophthalmol Vis Sci*. 1993;34:108-119.
18. Raasch TW, Bailey IL, Bullimore MA. Repeatability of visual acuity measurement. *Optom Vis Sci*. 1998;75:342-348.
19. De Valois RL, De Valois KK. *Spatial Vision*. New York, NY: Oxford University Press; 1988:147-175.
20. Elliott DB. Contrast sensitivity and glare testing. In: WJ Benjamin, ed. *Borish's Clinical Refraction*. Philadelphia, Pa: WB Saunders; 1998:203-241.
21. Miller DT. Retinal imaging and vision at the frontiers of adaptive optics. *Physics Today*. 2000;53:31-36.
22. Regan D, Neima D. Low-contrast letter charts as a test of visual function. *Ophthalmology*. 1983;90:1192-1200.
23. Bailey IL, Lovie JE. New design principles for visual acuity letter charts. *Am J Optom Physiol Opt*. 1976;53:740-745.
24. Bailey IL. Visual acuity. In: WJ Benjamin, ed. *Borish's Clinical Refraction*. Philadelphia, Pa: WB Saunders; 1998:179-202.
25. Verdon W, Bullimore MA, Maloney RK. Visual performance after photorefractive keratectomy. *Arch Ophthalmol*. 1996;114:1465-1472.
26. Bullimore MA, Olson MD, Maloney RK. Visual performance after photorefractive keratectomy with a 6-mm ablation zone. *Am J Ophthalmol*. 1999;128:1-7.
27. Hilmantel G, Applegate RA, Tu EY, Starck T, Howland HC. Low contrast acuity: a substitute for contrast sensitivity? *Invest Ophthalmol Vis Sci*. 1999;40(Suppl):S534.
28. Rabin J, Wicks J. Measuring resolution in the contrast domain: the small letter contrast test. *Optom Vis Sci*. 1996;73:398-403.
29. Smith WJ. *Modern Optical Engineering: The Design of Optical Systems*. New York, NY: McGraw-Hill, Inc; 1990:327-363.
30. Bradley A, Hong S, Chung L, Thibos LN. The impact of defocus-induced phase reversals on letter recognition is different for hyperopes and myopes. *Invest Ophthalmol Vis Sci*. 1999;40(Suppl):S35.
31. Applegate RA, Sarver EJ, Khemsara V. Are all aberrations equal? *J Refract Surg*. 2002;18:S556-S562.
32. Applegate RA, Marsack J, Ramos R. Interaction between aberrations can improve or reduce visual performance. *J Cataract Refract Surg*. 2003;29:1487-1495.
33. Applegate RA, Ballentine C, Gross H, Sarver EJ, Sarver CA. Visual acuity as a function of Zernike mode and level of RMS error. *Optom Vis Sci*. 2003;80:97-105.
34. Applegate RA. Wavefront sensing, ideal corrections and visual performance. *Optom Vis Sci*. In press.

Chapter 8

Metrics to Predict the Subjective Impact of the Eye's Wave Aberration

David R. Williams, PhD; Raymond A. Applegate, OD, PhD; and Larry N. Thibos, PhD

Introduction

The advent of rapid, automated wavefront sensing in the eye now provides the clinician with a much richer description of the optics of each patient's eye than has been available before. Numerous methods have been developed to measure the wave aberration, some of which are objective, such as the Shack-Hartmann wavefront sensor,[1] while others are subjective, such as the spatially resolved refractometer.[2] In either case, these devices measure only optical characteristics of the eye. This is all that is required for some applications, such as correcting the optics of the eye for imaging the retina. But in the case of correcting the optics of the eye for improving vision, neural processing as well as optical image formation is also important. As the technology for measuring the wave aberration matures, there is a need to discover better ways of using the wave aberration to improve vision.

> A key issue is how to transform the wave aberration into a succinct description of how it will affect the patient's vision, which is the focus of this chapter.

The ability to predict the visual impact of a given wave aberration is important for several reasons. First, this information can be used to evaluate quality of vision and expected visual performance. Such information could be used in screening individuals for driver's licenses, disability claims, or evaluating quality of life issues such as the ability to recognize faces. Second, a metric derived from the wave aberration can guide the clinician in selecting the best strategy for improving vision in each patient. For example, are the higher-order aberrations in the patient's wave aberration severe enough to warrant customized refractive surgery, or is he or she likely to benefit just as much from conventional refractive surgery? If the patient is complaining of halos, flares, monocular diplopia, or other visual defects, can the problem be linked to the eye's optical performance, is the patient unusually sensitive to small defects in vision, or are other neural factors implicated? Third, metrics to predict the subjective impact of the wave aberration can be incorporated into algorithms to compute the best vision correction given a particular wave aberration.[3,4] Methods of vision correction such as contact lenses, spectacles, and refractive surgery generally correct fewer aberrations than can be measured with wavefront sensing technology. For example, spectacles can correct only prism, sphere, and cylinder, whereas wavefront sensors can reliably measure tens or even hundreds of aberrations in normal human eyes. The higher-order aberrations can influence the values of defocus and astigmatism that provide the best subjective image quality.

> The development of metrics for subjective image quality that include the effects of higher-order aberrations will allow us to optimize vision correction.

The common practice today is to rely on the patient's responses to refract the eye. These measurements are time-consuming, with a typical subjective refraction taking several minutes per eye to perform. A wavefront sensor measurement can be performed in a matter of seconds. A conventional subjective refraction involves adjusting three aberrations (sphere, cylinder, and axis) simultaneously to optimize visual performance. However, wavefront technology allows more than three aberrations to be corrected. Moreover, conventional refraction is subject to the variability in the patient's response. If an objective metric could be developed that adequately mimics the behavior of the average visual system, one can average the results of multiple objective measurements in the time it takes to perform a single subjective refraction, reducing the variability in the correction and achieving a better visual outcome.

> A subjective procedure to identify the best values of more than three aberrations is not practical. For this reason, higher-order corrections must depend on algorithms to optimize vision rather than on the subjective response of the patient.

The Role of Individual Aberrations in Visual Performance

Just as the conventional refraction can be decomposed into prism, sphere, cylinder, and axis, we can also break "irregular astigmatism" into individual aberrations, or Zernike modes, with a process called *Zernike decomposition*. Zernike decomposition can provide valuable insight into the relative importance of different aberrations for vision. It is useful in diagnosing the

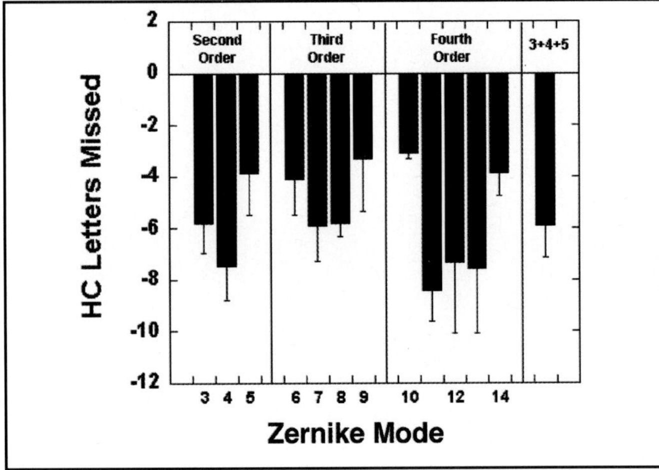

Figure 8-1. Average high contrast letters missed as a function of Zernike mode. The far right panel of each graph (labeled 3 + 4 + 5) displays the result for the experimental chart where the RMS error was equally distributed across C^{-2}_2, C^0_2, C^2_2 (sphere and cylinder modes) such that the total RMS error was 0.25 micrometers (μm) over a 6 mm pupil, λ = 555 nanometers (nm). Error bars are 1 standard deviation (SD).

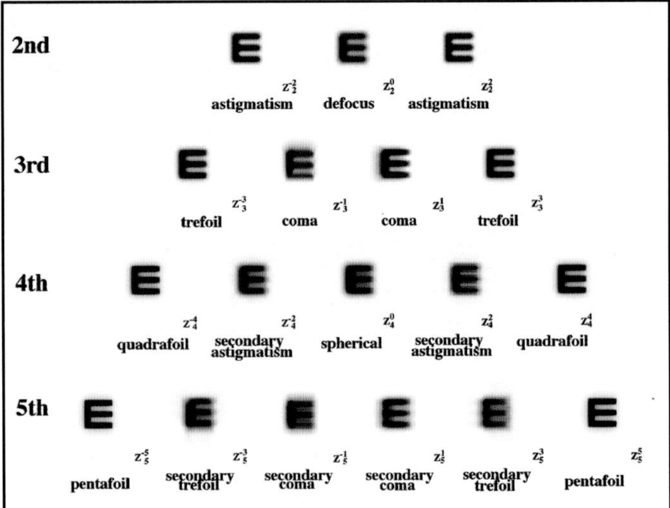

Figure 8-2. Image simulations of the impact of 0.25 μm of RMS error for the individual modes of the Zernike expansion through the fifth radial order over a 6 mm pupil, λ = 555 nm. Notice that modes in the center of the pyramid have bigger effect than modes along the edge of the pyramid.

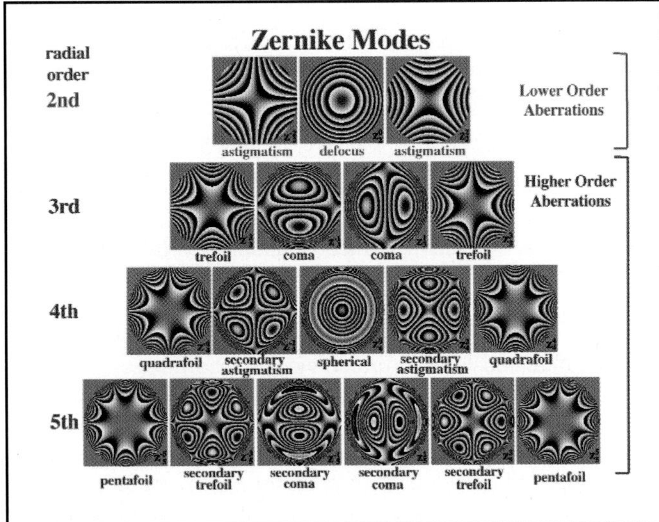

Figure 8-3. Wavefront error for Zernike modes through the fifth radial order (6 mm pupil, λ = 555 nm).

cause of a particular wave aberration as well as visual complaints. For example, a refractive surgery patient who presents postoperatively with an increase of vertical coma and complains of a vertical flare on car headlights at night very likely suffered some vertical decentration during laser ablation.

The evaluation of individual Zernike modes reveals large differences in their subjective impact. Applegate et al[5,6] aberrated log minimum angle of resolution (MAR) acuity charts by convolving the chart with the point spread functions (PSFs) corresponding to individual Zernike modes. They studied the visual impact of each Zernike mode in second through fourth radial order. A fixed level of root mean square (RMS) error (0.25 millimeter [mm] over a 6 mm pupil—a dioptric equivalent of 0.19 diopters [D]) was used in each case. They then asked subjects with 20/15 or better visual acuity and best-corrected vision to read each of the aberrated charts. The total number of letters read correctly up to the fifth miss was recorded for each chart. The number of letters lost was calculated by subtracting the number of letters read correctly for a perfect (unaberrated) chart. Figure 8-1 shows the number of high contrast letters lost as a function of Zernike Mode. Note that more letters are lost for modes in the middle of a given Zernike order than those at either the beginning or the end of each order. For example, in the second radial order, defocus (labeled 4 in the figure) degrades performance more than either astigmatism mode (3 and 5). Similarly in the third radial order, coma (modes 7 and 8) decreases acuity more than trefoil (modes 6 and 9). Despite the fact that the total aberration as expressed by RMS error was constant, acuity varied by up to 10 letters (two lines) depending on which Zernike mode contained the wavefront aberration. Figure 8-2 shows a simulation that captures the essence of Applegate's conclusion. The letter E at a size corresponding to 20/40 has been convolved with the PSF corresponding to each Zernike mode. The RMS wavefront error of each Zernike mode was fixed at 0.25 μm. Wavelength was 555 nm and the pupil size was 6 mm. Figure 8-3 shows the corresponding Zernike modes for comparison. Note that the letters at the center of the pyramid are more blurred than those along the flanks. Inspection of the original modes in Figure 8-3 shows why this is true. The flanking modes share the common feature that the wave aberration is flat (uniform gray in the figure) over much of the pupil. The light that passes through these regions of the pupil will form sharp images on the retina. The aberrations that blur strongly, on the other hand, tend to have nonzero slope over a larger contiguous fraction of the pupil.

Williams[7] obtained similar results to those of Applegate et al,[5,15] using a deformable mirror to produce aberrations instead of convolution. They used the deformable mirror to blur the subject's vision with a single Zernike mode, one at a time, while all other aberrations were corrected across a 6 mm pupil. The subject adjusted the coefficient associated with this Zernike mode to produce an amount of blur that equaled a standard amount of blur. They also found that aberrations in the center of the pyramid blurred more than those at the edge, and that this was true for fifth-order aberrations as well as second, third, and fourth order. See Figure 8-3 to see which modes belong to each order.

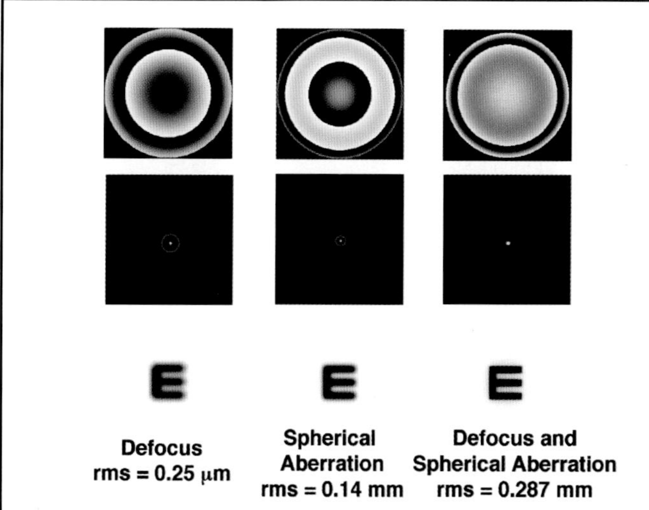

Figure 8-4. The interaction between defocus and spherical aberration. Each column represents a hypothetical eye with wave aberration over a 6 mm pupil, a PSF at 555 nm, viewing a 20/40 letter. The left column shows an eye suffering only from defocus at 0.25 mm RMS. The middle column shows an eye suffering only from spherical aberration at 0.14 mm RMS. The right column shows an eye suffering from both defocus and spherical aberration in the same amounts as in the other two eyes, for a total RMS of 0.287 mm. The eye on the right has the best image quality even though the RMS wavefront error is the highest.

The Problem With Zernike Decomposition

By analogy with the success in chemistry of reducing molecules to their atomic constituents, it is tempting to think that reducing the wave aberration to its fundamental components might provide the path to subjective image quality. However, experiments from our laboratories cast doubt on the value of this reductionist approach because Zernike modes can interact strongly with each other to determine final image quality. Their subjective effects do not add together in a simple way, as illustrated in Figure 8-4. Shown are the retinal images of the letter E for three hypothetical eyes, one suffering only from defocus, one suffering from spherical aberration, and one suffering from both defocus and spherical aberration in the same amounts as present in the first two eyes. (When adding aberrations, it is the variance, which is the RMS squared, that adds, not the RMS itself. For example, in this case $0.252^2 + 0.142^2 = 0.287^2$). Strikingly, the image quality is obviously best in the eye that suffers from both aberrations rather than the eyes than suffer from only one of them. Consistent with this demonstration, Applegate et al[8] have measured the interactions between Zernike modes and found that pairs of aberrations can sometimes increase acuity more than would be expected from the individual components or they can sometimes lead to a larger reduction in acuity than expected. Modes two radial orders apart and having the same sign and angular frequency tend to combine to increase visual acuity compared to loading the same magnitude RMS error into either component individually. Modes within the same radial order tend to combine to decrease acuity compared to loading the same magnitude RMS error into either component individually.

> Zernike modes can interact strongly with each other to determine final image quality.

> The complexity of the interactions between Zernike modes in subjective blur means that Zernike decomposition is unlikely to be a productive avenue for deriving a metric of subjective image quality.

Principles for Constructing a Metric

The purpose of incorporating an image quality metric into a wavefront sensor is to summarize the visual impact of each patient's wave aberration. Unfortunately, the number of metrics that one might explore is infinite. To make this problem tractable, one must restrict the search to those domains that are most likely to yield the best solutions. Therefore, we propose that biological plausibility should be the criterion for restricting the search for good metrics of image quality. That is, we seek a fast algorithm that mimics those steps that the patient's eye and brain actually take in order to see. The more realistically the model captures the processing stages in the human visual system, the more successful the metric will be. For example, the optics of the eye forms a retinal image through a process that is well understood and can be accurately described mathematically. The retinal image is then processed by a nervous system, the properties of which are also reasonably well understood. Another strength of building the metric around a model of vision is that additional factors can be added to the model as their significance is assessed. For example, the model might initially incorporate only blur from aberrations and neural blur. As the model develops, incorporating factors such as the Stiles-Crawford effect, light scatter, and/or neural plasticity should increase predictive power.

> Biological plausibility should be the criterion for restricting the search for good metrics of image quality.

Image Quality Metrics

Pupil Plane Metrics

Currently, the most commonly used metric is the RMS wavefront error, defined as the square root of the sum of the squares of the deviation of the actual wavefront from the ideal wavefront (Figure 8-5). This is the same as the standard deviation of the wave aberration. Unfortunately, RMS wavefront error is not an especially useful metric for describing the subjective impact of the eye's wave aberration.[4,5,9] For example, Figure 8-4 shows that the eye with the best image quality can sometimes have the highest RMS.[7,8] This is because metrics defined in the pupil plane, such as RMS, do not take into account the interaction of light entering through different parts of the pupil as they form the retinal image. Moreover, the retinal image is processed by neural stages that are not incorporated in pupil plane metrics.

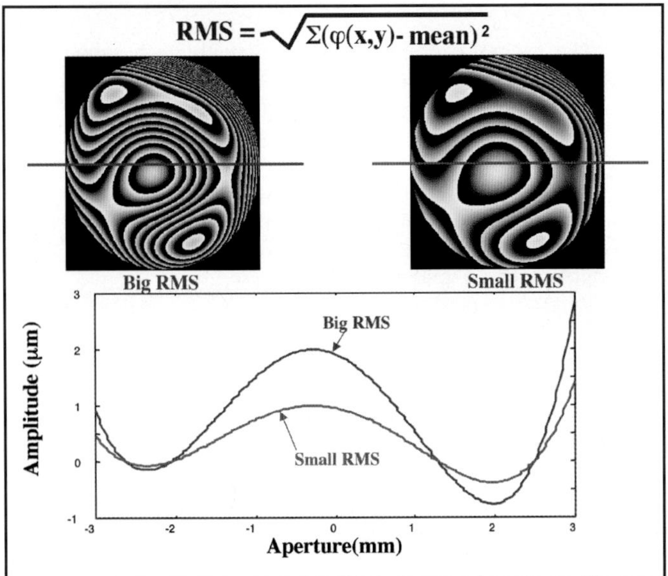

Figure 8-5. RMS wavefront error is a pupil plane measure of optical quality that is equal to the square root of wavefront variance. The contour map at the left indicates a relatively large RMS error whereas the contour map at the right indicates a relatively small wavefront error. The bottom graph shows the amplitude of wavefront error for a horizontal trace across the pupil.

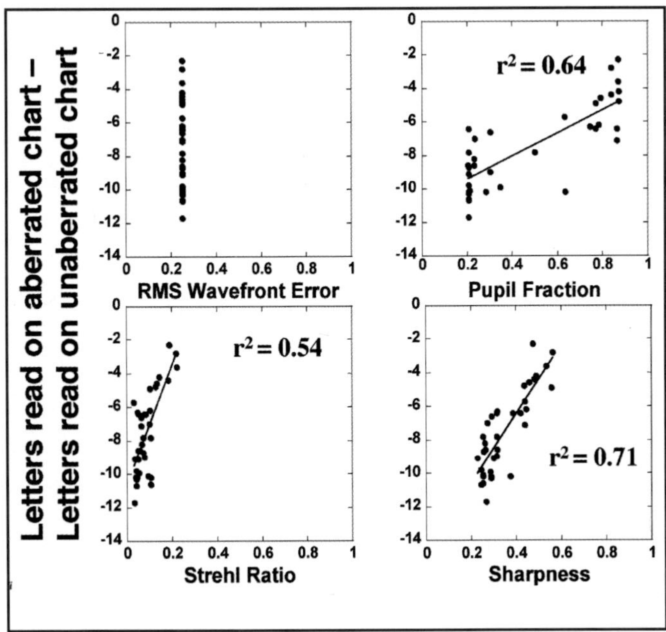

Figure 8-7. Different image quality metrics have different abilities to predict the loss of visual performance caused by optical aberrations in the experiments of Applegate et al.[8]

RMS wavefront error is not an especially useful metric for describing the subjective impact of the eye's wave aberration.

The retinal image is processed by neural stages that are not incorporated in pupil plane metrics.

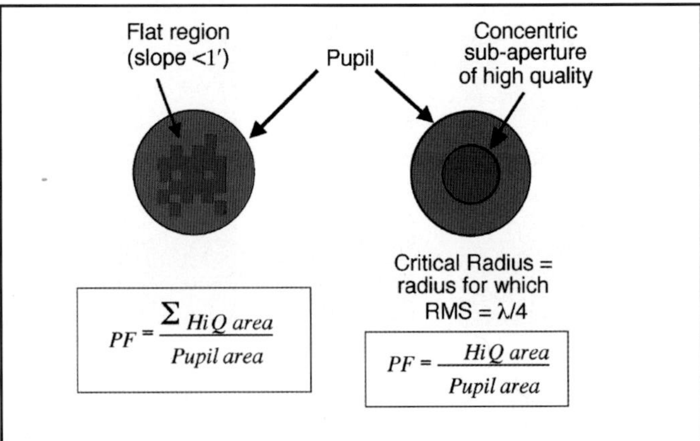

Figure 8-6. Two methods for determining PF. In the left diagram, we compute the total amount of pupil area for which the slope of the wavefront aberration function is less than some criterion (eg, 1 minute of arc) and divide the result by pupil area. In the right diagram, we compute the area of that subaperture for which the total RMS error is less than some criterion (eg, one-fourth wavelength of light) and divide the result by pupil area.

A better pupil plane metric, called pupil fraction (PF), quantifies what fraction of the eye's pupil has good optical quality. It is equal to the fraction of pupil area for which optical quality is reasonably good. There are many ways to locate the portion of the pupil that is optically good. For example, one criterion is that the RMS wavefront error is less than some criterion, such as one-fourth wavelengths of light, as illustrated in Figure 8-6. Another method, suggested by Stan Klein, is based on wavefront slope. Regardless of which method is used, a large PF is preferred because it means that most of the light entering the pupil is used to form a high quality retinal image. The range of possible values of PF is 0 to 1. PF accounts for 64% of the variance in acuity, whereas RMS error could not account for any of the variation in acuity because RMS was intentionally held constant (Figure 8-7).[8] PF was also an effective metric for calculating subjective refraction in the Indiana aberration study.[8] However, the data are not evenly distributed over the range of possible values, which reduces its usefulness.

Image Plane Metrics

Image plane metrics are computations performed on the retinal image rather than directly on the wave aberration. These metrics have the advantage that they take into account the interaction of light entering different parts of the pupil. The wave aberration measured by a wavefront sensor remains the input to the process, but image plane metrics incorporate the computations that transform the wave aberration into the retinal image.

Image plane metrics are computations performed on the retinal image rather than directly on the wave aberration. These metrics have the advantage that they take into account the interaction of light entering different parts of the pupil.

In optics, there are two general strategies for describing the quality of an imaging system: one based on the image formed of a point of light, like a star, and another based on the image formed of a set of sine wave gratings. These two descriptions

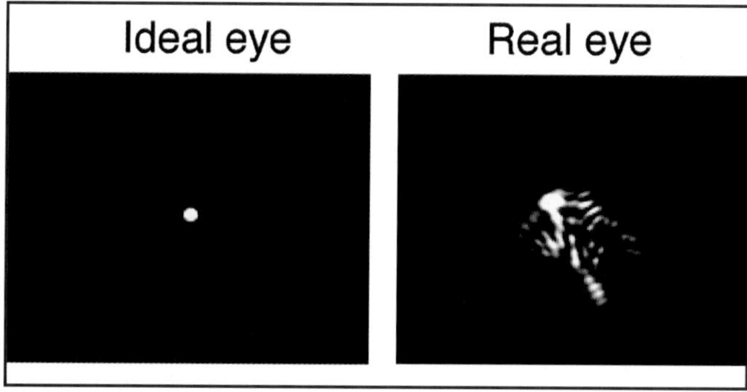

Figure 8-8. PSF examples for an eye that has no aberrations and is blurred only by diffraction (left, 6.00 mm pupil, 555.00 nm) and a typical PSF from a normal eye (right). The real eye light distribution is extremely complicated in its structure and the challenge for making a metric of image quality is to reduce this distribution to a single number that best captures its visual impact.

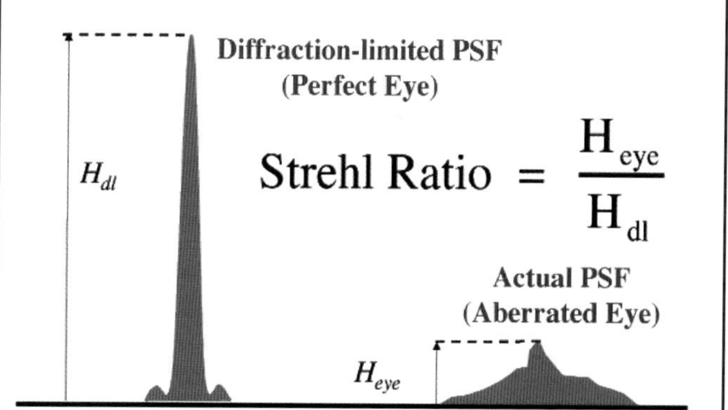

Figure 8-9. The Strehl ratio is equal to the maximum intensity in the PSF divided by the maximum intensity that would have been obtained in an optically perfect system. The range of possible values of Strehl ratio is 0 to 1. (Courtesy of Austin Roorda.)

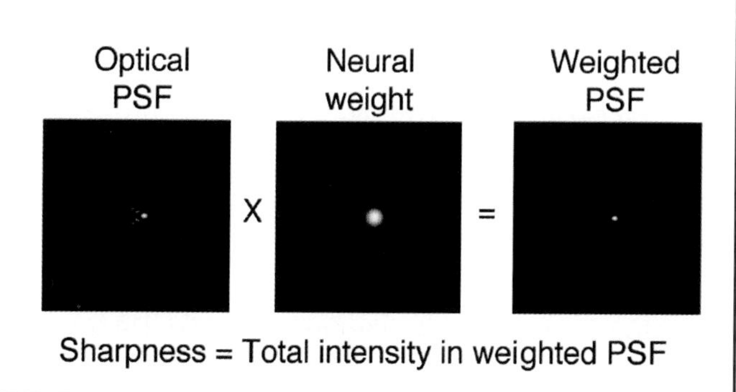

Figure 8-10. Sharpness of the PSF is computed by multiplying the PSF by a Gaussian weighting function and summing the result. A similar metric called *visual Strehl* uses a neural weighting function derived from the human contrast sensitivity function for interference fringes. On a scale of 0 to 1, sharpness = 0.35 and visual Strehl = 0.25 in this example (6 mm pupil, 0.25 mm coma).

turn out to be exactly equivalent to one another in terms of the information they contain, though often the description based on gratings is easier to compute. Of course, the visual environment is composed of many objects that are more interesting to people than points of light and gratings. However, it is possible to compute the retinal image of any object once the image of a point or the images of a number of gratings is known. The intuition behind the computation based on the PSF (convolution) is that any object can be thought of as a collection of points of light, each of which produces its own blurred image. The retinal image of the object is then the sum of all these blurred images, one from each point in the object. Similarly, the object can be described as the sum of many sine wave gratings, each of which produces a sine wave grating in the retinal image that is reduced in contrast (reduced modulation) and shifted in location (phase shift) (see Chapters 2 and 7). Believe it or not, these contrast reductions and phase shifts completely describe the optical quality of the eye and contain exactly the same information as the PSF.

Figure 8-8 shows examples of a typical PSF from a normal eye compared with the ideal PSF from an eye that has no aberrations and is blurred only by diffraction. The light distribution for the real eye is extremely complicated in its structure and the challenge is to reduce this distribution to a single number that best captures its visual impact. The goal of an ideal correction is to redirect the light so that it is concentrated as much as possible into a single spot. This will increase the compactness of the PSF, which increases its intensity at the center, and also reduces asymmetries. PSF metrics are attempts to capture these aspects of a good PSF with a single number. One common PSF metric based on the intensity of the PSF is the Strehl ratio, illustrated in Figure 8-9. The Strehl ratio is equal to the maximum intensity in the PSF divided by the maximum intensity that would have been obtained in an optically perfect system. The range of possible values of Strehl ratio is 0 to 1. Strehl ratio accounted for 54% of the variation in the acuity in blurred letter charts in the experiment of Applegate et al[8] as shown in Figure 8-7. Though this is better than the predictive power of RMS, it is not as good as the PF metric introduced earlier, which accounted for 64% of the variance.

> The goal of an ideal correction is to redirect the light so that it is concentrated as much as possible into a single spot. This will increase the compactness of the PSF, which increases its intensity at the center, and also reduces asymmetries. PSF metrics are attempts to capture these aspects of a good PSF with a single number.

One of us (Williams) introduced another metric called *sharpness*, illustrated in Figure 8-10, that is similar to the Strehl ratio, except that it includes a component intended to capture neural processing of the retinal image. Sharpness of the PSF is computed by multiplying the PSF by a Gaussian weighting function located in that retinal area over which the nervous system averages light. This averaging process is a form of neural blurring in addition to the optical blurring that is captured by the PSF alone. The total intensity in the weighted PSF indicates the compactness of the optical PSF. It is convenient to normalize this value by the corresponding value computed for an optically perfect eye so that the range of possible values of the sharpness metric is 0 to 1. A similar metric called *visual Strehl*, introduced by Thibos and Applegate, uses the neural PSF as a neural weighting function. This neural PSF is equal to the inverse Fourier transform of the neural contrast sensitivity function for interference fringes. Interference fringes bypass the optical aberrations of the eye, thereby isolating the neural factors that determine visual sensitivity to patterns.

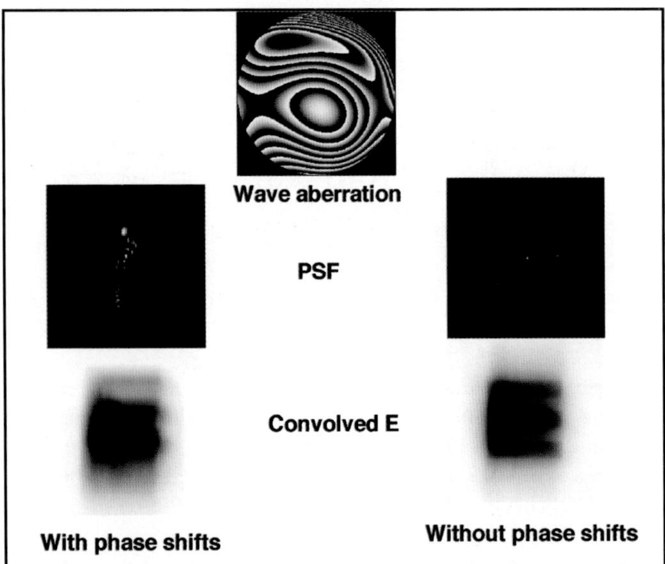

Figure 8-11. The importance of phase fidelity. The wave aberration of a post-LASIK patient (top) was used to compute the PSF (middle left), which was then convolved with the letter E to simulate the retinal image (bottom left). The calculation was then repeated assuming zero phase shifts to produce a much improved PSF (middle right) and consequently an improved retinal image of the letter E (bottom right). The letter subtended 40 degrees of arc.

Figure 8-7 shows the sharpness metric applied to the data of Applegate et al.[8] Sharpness accounts for 71% of the variance of visual acuity data of Applegate et al[8]and visual Strehl accounts for 81% of the variance, which is more than the PF metric, the Strehl ratio, or RMS wavefront error. We have also explored a number of variations of these metrics, all based on the premise of an image formation stage followed by a neural processing stage. As a practical matter, many of these variations are implemented more easily in the frequency domain (for grating images) instead of the spatial domain (for images of point sources). These metrics can also account for a large fraction of the variance in our experimental data for a variety of visual tasks. Further work will be required to identify the optimum metric or combination of metrics.

Future Directions

The results of our analysis of data from three different sites obtained with different experimental procedures supports the principle that metrics based on the optical and neural processes known to occur in human vision are superior to the most common metric in current use, RMS wavefront error. It seems highly likely that improvements in metric performance will be realized by building additional features into the model of human vision. For example, it is known that the eye is less sensitive to edges at oblique orientations than to those oriented horizontally or vertically,[10] and a metric that incorporated that feature might perform better than the isotropic metrics we have implemented so far.

Phase

Another aspect of the quality of any imaging system is its ability to preserve in the retinal image the spatial relationships between the grating components that make up the original object. Any failure to preserve these spatial relations is called a *phase shift*. The PTF describes the phase shift for all possible grating components (spatial frequency). A perfect optical system produces no phase shifts, but the real eye is not perfect[11] in this respect, especially when the pupil is large. It is well known that changes in the phase spectrum of an image can often be more disruptive than changes in image contrast.[12] The importance of phase fidelity is illustrated in Figure 8-11 (see also Chapter 7) which shows the wave aberration of a post-laser in-situ keratomileusis (LASIK) patient, the PSF with and without phase shifts, and the convolution of the PSF with the letter E. Note the difference in the retinal image when phase shifts are included. We suspect that the best metrics will include the phase shifts that the eye's optics can introduce.

Polychromatic Metrics

The metrics we have described to date are defined for a single wavelength of light. However, the world is composed of objects that generally reflect all wavelengths of light, albeit by different amounts. The retinal image quality depends on the spectral nature of light because of chromatic aberration in the eye (see Chapter 10). Our image plane metrics can be generalized to include chromatic aberration, and this will probably be important because chromatic aberration interacts with the eye's monochromatic aberrations in determining the overall image quality.

Metric Normalization

The metrics we have devised to date are generally normalized to the ideal optical system for the same pupil size. This is a good way to formulate the metric if one is interested in how sharp the image is compared with the sharpest it could be for that particular pupil size. In other circumstances, it would be useful to develop a metric that was robust across all pupil sizes. The advantage of such a metric is that it would capture the absolute quality of vision regardless of the pupil size.

Multivariate Metrics

The metrics described here are univariate: only one number is used to describe image quality. However, loss of image quality can arise from multiple causes that are perceptually distinct. For example, image quality declines when edges become blurred, but also when the overall contrast of the image is reduced. Alternatively, flaring in a particular direction or multiple ghost images can greatly reduce image quality and visual performance. A combination of metrics, each of which is sensitive to a different aspect of image quality, should be superior to any single metric on its own. Moreover, it would provide the clinician with an indication of how the retinal image is disrupted. For example, a retinal image with a strong flare in one direction could not be distinguished from a retinal image that suffered from an equivalent amount of symmetric blur. However, this would be revealed by a metric sensitive to the symmetry of the PSF. One strategy is to adopt a tripartite metric with separate numbers for contrast, sharpness, and symmetry in the retinal image. Even a tripartite scheme may not be sufficient to capture the important variations that can arise in the eye's PSF. For example, multiple ghost imagery could require a fourth metric. The number of metrics adopted may eventually be a compromise between simplicity and accuracy. Given the speed of modern computation, these additional metrics can be provided at little additional cost. Ultimately, psychophysical experiments will determine the

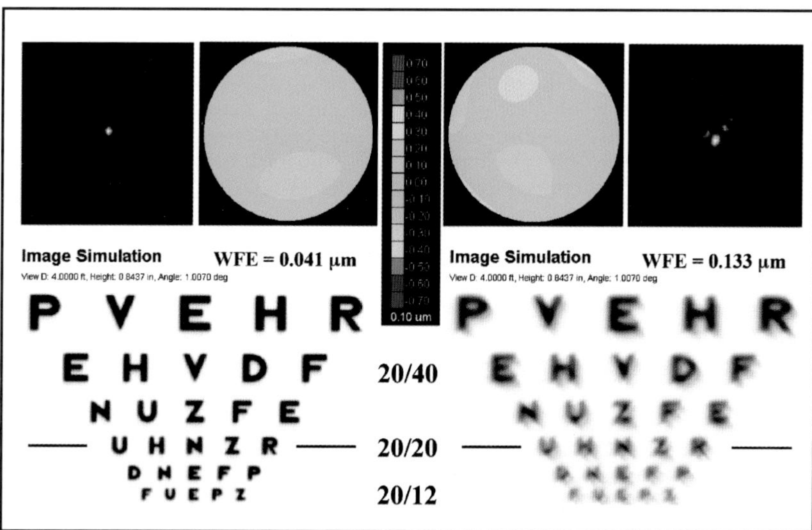

Figure 8-12. Two different wave aberrations for which high contrast visual acuity was the same (20/15) but subjective image quality was quite different. In this case, the value of a metric based on visual acuity would be different than the value of a metric based on a judgment of subjective image quality. Best spectacle correction, 3.00 mm pupil diameter. The eye on the left is a typical, nonsurgical eye. he eye on the right is a successful, post-LASIK patient after 1 year. The computed PSFs, wavefront error maps, and simulations of the retinal image were computed with CTView (Sarver & Associates, Celebration, Fla).

importance of each of these metrics in subjective image quality and visual performance.

Population Norms

One would probably choose to convert metric values into scores that reflect population norms. For example, if the metric were transformed to a percentile, the clinician would know what fraction of the patient population has worse optics than the patient in question.

Task Dependence

One of the fundamental difficulties in choosing an optimum metric is that it is highly dependent on the visual task. For example, a task that requires detecting relatively large features in a low contrast environment would demand a different metric than detecting tiny features at very high contrast. Other factors associated with the task can influence the optimum metric, such as luminance, pupil size, and object distance. Figure 8-12 shows an example of two different wave aberrations that generated indistinguishable visual acuity but different subjective image quality. In this case, a metric based on visual acuity would be different than a metric based on a judgment of subjective image quality.

One of the fundamental difficulties in choosing an optimum metric is that it is highly dependent on the visual task.

Plasticity and Vision Correction

Metrics might also need to incorporate the fact that neural processing is plastic, changing its performance depending on the wave aberration used to view the world. There is a long history of research revealing neural plasticity. Distortions in the visual field, introduced with prisms, disappear with time, as do the chromatic fringes caused by chromatic aberration.[13] Recent experiments by Pablo Artal reveal that this plasticity extends to the monochromatic aberrations of the eye as well. Artal used the Rochester Adaptive Optic System to remove the wave aberration from a subject. He then replaced the wave aberration, either in its original orientation or rotated by some amount. Despite the fact that the rotation only changes the orientation of the aberrations and not the objective amount of retinal blur, the subjective blur changed dramatically. Subjects viewing the world through their own wave aberration reported that it was much sharper than when the wave aberration was rotated. These observations support clinical wisdom that patients will often reject astigmatic corrections that improve image quality, but cause too large a departure from their normal experience of the world. The effect has far-reaching implications for vision correction, since it means that subjects who receive an aberration-free view of the world through customized correction may require time to adjust to the benefit. Alternatively, vision correction might best be accomplished through a multiple step process that ultimately converges on the desired correction.

Metrics might also need to incorporate the fact that neural processing is plastic, changing its performance depending on the wave aberration used to view the world.

Metric Customization

Though the development and validation of metrics based on the typical patient is the obvious first goal, the metrics might also be customized depending on the specific needs and characteristics of each patient. For example, older patients are likely to have more light scatter, their pupil sizes are smaller on average, their accommodation range is reduced, and they will probably tolerate large changes in vision correction less readily. A metric that included patient age as a parameter would help to ensure the optimum vision correction. For example, the optimum metric for someone with a poor neural contrast sensitivity will be different than the metric for someone with exquisite neural sensitivity. It may ultimately be possible to build known features of an individual patient's nervous system into the metric. For example, with laser interferometry, it is possible to measure the neural performance of the eye independent of its optical quality. There are large variations in the neural performance of normal eyes,[14] and the metric could be customized to each patient accordingly. One could also customize the metric based on lifestyle. For example, patients with reduced accommodation or whose lifestyle required good focus over a large range of viewing distances might benefit from a increase in spherical aberration, compared with a patient, such as a pilot, who would prefer to optimize performance at infinity. Any metric needs to incorporate the depth of field of the eye and how it varies with pupil size, accommodation, and aberrations to correct the eye in such a way as to maximize the range of viewing distances over which optical quality is acceptable. It is well known that some patients prefer a "softer" image than others, and a customized metric may offer patients a choice along this or other aesthetic dimensions.

Metrics might also be customized depending on the specific needs and characteristics of each patient.

Fully Automated Refraction

Autorefractors have not replaced subjective refraction as the ultimate method to prescribe vision correction. The advent of wavefront sensing reopens the possibility of fully automated and improved refraction. This is because wavefront sensors provide much more information than autorefractors, since they indicate the fate of light as it passes through every point in the pupil. A consortium of investigators from Lawrence Livermore National Laboratories, University of Rochester, Bausch & Lomb, Wavefront Sciences, and Sandia National Laboratories has developed a compact phoropter equipped with adaptive optics. This device, which incorporates a wavefront sensor, can provide a refraction and/or a prescription for correcting higher order aberrations in a fraction of a second. The incorporation of a deformable mirror also allows subjective image quality to be assessed with any of a broad range of customized vision corrections. Metrics of the kind discussed in this chapter will be required to find the endpoint of refraction based on a variety of criteria before choosing the best customized correction. Guirao and Williams[4] describe a fast algorithm to compute the optimum vision correction for any metric from wave aberration data. Further work will improve the clinical use of these metrics. Coupled with a biologically plausible metric designed to mimic the eye and brain of each patient, wavefront sensors may ultimately surpass the clinical refraction as the preferred method for choosing the best correction, whether the correction is implemented with refractive surgery, spectacles, contact lenses, intraocular lenses, or any other method.

The advent of wavefront sensing reopens the possibility of fully automated and improved refraction.

Coupled with a biologically plausible metric designed to mimic the eye and brain of each patient, wavefront sensors may ultimately surpass the clinical refraction as the preferred method for choosing the best correction, whether the correction is implemented with refractive surgery, spectacles, contact lenses, intraocular lenses, or any other method.

References

1. Liang J, Grimm B, Goelz S, Bille J. Objective measurement of the wave aberrations of the human eye using a Hartmann-Shack wavefront sensor. *J Opt Soc Am A*. 1994;11:1949-1957.
2. Webb RH, Penney CM, Thompson KP. Measurement of ocular wavefront distortion with a spatially resolved refractometer. *Appl Opt*. 1992;31:3678-3686.
3. Charman WN, Olin A. Image quality criteria for aerial camera systems. *Phot Sci Eng*. 1965;9:385-397.
4. Guirao A, Williams DR. A method to predict refractive errors from wave aberration data. *Optom Vis Sci*. 2003;80(1):36-42.
5. Applegate RA, Sarver EJ, Khemsara V. Are all aberrations equal? *J Refract Surg*. 2002;18:S556-S562.
6. Applegate RA, Ballentine C, Gross H, Sarver EJ, Sarver CA. Visual acuity as a function of zernike mode and level of RMS error. *Optom Vis Sci*. 2003;80:97-105.
7. Williams DR. What adaptive optics can do for the eye. *Review of Refractive Surgery*. 2002;3(3):14-20.
8. Applegate RA, Marsack J, Ramos R. Interaction between aberrations can improve or reduce visual performance. *J Cataract Refract Surg*. 2003;29:1487-1495.
9. Thibos LN, Hong X, Bradley A, Cheng X. Statistical variation of aberration structure and image quality in a normal population of healthy eyes. *J Opt Soc Am A*. 2002;19:2329-2348.
10. Campbell FW, Kulikowski JJ, Levinson J. The effect of orientation on the visual resolution of gratings. *J Physiol*. 1967;187:427-436.
11. Charman WN. Wavefront aberrations of the eye: a review. *Optom Vis Sci*. 1991;68:574-583.
12. Oppenheim AV, Lim JS. The importance of phase in signals. *Proceedings of the IEEE*. 1981;69:529-541.
13. Held R. The rediscovery of adaptability in the visual system: effects of extrinsic and intrinsic chromatic dispersion. In: Harris CS, ed. *Visual Coding and Adaptability*. Hillsdale, NJ: Lawrence Erlbaum Associates; 1980.
14. Williams DR. Visibility of interference fringes near the resolution limit. *J Opt Soc Am A*. 1985;2:1087-1093.

Chapter 9

Wavefront Information Sampling, Fitting, and Conversion to a Correction

Jim Schwiegerling, PhD

WAVEFRONT SAMPLING

The goal of aberrometry is to accurately measure the shape of an individual's wavefront error so that this information can be used to correct the optics of his or her eye. Wavefront error is the deviation of this individual's actual wavefront from an ideal shape. In terms of outgoing wavefronts, the ideal wavefront is perfectly planar and has a boundary defined by the edge of the pupil. In this manner, a point of light on the retina would map to a point at an infinite distance from the person, giving him or her diffraction-limited distance vision. In terms of ingoing wavefronts, the ideal wavefront is perfectly spherical and converges to a point on the retina. Again, the edge of the ideal wavefront is limited by the pupil margin. Wavefront error arises from distortions in the shape of the actual wavefront in comparison to the ideal wavefront. In other words, the actual wavefronts are continuous surfaces over the region of the pupil that have ripples and undulations. It is these variations that need to first be accurately measured and then corrected in order to enhance the optical performance of the eye.

> *Diffraction-limited*: Describes an aberration-free optical system whose only limit to image quality is the diffraction of light, which occurs at the aperture edges. In an optical system with a circular aperture, the diffraction-limited image of a point source is an Airy pattern, which limits spatial resolution. The diameter of an Airy disk increases (spatial resolution decreases) as pupil size decreases based on the following simple formula:
> Airy disk diameter = $2.44\ \lambda \times f/D$
> where λ = the wavelength of light, f = the focal length of the optical system, and D = pupil diameter.

Different techniques such as Shack-Hartmann, Tscherning, retinal ray tracing, and spatially-resolved refractometry have been proposed to measure the wavefront error. Each of these techniques only measures the slope of the wavefront error at a discrete set of points from which the shape of the wavefront is calculated. These sampling points are usually distributed across a rectangular, polar, or hexagonal grid pattern across the pupil. If the oscillations and undulations in the wavefront vary slowly compared to the spacing between the grid points, then the wavefront can be accurately measured. However, if the wavefront error varies wildly between grid points, then misinformation about the shape of the wavefront is obtained. Sampling theory is used to determine what density of measurement points is sufficient to accurately reproduce the shape of the wavefront error.

> Shack-Hartmann, Tscherning, spatially-resolved refractometry, and retinal ray tracing techniques only measure the slope of the wavefront error at a discrete set of points from which the shape of the wavefront is calculated.

Digital cameras are useful for illustrating some of the aspects of sampling theory. In photographing the scene of a pine forest, three levels of sampling occur: spatial sampling, spectral sampling, and temporal sampling. Spatially, the pine forest represents a continuous variation in intensity (brightness) levels from the dark tree bark in the shadows to moderately bright pine needles to bright sky in the background and all shades in between. Spectrally, the scene varies in a continuous fashion. There are an infinite number of colors present, from the brown bark to the green needles to the blue sky and all hues in between. Finally, the forest scene varies continuously in time. The trees sway in the wind, the branches grow, and the sky changes from dark to light to dark throughout the course of a day. To capture a perfect snapshot of this scene, an infinite number of brightness measurements at all wavelengths would need to be captured instantaneously. Obviously this is impossible, since the digital camera could not store this vast amount of data and could not operate quickly enough to capture it. Therefore, to photograph the scene, the image needs to be digitized or sampled into discrete units in order to limit the amount of data that need to be stored and the time needed to capture this information. In terms of spatial sampling, the sensor inside the camera is composed of discrete light-sensitive pixels. The number of samples corresponds to the "megapixel" or millions of pixels designation on the camera. There are pixels sensitive to the red, green, and blue portion of the visible spectrum (RGB). These pixels record the brightness at various points in the scene, and reduce the color at these points to a discrete combination of red, green, and blue wavelengths. The camera also samples the scene in time, recording over the time span that the shutter is open.

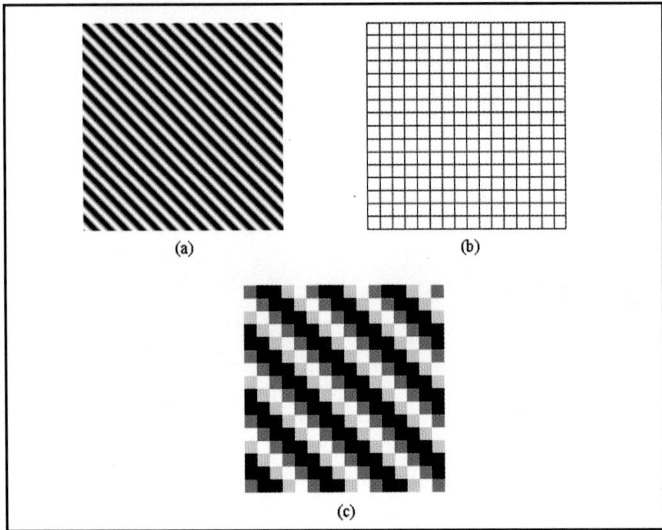

Figure 9-1. (A) A high frequency sinusoidal image. (B) A 32 x 32 sampling grid. Each pixel gives the average intensity of the image falling onto it. (C) Aliased sampled image of (A), which results in a lower frequency sinusoidal pattern.

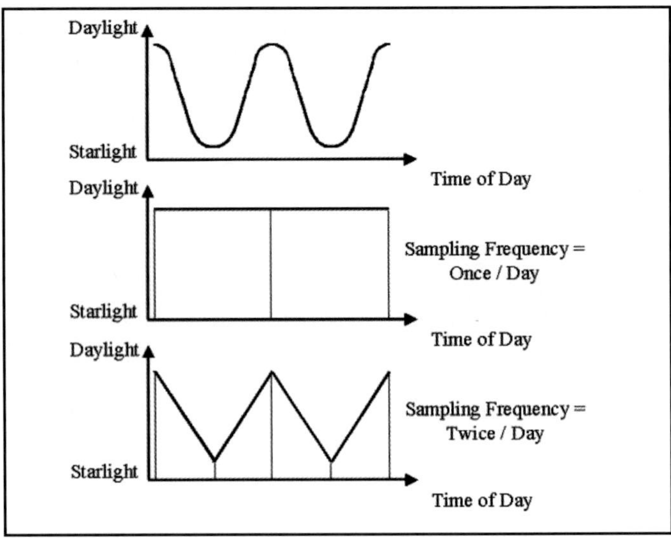

Figure 9-2. Example of temporal aliasing. If the scene is sampled once per day at noon, then there is a constant brightness to the scene. Increasing the sample to twice per day allows the diurnal variations to be seen.

Aliasing occurs if there are insufficient intervals between the samples.[1] Spatial aliasing occurs when the fluctuations in the intensity values in an image vary at a faster rate than the spacing between pixels. For example, if a series of alternating black and white bars are photographed with the digital camera described above, then the camera sensor needs at least one pixel on each of the black bars, with a single white-bar pixel in between in order to accurately reproduce the image. If the spacing between the pixels does not meet this criterion, then aliasing occurs. The consequence of spatial aliasing is that slower-varying intensity variations occur in the image that do not exist in the original scene. Figure 9-1 illustrates spatial aliasing. The sinusoidal pattern in Figure 9-1A represents the original image to be photographed by the digital camera. The grid pattern in Figure 9-1B is a 32 x 32-pixel sampling array that represents the sensor in a digital camera. The oscillations in the sine pattern in Figure 9-1A vary more quickly than the pixel spacing in Figure 9-1B. When the pattern is photographed, each pixel can only record the average intensity falling onto it. Figure 9-1C shows the "sampled" image. Aliasing has occurred because of the inadequate pixel size, resulting in a pattern that varies at a lower frequency (ie, fewer oscillations across the diagonal of the image). In addition to spatial aliasing, spectral aliasing can also occur when the spectrum reflected from an object is not adequately sampled. Aliasing in this case means that dramatically different spectral distributions can be mapped to the same RGB values. Finally, temporal aliasing can occur. In the case of a snapshot, any fluctuations that occur while the shutter is open will be "time-averaged." This type of aliasing is routinely seen in action photographs with slow shutter speeds. The motion blur is a result of the insufficient temporal sampling. Temporal aliasing also occurs when repeated measurements are taken, as is the case with a videocamera. If the scene changes too quickly between frames, then inaccurate information regarding the motion of objects is obtained.

> Spatial aliasing occurs when the fluctuations in the intensity values in an image vary at a faster rate than the spacing between pixels.

In general, aliasing occurs if there is some oscillation within the image that varies more quickly than the sampling frequency. Figure 9-1 illustrated spatial aliasing or the introduction of intensity variations that are not in the original image. Making decisions about the scene based on aliased data can be dangerous. If Figure 9-1A represented ripples on the surface of the cornea that need to be removed, then treating this cornea based on the sample pattern provided in Figure 9-1C would give horrendous results. This danger can also be illustrated with temporal aliasing. Suppose the digital camera is set up to automatically take a photograph of the pine forest every day at noon. Based on the information that is presented in the photographs, we could state that it is always light out and never gets dark. This is an incorrect assumption based on data that are temporally aliased. If we adjust our camera to take photographs at noon and midnight, then the oscillations from daylight to starlight are minimally sampled, and based on these photographs, we can correctly assume that the lighting varies in the pine forest but cannot resolve the gradual change. Figure 9-2 illustrates temporal aliasing. The top graph shows the daily variation in light levels. If this curve is measured with a sampling frequency of once per day at noon, then it appears that the light level is always bright. Increasing the sampling frequency to twice per day allows the diurnal fluctuations to be measured. In general, the oscillations need to be measured at least twice per cycle (twice per day, in the preceding example) to adequately sample them. Typically, four samples per cycle give more robust results.

> The definition of alias is "otherwise known as." It is used in sampling theory to mean the image of the object being sampled has changed its appearance and is no longer a good quality rendition of the original object.

Wavefront sensors all potentially suffer from aliasing. Wavefront sensors measure aberrations at discrete locations within the pupil. Fluctuations in the wavefront error that vary more quickly than the spacing between these samples will be

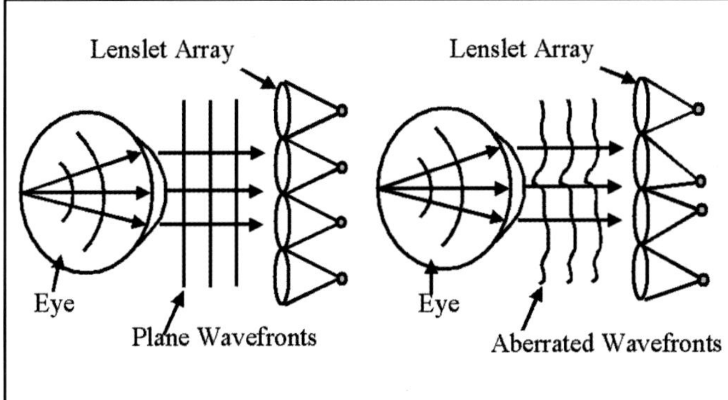

Figure 9-3. A Shack-Hartmann aberrometer. Unaberrated wavefronts are focused to a regular array of spots. Aberrated wavefronts form a distorted grid of spots.

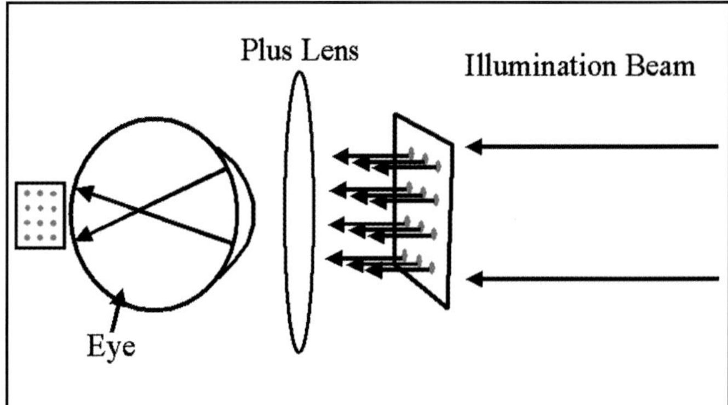

Figure 9-4. A Tscherning aberrometer. A mask is used to create a series of discrete collimated beams. An aberroscope lens forces these beams to focus in front of the retina and diverge to create a shadow of the mask on the retina. Aberrations distort this retinal grid pattern.

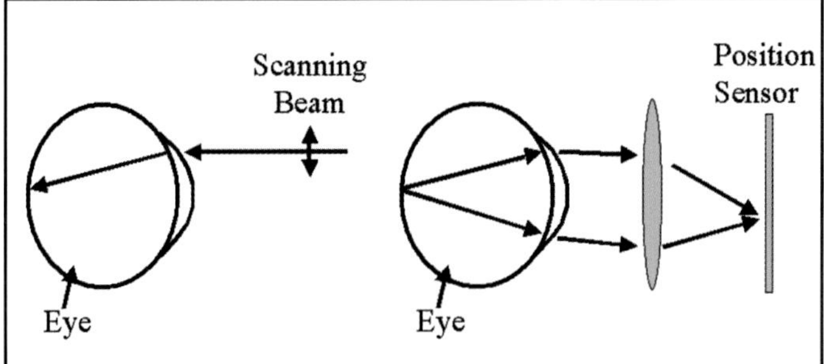

Figure 9-5. A retinal ray tracing aberrometer. A scanning beam probes different portions of the pupil. The positions at which these beams strike the retina are recorded and used to reconstruct the wavefront.

aliased. Spectral aliasing can occur because these devices typically operate at a single wavelength. Any variation in the aberration structure with wavelength will therefore be nonmeasurable. Finally, temporal aliasing can occur if the fluctuation in the aberration structure varies over the time period of the measurement. The different techniques for measuring aberrations have their intrinsic limitations on sampling density and these will be described in some detail below.

Shack-Hartmann wavefront sensing is a technique in which the wavefront emanating from the entrance pupil of the eye is superimposed onto a lenslet array.[2,3] These lenslets are typically set in a rectangular array. Each lenslet samples the wavefront falling onto its aperture and focuses the local section of wavefront to a point. Deviations in the locations of these focus points are related to the aberrations in the wavefront. Figure 9-3 shows an example of the lenslet sampling. Typical lenslet spacing (sampling spacing) for commercially available devices is 200 to 600 microns (µm).[4] These commercial devices also typically operate in the near infrared to allow for natural dilation of the pupil. Measurement time for these types of systems is typically 30 ms or a single video frame, although multiple images are sometimes captured and averaged or integrated to reduce noise.

> Over a 6 millimeter (mm) circular pupil, a rectilinear lenslet array with a lenslet spacing of 200 and 600 µm would have approximately 640 and 55 lenslets fully filled, respectively.

Tscherning aberrometry is a technique where a grid mask is used to generate multiple parallel beams entering the eye at different locations.[5,6] The grid pattern is typically rectangular with a central point missing to avoid corneal back-reflections. An aberroscope lens is used to force the beams to focus in front of the retina and then diverge again prior to striking the retina. A photograph, the grid pattern on the retina, is then captured and analyzed to extract aberration information. Each individual beam samples the optics of the eye through the local region it passes through on its journey to the retina. Aberrations will affect the path of each beam and ultimately distort the retinal grid pattern. Figure 9-4 illustrates the sampling of the Tscherning device. The sample spacing for the commercially available version of this device is 769 mm, and measurements are made at a wavelength of 532 nanometers (nm), with a total acquisition time of 40 ms.[7]

Retinal ray tracing measures the slope of beams of light entering the eye at different locations are generated in series, instead of in parallel.[8,9] In other words, retinal ray tracing probes the aberrations of the eye one beam at a time and measures the deviation in the position at which the beam strikes the retina from a reference chief ray. The beam is typically scanned in a polar grid, entering the eye at 64 different locations. Figure 9-5 illustrates retinal ray tracing. Commercially, the spacing between samples in the radial direction is 330 to 890 µm for pupils ranging from 3 mm to 8 mm. The total acquisition time is less than 50 ms, and the operating wavelength is 650 nm. The sample spacing and number of samples are adjustable. However, higher resolution measurements require longer measurement times.

Spatially-resolved refractometry is another ray tracing technique.[10,11] Individual beams of light are again used to probe different locations in the pupil. In this case, however, the subject adjusts the angle at which the beam enters the eye to force it to coincide with a reference chief ray striking the fovea. Figure 9-6 shows the setup for the spatially-resolved refractometer. Typical sample spacing for this device is 857 µm and a wavelength of 543 nm is typically used.[12] A series of wavelengths from 460 nm to 650 nm have been used with this device to explore the effects of chromatic aberration in the eye.[13] The measurement time for this type of system is usually several minutes because it requires feedback from the subject.

The Shack-Hartmann and Tscherning systems are inherently prone to spatial aliasing. This is because they measure different entry points within the pupil simultaneously. There is, therefore,

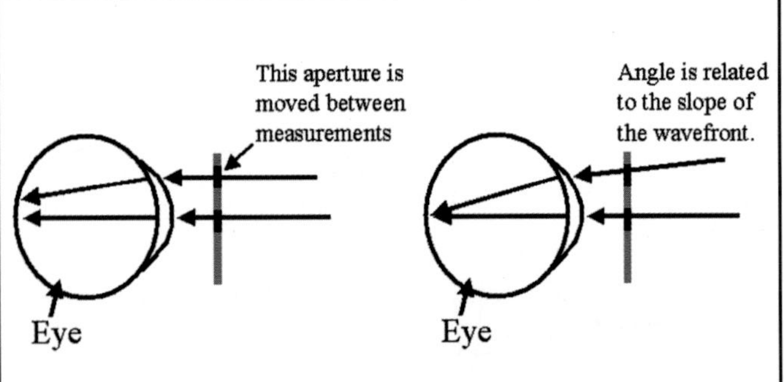
This aperture is moved between measurements
Angle is related to the slope of the wavefront.
Eye
Eye

Figure 9-6. A Spatially-Resolved Refractometer. A psychophysical test in which the subject simultaneously views two beams entering the eye. The subject adjusts the incident angle of one beam to make the beams coincide on the retina. The process is repeated for multiple pupil locations.

a limit to how closely spaced the lenslets or grid mask apertures can be made, while maintaining the ability to distinguish the individual points in their respective grid images. Based on the commercially available system, wavefronts with features smaller than 1 to 2 mm will probably give inaccurate or aliased results. Thus, features like central islands following refractive surgery as well as power changes from bifocal contact and intraocular lenses (IOLs) are not likely to be adequately measured with these systems. The Shack-Hartmann and Tscherning systems are not likely to suffer from temporal aliasing since they capture a single video frame. Small fluctuations in the aberration structure that occur at a rate faster than the video frame rate are unlikely to cause any foveal visual effects since the visual system does not respond at this frequency.

The current implementations of the retinal ray tracing and spatially-resolved refractometer systems have similar spatial sampling resolution as the Shack-Hartmann and Tscherning systems. They therefore will have similar limitations on the aberration structures they can measure. However, since these systems measure aberrations at sequential locations in the pupil, they can in theory provide a much higher resolution sampling of the wavefront error. The drawback to this increased resolution is an increase in measurement time. Longer measurement times increase the risk of temporal aliasing in these systems. Fluctuations in the aberration structure due to eye movements, ocular pulse, and accommodation changes can affect the measurements at longer acquisition times.[14]

Wavefront Reconstruction

In general, aberrometry measures the slope of the wavefront in the eye. The Shack-Hartmann and spatially-resolved refractometry techniques measure wavefront slope directly and the Tscherning and retinal ray tracing techniques measure the transverse ray error, which is proportional to wavefront slope. The slope measurements are the local tilt of the wavefront and can be in both the horizontal and vertical directions. For a wavefront error given by W(x,y), aberrometers give a set of slope measurements $\{dW(x_i,y_i)/dx\}$ and $\{dW(x_i,y_i)/dy\}$. The value of i ranges from 1 to the total number of sample points, N. The points (x_i,y_i) represent the locations within the pupil of the individual samples. The most common method of reconstructing the wavefront error is fitting the data to a set of polynomials $\{V_j\}$ with a least squares technique, where j ranges from unity to the total number of polynomials in the fitting set, J. Typically, the polynomial set for wavefront fitting has been either the Zernike polynomials or the Taylor polynomials. These sets have traditionally been chosen because they have properties that represent familiar concepts in ophthalmic optics. However, other polynomial sets can also be used. The least squares technique minimizes the absolute error between the sampled points and the reconstructed wavefront. To perform this fit, a matrix equation is set up, such that:

$$\overleftrightarrow{V}\,\vec{a} = \overleftrightarrow{W}, \tag{1}$$

where

$$\overleftrightarrow{V} = \begin{bmatrix} dV_1(x_1,y_1)/dx \ldots & dV^2(x_1,y_1)/dx & \ldots & dV_J(x_1,y_1)/dx \\ dV_1(x_2,y_2)/dx \ldots & dV_2(x_2,y2)/dx & \ldots & dV^J(x_2,y_2)/dx \\ \vdots & \vdots & \vdots & \vdots \\ dV_1(x_N,y_N)/dx \ldots & dV_2(x_N,y_N)/dx & \ldots & dV_J(x_N,y_N)/dx \\ dV_1(x_1,y_1)/dy \ldots & dV_2(x_1,y_1)/dy & \ldots & dV_J(x_1,y_1)/dy \\ dV_1(x_2,y_2)/dy \ldots & dV_2(x_2,y_2)/dy & \ldots & dVJ(x_2,y_2)/dy \\ \vdots & \vdots & \vdots & \vdots \\ dV_1(x_N,y_N)/dy \ldots & dV_2(x_N,y_N)/dy & \ldots & dV_J(x_N,y_N)/dy \end{bmatrix} \tag{2}$$

$$\vec{a} = \begin{bmatrix} a_1 \\ a_2 \\ \vdots \\ a_J \end{bmatrix} \tag{3}$$

$$\overleftrightarrow{W} = \begin{bmatrix} dW(x_1,y_1)/dx \\ dW(x_2,y_2)/dx \\ \vdots \\ dW(x_N,y_N)/dx \\ dW(x_1,y_1)/dy \\ dW(x_2,y_2)/dy \\ \vdots \\ dW(x_N,y_N)/dy \end{bmatrix} \tag{4}$$

Essentially, the $\overleftrightarrow{V}$ matrix contains slope information for the fitting polynomials. The top half of the matrix is the x derivative of the fitting polynomials and the lower half is the y derivative of the fitting functions. Each row in the matrix is for a given sample point (x_i,y_i). Each column in this $\overleftrightarrow{V}$ matrix is for a different fitting polynomial V_j. The $\vec{a}$ vector is a series of weighting coefficients that describes how much of each fitting polynomial contributes to the reconstructed wavefront. The $\overleftrightarrow{W}$ matrix contains the data measured from the aberrometer. The upper half of this matrix contains the x derivative information, while the lower half of the matrix describes the y derivative data. Each row in the $\overleftrightarrow{W}$ matrix is for a different sample point (x_i,y_i). The goal of the reconstruction is to determine the values of the coefficients in the $\vec{a}$ vector. Since there are usually many more sample points (N) than there are polynomials (J) to fit the wavefront, an exact solution to equation 1 cannot be obtained. Instead, a least squares solution is calculated. The solution is given by:

$$\vec{a} = \left[\overleftrightarrow{V}^T\overleftrightarrow{V}\right]^{-1}\overleftrightarrow{V}^T\overleftrightarrow{W} \tag{5}$$

where $\overleftrightarrow{V}^T$ is the transpose of $\overleftrightarrow{V}$, and []-1 is the inverse matrix operation. Equation 5 allows for the calculation of the fitting coefficients. The final reconstructed wavefront W(x,y) is then given by:

$$W(x,y) = \sum_{j=1}^{J} a_j V_j(x,y) \tag{6}$$

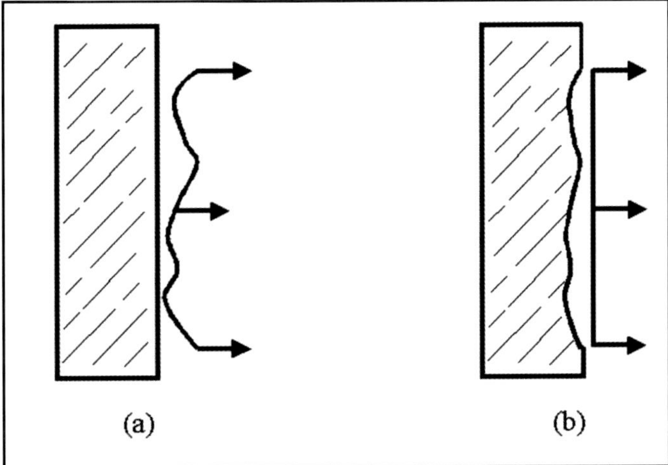

Figure 9-7. Thin phase plate model. (A) An aberrated wavefront exiting a slab of material. (B) The slab is modified to let lagging portions of the wavefront catch up to accelerated portions.

Thus, once the slope information is obtained from the aberrometer, straightforward matrix calculations are all that are required to reconstruct the wavefront.

Correction Creation

Once the wavefront error has been reconstructed from the aberrometry data, a correction for this error needs to be determined. In the corneal plane, this correction can then be imparted to either the cornea in a custom refractive surgery procedure or to the front of a contact lens in a custom lens application. The simplest model for calculating the required correction is the thin phase plate model.[15] Figure 9-7A shows an aberrated wavefront at the interface of a slab of material of index of refraction n. Portions of the aberrated wavefront are accelerated (ahead of the ideal planar wavefront), while other portions are retarded (lag behind the ideal). The goal of the custom correction is to modify the aberrated wavefront into the ideal wavefront. To accomplish this, the accelerated portion of the aberrated wavefront needs to be slowed down, while the lagging portion of the aberrated wavefront needs to be sped up. In customized techniques where tissue or lens material is being removed, only the lagging portions of the wavefront can be sped up relative to the accelerated portion of the wavefront. This speeding up is accomplished by forcing the lagging portions of the wavefront to pass through less material than the accelerated portions of the wavefront. Figure 9-7B shows the modification to the surface of the interface that is required to correct the aberrated wavefront. In general, if the wavefront error is given by W(x,y) (ie, the difference in the shapes of the ideal and aberrated wavefronts), then the thickness t(x,y) of the material that needs to be removed is given by:

$$t(x,y) = (n - 1)\, W(x,y) \qquad (7)$$

> The simplest model for calculating the required correction is the thin phase plate model.[15]

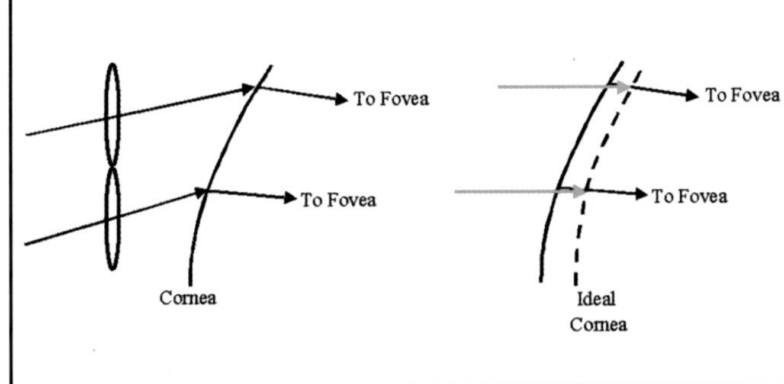

Figure 9-8. Backward ray tracing model. Light is traced backward through the lenslets of a Shack-Hartmann aberrometer. The intersection of these rays with the cornea is determined. The ideal cornea refracts collimated light so that the rays follow the same path as the refracted rays in the aberrated cornea.

For custom refractive surgery procedures, the index of refraction, *n*, will be the index of the cornea. For custom contact lens applications, the index *n* will be the index of refraction of the contact lens material. The thin phase plate model assumes that the refraction that occurs at the interface is negligible. This assumption is reasonable for small levels of wavefront error, but will break down for more substantial aberrations levels. Another assumption of this model is that the thickness in equation 7 can be draped over the curved surface of the cornea or a contact lens. Again, this approximation is reasonable for small aberrations but is inaccurate for larger aberrations.

> The thin phase plate model assumes that the refraction that occurs at the interface is negligible.

Klein[16] demonstrated a backward ray tracing technique for calculation of the ablation pattern required to correct an aberrated Shack-Hartmann measurement. This technique can also be used to design custom contact lenses. In Shack-Hartmann aberrometry, a spot of light is placed on the fovea. This light scatters from the retina and emanates out of the eye. The light is captured by a lenslet array and each individual lenslet focuses the locally sampled wavefront down to a point. The path of the rays of light in this setup can be reversed and traversed backward. In other words, a ray starting from the lenslet focal spot traced back through the appropriate lenslet will ultimately strike the fovea. This concept is employed to determine the required corneal ablation. Figure 9-8 shows a Shack-Hartmann lenslet array near an eye. If a ray is traced from the focal spot backward through the lenslet, an intersection between the ray and the cornea can be determined. By knowing the slope of the cornea at this intersection point, the ray can be refracted via Snell's law as it passes through the cornea. As stated earlier, this same ray will continue through the various ocular elements and ultimately strike the fovea. To calculate the required ablation pattern, the new cornea must refract a ray from infinity such that it follows the path of the original refracted ray. To accomplish this modification, both the slope and the depth of the surface may be modified, and a continuum of possible combinations of slope and depth exist.

However, in going from lenslet to lenslet, a unique, contiguous surface can be created that represents the final corneal shape. The difference between the original corneal surface and this new shape is the amount of tissue that needs to be removed.

Conclusion

Customized laser treatment and contact lenses represent an advance in the treatment of ocular aberrations. The potential for improvement of vision based on these technologies is large. In order to accomplish such corrections, three stages are necessary. The first stage is to accurately measure the shape of the wavefront aberration in the eye. As shown here, adequate sampling of the wavefront error is required for accurate results. If the wavefront error is inadequately sampled, then aliasing will occur and treatments will be based on false data. The current limitation based on commercial aberrometers is to treat aberration structures no smaller than roughly 1 to 2 mm in lateral dimension. The second stage is to reconstruct the wavefront based on aberrometer data. A least squares technique has been shown to perform this task. In performing least squares fit, there is always a danger of either using too many or not enough fitting polynomials. If too many fitting polynomials are used, then the reconstructed wavefront begins fitting the measurement noise and artificial wiggles will appear in the reconstruction. If too few polynomials are used to fit the data, then a poor and inaccurate fit will result. Somewhere between 15 and 36 (fourth to sixth order) Zernike polynomials are sufficient to fit wavefront errors found in the normal human eye. The final stage is to convert the wavefront error data into a treatment pattern. For small aberrations, the thin phase plate model, where the ablation pattern is directly proportional to the wavefront error, simplifies the process. In cases where aberrations are larger, a reverse ray tracing technique can be used to determine the appropriate wavefront correction.

The potential for improvement of vision based on these technologies is large.

References

1. Gaskill JD. *Linear Systems, Fourier Transforms, and Optics*. New York, NY: John Wiley & Sons; 1978.
2. Shack RV, Platt BC. Production and use of a lenticular Hartmann screen. *J Opt Soc Am A*. 1971;61:656.
3. Liang J, Grimm W, Geolz S, Bille JF. Objective measurement of the wave aberrations of the human eye using Shack-Hartmann wavefront sensor. *J Opt Soc Am A*. 1994;11:1949-1957.
4. Pettit GH. How Alcon/Summit/Autonomous answers six important questions about their customized laser platform. *J Refract Surg*. 2001;17:S613-S615.
5. Tscherning M. Die monochromatischen aberrationen des menschlichen auges. *Z Psychol Physiol Sinne*. 1894;6:456-471.
6. Mrochen M, Kaemmerer M, Mierdel P, Krinke HE, Seiler T. Principles of Tscherning aberrometry. *J Refract Surg*. 2000;16:S570-S571.
7. Mrochen M, Kaemmerer M, Mierdel P, Seiler T. Wavefront-guided LASIK using a Tscherning wavefront analyzer. In: MacRae SM, Krueger RR, Applegate RA, eds. *Customized Corneal Ablation: The Quest for Super Vision*. Thorofare, NJ: SLACK Incorporated; 2001: 185-191.
8. Molebny VV, Pallikaris IG, Naoumidis LP, Chyzh IH, Molebny SV, Sokurenko VM. Retinal ray tracing technique for eye refraction mapping. *Proc SPIE*. 1997;2971:175-183.
9. Molebny VV, Panagopoulou SI, Molebny SV, Wakil YS, Pallikaris IG. Principles of ray tracing aberrometry. *J Refract Surg*. 2000;16:S572-S575.
10. Smirnov HS. Measurement of the wave aberration in the human eye. *Biophys*. 1961;6:52-66.
11. Webb RH, Penny CM, Thompson K. Measurement of the ocular local wavefront distortion with a spatially resolved refractometer. *Appl Opt*. 1992;31:3678-3686.
12. He JC, Marcos S, Webb RH, Burns SA. Measurement of the wavefront aberration of the eye by a fast psychophysical procedure. *J Opt Soc Am A*. 1998;15:2449-2456.
13. Marcos S, Burns SA, Moreno-Barriuso E, Navarro R. A new approach to the study of ocular chromatic aberrations. *Vision Res*. 1999;39:4309-4323.
14. Hofer H, Artal P, Singer B, Aragon JL, Williams DR. Dynamics of the eye's wave aberration. *J Opt Soc Am A*. 2001;18:497-506.
15. Goodman JW. *Introduction to Fourier Optics*. New York, NY: McGraw-Hill; 1968.
16. Klein SA. Optimal corneal ablation for eyes with arbitrary Hartmann-Shack aberrations. *J Opt Soc Am A*. 1998;15:2580-2588.

Chapter 10

Chromatic Aberration and Its Impact on Vision

Larry N. Thibos, PhD and Arthur Bradley, PhD

Three Aspects of Ocular Chromatic Aberration

The human eye suffers from significant amounts of chromatic aberration caused by chromatic dispersion, which is caused by the variation of refractive index n of the eye's refractive media with wavelength λ. Chromatic dispersion causes the focus, size, and position of retinal images to vary with wavelength as illustrated in Figure 10-1. Variation in the focusing power of the eye with wavelength is called *longitudinal* (or *axial*) *chromatic aberration* (LCA) and is measured in diopters. In effect, the eye's far-point varies with wavelength, which means that only one wavelength of light emitted by a point source can be well-focused on the retina at any moment in time. Retinal image size for extended objects also varies with wavelength, which is called *chromatic difference of magnification* (CDM) and is specified as a fractional change. For any given point on an extended object, the position of the image on the retina varies with wavelength. This phenomenon is called *transverse* (or *lateral*) *chromatic aberration* (TCA) and is specified as a visual angle subtended at the nodal point, N.

> Chromatic dispersion causes the focus, size, and position of retinal images to vary with wavelength.

> In general, the shorter the wavelength, the slower light travels in an optical medium. Consequently, the refractive index varies with wavelength. Refractive index is defined as:
>
> $$n = \frac{c}{v}$$
>
> where c is the speed of light in a vacuum and v is the speed of light for a particular wavelength of light in the optical media of interest. Using Snell's law, n sin i = nλ 'sin iλ', we can see that for a fixed angle of incidence (i) of white light at an optical interface for each wavelength, the angle of refraction will vary with wavelength, causing the white light to be dispersed.

Approximate relationships between the three aspects of chromatic aberration illustrated in Figure 10-1 can be derived from a reduced-eye model that represents the eye's complicated optical system with a single refracting surface separating air from the watery ocular medium.[1] For this simplified model, called the Indiana Eye, the longitudinal chromatic aberration is due entirely to the variation in optical power with wavelength of the refracting surface. LCA is calculated as:

$$LCA = DFocus = K_\lambda = \frac{n(\lambda_1) - n(\lambda_2)}{rn_0} \qquad (1)$$

where r is the apical radius of curvature of the model's surface and n_0 is the refractive index for the in-focus reference wavelength.

> Nodal points in an optical system are important because incoming light directed toward the primary nodal point leaves the secondary nodal point undeviated (having the same angle as the incoming light).

The fractional change of magnification with wavelength for extended objects (see Figure 10-1B) is directly proportional to chromatic difference in focus:

$$CDM = \Delta\ Magnification = zK_\lambda \qquad (2)$$

where the constant of proportionality z is the axial separation between the eye's entrance pupil and the eye's nodal point.[2] Equation 2 implies that retinal image size would be the same for all wavelengths if the eye's pupil were centered on the eye's nodal point. The explanation for this special case is that the chief ray for every wavelength emitted by any point on the object would pass through the nodal point (and, therefore, would be undeviated) and would intersect the retina at the same location.

> The entrance pupil is the image of the limiting aperture as seen from object space (ie, from the incoming side of the optical system).

The TCA of the eye is defined only for point objects and depends on the location of the point in the visual field (see Figure 10-1C):

$$TCA = \Delta\ Position = \tau = K_\lambda z \sin\omega \qquad (3)$$

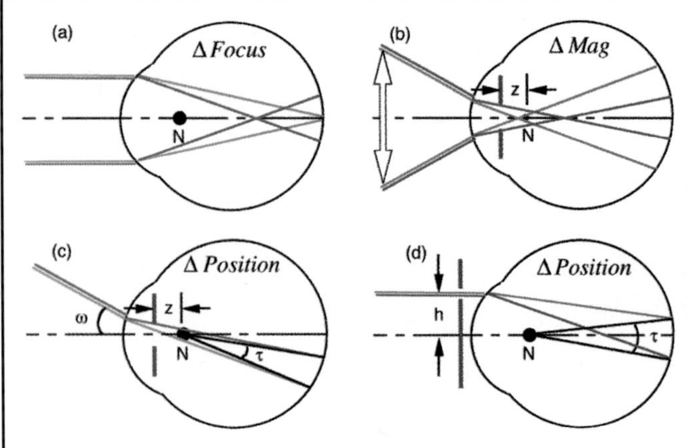

Figure 10-1. Ocular chromatic aberration takes the form of chromatic difference of focus (A), magnification (B), or position (C, D). Short-wavelength rays are shown in blue, long-wavelength rays are in red. (Adapted from Thibos LN. Formation and sampling of the retinal image. In: De Valois K, ed. *Seeing Handbook of Perception and Cognition.* London: Academic Press; 2000:1-54.)

where ω is the field angle of the object point relative to the eye's achromatic axis. The achromatic axis connects the nodal point with the center of the pupil and represents the path rays must follow if they are to avoid the effects of chromatic dispersion. A ray following the achromatic axis is a chief ray (because it passes through the pupil center) and therefore locates the center of the retinal image even if the image is blurred by LCA. Such a ray is also undeviated (because it passes through the nodal point) and therefore has zero transverse chromatic aberration, as indicated by equation 3 when $\omega = 0$. Notice that for small field angles, $\sin \omega = \omega$ and the ratio τ/ω by equation 3 is the same as CDM by equation 2. In other words, chromatic difference of magnification is equal to the rate of change of TCA with field angle.

The *chief ray* is the ray of light from an object point directed toward the center of the entrance pupil.

Field angle is the angle defined by the achromatic axis of the system and the line connecting an off-axis point with the center of the entrance pupil.

Although central vision may be spared the effects of TCA in the naked eye, the fovea becomes highly vulnerable when viewing through an optical instrument or an artificial pupil located in front of the eye. This situation is depicted in Figure 10-1D. If the limiting aperture is displaced by amount *h* from the visual axis (defined as the line containing the fovea, nodal point, and fixation point), then the magnitude of TCA present at the fovea is given by the approximate formula:

$$TCA = \Delta\ Position = \tau h K_{\lambda} \qquad (4)$$

Although central vision may be spared the effects of TCA in the naked eye, the fovea becomes highly vulnerable when viewing through an optical instrument or an artificial pupil located in front of the eye.

Comparing equations 3 and 4 indicates that each millimeter of displacement of the entrance pupil is equivalent to 15 degrees of eccentricity in the visual field, in the sense that they both generate the same amount of TCA.

The angular diameter of a blur circle (in radians) is the product of pupil diameter (in meters) and refractive error (in diopters).

A simulation of the combined effects of LCA and TCA on the foveal image of a point source of light is shown in Figure 10-2. For simplicity, we assume the source contains just three wavelengths of light. Each monochromatic component of the source forms a blur circle that is more or less out-of-focus. To first approximation, the diameter of the blur circle expressed as a visual angle (in radians) is the product of pupil diameter (in meters) and refractive error (in diopters). Since refractive error varies with wavelength according to equation 1, so will the size of the blurred retinal image. Two cases are illustrated. In the top row of images, the pupil is assumed to be well-centered on the visual axis so that TCA = 0 and the various blur circles are concentric. Notice how the dark gaps in the image for one wavelength tend to be filled in by light from a different wavelength. This tendency has two effects. First, the composite image has distinctly different colored-bands. Second, the luminance of the composite image is smoother than any of its monochromatic components. The bottom row of Figure 10-2 is the more general case in which the eye's pupil is displaced from the visual axis. Pupil displacement induces TCA that causes the colored blur circles to spread across the retina by an amount specified by equation 3. Superimposing these displaced, blurred images yields a complicated distribution of light intensity with multi-colored fringes.

Pupil displacement induces TCA that causes the colored blur circles to spread across the retina like a rainbow.

The Magnitude of Ocular Chromatic Aberration in Human Eyes

The variation of focal power of the eye with wavelength has been widely studied in human eyes, and the results are summarized in Figure 10-3. Various symbols show the refractive error measured in human eyes in 13 different studies over the past 50 years using a wide variety of experimental methods.[1] The sign convention is best illustrated by example: the human eye has too much power (ie, is myopic) for short wavelengths, and so a negative spectacle lens is required to correct this focusing error. The good agreement between these various studies is testimony to

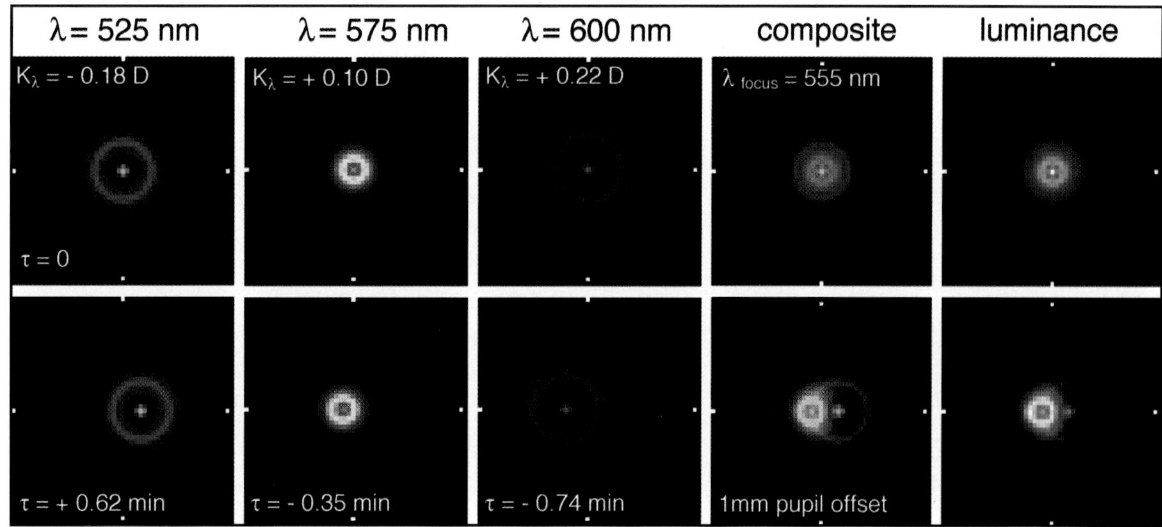

Figure 10-2. Image formation for a polychromatic source in the presence of chromatic aberration. Top row is for an eye with LCA only. Bottom row is for an eye with LCA and TCA produced by 1 millimeter (mm) of horizontal pupil offset from the visual axis (or, equivalently, 15 deg of eccentricity). Point source emits three wavelengths of light (500 nm, 575 nm, 600 nm) and the eye is assumed to be focused for 550 nm. Chromatic errors of focus and position indicated for each image are derived from the analysis of the Indiana Eye model of chromatic aberration shown in Figure 10-1. Monochromatic images in the top row are well centered on the origin (coordinate axes are indicated by the small white dots at the edge of each image) and therefore are concentric when superimposed to form the composite, polychromatic image. Images in the bottom row are displaced horizontally and therefore are not concentric when superimposed. Colored images are rendered with a hue that is indicative of the corresponding wavelength. Luminance image shows only the luminance component of the colored image. Luminances of the three monochromatic images are not to scale.

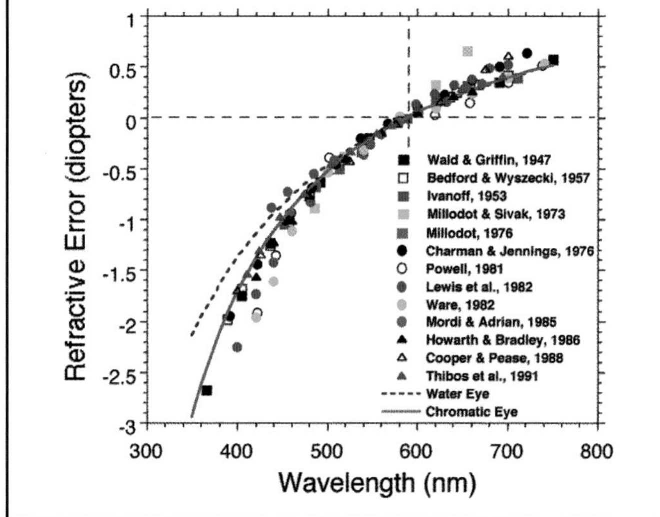

Figure 10-3. Comparison of published measurements of ocular chromatic aberration. Data were put on a common basis by translating data points vertically until the refractive error was zero at the reference wavelength (589 nm). (Adapted from Thibos LN, Ye M, Zhang X, Bradley A. The chromatic eye: a new reduced-eye model of ocular chromatic aberration in humans. *Appl Opt.* 1992;31: 3594-3600.)

the fact that, unlike the monochromatic aberrations of the eye, there is little variability between individuals with regard to LCA. Likewise, LCA does not change significantly over the life span.[3]

As predicted by analysis of the reduced eye (equation 2), the chromatic difference of magnification is strongly affected by axial pupil location. As the separation of entrance pupil from nodal point increases, the rays admitted by the pupil from an eccentric point of the object will enter the eye with greater angle of incidence. Consequently, these rays will be subjected to stronger chromatic dispersion and a larger CDM. Measurements indicate that the difference in retinal image size is less than 1% for the natural eye but can increase significantly when viewing through an artificial pupil placed in front of the eye, as may occur with some clinical instruments.[4]

Examples of instruments that can amplify CDM include ophthalmoscopes, slit-lamp microscopes, and fundus cameras.

Since the magnitude of TCA depends on the field angle of the object (equation 3), it is different for every point in the visual field. Unfortunately, the poor spatial resolution of the peripheral retina hampers the subjective measurement of TCA, and objective methods have not been widely used. Consequently, detailed information is available only for foveal vision.[5-7] A statistical study of young adult eyes found that foveal TCA is randomly distributed about a mean value of zero, which indicates that on average the pupil tends to be centered on the visual axis.[8] This remarkable result suggests that human eyes have evolved, or responded, to some active process, such that retinal image quality is maximized at that singular location where it will do the most good: the fovea. Although positive and negative aberration values tend to cancel when averaged across the population, TCA is rarely zero for any given eye as shown in Figure 10-4. This frequency distribution documents the proportion of eyes with different magnitude of TCA. It is well described by a theoretical Rayleigh distribution derived under the assumption that the two-dimensional distribution of TCA is normally distributed

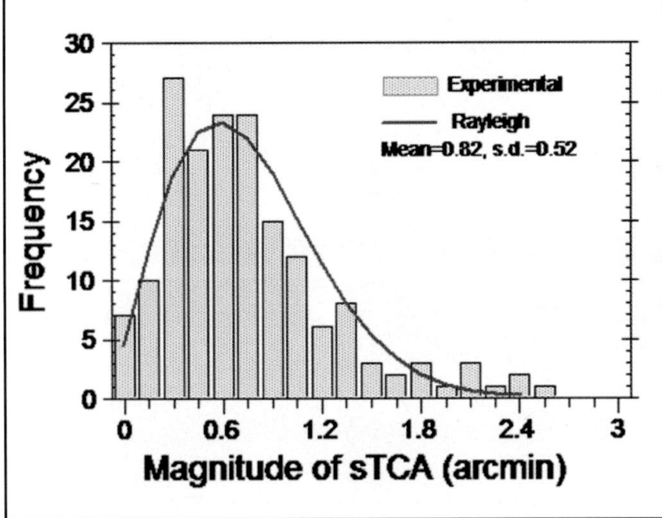

Figure 10-4. Frequency distribution (N = 170 eyes) of the magnitude of TCA measured subjectively for the red and blue light emitted by a typical computer monitor (mean wavelengths 605 nm and 497 nm, respectively). (Adapted from Rynders MC, Lidkea BA, Chisholm WJ, Thibos LN. Statistical distribution of foveal transverse chromatic aberration, pupil centration, and angle psi in a population of young adult eyes. *J Opt Soc Am A.* 1995;12:2348-2357.)

about zero. The mean magnitude of foveal TCA for the red and blue light produced by a color computer monitor was 0.82 arcmin of visual angle, which is slightly less than the width of individual strokes in a 20/20 letter of a visual acuity chart.

> Human eyes have evolved, or have responded, to some active process, such that retinal image quality is maximized at that singular location where it will do the most good: the fovea.

Visual Impact of Chromatic Differences of Focus

At first glance, the more than 2 diopter (D) range of LCA indicated by Figure 10-3 would seem to be a major problem. In clinical terms, 2 D of uncorrected refractive error would be a serious visual handicap. However, the situation is not as bad as it seems. If the eye accommodates so that a wavelength in the middle of the spectrum is well-focused, then the range of refractive error is effectively halved to ±1 D. Then, recalling that the extremes of the visible spectrum have less luminosity, we realize that the greatest amount of chromatic defocus will affect those wavelengths that are least visible. Indeed, when the peak of the luminance spectrum is in focus, most of the light is only slightly defocused.[9] When all the images of different wavelengths are superimposed to form a composite retinal image, visibility of the target will be dominated by wavelengths that are only slightly defocused. Quantitative development of this argument indicates that the effect of LCA on image contrast is roughly equivalent to about 0.20 D of defocus.[10] Visually, this is a relatively minor amount of defocus that is comparable in magnitude to the depth of focus of the human eye or to the residual refractive error expected after routine spectacle correction. Thus, it is not surprising that contrast sensitivity for white and for monochromatic lights over a 10 to 40 cycles per degree (c/deg) range of spatial frequencies differ by less than 0.2 log units.[11] Furthermore, because the neural contrast threshold rises steeply at high spatial frequencies,[12] large losses of image contrast have relatively little effect on visual acuity. Consequently, visual acuity for polychromatic grating stimuli is only 5% less than acuity for monochromatic gratings.[11]

> The greatest amount of chromatic defocus will affect those wavelengths that are least visible.

Visual Impact of Chromatic Difference of Magnification

Theory predicts that CDM is less than 1%, a value generally believed to be insignificant for monocular vision. However, even this small amount of magnification difference can have dramatic effects on depth perception if one eye is viewing short wavelength light while the other eye is viewing long wavelength light. Depending on the nature of the visual target, the visual system may interpret the different sized retinal images as a difference in relative depth, resulting in a distorted perception of the three-dimensional world. Experimental measurements of this perceptual distortion have been used to measure CDM psychophysically.[4] The results indicated large individual differences between eyes but confirmed that the value is typically less than 1%. By repeating the measurements for a range of z-axis locations of an artificial pupil, those experiments also confirmed the linear relationship embodied in equation 2. This latter result emphasizes the importance of axial separation between aperture and nodal point. Any optical or clinical instrument that moves the entrance aperture outside the eye has the potential to greatly amplify the eye's chromatic magnification differences and to introduce correspondingly large amounts of spatial distortion. This has potential implications for vision through differently colored spectacles or contact lenses that are sometimes prescribed for people with anomalous color vision.[13]

> Any optical or clinical instrument that moves the entrance aperture outside the eye has the potential to greatly amplify the eye's chromatic magnification differences and to introduce correspondingly large amounts of spatial distortion.

Impact of Chromatic Difference of Position

The visual impact of TCA is understood best for grating objects viewed under two different but equivalent conditions: when viewing an eccentric target through a pupil centered on the visual axis or when viewing a foveal target through a displaced pupil. Fourier optics theory tells us that any visual target may be decomposed into a multitude of sinusoidal gratings, each of a different wavelength, luminance, contrast, spatial frequency, phase, and orientation.[14] The only effect of a shift in image position on these elemental gratings due to TCA will be to alter spa-

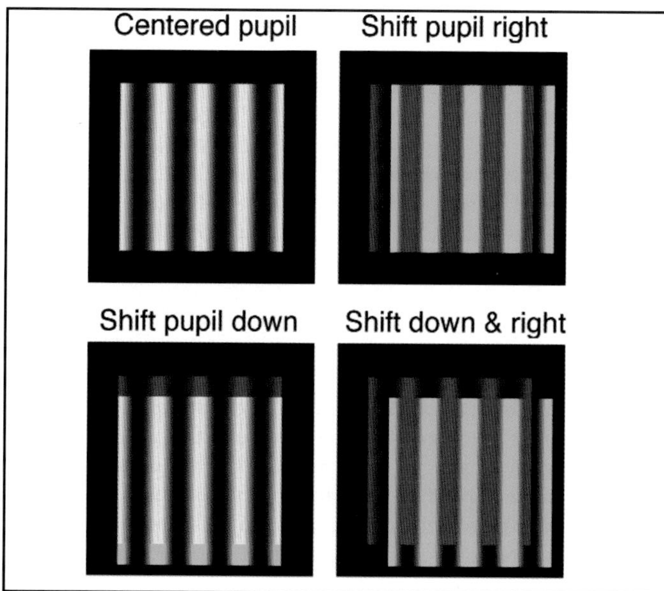

Figure 10-5. Simulation of the effect of TCA induced by pupil decentration on the retinal image of a polychromatic grating containing two wavelengths of light.

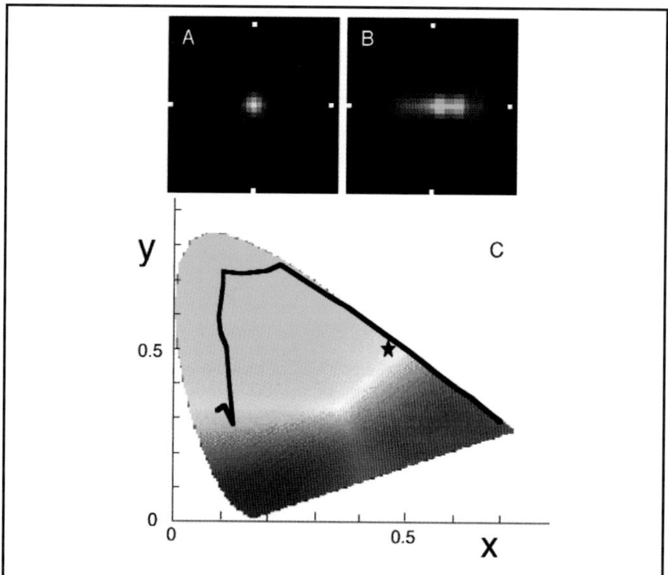

Figure 10-6. Effect of chromatic aberration on the image of a white point of light with equal-energy spectrum. Foveal retinal image was computed for normal amount of LCA assuming a 3 mm pupil is either well-centered on the visual axis (panel A) or displaced horizontally by 2 mm (panel B). Color artifacts present in a horizontal trace through the middle of the images in panels A and B are specified in CIE chromaticity coordinates in panel C by the star symbol and black line, respectively. Wavelength-in-focus = 570 nm.

tial phase, with all other attributes unchanged. The amount of phase shift produced by a given amount of image displacement depends on the orientation and frequency of the grating. Maximum phase shift occurs when high-frequency gratings are oriented perpendicular to the direction of displacement of the image, as illustrated in Figure 10-5. Zero phase shift occurs when the grating is parallel to the direction of displacement.

There are several ways in which chromatic phase shifts could affect visual performance. For example, judgments of hue, saturation, or brightness could each be affected by differential smearing of the spectrum. Perhaps the most important consequence of TCA is that phase shifts can destroy luminance contrast in the image. For example, if two chromatic components of a white sinusoidal grating have the same contrast and mean luminance but are shifted by 180 degrees, they would completely cancel each other out, leaving zero luminance contrast. This is the case depicted in the top right panel of Figure 10-5. In addition to the loss of luminance contrast, the misregistration of the red and green images induces obvious color artifacts.

Perhaps the most important consequence of TCA is that phase shifts can destroy luminance contrast in the image.

Combined Impact of Longitudinal and Transverse Chromatic Aberration

The intersection of the eye's achromatic axis with the retina is the only location of the retinal image that is always free of the transverse effects of chromatic aberration. Fortunately, this singular location is typically close to the fovea in most eyes.[8] All other points in the retinal image will suffer from the combined effects of LCA and TCA. These individual and combined effects are illustrated in Figure 10-6. The colored image shown in Figure 10-6A was computed for a point source of white light with equal energy spectrum sampled every 20 nm, viewed through a 3 mm pupil by an eye suffering only from LCA. The compact, radial symmetry of this image is due to the lack of TCA. The image shown in Figure 10-6B is for the same conditions except the pupil is displaced 2 mm horizontally from the visual axis. A large amount of TCA results from the pupil displacement, causing the image to be spread out horizontally like a tiny rainbow. The center of the rainbow is well focused for the emmetropic wavelength, but the ends are blurred by the myopic and hyperopic defocus of LCA. These color artifacts can be quantified by plotting the chromaticity coordinates of a horizontal trace through the images, as shown in Figure 10-6C. The result is a trajectory (marked by the heavy dark curve) through the diagram from the left (red) side of the point image in B to the right (blue) side of the point image. In the middle of this trajectory lies the chromaticity for image A, indicated by a star in the diagram. The chromaticity diagram in C documents major artifacts of hue and saturation caused by ocular chromatic aberration. Luminance artifacts are not shown in the chromaticity diagram, but are typically quantified in the spatial frequency domain of grating objects as described next.[15]

The intersection of the eye's achromatic axis with the retina is the only location of the retinal image that is always free of the transverse effects of chromatic aberration.

The impact of chromatic aberration on luminance of the retinal image is quantified in the spatial frequency domain by computing the Fourier transform of the luminance component of the

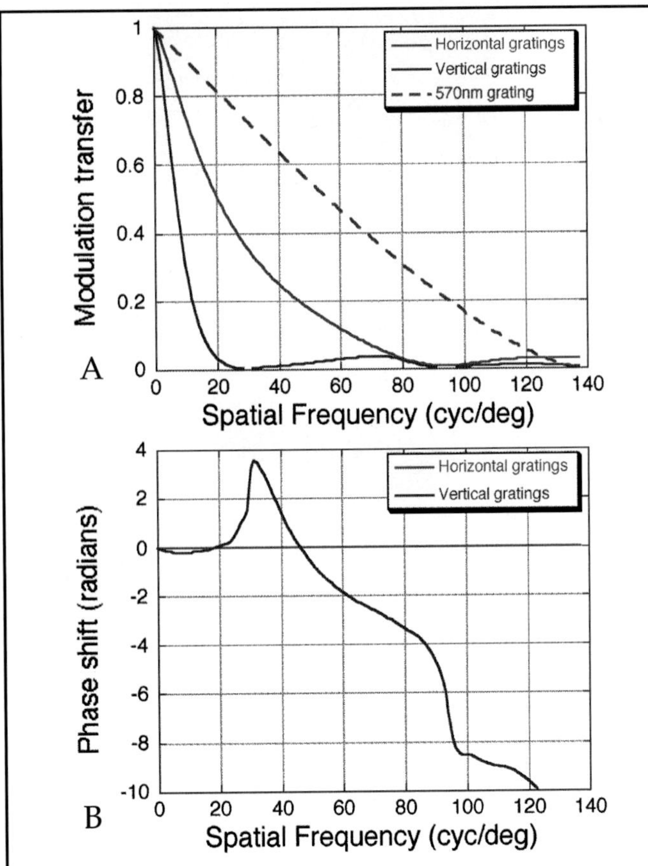

Figure 10-7. Optical transfer functions (OTF) computed from the luminance component of polychromatic point images of Figure 10-6. Magnitude and phase portions of the OTF are shown separately as modulation transfer functions (MTF, panel A) and phase transfer functions (PTF, panel B). Red curves were computed from image in Figure 10-6A and pertain to gratings of all orientations. Blue curves were computed from image in Figure 10-6B and pertain to vertical gratings only, whereas OTF for horizontal gratings is the same as the red curves. Dashed curve in A is a diffraction-limited MTF for 570 nm light.

polychromatic point images shown in Figure 10-6. The result of such a calculation is a polychromatic, optical transfer function (OTF) shown in Figure 10-7. The magnitude of the OTF, called the *modulation transfer function* (MTF), describes how luminance contrast of the image varies with spatial frequency of a grating object. The phase portion of the OTF, called the *phase transfer function* (PTF), describes how the spatial phase of the image varies with spatial frequency. The longitudinal and transverse aspects of chromatic aberration both affect both parts of the OTF. LCA reduces image contrast by blurring the image, and TCA reduces contrast by inducing phase shifts that lead to cancellation of image components. LCA can induce phase reversals of 180 degrees only, whereas TCA can produce any amount of phase shift.

LCA reduces image contrast by blurring the image and TCA reduces contrast by inducing phase shifts that lead to cancellation of image components.

The MTF and PTF computed from the luminance component of images in Figure 10-6A (TCA = 0) are indicated by the red curves in Figures 10-7A and 10-7B, respectively. Because of the radial symmetry of the point image in Figure 10-6A, the red curves in Figure 10-7 apply to gratings of any orientation. To the contrary, the point image in Figure 10-6B (TCA $\neq$ 0) is elongated horizontally; therefore, the MTF and PTF will vary with grating orientation. The computed OTF for vertical gratings is shown by the blue curves in Figure 10-7 (the OTF for horizontal gratings are the same as the red curves). One implication of these calculations is that image contrast can be reduced more by TCA than by LCA. Psychophysical experiments confirmed that inducing TCA causes a dramatic loss of polychromatic contrast sensitivity.[16] Also, the fact that the drop in contrast sensitivity associated with pupil decentration is much greater for polychromatic gratings than for monochromatic gratings[17] confirms that chromatic aberration is the major cause of poor vision through small, displaced pupils. In addition, the phase shifts associated with TCA would be expected to greatly reduce retinal image quality for objects with rich Fourier spectra (eg, letters, faces).

Image contrast can be reduced more by TCA than by LCA.

The effect of chromatic aberration on visual acuity for gratings may be estimated by locating the intersection of polychromatic MTFs with the neural contrast threshold function. Such analysis predicts that TCA alone should produce a two-fold loss of acuity (from 50 to 25 c/deg) when viewing a white test grating through a 2.5 mm pupil displaced laterally by 3 mm.[18] Accurate predictions depend upon the precise wavelength that is in-focus on the retina and upon the degree of other off-axis aberrations. Nevertheless, experiments show that polychromatic visual acuity drops by approximately the predicted amount when viewing through a displaced pupil.[19,20] Similar predictions apply to acuity measured with clinical instruments designed to avoid ocular aberrations, such as the potential acuity meter or the polychromatic interferometer.[21,22] We have experimentally verified these theoretical predictions by showing that polychromatic acuity drops from 20/20 to 20/60 when the test instrument is displaced 3 mm from the visual axis.[23,24]

One consequence of TCA is that a point object emitting two wavelengths of light will produce a double retinal image that gives rise to the perception of a double object, a condition called *chromatic diplopia*. This phenomenon is the basis for chromostereopsis, a stereoscopic illusion in which differently colored objects located at the same viewing distance appear to lie at different distances. This intensively studied effect of chromatic aberration on vision is accounted for precisely by the interocular difference in monocular TCA.[25-27] Furthermore, interocular differences in chromatic diplopia caused by TCA can account for seemingly paradoxical reversals of color-depth illusions for complex objects on colored backgrounds.[28,29]

One consequence of TCA is that a point object emitting two wavelengths of light will produce a double retinal image that gives rise to the perception of a double object, a condition called *chromatic diplopia*.

Impact of Chromatic Aberration in the Presence of Monochromatic Aberrations

In this chapter, we have described chromatic aberration in isolation, as if chromatic dispersion were the only optical defect present in human eyes. In fact, all eyes suffer from various kinds and amounts of monochromatic aberration.[30,31] Therefore, a complete account requires an assessment of the combined effects of chromatic and monochromatic aberrations on the quality of the retinal image. Until very recently, this account was based on theoretical calculations without the benefit of experimental confirmations. For example, in the first edition of this book, we predicted that correcting typical amounts of spherical aberration would yield a larger increase in contrast sensitivity than could be achieved by correcting chromatic aberration.[32] That prediction has now been extended to include all of the higher-order, monochromatic aberrations and has been verified experimentally with the aid of an adaptive optical system.[33] Using contrast sensitivity for white-light gratings as a reference standard, experiments demonstrated a small improvement in contrast sensitivity for monochromatic light (thereby avoiding the effects of chromatic aberration). A slightly greater improvement was obtained for polychromatic gratings by correcting the monochromatic aberrations of the subject's eye with the adaptive optical system. However, a much larger increase in contrast sensitivity was measured for monochromatic stimuli viewed through the adaptive optical system. This latter condition avoided chromatic aberration and actively corrected monochromatic aberration to produce retinal images with super-normal optical quality. These results demonstrate that to achieve an optically superior eye requires the correction of monochromatic and chromatic aberrations. Correcting one but not the other leaves the eye aberrated and image quality far from perfect.

> To achieve an optically superior eye requires the correction of monochromatic *and* chromatic aberrations. Correcting one but not the other leaves the eye aberrated and image quality far from perfect.

Impact of Patient's Chromatic Aberration on Clinical Ophthalmoscopy

Improving vision of the patient is only one possible use for technologies that aim to reduce the eye's optical aberrations. Another major advantage of reducing the patient's aberrations, even temporarily, is the anticipated improvement in the clinician's view of the internal structures of the patient's eye by ophthalmoscopy. Modern ophthalmoscopes and fundus cameras may be characterized as extremely well-designed optical instruments that use the eye's mediocre optical system as the objective lens. Consequently, the clinician's view is limited not by the instrument, but by the aberrations of the patient's eye. By improving the optical quality of the patient's eye, significant improvements in the quality of ophthalmoscopic images should be realized, with corresponding improvements in diagnostic value. Recent advances in the application of adaptive-optics technology to the scanning laser ophthalmoscope has demonstrated superior fundus images obtained by correcting the monochromatic aberrations of the eye.[34] Correcting chromatic aberrations as well should make it possible to obtain significant improvement in colored ophthalmoscopic images in the future (see Chapter 5).

Beneficial Effects of Chromatic Aberration

As a general rule, aberrations of any kind reduce image quality when they act in isolation. However, the loss of image quality caused by one kind of aberration can often be recovered partially by the addition of a different kind of aberration. This phenomenon is exploited by lens designers who deliberately introduce aberrations in order to compensate for other, unavoidable aberrations. In vision, Applegate et al have demonstrated a reduction of the adverse effects of spherical aberration on visual acuity by adding an appropriate amount of defocus.[35] A similar phenomenon occurs for chromatic aberration of the eye. As shown in Figure 10-5, TCA reduces image quality for polychromatic gratings because phase shifting of individual wavelength components causes the gratings to counteract each other, thereby reducing luminance contrast. However, the blurring effect of LCA reduces the contrast of those same components, thereby reducing their ability to counteract. As a result, contrast is higher when both TCA and LCA are present than when the TCA acts alone. In effect, LCA protects the eye against the deleterious effects of TCA by defeating the mechanism by which TCA attenuates contrast.[36] Similarly, recent experiments suggest that the predicted loss of image quality seen by the short wavelength-sensitive (blue) cones due to chromatic blur may be recovered partially by the eye's natural monochromatic aberrations.[37] It is worth noting in this context that fundus cameras and other ophthalmic instruments that record the retinal features of a patient's eye may not receive the same level of protection against chromatic blur as does the human clinician's eye. This is because protection is determined by the instrument's spectral sensitivity, which might be broader and flatter than the retina's spectral sensitivity.

> LCA protects the eye against the deleterious effects of TCA by defeating the mechanism by which TCA attenuates contrast.

Prospects for Correcting Chromatic Aberration

The evidence reviewed above suggests that little improvement in visual performance for white light should be anticipated by any attempt to correct the eye's LCA. Not only are the potential benefits small, but new problems surface when attempting to achromatize the human eye, which can actually make the situation worse. We have already described how image quality may suffer by such correction if the eye has a significant amount of TCA. In addition, the introduction of achromatizing spectacle lenses to compensate for the eye's LCA has the potential to introduce a new phenomenon—chromatic parallax—that reduces image quality by the same phase-shifting mechanism described above for TCA. Parallax arises because the achromatizing lens creates numerous virtual images of a polychromatic object, one image for every wavelength. Each virtual image lies at the eye's far point for the corresponding wavelength and thus becomes a virtual object that is optically conjugate with the retina. The problem is that this collection of virtual objects occupies a range of visual space and is therefore subject to parallax, which can displace the objects laterally, thereby introducing phase shifts that attenuate image contrast. Theory and experiments have demonstrated that misalignments between lens and the eye as small as 0.4 mm is enough to offset any visual benefit expected from the correction of chromatic errors of focus.[16]

> Achromatizing spectacle lenses must be carefully aligned with the eye to avoid introducing chromatic parallax that reduces image quality.

Chromatic difference of magnification is also affected by achromatizing lenses. Theoretical calculations and experiments have shown a seven-fold increase in CDM when the eye's LCA is corrected by an achromatizing lens of compact design.[38] Consequently, any gains in polychromatic image quality yielded by these lenses are restricted to a small region of the retina that may, or may not, include the fovea.

A polychromatic interferometer is a clinical instrument designed to avoid chromatic errors of focus and other monochromatic aberrations when testing vision.[39] This ingenious device casts a multitude of interference fringes directly onto the retina without the aid of the normal, image-forming properties of the eye's optical system. When well aligned to the eye's visual axis, these monochromatic fringes overlap precisely to produce a high-contrast, white grating. However, even small misalignments can introduce significant phase shifts caused by TCA.[21] The result is a loss of grating contrast that can lead to a three-fold reduction in visual acuity when the beam enters the eye near the pupil margin.[24] A similar problem arises also with the clinical instrument known as the *potential acuity meter*.[23]

> A unique feature of diffractive contact lenses with positive power is that they compensate for the chromatic aberration of the eye.

It is difficult to conceive how corneal refractive surgery could be used to correct the eye's chromatic aberration. However, contact lenses or intraocular lenses have the potential for correcting the eye's LCA without introducing excessive amounts of TCA or CDM.[38] A unique feature of diffractive lenses with positive power is that they produce a large amount of chromatic aberration that is opposite in sign to that of human eyes. For example, a +2 D diffractive lens has enough negative chromatic aberration to cancel about half of the eye's natural LCA.[40] Problems of chromatic parallax and chromatic difference of magnification for a well-centered lens should be smaller than for achromatizing spectacle lenses because the contact lens will lie much closer to the eye's nodal point.

Summary

The chromatic aberration of the eye can be measured with relatively simple methods compared to those needed for measurement of the higher-order monochromatic aberrations. For this reason, the chromatic aberration of human eyes was well documented prior to the recent explosion of research on monochromatic aberrations. That documentation indicates that chromatic aberration is manifest in several ways, each of which can have detrimental effects on vision for everyday objects. Although special lenses for correcting chromatic errors of focus have been available for more than 50 years,[41] they have not been widely used because of limited benefits and the potential for reducing retinal image quality rather than enhancement. However, as technology develops for correcting the monochromatic aberrations of the eye, the significance of ocular chromatic aberration will grow because it will be the only remaining barrier to attaining "super vision." Thus, new strategies for correcting chromatic aberration may be required in the future to achieve the full potential of customized corneal ablation or any other technique for reducing ocular aberrations.

> As technology develops for correcting the monochromatic aberrations of the eye, the significance of ocular chromatic aberration will grow because it will be the only remaining barrier to attaining "super vision." Thus, new strategies for correcting chromatic aberration may be required in the future to achieve the full potential of customized corneal ablation, or any other technique for reducing ocular aberrations.

References

1. Thibos LN, Ye M, Zhang X, Bradley A. The chromatic eye: a new reduced-eye model of ocular chromatic aberration in humans. *Appl Opt.* 1992;31:3594-3600.
2. Zhang X, Thibos LN, Bradley A. Relation between the chromatic difference of refraction and the chromatic difference of magnification for the reduced eye. *Optom Vis Sci.* 1991;68:456-458.
3. Howarth PA, Zhang X, Bradley A, Still DL, Thibos LN. Does the chromatic aberration of the eye vary with age? *J Opt Soc Am A.* 1988;5:2087-2092.
4. Zhang X, Bradley A, Thibos LN. Experimental determination of the chromatic difference of magnification of the human eye and the location of the anterior nodal point. *J Opt Soc Am A.* 1993;10:213-220.
5. Campbell MCW, Harrison EM, Simonet P. Psychophysical measurement of the blur on the retina due to optical aberrations of the eye. *Vision Res.* 1990;30:1587-1602.
6. Simonet P, Campbell MCW. The optical transverse chromatic aberration on the fovea of the human eye. *Vision Res.* 990;30:187-206.
7. Thibos LN, Bradley A, Still DL, Zhang X, Howarth PA. Theory and measurement of ocular chromatic aberration. *Vision Res.* 1990;30:33-49.
8. Rynders MC, Lidkea BA, Chisholm WJ, Thibos LN. Statistical distribution of foveal transverse chromatic aberration, pupil centration, and angle psi in a population of young adult eyes. *J Opt Soc Am A.* 1995;12:2348-2357.
9. Bradley A, Glenn A. Fry Award Lecture 1991: Perceptual manifestations of imperfect optics in the human eye: attempts to correct for ocular chromatic aberration. *Optom Vis Sci.* 1992;69:515-521.
10. Thibos LN, Bradley A, Zhang XX. Effect of ocular chromatic aberration on monocular visual performance. *Optom Vis Sci.* 1991;68:599-607.
11. Campbell FW, Gubisch RW. The effect of chromatic aberration on visual acuity. *J Physiol.* 1967;192:345-358.
12. Campbell FW, Green DG. Optical and retinal factors affecting visual resolution. *J Physiol.* 1965;181:576-593.

13. Zeltzer H. The X-chrome lens. *Journal of the American Optometry Association.* 1971;42:933-939.
14. Thibos LN. Formation and sampling of the retinal image. In: De Valois K, ed. *Seeing Handbook of Perception and Cognition.* London: Academic Press; 2000:1-54.
15. Bradley A, Zhang X, Thibos LN. Failures of isoluminance caused by ocular chromatic aberrations. *Appl Opt.* 1992;31:3657-3667.
16. Zhang X, Bradley A, Thibos L. Achromatizing the human eye: the problem of chromatic parallax. *J Opt Soc Am A.* 1991;8:686-691.
17. Artal P, Marcos S, Iglesias I, Green DG. Optical modulation transfer and contrast sensitivity with decentered small pupils in the human eye. *Vision Res.* 1996;35:3575-3586.
18. Thibos LN. Calculation of the influence of lateral chromatic aberration on image quality across the visual field. *J Opt Soc Am A.* 1987;4:1673-1680.
19. Green DG. Visual resolution when light enters the eye through different parts of the pupil. *J Physiol.* 1967;190:583-593.
20. van Meeteren A, Dunnewold CJW. Image quality of the human eye for eccentric entrance pupil. *Vision Res.* 1983;23:573-579.
21. Thibos LN. Optical limitations of the Maxwellian-view interferometer. *Appl Opt.* 1990;29:1411-1419.
22. Thibos LN, Bradley A. Use of interferometric visual stimulators in optometry. *Ophthalmic Physiol Opt.* 1992;12:206-208.
23. Bradley A, Thibos LN, Still DL. Visual acuity measured with clinical Maxwellian-view systems: effects of beam entry location. *Optom Vis Sci.* 1990;67:811-817.
24. Thibos LN, Bradley A, Still DL. Interferometric measurement of visual acuity and the effect of ocular chromatic aberration. *Appl Opt.* 1991;30:2079-2087.
25. Simonet P, Campbell MCW. Effect of illuminance on the directions of chromostereopsis and transverse chromatic aberration observed with natural pupils. *Ophthalmic Physiol Opt.* 1990;10:271-279.
26. Ye M, Bradley A, Thibos LN, Zhang X. Interocular differences in transverse chromatic aberration determine chromostereopsis for small pupils. *Vision Res.* 1991;31:1787-1796.
27. Ye M, Bradley A, Thibos LN, Zhang XX. The effect of pupil size on chromostereopsis and chromatic diplopia: interaction between the Stiles-Crawford effect and chromatic aberrations. *Vision Res.* 1992;32:2121-2128.
28. Flaubert J. Seeing depth in colour: more than just meets the eyes. *Vision Res.* 1994;34:1165-1186.
29. Winn B, Bradley A, Strang NC, McGraw PV, Thibos LN. Reversals of the colour-depth illusion explained by ocular chromatic aberration. *Vision Res.* 1995;35:2675-2684.
30. Porter J, Guirao A, Cox IG, Williams DR. Monochromatic aberrations of the human eye in a large population. *J Opt Soc Am A Opt Image Sci Vis.* 2001;18:1793-103.
31. Thibos LN, Hong X, Bradley A, Cheng X. Statistical variation of aberration structure and image quality in a normal population of healthy eyes. *J Opt Soc Am A.* 2002;19:2329-2348.
32. Applegate RA, Hilmantel G, Thibos LN. Visual performance assessment. In: MacRae SM, Krueger, RR, Applegate RA, eds. *Customized Corneal Ablation: The Quest for Super Vision.* Thorofare, NJ: SLACK Incorporated; 2001.
33. Yoon GY, Williams DR. Visual performance after correcting the monochromatic and chromatic aberrations of the eye. *J Opt Soc Am A Opt Image Sci Vis.* 2002;19:266-275.
34. Roorda A, Romero-Borja F, Donnelly III WJ, Hebert TJ, Queener H. Dynamic imaging of microscopic retinal features with the adaptive optics scanning laser ophthalmoscope. Presentation 4377 at: ARVO; May 9, 2003; Ft. Lauderdale, Fla.
35. Applegate RA, Marsack J, Ramos R. Interaction between aberrations can improve or reduce visual performance. *J Cataract Refract Surg.* 2003;29:1487-1495.
36. Thibos LN, Bradley A. Modeling the refractive and neuro-sensor systems of the eye. In: Mouroulis P, ed. *Visual Instrumentation: Optical Design and Engineering Principle.* New York: McGraw-Hill; 1999:101-159.
37. McLellan JS, Marcos S, Prieto PM, Burns SA. Imperfect optics may be the eye's defense against chromatic blur. *Nature.* 2002;417:174-176.
38. Bradley A, Zhang XX, Thibos LN. Achromatizing the human eye. *Optom Vis Sci.* 1991;68:608-616.
39. Lotmar W. Apparatus for the measurement of retinal visual acuity by moire' fringes. *Invest Ophthalmol Vis Sci.* 1980;19:393-400.
40. Atchison DA, Ye M, Bradley A, et al. Chromatic aberration and optical power of a diffractive bifocal contact lens. *Optom Vis Sci.* 1992;69:797-804.
41. van Heel ACS. Correcting the spherical and chromatic aberrations of the eye. *J Opt Soc Am.* 1946;36:237-239.

Chapter 11

Optical Quality of the Eye and Aging

Susana Marcos, PhD; Sergio Barbero, MSc; James S. McLellan, PhD; and Stephen A. Burns, PhD

Introduction

Visual performance declines with age. Several cross sectional studies show a progressive decrease in contrast sensitivity with normal aging.[1,2] While some of these changes are neural, an important part of contrast loss is due to degradation of the eye's optical quality. There are several reasons to study how the optical properties of the eye change with age:

1. Objective measurements of the degradation due to optics allow the subtraction of the contribution of the changes in the optics, revealing the effect of neural changes. This is important to understanding basic and clinical questions underlying the aging of the human nervous system
2. Changes in the ocular wave aberrations must result from changes in the physical, optical, structural, and biometric properties of the ocular components in the eye, and in particular, the crystalline lens.[3] Several studies report in vivo and ex vivo measurements of lens thickness, curvatures, asphericities, and effective refractive index with age, but the studies differ in detail.[4-8] These data are important to understanding the causes of presbyopia. Accurate measurements of age-related changes in the aberrations of the crystalline lens should help shed light onto some of the controversies in this field
3. Retinal ophthalmoscopy is likely to benefit clinical practice by utilizing recent advances in static and dynamic correction of aberrations. Promising results show a significant increase in the contrast of retinal features and visualization of new structures using scanning laser ophthalmoscopy in combination with phase plates[9] or adaptive optics,[10] which correct individual higher-order aberrations. These preliminary results are generally obtained in young or middle-aged subjects, while the sector of the population most in need of retinal examination is predominantly old (ie, age-related macular degeneration, diabetic retinopathy). It is important to study the optical degradation in older eyes to assess the limits of these emerging technologies
4. Ninety percent of the population above 75 years suffer from cataracts. In developed countries, the aging crystalline lens is typically replaced by an artificial intraocular lens (IOL). Knowledge of the optical aberrations of the aging eye, in comparison to the young, as well as the optical aberrations of the aging cornea, are important both for an appropriate evaluation of the cataract surgical outcomes and improved IOL designs[11]
5. The increasing popularity of laser in-situ keratomileusis (LASIK) surgery as an alternative treatment for refractive errors is expanding both the percentage and the age-span of the population undergoing this procedure. The knowledge of the changes of the aberrations of the ocular components with aging, and particularly close to the onset of presbyopia, may be important to optimize standard procedures for a particular age range. Standard refractive LASIK procedures are known to increase the amount of spherical aberration of the eye. Knowledge of the typical change of aberrations with aging will help to predict long-term optical quality expectations[12]

Customized refractive surgery aims at correcting both lower- and higher-order aberrations by ablating the cornea with the appropriate shape to compensate for the individual aberrations.[13] Given that the optical properties of the eye change with age, it is important to determine whether the changes provide an adequate time period over which improved optics could be enjoyed. In the present chapter, we review the state-of-the-art on changes of the optical aberrations with aging. The potential sources of the age-related change of aberrations are discussed. The study is restricted to monochromatic aberrations and only foveal measurements with relaxed accommodation. Cataract formation affects most of the population beyond a certain age, and despite being considered a pathology in the studies on normal eyes reported in this chapter, it can be regarded as a normal consequence of aging. The change of aberrations with cataract surgery is discussed in the last section of this chapter.

> The knowledge of the changes of the aberrations of the ocular components with aging, particularly close to the onset of presbyopia, may be important to optimize standard procedures for a particular age range.

Optical Monochromatic Aberrations as a Function of Age

Cross sectional studies show an increase in optical aberrations of the eye with age. Figure 11-1 shows results from the study by

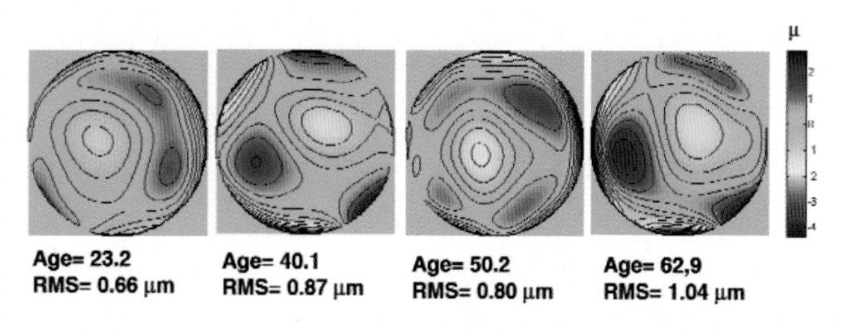

Figure 11-1. Wave aberration maps (for third- and higher-order aberrations) for four typical subjects of different ages. Data from McLellan et al[14] using a spatially resolved refractometer. Pupil size was 7.32 millimeters (mm); contour spacing was 0.50 mm.

McLellan et al[14] in a group of 38 normal subjects (from 22.9 to 64.5 years), using a spatially resolved refractometer.[15] Pupils were dilated by a mydriatic agent. The pupil was sampled by 37 1 mm apertures forming a rectangular sampling with 1 mm steps. Data were fit to a seventh-order Zernike expansion. Computations were done using pupil size of 7.32 mm. Figure 11-1 shows examples of four wave aberration maps of subjects selected to be representative of their age groups. Figure 11-2 represents the root mean square (RMS) wavefront error as a function of age for different orders of the Zernike expansion: (A) Third- and higher-order aberrations (ie, all nonconventional aberrations); (B) Third-order aberrations; (C) Fourth-order aberrations; and (D) Fifth- through seventh-order aberrations. Despite the large intersubject variability, the increase of ocular aberrations (excluding tilt, defocus, and astigmatism) was found to be statistically significant: ($r = 0.33$, $p = 0.042$). The correlations with age were found to increase as the order of aberrations increase. Third-order aberrations were not significantly correlated with age ($r = 0.18$, $p = 0.28$). Fourth-order aberrations were significantly correlated with age ($r = 0.47$, $p = 0.003$) as were the higher-order (fifth through seventh) aberrations ($r = 0.57$, $p = 0.0002$).

Cross sectional studies show an increase in optical aberrations of the eye with age.

Other studies in the literature reporting optical aberrations measured through different techniques showed similar trends. Calver et al[16] compared the aberrations (measured using a cross-cylinder aberroscope[17,18]) in a group of young subjects (n = 15, mean age = 24.2 years) and a group of older subjects (n = 15, mean age = 68.0). Their analysis is restricted to 14 terms in the Zernike expansion (fourth order). For matched pupil diameters (both 4.00 and 6.00 mm), they found that some particular third- and fourth-order Zernike coefficients were significantly higher in the older group. While third- and fourth-order RMS values were also higher in the older group, this difference was not statistically significant (which they attributed to a lack of statistical power in the sample). Interestingly, when measurements were made under natural pupils (typically larger in the young than in the old group), RMS was not larger for the older group and third-order RMS was actually smaller, indicating that age-related miosis is an important attenuating factor of the optical degradation occurring with age.

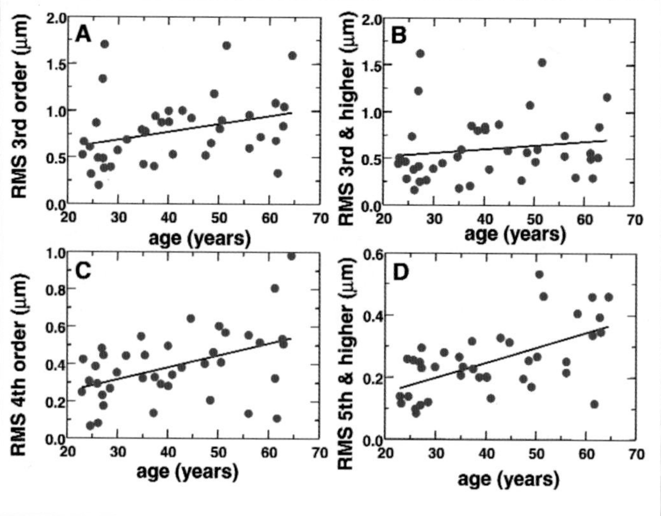

Figure 11-2. Relation between age and RMS wavefront error. (A) Third-order terms. (B) All terms except tilt, defocus, and astigmatism. (C) Fourth-order terms. (D) Fifth- thru seventh-order terms. Data from McLellan et al[14] for a 7.32 mm pupil.

RMS was not larger for the older group and third-order RMS was actually smaller, indicating that age-related miosis is an important attenuating factor of the optical degradation occurring with age.

Artal et al[19] reported ocular aberrations measured with a Shack-Hartmann wavefront sensor in a group of 17 normal subjects (ages ranging from 20 to 70 years). They found a significant increase of the third and higher RMS ($r = 0.73$, $p = 0.0007$), for 5.9 mm pupil diameters. Third- and fourth-order RMS considered separately also seemed to increase significantly with age, although correlation and significance values were not included.

A recent abstract by Brunette et al[20] reports ocular aberrations as a function of age for a sample of 38 subjects, using a Shack-Hartmann technique, and a 5 mm dilated pupil. This study expands the age range from previous studies: 8 to 80 years. They also found a significant increase of the monochromatic aberrations with age, although they found it more prominent after age 50. Interestingly, ocular aberrations decreased during adolescence and reached a minimum around age 20.

Figure 11-3 shows the spherical aberration Zernike coefficient as a function of age, from different studies. Data from McLellan et al[14] and from Smith et al[21] are for 7.32 mm pupils, data from Calver et al[16] are for 6 mm pupils, and data from Artal et al[19] are for 5.9 mm pupils. In all studies, the spherical aberration of the eye shows a slight increase toward more positive values with age.

All the data reported below were collected using monochromatic light, either visible or infrared. A recent study shows that both wavelengths provide similar higher-order aberrations in both normal, young subjects and old/pathological eyes.[22] These results refer to monochromatic image quality. Longitudinal chromatic aberrations (LCA) and transverse chromatic aberrations (TCA) combine with monochromatic aberration, when using white light.[23,24] Some studies have found a decrease in LCA with age,[25,26] but many studies have not been able to replicate this finding.[16,27,28]

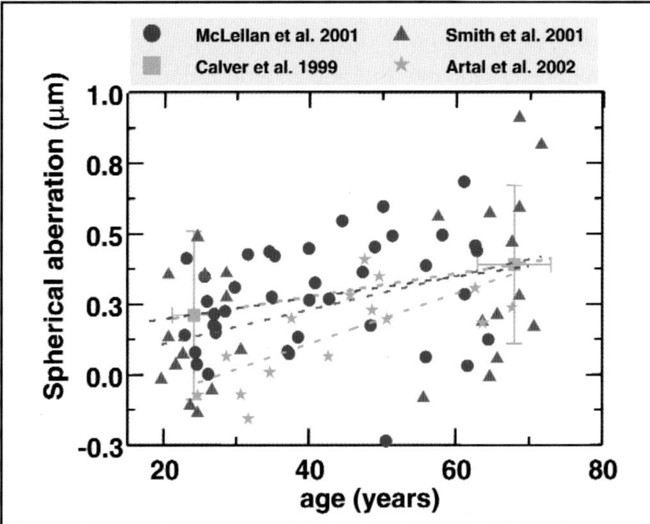

Figure 11-3. Spherical aberration of the eye as a function of age (coefficient Z_4^0 following the Optical Society of America (OSA) standard notation) from different studies. Blue circles from McLellan et al[14] for a 7.32 mm pupil, red triangles estimated from Smith et al[21] for a 7.32 mm pupil, green squares are averages across two different age groups from Calver et al[16] for a 6 mm pupil (horizontal and vertical bars represent the age and spherical aberration standard deviations), and orange stars are data from Artal et al[19] for a 5.9 mm pupil.

Why Do the Ocular Aberrations Change With Age?

Corneal Changes With Age

An increase of prevalence of astigmatism with age has been reported (see, for example, reference 29 for a review). In young eyes, the anterior cornea is typically steeper in the vertical than in the horizontal meridian, but this asymmetry tends to reverse with increasing age[30] (ie, corneal astigmatism changes from "with-the-rule" to "against-the rule" with age). In general, the cornea becomes more curved with age.

Oshika et al[31] estimated corneal aberrations from corneal elevation maps obtained with a videokeratoscope on 102 subjects and found a significant increase in third- and higher-order corneal aberrations ($r = 0.552$; $p < 0.001$) and third-order terms ($r = 0.561$; $p < 0.001$), but not for fourth order (7 mm pupils). Guirao et al[32] conducted a similar measurement on 59 eyes. They found higher amounts of fourth-order spherical aberration in middle-aged and older corneas and attributed this to a decrease in the radius of curvature. Guirao et al[32] also found that coma and other higher-order aberrations were correlated with age. Both studies show a moderate increase of corneal aberrations with age, and corneal changes alone are not sufficient to explain the measured increases in ocular aberrations with age.

Recent data by Dubbelman et al[33] show, for the first time, cross sectional data of the radius of curvature and asphericities of both anterior and posterior corneal surfaces as a function of aging. Measurements were based on corrected Scheimpflug images. They found a slight decrease in the radius of the anterior corneal surface with age. The only statistically significant change measured as a function of age was the decrease of posterior corneal asphericity with age. Assuming that the corneal refractive index remains constant with age, we used those data to estimate, by virtual ray tracing, the theoretical impact of these age-related physical changes on the change of corneal aberrations with age (25 to 66 years, on average). We computed only a minor increase in the spherical aberration of the anterior corneal surface (from 0.294 to 0.317 mm). While according to Dubbelman et al[33] the most significant changes occur on the posterior corneal surface, its contribution to changes in the spherical aberration of the posterior corneal surface are negligible (-0.0108 mm in the young group, and -0.0114 mm in the older group).

Crystalline Lens Changes With Age

To date, several methods have been used to measure the aberrations of the crystalline and, in particular, its spherical aberration: 1) in vitro measurements of spherical aberration (along one meridian) of donor lenses, using a scanning laser apparatus,[34] 2) neutralization of the cornea and measurement of the aberrations of the eye,[35,36] and 3) measurement of total and anterior corneal aberrations, and computation of the internal aberrations by subtraction of the two measurements.[37,38] Glasser and Campbell[5] used the first method to assess the spherical aberration of the crystalline lens in a group of 27 human donor lenses (ages ranging from 10 to 87 years) and found dramatic changes in the spherical aberration going from negative to positive with aging. It should be noted that parallel beams were used in the experimental ray tracing rather than converging rays used in the other studies (for most distances, the cornea converges light from a target onto the lens). Artal et al[19] used a subtraction method to estimate the aberrations of the crystalline lens as a function of age. They found an increase in the RMS of the aberrations of the crystalline lens with aging. Smith et al[21] measured the total and corneal spherical aberration (and the crystalline lens' by subtraction) in two groups of young and older eyes, respectively. They found that the spherical aberration of the crystalline lens was negative in both young and old adults, although it was less negative in the older group. The increase of spherical aberration with age found in the study by McLellan[14] is also suggestive of an absolute increase of the spherical aberration of the crystalline lens.

The optical and physical properties of the lens change with age, and they should be directly related to changes in the aberrations of the crystalline lens with aging. There is extensive literature on the changes in the shape and refractive index of the aging crystalline lens in relation to presbyopia. Many of the studies are mutually contradictory. Using Scheimpflug photography in a cross sectional study of 100 subjects, Brown showed that the radius of the anterior lens decreases with age.[4] A similar trend was found in later experiments by Koretz et al.[8] These results disagree with results from excised lenses from Glasser and Campbell,[3] who found an increased radius of curvature of the anterior surface of the lens (at least up to age 65) and no significant change in the posterior radius of curvature. An increase in the lens power should imply a shift toward myopia. However, an age-related hypermetropic shift is typically observed.[39-41] This contradiction (known as the *lens paradox*) was explained by assuming a decrease in the effective refractive index of the lens.[42,43] In vivo measurements of the lens radius of curvature using phacometry (by recording Purkinje images) also support the concept that index of refraction changes of the aging lens are needed to compensate for changes in the surface curvatures.[6] Dubbelman and Van de Heijde[7] applied corrected images of the anterior segment provided by a Scheimpflug lamp from the dis-

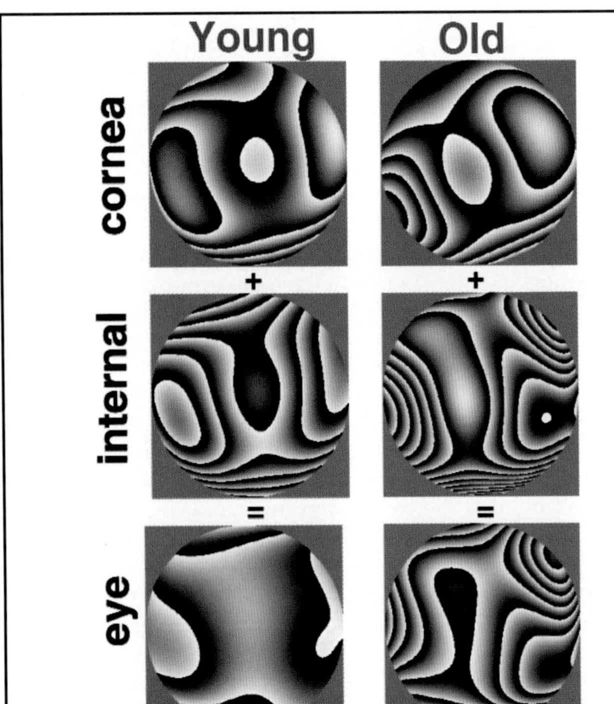

Figure 11-4. Examples of corneal, internal, and total aberrations for a young (showing a good corneal/internal compensation) and an old subject (with little cancellation of corneal aberrations by the internal aberration). (Courtesy of Pablo Artal.)

tortion produced by the refractive ocular surfaces and the geometry of the Scheimpflug configuration. They found a decrease in the anterior and posterior lens radius (but much less pronounced than found by Brown[4]), a consequent decrease in the equivalent refractive index with age, and no significant change in the asphericities of anterior and posterior lens surfaces. Some empirical studies on in vitro eyes did not report age-related changes of the index of refraction.[3,44] However, recent measurements[45] of the gradient refractive index of excised lenses (ages ranging from 14 to 82 years) using magnetic resonance microimaging provides evidence for a change in the refractive index distribution as a function of age, which offsets the changes in lens curvature. In addition, lens thickness has been reported to increase with age.[46]

Smith and Atchison[47] discussed the idea that changes in the gradient refractive index distribution with age could result in a shift of the spherical aberration of the crystalline lens in the positive direction. This increase should, at least in the paraxial approximation, result predominantly from changes in the equatorial quadratic terms of a gradient index distribution (N2j). However, recent data from Moffat et al[45] show no significant trend as a function of age for these particular terms, although there is a great deal of intersubject variability.

In order to study the sources of changes in spherical aberration in the crystalline lens, we performed some simulations using the most recent parameters available in the literature and comparing the results with reported changes in internal spherical aberration for different age groups. Surface shape and position data were obtained from anterior and posterior lens radii of curvature and asphericities reported by Dubbelman and Van der Heijde[7] and lens thickness changes from Dubbelman et al.[46]

Convergence of the light rays onto the crystalline lenses was ensured by modeling the cornea with average radii of curvature and asphericities of the anterior and posterior surface of the cornea for the different age groups based on data by Dubbelmann et al.[33] The refractive index distribution with age was modeled in several ways: 1) using changes in the gradient index with age reported by Moffat et al;[45] 2) assuming a constant refractive index (n = 1.426) with age; and 3) assuming an age-related change in the effective refractive index of the crystalline lens, as reported by Dubbelman et al[7] (from n = 1.435 to n = 1.415). The internal spherical aberration was estimated in all cases using the same procedure as in the experimental measurements (ie, subtracting the corresponding corneal aberration from the estimated total aberration). Using Moffat et al's index of refraction[45] 1) we did not find a clear tendency of internal spherical aberration with age, although the influence of these changes is considerable large in the computation. Assuming no change in the index of refraction with age 2), we calculated that the internal aberration changed from -0.018 mm to 0.114 mm on average. The simulated results are in good agreement with the experimental data reported by Smith for the same age groups and corrected by the posterior corneal data reported by Dubbelman[33]: -0.045 to 0.112 mm, for the young and old groups, respectively. Assuming a change of the effective refraction index 3) does not have a significant impact on the estimated internal spherical aberration: -0.032 and 0.114 mm, respectively. The simulations of (2) and (3) suggest the observed change in lens curvatures and asphericities could be sufficient to explain the observed changes in the spherical aberration of the crystalline lens. However, the simulations in (1) showed that slight changes in the gradient refractive index can modify significantly spherical aberration, although no significant trend was found with age. Therefore, more research on changes in the refractive index structure with age, with various techniques, and on a larger sampler of eyes is needed to understand age-related optical changes in the crystalline lens.

Cornea/Internal Aberration Compensation

Several studies in the literature report a compensation of the aberrations of the anterior cornea by the aberrations of the crystalline lens, particularly the spherical aberration.[38,48,49] Artal et al[19] reported that this balance of aberrations between cornea and lens, which is frequent in young adults, decreases with age. They argued that decreased compensation in older eyes is a major cause for the increase of the aberrations of the eye with age. In the previous section, we described the shift of the spherical aberration of crystalline lens toward positive or at least less negative values. This limits the compensation of the generally positive spherical aberration of the cornea. Surprisingly, Artal et al[19] found that the disruption of corneal and internal balance also occurred with coma-like terms, although the mechanisms of how this occurs are not understood. Figure 11-4 shows examples of corneal, internal, and total aberrations for a young and an old subject, illustrating the positive addition of aberrations of the ocular components in the older subject, as opposed to the partial balance of aberrations in the young subject.

> The balance of aberrations between cornea and lens, which is frequent in young adults, decreases with age.

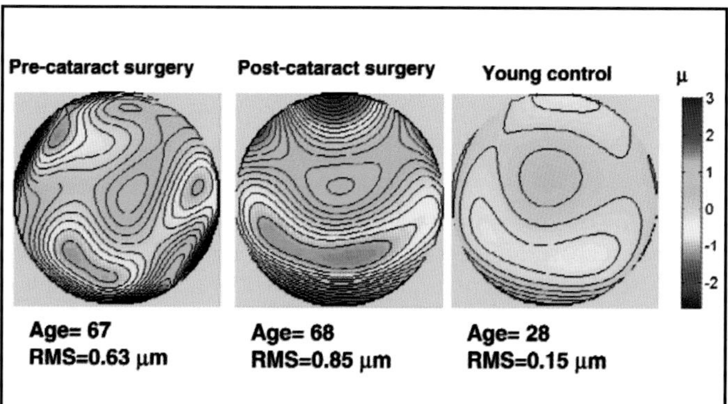

Figure 11-5. Examples of wave aberration maps (third- and higher-order aberrations) for an old patient before cataract surgery, a patient after cataract surgery (with an implanted IOL), and a young adult. Data from Barbero et al[61] for a 5 mm pupil. Contour spacing was 0.25 mm.

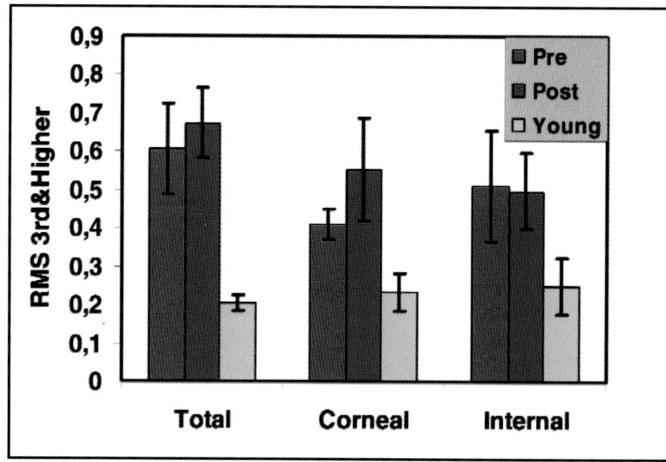

Figure 11-6. Comparison of average RMS wavefront error (for third- and higher-order aberrations) between old subjects before cataract surgery; old subjects after cataract surgery (with implanted IOLs); and young, normal eyes. Data from Barbero et al[16] for a 5 mm pupil.

Ocular Scattering and Aging

Forward and backward scattering has been shown to increase with age, most of which is due to changes in the crystalline lens. Ijspeert et al[50] measured intraocular straylight in a group of 129 healthy eyes, ranging between 20 and 82 years of age. Despite intersubject variability, they found that forward scattering increased significantly with age (with the fourth power of age) and doubled between the ages of 20 and 70. Hemenger[51] argued, using mathematical analysis, that intraocular light scatter could fully explain the decrease in contrast sensitivity with age.

> Forward and backward scattering has been shown to increase with age, most of which is due to changes in the crystalline lens.

Comparisons of double-pass modulation transfer function (MTF) measurements (which should incorporate scattering effects)[52,53] with MTFs estimated from wave aberration measurements[14] show that both an increase in aberrations and intraocular scattering are responsible for the degradation of optical quality with age. In the older groups, double-pass MTFs typically decrease more with age than do the wave aberration measurements, supporting the increased importance of intraocular backscattering with age (captured in double-pass measurements[54,55] but not by wavefront sensors). The decrease in the double-pass MTF with age seems to agree with reported decrease in contrast sensitivity function (CSF), indicating that a degradation of the optical quality (through aberrations and scattering) is a major contributor to the degradation of visual performance.[52] In vitro measurements of light scattering in normal and cataractous donor lenses (21 to 86 years) by van den Berg and Ijspeert[56] showed a monotonic increase of scattering between 700 and 400 nanometers (nm) of illumination. Scattering also increased with age and with the severity of the cataract. Along with an increase of scattering, retinal illumination also decreases drastically with age and progressive cataract. Said and Weale found that the transmittance of the lens decreased by about 25% between the ages of 20 and 60.[57] Delori and Burns[58] measured lens density differences through fundus reflectometry in a group of 81 normal eyes between the ages of 15 and 80 and found a monotonical increase with age, while eyes with IOLs showed substantially lower values than phakic individuals of the same age.

Change of Aberrations With Standard Cataract Surgery

In western societies, cataractous lenses are normally replaced by artificial IOLs, eliminating the glare, light loss (particularly at shorter wavelengths), and decreasing contrast sensitivity produced by scattering (see previous section). However, several data in the literature suggest that optical quality is not restored to normal levels for young adults after cataract surgery.

> Optical quality is not restored to normal levels for young adults after cataract surgery.

MTF double-pass measurements after IOL implantation are lower than those of young adults.[59,60] We measured ocular aberrations (both corneal and total aberrations) in patients before (n = 6, mean age = 70.7 ± 10.7)) and after (n = 7, mean age = 70.6 ± 9.0) cataract surgery, and compared them with the aberrations in a group of normal, young adults (n = 14, mean age = 29.0 ± 3.7).[11,61] Surgery consisted of phacoemulsification with a 4.1 mm incision and insertion of spherical IOLs. Figure 11-5 shows examples of wave aberration maps in an old subject before cataract surgery, a pseudoaphakic eye, and young adult. Figure 11-6 shows average RMS wavefront errors (corneal and total): (a) third and higher, (b) third-order, (c) fourth-order, and (d) fourth-order spherical aberration in the three groups. Aberrations in young eyes are typically much lower than in the other two groups. The amount of aberration is not lower in patients after cataract surgery than their natural lens age-matched counterparts. We found several reasons why the IOLs failed to provide a higher optical quality: 1) The spherical aberration of the IOL was positive (as was confirmed by in vitro measurements that we conducted using an eye model), which added to the positive spherical aberration of the cornea. In young eyes, however, the spherical aberration of the crystalline lens was negative, partially balancing the corneal spherical aberration. 2) Third-order aberrations were high in eyes with implanted IOLs and consistent with tilts and decentrations produced in the eye model, which produced increased amounts of coma. 3) Certain eyes showed a significant increase of corneal aberrations after surgery, probably due to the incision (as has been reported earlier as a cause for increased corneal astigmatism[62]). If deleterious tilts and decentrations can be avoided, IOLs with negative rather than positive spherical aberration[63] (or even customized to correct for corneal aberrations) could be conceived. Accurate positioning of these lenses is critical to getting the expected benefit. Atchison[64] concluded that if these lenses are not well-centered, the asphericity that eliminates spherical aberration may result in poorer performance than that occurring with purely spherical surfaces.[65] These results also allow reinterpretation of some speculations in the literature about the role of the crystalline lens in the spatial vision loss of the elderly. Owsley et al[66] measured contrast sensitivity in three groups of young, healthy, older eyes (ie, with transparent lenses and no ocular disease) and older eyes after IOL implantation. In keeping with our results based on aberration measurements, they found significantly higher performance in young eyes than in the two older groups, even after IOL implantation. They did not find higher contrast sensitivities in eyes after IOL implantation, compared to their age-mates who had no history of lens opacity or ocular disease. They then concluded that the crystalline lens is not primarily responsible for the spatial sensitivity loss of healthy older adults. From our results, it should be said that the optical quality of the cornea and IOL in patients after cataract surgery is not better than that of the cornea and aged crystalline lens in old adults. Thus, these patients do not represent a good control group for studies of neural deficits in contrast sensitivity.

Summary

There is a significant increase of ocular aberrations with aging. Part of this increase is due to an increase in the corneal aberrations with aging. This produces a decrease in the balance between corneal spherical aberration (typically positive) and the spherical aberration of the crystalline lens, and therefore an increase in the overall aberration. The optical quality is further degraded by an increase in intraocular scattering with age, which impairs vision when a cataract develops. Implantation of an IOL restores transparency but not optical quality to young levels.

> Changes in surface shape and refractive index of the crystalline lens lead to an increase in the spherical aberration (toward less negative values) of the crystalline lens with age.

Customized aspheric IOLs could be particularly useful in patients that underwent corneal surgery at an earlier age and suffer for abnormally increased corneal spherical aberration.[49] Current efforts in corneal refractive surgery aim at canceling not only second-order aberrations, but also naturally occurring higher-order aberrations. It should be kept in mind, however, that given the changes of aberrations with age, this "perfect correction" will not last forever. Also, if aberrations of the crystalline lens have been corrected by modifying the corneal shape, those are likely to reappear when the lens is replaced by a conventional or aspheric IOL.

> Optimized IOL lens designs could improve optical performance if their spherical aberration matched the spherical aberration of the cornea, with opposite sign, provided that tilts and decentrations are avoided.

The impact of some of the problems mentioned associated with an increase of aberrations may be attenuated by pupillary miosis, the decreased natural pupil size with age.[67] In addition, a larger amount of aberrations results in larger depth-of-field,[68] which may help to gain some "multifocality" in eyes with no accommodation capability. Even if an ideal compensation of aberrations was possible in the elderly eye, it is questionable that this may be beneficial. Perfect optical systems have a much narrower depth of field than aberrated systems. For a certain range of focus, the absolute defocused performance can be even worse. A certain level of tolerance to defocus is desirable in eyes that lack accommodation. An increase in optical contrast may help in eyes with reduced visual sensitivity from neural factors.[69] However the loss of photoreceptors occurring with aging (although the decline is much more marked for rod than for cones),[70,71] or the degradation of visual pathways critical for visual acuity[72] makes it unlikely that those eyes can fully benefit from the potential increased spatial resolution provided by an optimized optics.

> Even if an ideal compensation of aberrations was possible in the elderly eye, it is questionable that this may be beneficial. Perfect optical systems have a much narrower depth of field than aberrated systems. For a certain range of focus, the absolute defocused performance can be even worse.

Acknowledgments

We thank Rob Van der Heijde and Michael Dubbelman for providing us with physical parameters of the cornea and lens; Brad Moffat, David Atchison, and Jim Pope for providing coefficients for the gradient refractive index of the crystalline lens; and Pablo Artal for providing ocular spherical aberration data and graphic material. Susana Marcos acknowledges grants BFM2002-0268, Ministerio de Ciencia y Tecnología, Spain and CAM08.7/004.1/2003, Comunidad Autônoma de Madrid. Stephen A. Burns acknowledges EYO4395 from the National Insitutes of Health.

References

1. Elliott D, Whitaker D, MacVeigh D. Neural contribution to spatiotemporal contrast sensitivity decline in healthy aging eyes. *Vision Res.* 1990;30:541-547.
2. Owsley C, Sekuler R, Siemsen D. Contrast sensitivity throughout adulthood. *Vision Res.* 1983;23:689-699.
3. Glasser A, Campbell M. Biometric, optical and physical changes in the isolated human crystalline lens with age in relation to presbyopia. *Vision Res.* 1999;39:1991-2015.
4. Brown N. The change in lens curvature with age. *Exp Eye Res.* 1974;19:175-183.
5. Glasser A, Campbell M. Presbyopia and the optical changes in the human crystalline lens with age. *Vision Res.* 1998;38(2):209-229.

6. Hemenger H, Garner F, Ooi S. Change with age of the refractive index gradient of the human ocular lens. *Invest Ophthalmol Vis Sci.* 1995;36(3):703-707.
7. Dubbelman M, Heijde V. The shape of the aging human lens: curvature, equivalent refractive index and the lens paradox. *Vision Res.* 2001;41:1867-1877.
8. Koretz J, Cook C, Kaufman P. Aging of the human lens: changes in lens shape at zero-diopter accommodation. *J Opt Soc Am A.* 2001;18:265-272.
9. Burns SA, Marcos S, Elsnser AE, Bará S. Contrast improvement for confocal retinal imaging using phase correcting plates. *Optics Letters.* 2002;27:400-402.
10. Roorda A, Romero-Borja F, Donnelly IWJ, Queener H, Hebert TJ, Campbell MCW. Adaptive optics scanning laser ophthalmoscopy. Optics Express [serial online]. http://www.opticsexpress.org/abstract.cfm?URI=OPEX-10-9-405 2002;10:405-12.
11. Barbero S, Marcos S, Llorente L. Optical changes in corneal and internal optics with cataract surgery. 2002 Annual Meeting Abstract and Program Planner accessed at www.arvo.org. Association for Research in Vision and Ophthalmology. Abstract 388 2002;73.
12. Marcos S. Are changes in ocular aberrations with age a significant problem for refractive surgery? *J Refract Surg.* 2002;18(5):S572-S578.
13. MacRae SM, Schwiegerling J, Snyder R. Customized corneal ablation and super vision. *J Refract Surg.* 2000;16:230-235.
14. Mclellan J, Marcos S, Burns S. Age-related changes in monochromatic wave aberrations in the human eye. *Invest Ophthalmol Vis Sci.* 2001;42:1390-1395.
15. He JC, Marcos S, Webb RH, Burns SA. Measurement of the wavefront aberration of the eye by a fast psychophysical procedure. *J Opt Soc Am A.* 1998;15:2449-2456.
16. Calver R, Cox M, Elliott D. Effect of aging on the monochromatic aberrations of the human eye. *J Opt Soc Am A.* 1999;16:2069-2078.
17. Howland HC, Howland B. A subjective method for the measurement of the monochromatic aberrations of the eye. *J Opt Soc Am A.* 1977;67:1508-1518.
18. Walsh G, Cox M. A new computerized video-aberroscope for the determination of the aberration of the human eye. *Ophthalmic Physiol Opt.* 1995;15:403-408.
19. Artal P, Berrio E, Guirao A, Piers P. Contribution of the cornea and internal surfaces to the change of ocular aberrations with age. *J Opt Soc Am A.* 2002;19:137-143.
20. Brunette I, Parent M, Hamam H. Monochromatic Optical Aberration as a function of Age. 2002 Annual Meeting Abstract and Program Planner accessed at www.arvo.org. Association for Research in Vision and Ophthalmology. Abstract 437 2002.
21. Smith G, Cox M, Calver R, Garner L. The spherical aberration of the crystalline lens of the human eye. *Vision Res.* 2001;15:235-243.
22. Llorente L, Diaz-Santana L, Lara-Saucedo D, Marcos S. Aberrations of the human eye in visible and near infrared illumination. *Optom Vis Sci.* 2003;80:26-35.
23. Marcos S, Burns SA, Moreno-Barriuso E, Navarro R. A new approach to the study of ocular chromatic aberrations. *Vision Res.* 1999;39:4309-4323.
24. McLellan JS, Marcos S, Prieto PM, Burns SA. Imperfect optics may be the eye's defense against chromatic blur. *Nature.* 2002;417:174-176.
25. Millodot M. The influence of age on the chromatic aberration of the eye. *Graefes Arch Clin Exp Ophthalmol.* 1976;198:235-243.
26. Mordi J, Adrian W. Influence of age on chromatic aberration of the human eye. *Am J Optom Physiol Opt.* 1985;62:864-869.
27. Howarth PA, Zhang XX, Bradley A, et al. Does the chromatic aberration of the eye vary with age? *J Opt Soc Am A.* 1988;5:2087-2092.
28. Morrell A, Whitefoot H, Charman W. Ocular chromatic aberration and age. *Ophthal Physiol Opt.* 1991;11:385-390.
29. Pierscionek BK. Aging changes in the optical elements of the eye. *J Biomed Opt.* 1996;1:147-157.
30. Hayashi K, Hayashi H, Hayashi F. Topographic analysis of the changes in corneal shape due to aging. *Cornea.* 1995;14:527-532.
31. Oshika T, Klyce SD, Applegate RA, Howland HC. Changes in corneal wavefront aberrations with aging. *Invest Ophthalmol Vis Sci.* 1999;40:1351-1355.
32. Guirao A, Redondo M, Artal P. Optical aberrations of the human cornea as a function of age. *J Opt Soc Am A.* 2000;17:1697-1702.
33. Dubbelman M, Weeber H, Van Der Heijde R, Volker-Dieben H. Radius and asphericity of the posterior corneal surface determined by corrected Scheimpflug photography. *Acta Ophthalmol Scand.* 2002;80:379-383.
34. Sivak JG, Kreuzer RO. Spherical aberration of the crystalline lens. *Vision Res.* 1983;23:59-70.
35. Millodot M, Sivak J. Contribution of the cornea and lens to the spherical aberration of the eye. *Vision Res.* 1979;19:685-687.
36. Artal P, Guirao A. Contributions of the cornea and the lens to the aberrations of the human eye. *Optics Letters.* 1998;23(21):1713-1715.
37. El Hage SG, Berny F. Contribution of the crystalline lens to the spherical aberration of the eye. *J Opt Soc Am A.* 1973;63(2):205-211.
38. Artal P, Guirao A, Berrio E, Williams DR. Compensation of corneal aberrations by the internal optics in the human eye. *Journal of Vision.* 2001;1:1-8. http://journalofvision.org/1//, DOI 10.1167/ 1.1.1.
39. Slataper F. Age norms of refraction and vision. *Arch Ophthalmol.* 1950;43:466-481.
40. Saunders H. Age-dependence of the human refractive errors. *Ophthal Physiol Opt.* 1981;1:159-174.
41. Saunders H. A longitudinal study of the age dependence of human ocular refraction: 1. Age-dependent changes in the equivalent sphere. *Ophthal Physiol Opt.* 1986;6:39-46.
42. Koretz J, Handelman G. The lens paradox and image formation in accommodating human lenses. *Topics in Aging Research in Europe.* 1986;6:57-64.
43. Smith G, Atchison D, Pierscionek B. Modeling the power of the aging human eye. *J Opt Soc Am A.* 1992;9:2111-2117.
44. Pierscionek B. Refractive index contours in the human lens. *Exp Eye Res.* 1997;64:887-893.
45. Moffat B, Atchison D, Pope J. Age-related changes in refractive index distribution and power of the human lens as measured by magnetic resonance micro-imaging in vitro. *Vision Res.* 2002;1683-1693.
46. Dubbelman M, van der Heijde G, Weeber H. The thickness of the aging human lens obtained from corrected Scheimpflug images. *Optom Vis Sci.* 2001;78:411-416.
47. Smith G, Atchison D. The gradient index and spherical aberration of the lens of the human eye. *Ophthalmol Physiol Opt.* 2001;21(4):317-326.
48. Marcos S, Barbero S, Llorente L. The sources of optical aberrations in myopic eyes. 2002 Annual Meeting Abstract and Program Planner accessed at www.arvo.org. Association for Research in Vision and Ophthalmology. Abstract 1510 2002.
49. Marcos S, Barbero B, Llorente L, Merayo-Lloves J. Optical response to LASIK for myopia from total and corneal aberrations. *Invest Ophthalmol Vis Sci.* 2001;42:3349-3356.
50. IJspeert JK, de Waard PW, van den Berg TJ, de Jong PT. The intraocular straylight function in 129 healthy volunteers: dependence on angle age and pigmentation. *Vision Res.* 1990;30:699-707.
51. Hemenger R. Intraocular light scatter in normal vision loss with age. *Appl Opt.* 1984;23:1972-1974.
52. Artal P, Miranda I, Navarro R. Effects of aging in retinal image quality. *J Opt Soc Am A.* 1993;10:1656-1662.
53. Guirao A, Gonzalez C, Redondo M, Geraghty E, Norrby S, Artal P. Average optical performance of the human eye as a function of age in a normal population. *Invest Ophthalmol Vis Sci.* 1999;40:203-213.
54. Westheimer G, Liang J. Evaluating diffusion of light in the eye by objective means. *Vision Sci.* 1994;35:2652-2657.
55. Westheimer G, Liang J. Influence of ocular light scatter on the eye's optical performance. *J Opt Soc Am A.* 1995:1417-1424.

56. van den Berg T, Ijspeert JK. Light scattering in donor lenses. *Vision Res.* 1995;35:169-177.
57. Said F, Weale R. The variation with age of the spectral transmissivity of the living human crystalline lens. *Gerontologia.* 1959;3:213-231.
58. Delori F, Burns S. Fundus reflectance and the measurement of crystalline lens density. *J Opt Soc Am A.* 1996;13:215-226.
59. Artal P, Marcos S, Navarro R, Miranda, I, Ferro M. Through-focus image quality of eyes implanted with monofocal and multifocal intraocular lenses. *Optical Engineering.* 1995;34:772-779.
60. Guirao A, Redondo M, Geraghty E, Piers P, Norrby S, Artal P. Corneal optical aberrations and retinal image quality in patients implanted with monofocal IOLs. *Arch Ophthalmol.* 2002;120:1143-1151.
61. Barbero S, Marcos S, Llorente L, Jimenez-Alfaro I. Optical aberrations of intraocular lenses measured in vivo and in vitro. *J Opt Soc Am A.* 2003;20:1841-1851.
62. Jacobs B, Gaynes BL, Deutsch TA. Refractive astigmatism after oblique clear corneal phacoemulsification cataract incision. *J Cataract Refract Surg.* 1999;25:949-952.
63. Holladay JT, Piers A, Koranyi G, Van der Mooren M, Norrby NE. A new intraocular lens design to reduce spherical aberration of pseudophakic eyes. *J Refract Surg.* 2002;18:683-691.
64. Atchison DA. Design of aspheric intraocular lenses. *Ophthal Physiol Opt.* 1991;11:137-146.
65. Atchison DA. Design of aspheric intraocular lenses. *Ophthal Physiol Opt.* 1991;11(2):137-146.
66. Owsley C, Gardner T, Sekuler R, Lieberman H. Role of the crystalline lens in the spatial vision loss of the elderly. *Invest Ophthalmol Vis Sci.* 1985;26:1165-1170.
67. Said F, Sawires W. Age dependence of the changes in pupil diameter in the dark. *Optica Acta.* 1972;19:359-361.
68. Marcos S, Moreno E, Navarro R. The depth-of-field of the human eye from objective and subjective measurements. *Vision Res.* 1999;39:2039-2049.
69. Spear PD. Neural bases of visual defects during aging. *Vision Res.* 1993;33:2589-2609.
70. Panda-Jonas S, Jonas J, Jakobczyk-Zmija M. Retinal photoreceptor density decreases with age. *Ophthalmology.* 1995;102:1853-1859.
71. Curcio C. Photoreceptor topography in aging and age-related maculopathy. *Eye.* 2001;14:376-383.
72. Scialfa CT, Kline DW, Wood PK. Structural modeling of contrast sensitivity in adulthood. *J Opt Soc Am A.* 2002;19:158-165.

Chapter 12

Variation in Ocular Aberrations Over Seconds, Minutes, Hours, Days, Months, and Years

Larry N. Thibos, PhD and Arthur Bradley, PhD

The rapid transfer of ophthalmic aberrometry from the research laboratory to the clinic gives clinicians an extremely sensitive diagnostic tool with the potential to significantly impact ophthalmic practice. Aberrometers are essentially 21st-century optometers that are capable of measuring ocular aberrations smaller than the wavelength of light to produce a detailed map of the eye's optical imperfections over the entire pupil, not just the paraxial region typically measured by autorefractors. At the same time, advances in refractive surgery and new designs of custom contact lenses and intraocular lenses have suggested the possibility of creating an optically perfect eye, using the aberration map itself as a "prescription for perfection." On the other hand, our enthusiasm for optical perfection and its implication for supernormal vision is tempered by a nagging worry that the aberration map of a human eye may be a moving target. How will a clinician know if the aberration map measured this morning is different from the map measured this afternoon, tomorrow, next week, or next year? Does it make sense to even attempt a correction of small aberrations that oscillate from plus to minus and, on average, are zero? Even if aberrations are consistently non-zero, how can we treat them if they vary significantly over time?

> An aberrometer is an instrument that measures optical defects (optical aberrations).

> How will a clinician know if the aberration map measured this morning is different from the map measured this afternoon, tomorrow, next week, or next year?

In an attempt to provide answers to these questions, our group of visual optics researchers at Indiana University has repeatedly measured the monochromatic aberration of the same eyes over a variety of time scales ranging from seconds to years.[1] For example, in one experiment, the aberration map was measured five times in 1 second. Over this time span, the patient adopted a freeze position to stabilize the eye as much as possible by refraining from blinking, moving, and breathing. The resulting aberration maps are shown in the top row of Figure 12-1. Notice that the aberration pattern is virtually identical in all five maps, indicating a high degree of temporal stability over a time scale of 1 second. In another experiment, aberration maps were measured for the same eye every few minutes over a 30-minute period. Between measurements, the patient was allowed to blink and move about, with the aberrometer being realigned with the patient's eye prior to each measurement. The resulting aberration maps are shown in the middle row of Figure 12-1. These maps are still reasonably stable, but close inspection reveals some slight differences over time. Next, aberration maps were obtained from this eye at the same time of day, Monday through Friday, for 1 week. These aberration maps, shown in the bottom row of Figure 12-1, reveal obvious differences from day-to-day, although a common pattern remains recognizable. Using this same basic paradigm, we systematically increased the time between measurements from days to weeks, months, and for some patients, years. The results of these experiments indicated that the longer the time-span between measurements, the greater the variability.

> Monochromatic optical aberrations are present at every wavelength, are sometimes referred to as *geometrical aberrations*, and are distinct from the chromatic aberrations.

The aberration measurements shown in Figures 12-1 and 12-2 were obtained using the Complete Ophthalmic Analysis System (COAS) (Wavefront Sciences Inc, Albuequerque, NM) clinical aberrometer, which employs Shack-Hartmann principles to measure monochromatic aberrations. Each sampled aberration map (sampling rate of 288 microns [µm] determined by the Shack-Hartmann aberrometer) was fit by a series of Zernike radial polynomials.[2] The outcome of this analysis is a collection of numbers called *Zernike coefficients* that represent the amount of each polynomial required to fit the eye's aberrations. Three of these aberration coefficients are very familiar to clinicians since they describe the sphere, cylinder, and axis of ordinary refractive errors. Other coefficients indicate the amount of coma, spherical aberration, and other so-called "higher-order" aberration modes that clinicians often bring together under the umbrella of "irregular astigmatism." The collection of Zernike aberration coefficients is called a *Zernike spectrum*. A convenient way to visualize the Zernike spectrum graphically is to display a pyramid of values, rather like the chemist's periodic table of the elements.[2] Each row in the pyramid corresponds to a given order, and each column corresponds to a different meridional frequency. The order determines how rapidly the aberration accelerates from pupil

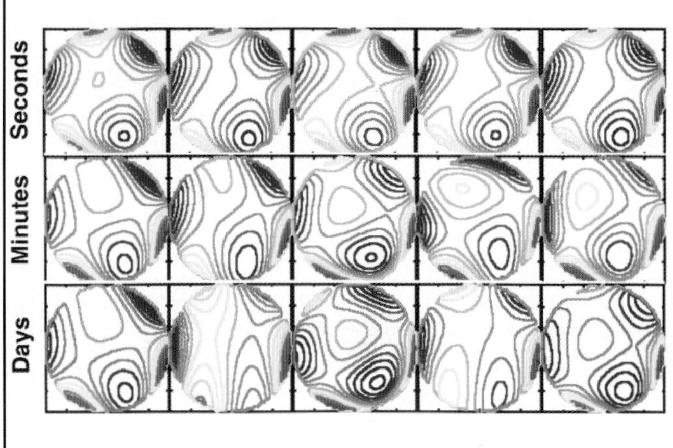

Figure 12-1. Aberration maps for patient CT determined over five different time scales. Contour interval = 0.10 millimeter (mm) map includes aberrations of third- and fourth-order only. Pupil size 6 mm. The top row of maps were collected in less than 1 second without instrument realignment. The middle row of maps were collected at intervals of a few minutes with instrument realignment between each measurement. The bottom row of maps was captured at the same time of day, Monday through Friday, of the same week.

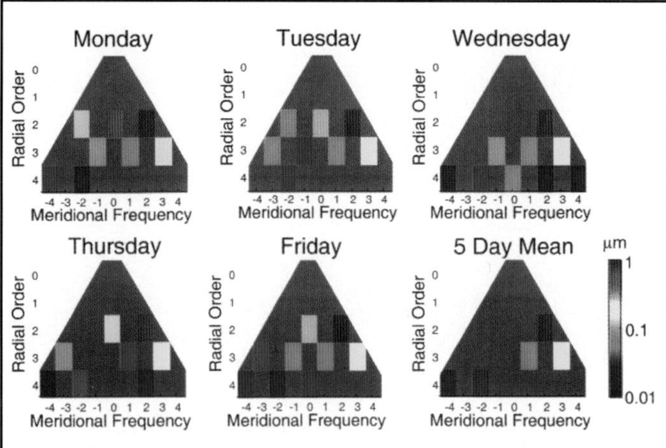

Figure 12-2. Average daily aberrations represented by pyramids of Zernike coefficients. The color of each rectangle indicates the log magnitude of the mean of five measurements of the corresponding coefficient obtained on the same day. The bottom right diagram shows the mean of all 25 measurements for those modes that were statistically significant on all 5 days. Orders 0 and 1 are omitted because they are not relevant to the quality of monochromatic images. The aberrometer was realigned to patient CT's eye before each measurement. It is a 6 mm pupil. Missing rectangles indicate statistically insignificant aberrations.

center to pupil margin, and the frequency determines how many times the aberration oscillates along the circular path around the pupil center. Once the aberration map is reduced to a spectrum of Zernike aberration coefficients, we can look at each type of aberration individually to ask the question, "Is this aberration large enough and stable enough to warrant treatment?"

If Zernike aberration coefficients are going to be used to design a custom cornea, contact lens, or intraocular lens, then it makes sense to exclude all coefficients that are zero. Given repeated measurements of the aberration map, we can use statistics to determine which aberration coefficients qualify for inclusion by this criterion. To illustrate the process, we performed Zernike analysis on the aberration maps in the middle row of Figure 12-1 to compute the mean values for N = five repetitions. We then used the t-test of statistics to determine which coefficients were significantly different from zero. These statistically significant coefficients are displayed graphically in the diagram labeled "Monday" in Figure 12-2. Each colored rectangle shows the magnitude of the mean aberration coefficient in the corresponding location of the Zernike pyramid. Higher-order aberrations tend to be small in magnitude, so for display purposes we use the logarithmic scale shown at the bottom right. Blank locations in the pyramid indicate the corresponding coefficient failed the t-test of significance. For example, on Monday, patient CT had a statistically significant amount of aberration for all three modes of the second-order, three of the four modes of the third-order, and two of the five modes in the fourth-order. Some of these modes were statistically significant also on Tuesday, but some were not. Slightly different patterns were observed on Wednesday, Thursday, and Friday. If a clinician adopted the conservative strategy that a given Zernike mode had to be statistically significant 5 days in a row before including that mode in a treatment plan, then only five of the 12 modes would be treated (see the diagram in the lower right hand corner of Figure 12-2), even though every mode was statistically significant at some time during the week.

In addition to requiring that individual Zernike coefficients be statistically significant, a conservative strategy would also require that the value of the Zernike coefficient be stable over time before including that mode in a treatment plan. To determine which aberrations are stable over 5 consecutive days, we used a statistical technique called *analysis-of-variance*. This test defines stability as a condition in which variability between days is relatively small compared to the variability within any given day. For patient CT, we found that only one aberration coefficient (horizontal coma: order = 3, frequency = +1) was statistically significant 5 days in a row and was stable for the entire week. Notice that several of the other aberration coefficients were larger, but also more variable from day-to-day, and therefore failed to pass the analysis-of-variance test of stability. The implication of these results is that day-to-day variability in this patient was large enough to preclude using the aberration coefficients obtained on any given day as adequately representing the values obtained on other days of the week. Given this outcome, a sensible strategy would be to average the aberration maps acquired over several days to obtain a more representative estimate of the patient's condition.

> *Analysis-of-variance* defines stability as a condition in which variability between days is relatively small compared to the variability within any given day.

Long-term stability of the aberration structure of eyes over a period of months or years should also be considered when planning treatment or monitoring outcome. Two of the subjects in our study have been examined with a laboratory Shack-Hartmann aberrometer repeatedly over the last 5 years. A summary of data for one of these individuals is shown in Figure 12-3. Although the

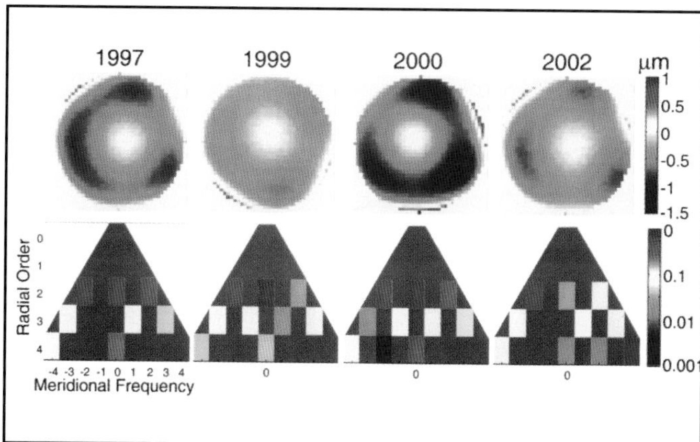

Figure 12-3. Long-term stability of the aberration map. Individual wavefront maps in the top row show the mean of five aberration measurements acquired on the same day; the bottom row shows log-magnitude Zernike spectra for the corresponding map. Right eye of patient AB, 6 mm pupil.

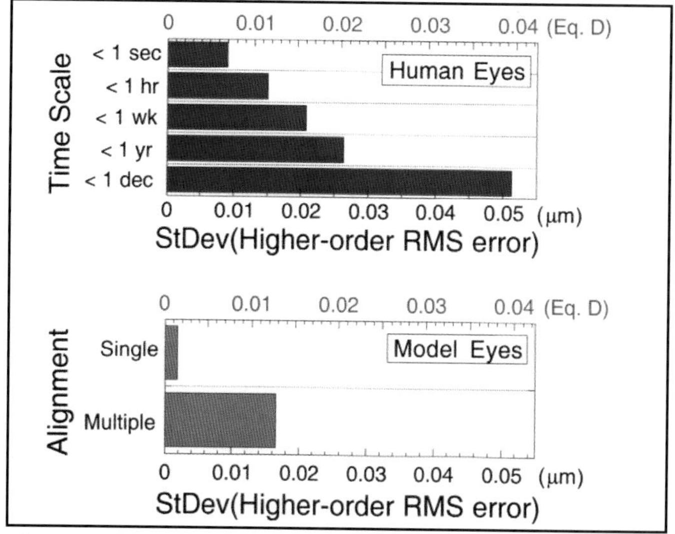

Figure 12-4. Top: summary of variability of total wavefront error in higher-order aberrations (orders three and four) over time scales ranging from seconds to decades. Bottom: variability of wavefront error in a physical model eye measured for the same alignment or for different alignments before each measurement. Dioptric scale indicates the amount of defocus that would generate the same level of wavefront root mean square (RMS) as the standard deviation in microns.

Zernike spectrum changes from year-to-year, the main features of the aberration maps appear remarkably stable over this 5-year period. However, formal statistical analysis revealed that only one mode is both statistically significant and stable over this time span. This is the third-order mode called *trefoil* (frequency = +3). Although several other modes were much larger in magnitude, they were not as stable over time. Statistical analysis-of-variance detected more variability between years than between repeated measures on the same day for all of the larger aberration coefficients. Lack of stability does not necessarily preclude these modes from treatment, but if they are to be included in a treatment plan, then we must be prepared for less-than-perfect outcome because the "prescription for perfection" obtained in the first year is only an approximation of what the aberration map would be like in subsequent years.

> Lack of stability does not necessarily preclude these modes from treatment, but if they are to be included in a treatment plan then we must be prepared for less-than-perfect outcome because the "prescription for perfection" obtained in the first year is only an approximation of what the aberration map would be like in subsequent years.

A summary of results from our study of temporal variability over a variety of time scales is presented in Figure 12-4. Each bar in the upper graph represents the average amount of statistical variability in the higher-order aberrations in the eyes of four patients. For each aberration map, the total amount of wavefront error was represented by RMS wavefront error, a single number describing how warped the aberration map is without concern for its exact shape. The standard deviation of five repeated measures of RMS error was determined five times over the indicated time span for each of the four patients. The average of these 20 estimates of temporal variability is indicated by the length of a bar in Figure 12-4. This graph indicates that variability in aberration measurements increases as the time scale used to assess variability increases. Only data from two subjects are available over multiple years (last bar in top histogram in Figure 12-4).

To judge the clinical significance of this trend, it is helpful to convert RMS wavefront error into units of diopters. Currently, most commercial aberrometers report aberration coefficients in physical units of microns, which makes clinical interpretation difficult. However, it is possible to convert from microns to the more familiar units of diopters by applying the concept of "equivalent defocus," which is defined as the amount of defocus needed to produce the same degree of wavefront error produced by one or more higher-order aberrations.[2] It is important to remember that 1 diopter (D)of a higher-order aberration defined in this way does not necessarily have exactly the same visual effect as 1 D of defocus.[3,4] Indeed, the same could be said of astigmatism: 1 D of astigmatism does not have exactly the same effect as 1 D of defocus, yet the use of a common physical unit helps us judge their relative importance. In this same way, the concept of equivalent defocus permits a loose comparison of the order of magnitude of different kinds of aberrations and judgment of their clinical significance. Applying this approach to Figure 12-4, we see that the variability of higher-order aberration in our patients was less than 0.04 D for any time scale from seconds to years. This value is extremely small by ordinary clinical standards but nevertheless is large enough to prevent the attainment of truly "perfect" optics with a single, static prescription.

> All aberrations are not equal. For example, 0.25 µm of RMS error loaded into secondary astigmatism over a 6 mm pupil (an equivalent defocus of 0.19 D) reduces high contrast acuity 3+ times more than the same error loaded into quadrafoil.[3]

The source of variability depicted in Figure 12-4 may be measurement noise or normal biological fluctuations. To determine which of these two factors is paramount, we examined temporal variability in a physical model eye that has a degree of spherical aberration similar to the human eye. When we collected multiple aberration maps after aligning the instrument just once, the variability was practically zero as shown in the lower graph of Figure

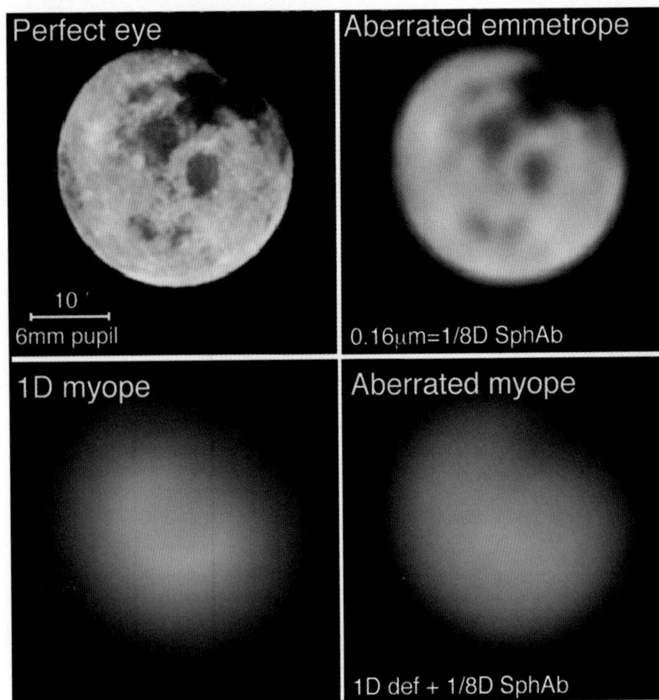

Figure 12-5. Simulation of the effect of ocular aberrations on the retinal image of the moon. Upper left: an optically perfect eye limited only by diffraction by a 6 mm pupil. Upper right: image for an eye suffering only from 0.16 μm (0.125 D equivalent defocus) of spherical aberration. Bottom left: image for an eye suffering only from 1 D of defocus. Bottom right: image for an eye suffering from 1 D of defocus and 0.16 μm of spherical aberration.

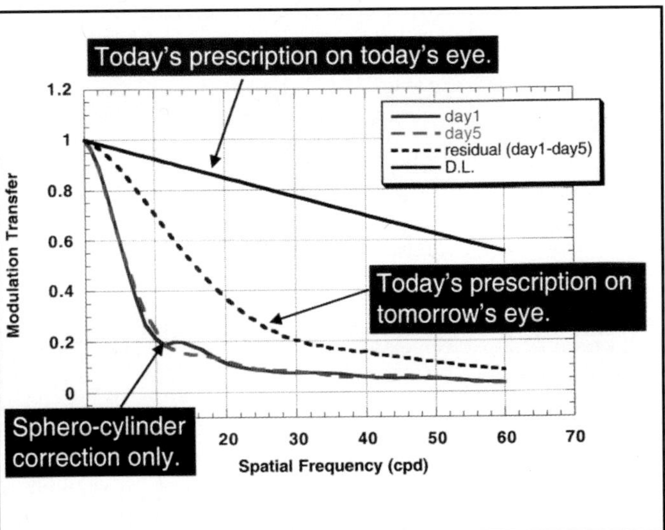

Figure 12-6. Effect of temporal variability in aberrations on retinal image quality. Modulation transfer functions (MTFs) for monochromatic light (6 mm pupil) are shown for patient CT assuming perfect correction of only the second-order components (defocus and astigmatism) of the aberration map obtained on day 1 (blue curve) and for the map obtained on day 5 (red curve). Perfect correction of the higher-order aberrations measured on day 1 would yield a perfect MTF (solid black curve) on day 1. However, using the measurements obtained on day 1 to correct the aberrations present on day 5 yields an imperfect MTF (dashed black curve) on day 5.

12-4. However, when we realigned the instrument to the model eye before each measurement, the variability was similar in magnitude to that obtained from human eyes over a time span of 1 hour. We conclude from this result that most of the variability we observed in human eyes on an hourly time scale could be accounted for by measurement noise associated with realigning the instrument. On the other hand, the gradual increase in variability observed on longer time scales probably reflects real biological changes in the patients' eyes.

Ultimately, we would like to know the impact of temporal variability of the aberration map on vision. We can gain some appreciation of this fact by considering the visual effect of spherical aberration on the simulated retinal image of the moon as shown in Figure 12-5. A relatively small amount of spherical aberration (equivalent to 0.125 D of defocus) significantly reduces the quality of the retinal image when added to a perfect (aberration-free) emmetropic eye, as shown in the top row of images. However, the same amount of aberration has very little effect when added to a myopic eye with 1 D of uncorrected refractive error, as shown in the bottom row of images.[4] In general, we can expect variability in higher-order aberrations to be visually insignificant if variability is small compared to the total amount of aberrations in the eye. Indeed, this was the case in our study. The standard deviation of RMS wavefront error for higher-order aberrations was about 10% of the mean for each of our four patients. This result suggests that the visual effect of temporal variability is negligible in the presence of the eye's normal level of aberrations. However, if the normal level of aberrations is greatly reduced by surgery or custom contact or intraocular lenses, then the visual impact of temporal variability in those aberrations will become increasingly important.

> If the normal level of aberrations is greatly reduced by surgery or custom contact or intraocular lenses, then the visual impact of temporal variability in those aberrations will become increasingly important.

To demonstrate the increasing importance of temporal variability as the eye approaches optical perfection, we used the aberration maps determined on two different days to compute the modulation transfer function (MTF) for one patient's eye. In performing this calculation, we assumed that the second-order aberrations of sphere and cylinder were perfectly corrected. The results, shown by the red and blue curves in Figure 12-6, are virtually identical, indicating that temporal variability has very little effect in the presence of normal levels of higher-order ocular aberrations. Now imagine that the higher-order aberrations of this eye are corrected by some surgical process or ophthalmic lens. The result would be an optically perfect eye that is limited solely by diffraction. The MTF for such an eye is shown by the solid black line in Figure 12-6. However, if we use the aberration map collected on one day to treat the patient's eye on the other day, the aberration map would have changed enough to prevent the attainment of an optically perfect eye. Theoretical calculations indicate that the anticipated ten-fold improvement in contrast sensitivity at 30 cycles per degree (c/deg) expected from correcting higher-order aberrations is reduced to only a two-fold increase, all because of a seemingly trivial degree of variability amounting to a small fraction of a diopter. Even this two-fold gain in contrast sensitivity is probably an overestimate because it assumes the unlikely event that ordinary spherocylindrical refractive errors are stable and perfectly corrected.

While it is instructive to look at the diffraction-limited case, it is important to remember that it is impossible to totally eliminate the aberrations of the eye and that if the therapy designed to reduce aberrations instead induces an increase in optical aberrations, retinal image quality will be decreased.

Summary

From a clinical perspective, the higher-order aberrations of the normal healthy eye are typically of the same order of magnitude as the residual sphere and cylinder present in an eye that is well-corrected by clinical standards. Variability in those higher-order aberrations is an order of magnitude smaller, on any time scale from seconds to years, and therefore is likely to have an insignificant impact on image quality in the normally aberrated eye. Nevertheless, this variability is large enough to significantly limit the potential gain in retinal image quality expected from a treatment method capable of fully correcting the higher-order aberrations of the eye. On the other hand, for clinically abnormal eyes (eg, keratoconus, or unsuccessful laser in-situ keratomileusis outcomes), aberrations can be orders of magnitude larger than in a normal eye and visually debilitating to the patient. In such cases, correction of higher-order aberrations would be expected to yield a major improvement in image quality even though the final result may be far from perfect due to variability.

References

1. Cheng, X, Hinebaugh N, Kollbaum, P, Thibos LN, Bradley A. Test-retest reliability of clinical Shack-Hartmann measurements. *Invest Ophthalmol Vis Sci*. In press.
2. Thibos LN, Applegate RA. Assessment of optical quality. In: MacRae SM, Krueger RR, Applegate RA, eds. *Customized Corneal Ablation: The Quest for Super Vision*. Thorofare, NJ: SLACK Incorporated; 2001:67-78.
3. Applegate RA, Sarver EJ, Khemsara V. Are all aberrations equal? *J Refract Surg*. 2002;18:S556-S562.
4. Applegate RA, Marsack J, Ramos R. Interaction between aberrations can improve or reduce visual performance. *J Cataract Refract Surgery*. 2003;29:1487-1495.

Chapter 13

Accommodation Dynamics and Its Implication on Customized Corrections

Vikentia J. Katsanevaki, MD, PhD; Sophia I. Panagopoulou, PhD; Sotiris Plainis, PhD; Harilaos Ginis, PhD; and Ioannis Pallikaris, MD, PhD

Introduction

The ability to see clearly at different distances is one of the most important functions of the human visual system. This is performed in daily life by the process of accommodation (ie, the change of the refractive power of the crystalline lens via the contraction of the ciliary muscle).

The study of the eye's optical quality with accommodation goes back at least 200 years,[1] revealing that the aberrations of the eye do not remain static but change upon accommodation. The quality of the retinal image for objects in focus is governed by the eye's optics and by diffraction. Since the eye undergoes substantial optical changes upon accommodation, the associated retinal image quality is expected to be modified.

The Effect of Accommodation on Ocular Aberrations

Changes in individual aberrations, as a function of accommodation, have been examined in a number of previous studies. The most studied monochromatic aberration, excluding defocus, has been spherical aberration.[1-4] Using different methodologies, including annular apertures,[1] the vernier acuity method,[2,3] or the knife-edge test,[4] investigators on the subject agree that positive spherical aberration in the unaccommodated eye changes toward zero or negative values during accommodation. Lu et al[5] refined Ivanoff's vernier acuity testing[2] and fitted aberration terms up to the sixth power along the horizontal meridian of the pupil for accommodation stimuli of up to 4 diopters (D). They reported the classical trend of decreased spherical aberrations with increasing accommodation in two of the four eyes they examined. The higher-order terms (fifth and sixth) were opposite in sign, balancing their primary terms (third and fourth, respectively).

The main drawbacks of these initial methods to identify and measure ocular aberrations were the reliance on subjective response, as well as the need for time-consuming recordings and data analysis. Furthermore, these methods suffered from lack of thorough validation, since they were limited to a one-dimensional analysis of the wave aberration. Advances in instrumentation (eg, dynamic infrared optometers, video-based systems) and the evolution of wavefront aberrometers, most notably the Shack-Hartmann wavefront sensor, have overcome these problems and can now provide a reliable and relatively rapid evaluation of ocular aberration changes with accommodation.

Atchison et al[6] made the first detailed attempt to describe the change of ocular aberrations as a function of accommodation. They investigated its effect on aberrations up to the fourth order for three states of accommodation (0, -1.5, and -3 D) in 15 eyes using the Howland principle-based aberroscope. The authors found no clear trend of variance of the wave aberration with change in accommodation. The classical trend of spherical aberrations toward negative values was only shown in half (8 out of 15) of the subjects they examined. They reported third-order coma as being the dominant aberration within their sample with no other information regarding its change with accommodation. In a more recent and detailed study, He et al[7] measured the monochromatic wavefront aberrations (35 Zernike terms) with increasing levels of accommodation ranging from 0 to -6 D using a spatially resolved refractometer. They reported substantial individual variations in the ocular aberration profile. Spherical aberration always decreases (becomes more negative) with increasing accommodation, whereas aberrations with orders higher than four are minimal near the resting state of accommodation. The change of coma shows a complex pattern that varies across individuals. The accommodation-induced change in wavefront aberration is not strongly related to the total amount of aberration in the eight eyes studied, but in general the optical quality of the eye improves from 0 to -1 D and then gradually decreases thereafter.

> In general, with accommodation the optical quality of the eye improves from 0 to -1 D and then gradually decreases thereafter.

Time-resolved measurements of accommodation have been possible since the 1930s,[8] providing considerable information on accommodation using dynamic infrared optometers[9,10] and video-based systems.[11] Newly released video-based autorefractors provide measurements with temporal resolution up to 60 hertz (Hz).[12] Using these modalities, dynamics of accommodation have been intensely investigated in terms of lower-order aberrations, namely defocus. However, little is known about the stability of the other monochromatic aberrations, such as spherical aberrations and coma, during near fixation as well as the dynamic sensitivities of these aberrations upon fixation from infinity to a near target.

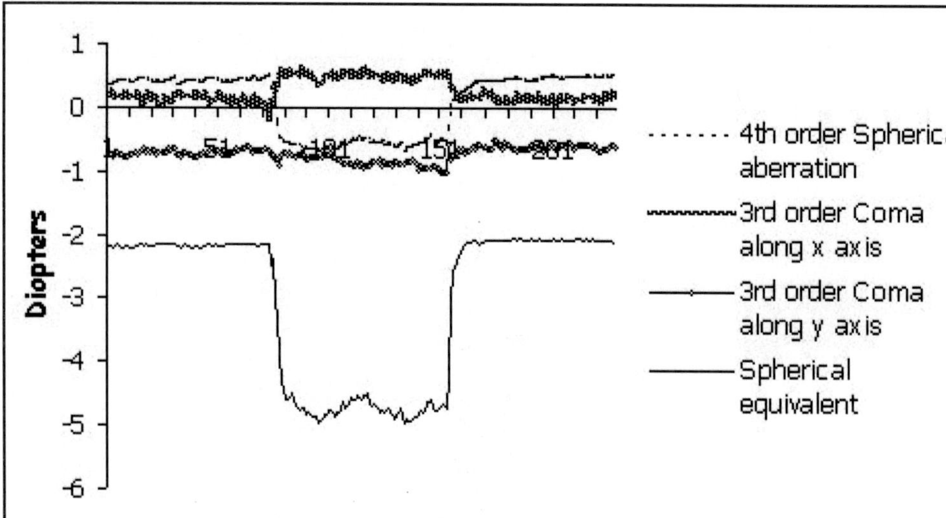

Figure 13-1. An example of plotted time-resolved measurements of fourth-order spherical, third-order vertical and horizontal coma aberrations, and spherical equivalent of a 32-year-old subject who fixated from a distant target to the near point of fixation and back to the distant target. The measurements were obtained at 7.7 Hz and the pupil aperture was of 5.5 millimeters (mm). The spherical aberrations showed the classical trend of obtaining negative sign with accommodation. Horizontal coma changed toward positive values, whereas vertical coma remained almost stable.

Hofer et al[13] were the first to obtain time-resolved measurements of higher-order aberrations up to the seventh order. They examined three normal subjects for 5 seconds at 25.6 captures/sec with natural and paralyzed accommodation using a Shack-Hartmann sensor-based device. With unparalyzed accommodation, subjects fixated on a complex target of 3.3 D, 2 D, and the far point. Their results indicate the presence of fluctuations among all of the eye's examined aberrations. The shape for higher-order aberrations was generally different from that for microfluctuations of accommodation, and the authors suggested that these changes upon accommodation were not only due to change of the lens shape when accommodated but also to other causes such as tear film instability, artificial eye movements, or changes in the axial length of the eye caused by the heartbeat. Using similar methodology, Artal et al[14] used a Shack-Hartmann sensor to obtain time-resolved measurements of two subjects when fixating from infinity to a near target (vergence of 2.5 D) at 25 Hz. They also found induced spherical aberrations as well as coma with accommodation. Uploading of their data on a customized optical software have shown that point spread function images could not be perfect for both near and distant vision after static corrections of either the far or the near wavefront, respectively.

The quality of the retinal image for objects in focus was also investigated by Lopez-Gil et al and estimated the changes of the retinal image quality in four young subjects (aged from 18 to 34 years) with a vergence of -4 to -5.5 D by using a near infrared double pass apparatus.[15] The specific differences in the modulation transfer function (MTF) obtained for near and far vision depended on subjects. In general, the MTFs of the unaccommodated eyes were slightly better. Their technique allowed for discounting the effect of the accommodative refractive error, which would also be expected to degrade retinal image of near vision under every day viewing conditions.

In the University of Crete, Greece we have used a commercially available Shack-Hartmann (Wavefront Aberration Supported Cornea Ablation [WASCA], Asclepion Meditec, Jena, Germany) sensor to dynamically assess accommodation in six subjects (aged from 24 to 48) when fixated from a distant target to the near point of fixation at 7.7 Hz. Change of spherical aberrations followed the classical trend toward negative values in all subjects, and their change was related to accommodation in a linear pattern. In agreement with previous reports,[7,15] coma-like aberrations were either increased or decreased in a nonrepeatable change pattern and were not related to the changes of the spherical equivalent (Figure 13-1). The variable changes of coma could be attributed to the lateral displacement of the lens relative to the cornea as it moves in the accommodation process.[7] Another possible explanation could be the lack of rotational symmetry of the cornea and/or the lens that would be expected to induce asymmetric aberrations of variable magnitude upon the forward movement of the accommodating lens. Regarding the retinal image quality, we found variable changes of the MTFs upon accommodation. In general, the retinal image quality of the accommodating eyes of younger subjects was worse than in the nonaccommodative state (Figure 13-2). Findings were more complex in older subjects: the retinal image may be improved, worsened only at lower spatial frequencies, or remain almost unaffected with accommodation. In our study, we compared examinations when subjects fixated at the near point of fixation, thus having targets of different vergences for the near task. The most probable reason for the different effect of the accommodation and induced aberrations in the quality of the retinal image seems to be the different amount of accommodation within the subjects we examined.

Change of spherical aberrations followed the classical trend toward negative values in all subjects, and their change was related to accommodation in a linear pattern.

The variable changes of coma could be attributed to the lateral displacement of the lens relative to the cornea as it moves in the accommodation process.[7] Another possible explanation could be the lack of rotational symmetry of the cornea and/or the lens that would be expected to induce asymmetric aberrations of variable magnitude upon the forward movement of the accommodating lens.

Steady-State Errors in Accommodation

It is now well accepted that steady-state errors are an intrinsic part of the accommodation control system. The system is characterized by over-accommodation for far targets ("leads" of accommodation) and under-accommodation for near targets ("lags" of accommodation). These defocusing errors are dependent on the

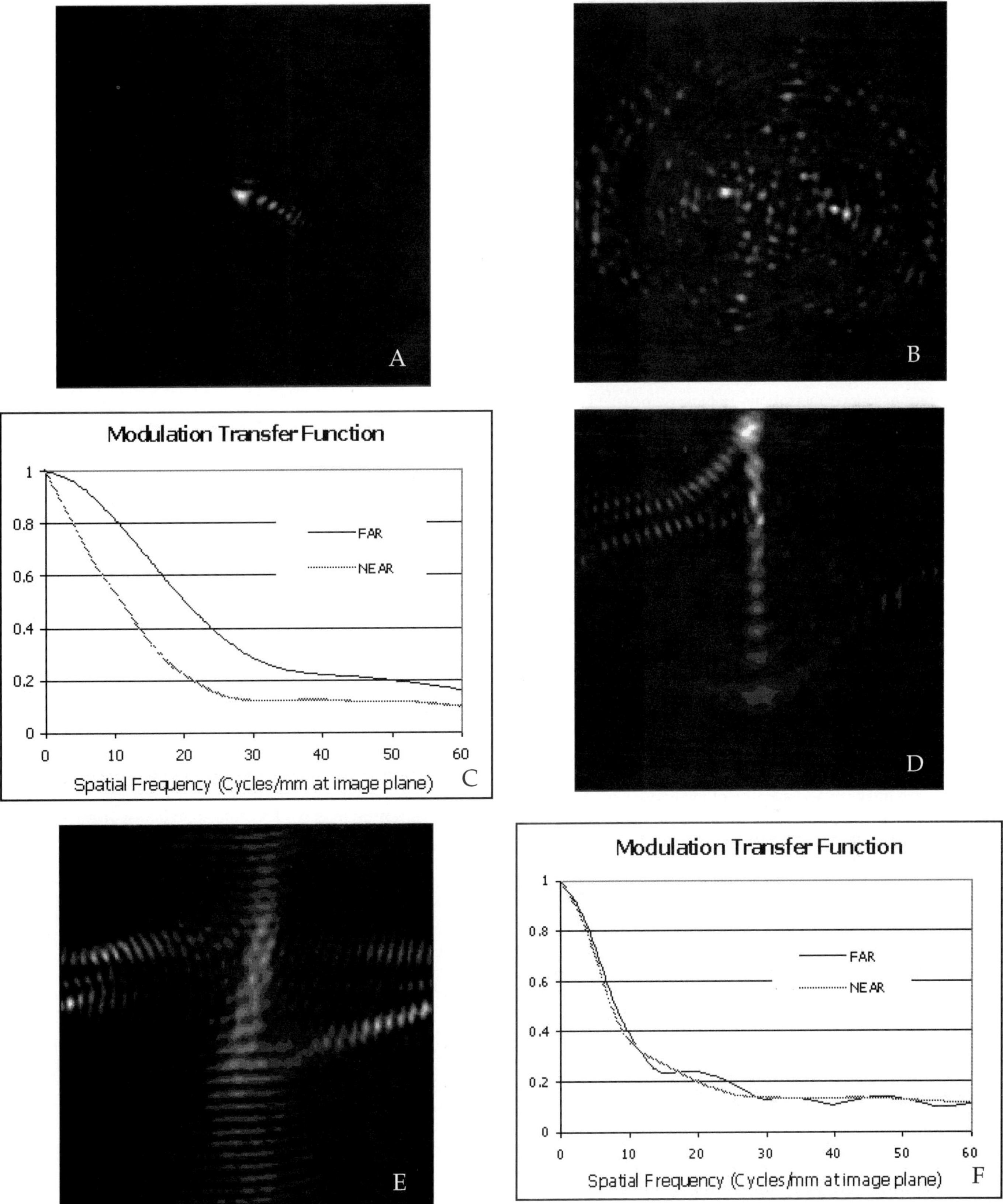

Figure 13-2. Calculated MTF (C and F) and point spread function (PSF) for the distant (A and D) and near (B and E) fixation of a subject 24 years old fixating at a target vergence of 4 D (A, B, and C) and a subject 48 years old fixating at a target vergence of 1 D (D, E, and F). The MTF of the younger subject (A) was slightly worse at the near fixation, whereas the MTF of the older subject (D) was almost unchanged with near fixation. The relevant PSF images of both subjects at near fixation were more scattered but still more symmetric as compared to that of distant vision. As has been previously suggested,[15] this could either be to the decrease in the amount of coma-like aberrations or to the increase of other symmetric aberrations such as spherical aberrations or defocus.

pupil size: small pupils allow large errors in accommodation due to increased depth-of-focus.[16]

Moreover, the stability of accommodative response is heavily affected at low light levels.[17] We have collected data from a small group of patients, highlighting the effect of accommodation on spherical aberration under different luminance conditions: spherical aberrations show the classical trend toward negative values; however, this effect is more pronounced for low light levels. This could be due to the increased pupil diameter and probably the reduced accommodation stability under scotopic conditions. These changes were also related to the accommodative amplitude of the examined subjects.

Additionally, under all conditions, the accommodation response is not steady but changes rapidly and continuously, showing small fluctuations. These small oscillations of dioptric power are called *microfluctuations* and have typical values of about 0.2 D.[18] These fluctuations, which are related to both pupil size and target vergence,[18,19] as already mentioned, are present in all of the eye's wave aberrations, not just defocus.[13] These fluctuations, although not considerable enough to degrade high contrast visual acuity, may affect retinal image quality as expressed by MTF and further complicate the effect of accommodation on the ocular wavefront profile changes.

Discussion: Implications on Wavefront-Guided Refractive Surgery

In summary, the optical performance of the eye at different accommodation conditions is not well characterized. The total range of accommodative states and final conclusions on the exact trends of different terms of higher-order aberrations is not yet fully understood.

The evolution of faster and more accurate devices (eg, the Shack-Hartmann wavefront sensor) for studying the optics of the eye seems to provide the technological platform to understand the change of imaging performance of the eye.

Recently applied excimer laser customized ablations[20-22] aim to achieve super vision, attempting to correct both lower-order (sphere and cylinder) and higher-order aberrations. Apart from encountered problems, such as laser in-situ keratomileusis (LASIK)-induced aberrations[23,24] and a number of parameters (eg diffraction, photoreceptor sampling,[25] chromatic aberration[26]) that limit the finest detail we can see, it is apparent that any small changes in accommodation may be of vast importance in wave-guided customized refractive surgery. The potential alterations of the ocular aberrations and respecting retinal image quality during accommodation are putting customized ablations for both distant and near vision under question. In other words, the higher-order static correction for distant vision would not be necessarily optimal for near work and vice versa. Hence, the "correction" of the aberrations can only be effective at one object distance.

Recent reports of dynamic corrections of the ocular aberrations using closed-looped adaptive optics showed effective correction of aberrations with a residual uncorrected wavefront of almost 0.12 microns (μm) for a 4.3 mm pupil diameter.[27] Using this methodology, Hofer et al[28] have shown that correction of the temporal variation of the eye's wave aberration increased the Strehl ratio of the PSF nearly three times, improving the contrast of images of the cone receptors by 33% compared with images taken with only static correction of the eye's higher-order aberrations.

We assume that dynamic correction of eye's aberrations would be most valuable in ophthalmic imaging systems (eg, charged-coupled device [CCD] fundus camera[29] and scanning laser ophthalmoscopy[30]) but in regard to photorefractive corrections, common experience indicates that there is no evident loss of visual performance when viewing distant and near objects at the same angular subtence. As been previously suggested,[14] it is most probable that static corrections, like customized ablations, would not provide optimal results for both near and distant visual performance but the clinical importance of this implication remains unclear.

Editor's note:
It is likely that the only place of clinical importance for super vision is at distance viewing, since the subtended angle of small distant objects cannot be altered as it can with near objects, which are just held closer to the viewer.
R. Krueger, MD, MSE

At present, commercially available laser vision correction platforms measure wavefront aberration with dilated pupils to gain the largest pupil capture of aberrations. No matter what extend accommodation may alter the aberration outcome, pupil size remains the most important variable that can affect the ocular wavefront map. Treatments based on maps obtained after pupil dilation are clearly the best modalities to perform customized laser treatments.

Editor's note:
This chapter raises the issue of the eye's wavefront higher-order aberration pattern changing moderately with accommodation. It seems that one wavefront pattern is not preferable under all conditions, but we are coming to understand that there are no "one size fits all" condition.

Currently, most surgeons are trying to minimize higher-order aberration measured when the eye is in focus at distance. This assumption seems reasonable given that most people prefer optimal sharpness at distance. Sharp distance vision is particularly relevant when driving at night when the pupils are more dilated, which increases the effect of higher-order aberration, and contrast is reduced by darkness. This is in contrast to near vision tasks generally, which mostly take place under bright light conditions, with good contrast, the pupil is more constricted, making higher-order aberration less prominent. In the future, we will learn how to "optimize the wavefront correction" so that both distance and near vision are considered. This "optimization of the wavefront correction" is an important area of future refinement in wavefront-corrected customization.
S. MacRae, MD

References

1. Koomen M, Tousey R, Scolnic R. The spherical aberration of the eye. *J Opt Soc Am A*. 1949;39:987-992.
2. Ivanoff A. About the spherical aberration of the eye. *JOSA*. 1956;46: 901-903.
3. Jenkins TCA. Aberrations of the human eye and their effects on vision: part I. *Br J Phys Opt*. 1963;20:59-91.

4. Berny F, Slansky S. Wavefront determination resulting from Foucault test as applied to the human eye and visual instruments. In: Dickson JH, ed. *Optical Instruments and Techniques.* Newcastle-upon Tyne: Oriel Press; 1969:375-386.
5. Lu C, Munger R, Campbell MC. Monochromatic aberrations in accommodated eyes. In: *Technical Digest Series, Ophthalmic and Visual Optics.* 1993;3:160-163. Washington DC: Optical Society of America.
6. Atchison DA, Collins MJ, Wildsoet CF, Christensen J, Waterworth MD. Measurement of monochromatic ocular aberrations of human eyes as a function of accommodation by the Howland aberroscope technique. *Vision Res.* 1995;35:313-323.
7. He JC, Burns SA, Marcos S. Monochromatic aberrations in the accommodated human eye. *Vision Res.* 2000;40:41-48.
8. Charman WN, Heron G. Fluctuations in accommodation: a review. *Ophthalmic Physiol Opt.* 1988;8:153-163.
9. Campbell F, Robson JC. High speed infrared optometer. *J Opt Soc Am.* 1959;49:268-272.
10. Charman WN, Heron G. A simple infrared optometer for accommodation studies. *Br J Physiol Opt.* 1975;30:1-12.
11. Schaeffel F, Wilhelm H, Zrenner E. Interindividual variability in the dynamics of natural accommodation in humans: relation to age and refractive errors. *J Physiol.* 1993;461:301-320.
12. Wolffson JS, Gilmartin B, Mallen EAH, Tsutjimura S. Continuous recording of accommodation and pupil size using the Shin-Nippon SRW-5000 autorefractor. *Ophthalmic Physiol Opt.* 2001;21:108-113.
13. Hofer H, Artal P, Singer B, Aragon JL, Williams DR. Dynamics of the eye's wave aberrations. *J Optom Soc Am A.* 2001;18:497-506.
14. Artal P, Fernandez EJ, Manzanera S. Are optical aberrations during accommodation a significant problem for refractive surgery? *J Refract Surg.* 2002;18:563-566.
15. Lopez-Gil N, Inglesias I, Artal P. Retinal image quality in the human eye as a function of accommodation. *Vision Res.* 1998;38:2897-2907.
16. Charman WN. Optics of the eye. In: Bass M, Van Stryland EW, Williams DR, Wolfe WL, eds. *Handbook of Optics.* Vol 1. 2nd ed. New York: McGraw Hill; 1995:24.3-24.54.
17. Johnson CA. Effects of luminance and stimulus distance on accommodation and visual resolution. *J Opt Soc Am A.* 1976;66:138-142.
18. Charman WN, Heron G. Fluctuations in accommodation: a review. *Ophthalmic Physiol Opt.* 1988;8:153-164.
19. Stark LR, Atchison DA. Pupil size, mean accommodation response and the fluctuations of accommodation. *Ophthalmic Physiol Opt.* 1997;17:316-323.
20. MacRae S, Schwiegerling J, Snyder R. Customized corneal ablations and super vision. *J Refract Surg.* 2000;16:230-235.
21. Panagopoulou SI, Pallikaris GI. Wavefront customized ablations with the WASCA Asclepion workstation. *J Refract Surg.* 2001;17:608-612.
22. Mrochen M, Kaemmerer M, Seiler T. Clinical results of wavefront-guided laser in situ keratomileusis 3 months after surgery. *J Cataract Refract Surg.* 2001;27:201-207.
23. Pallikaris, IG, Kymionis GD, Panagopoulou SI, Siganos CS, Theodorakis MA, Pallikaris AI. Induced optical aberrations following formation of a laser in situ keratomileusis flap. *J Cataract Refract Surg.* 2002;28:1737-1741.
24. Moreno-Barriuso E, Lloves JM, Marcos S, Navarro R, Llorente L, Barbero S. Ocular aberrations before and after myopic corneal refractive surgery: LASIK-induced changes measured with laser ray tracing. *Invest Ophthalmol Vis Sci.* 2001;42:1396-1403.
25. Curcio CC, Sloan KR, Kalina RE, Hendrickson AE. Human photoreceptor topography. *J Comp Neurol.* 1990;292:497-523.
26. Campbell FW, Gubisch RW. The effect of chromatic aberration on visual acuity. *J Physiol.* 1967;192:345-358.
27. Fernandez EJ, Inglesias I, Artal P. Closed-loop adaptive optics in the human eye. *Optics Letters.* 2001;26:746-748.
28. Hofer H, Chen L, Yoon GY, Singer B, Yamauchi Y, Williams DR. Improvement in retinal image quality with dynamic correction of the eye's aberrations. *Optics Express.* 2001;8:631-643.
29. Roorda A, Williams DR. The arrangement of the three cone classes in the living human eye. *Nature.* 1999;397:520-522.
30. Roorda A, Romero-Borja F, Donnely WJ, Queener H. Adaptive optics scanning laser ophthalmoscope. *Optics Express.* 2002;10:405-412.

Chapter 14
The Implications of Pupil Size and Accommodation Dynamics on Customized Wavefront-Guided Refractive Surgery

Sophia I. Panagopoulou, PhD; Sotiris Plainis, PhD; Scott M. MacRae, MD; and Ioannis Pallikaris, MD, PhD

Customized Refractive Surgery: Background

Since the application of excimer laser technology for the correction of the eye's simple refractive errors (ie, defocus and astigmatism), there has been a considerable debate concerning the visual impact of correcting the higher-order monochromatic aberrations of the eye (eg, spherical aberration, coma, and secondary astigmatism), which also degrade retinal image quality.[1-4] Advances in the measurement of the eye's wave aberration and the ability to accurately correct it using adaptive optics technology[5] have initiated the effort in exploring the possibility of eliminating ocular aberrations to give an enhanced visual acuity.[6,7]

Investigators have recently demonstrated that they can correct ocular aberrations with adaptive optics. They have already proven its value when incorporated in ophthalmic imaging systems (eg, charged-coupled device [CCD] fundus camera[8] and scanning laser ophthalmoscopy[9]). The success of adaptive optics has encouraged the implementation of higher-order correction through wavefront-guided refractive surgery, which suggests the potential of producing aberration-free human eyes. In principle, the eye's wavefront aberrations are measured using rapid and accurate devices, most notably the Shack-Hartmann wavefront sensor. This information would then be fed to the controlling computer, which in turn would modify the excimer laser's scanning pattern to allow simple refractive errors as well as higher-order aberrations to be corrected.

There is currently a major ongoing effort to refine laser refractive surgery for correcting higher-order aberrations. The first groups performing wavefront-guided customized ablation have recently reported preliminary data that are encouraging but still tentative: an increase in the overall root mean square (RMS) wavefront error has been observed postoperatively.[10-13] However, the increase in the magnitude of higher-order aberrations is less pronounced when compared with conventional laser in-situ keratomileusis (LASIK).[11,14] It seems reasonable that the target of the investigators would be first to minimize LASIK-induced higher-order aberrations and then to reduce them to preoperative levels, especially in highly aberrated eyes. In post-LASIK eyes, the most predominant aberrations are spherical aberration[15] (see below and Chapter 2) and coma-like aberrations along the flap's hinge axis.[14] For this reason, several of the excimer laser manufacturers are already planning to change their ablation profiles from spherical to aspherical to correct for spherical aberrations.

> In post-LASIK eyes, the most predominant aberrations are spherical (see below) and coma-like aberrations along the flap's hinge axis.

Although these ideas are simple in principle, the visual benefit we could receive from attempts to correct higher-order aberrations depends on a number of parameters that reduce retinal image quality and limit the finest detail we can see. Beside photoreceptor sampling[16,17]; cortical magnification,[18] which cannot be regulated and will always limit visual resolution; and chromatic aberration, which will always be present in white light,[19] other factors include pupil size and accommodation. Their possible implications on customized-refractive correction are discussed below.

The Effect of Pupil Size on Ocular Aberrations

The normal pupil varies in size depending on the amount of incident light. Most people in the modern world function under photopic conditions, which is defined as greater than 10^2 candelas/meter^2 (cd/m^2). Normal indoor lighting is roughly 10^2 cd/m^2 and the lighting increases to 10^5 cd/m^2 outdoors. When the sun goes down or we go into a partially illuminated environment, we are typically functioning under mesopic conditions that are between 0.01 to 10 cd/m^2, with both rod and cone systems enactive. Night driving and most low light activities are done under mesopic conditions where there is partial light, such as the dashboard lights or headlights that help increase the illumination. When the illuminance is further reduced, one is functioning under scotopic conditions, where the rods are primarily active. Most activities of daily living are not done under scotopic conditions.

> A recent large cohort study on 340 eyes found the mean mesopic pupil diameter was 5.69 ± 1.07 mm prior to customized LASIK surgery (see Figure 14-1). Interestingly, over 32% of eyes had pupillary diameters 6.00 mm or greater, indicating that larger effective ablation optical zones than 6.00 or even 6.50 mm may be indicated with such patients (see Figure 14-1).

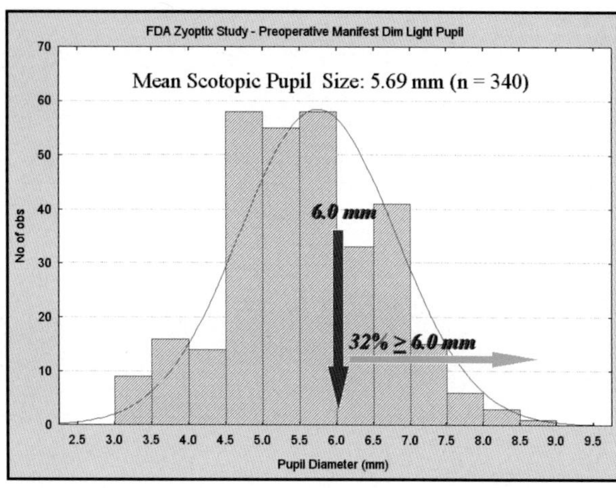

Figure 14-1. Mesopic pupil diameter of 340 eyes prior to LASIK. The mean preoperative pupil diameter was 5.69 mm. Thirty-two percent of eyes had pupil diameters of 6 mm or greater.

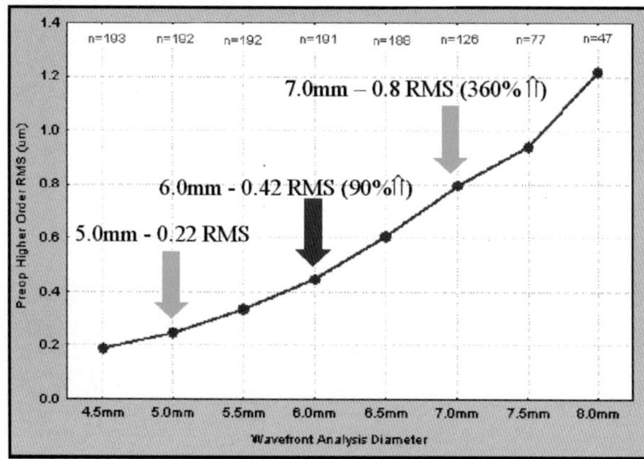

Figure 14-2. Mean RMS wavefront error for a large cohort of 340 normal eyes prior to LASIK demonstrating increasing RMS error as the wavefront analysis or aperture diameter increases. The wavefront analysis diameter simulates what occurs when the pupil dilates. Note that the mean RMS wavefront error almost doubles as the wavefront analysis diameter increases from 5 mm to 6 mm and it almost doubles again going from 6 mm to 7 mm.

A recent large cohort study on 340 eyes found the mean mesopic pupil diameter was 5.69 ± 1.07 millimeters (mm) prior to customized LASIK surgery (Figure 14-1). Interestingly, over 32% of eyes had pupillary diameters 6 mm or greater, indicating that effective ablation optical zones larger than 6 mm or even 6.5 mm may be indicated for such patients (see Figure 14-1). In that same study, the normal preoperative eyes received a noncycloplegic dilated wavefront sensing with the Zywave wavefront sensor (Bausch & Lomb, Rochester, NY). The increase in higher-order aberration was dramatic, as the pupil size (or wavefront aperture diameter) was increased (Figure 14-2). As the wavefront sensor aperture was opened to simulate pupillary enlargement from 5 to 6 mm., the RMS wavefront error increased from 0.22 to 0.42 mm (a 90% increase). When the wavefront sensor aperture was opened from 6 to 7 mm, there was almost another doubling from 0.42 to 0.80 mm of RMS wavefront error (a 90% increase). Thus, there was a 360% increase in RMS wavefront error as the wavefront aperture diameter increased from 5 to 7 mm in a normal untreated group of eyes. The clinical implications of this are important for three reasons:

1. There is a sharp rise in RMS wavefront error when the pupil (or wavefront aperture diameter) increases even 1 mm, in this case almost 100%. Thus, the wavefront analysis diameter (or clinically, pupil size) has a profound effect on the RMS value and should always be reported when reporting RMS values
2. If a RMS wavefront error is reported without the wavefront aperture diameter (or pupillary diameter), the RMS value is not meaningful, since it is ambiguous
3. There is a large increase in RMS wavefront error between 5 and 7 mm. Thus, patients with large ablation optical zones (5.5 mm and larger) are indeed less likely to have problems with their mesopic vision (related to higher-order aberrations) than individuals with smaller pupils

> There was a 360% increase in RMS wavefront error as the wavefront aperture diameter increased from 5.00 to 7.00 mm in a normal untreated group of eyes

> The wavefront analysis diameter (or clinically, pupil size) has a profound effect on the RMS value and should always be reported when reporting RMS values.

The size of the pupil controls the level of retinal illuminance and the depth-of-field of the eye. Due to diffraction-limited visual performance (ie, the Rayleigh criterion), the maximal benefit of correcting aberrations are greatest for the largest pupil diameters (ie, > 5.00 mm). However, there are several practical problems that may compromise visual benefit for large pupils. First, as a result of the spherical aberration, image quality will be reduced as the pupil dilates (Figure 14-3). This pattern is more pronounced in postsurgical eyes,[14,15] with the resulting image degradation being more serious in the peripheral field.[20]

Second, in a natural eye, such large diameters typically occur at low light levels (ie, low mesopic and scotopic conditions). Figure 14-3 demonstrates the effect of luminance on pupil size. However, at scotopic levels, visual performance is dictated by rods; thus, the fine detail available will not normally be used due to the reduced spatial resolution of rod vision. At photopic light levels, spherical aberration will be reduced because of the smaller pupil diameter, but visual performance will also be limited by diffractive effects when the pupil is 2 mm or smaller. Finally, due to directionality of the cones (ie, Stiles-Crawford effect[21]), light sensitivity is reduced to 60% at the edge of 4 mm pupil and 35% at the edge of a 6 mm pupil. The Stiles-Crawford effect on retinal image quality is believed to be important, as it ameliorates the detrimental effect of defocus and aberrations on visual performance.

The Effect of Accommodation on Ocular Aberrations

Optimal monochromatic performance will only be achieved if the eye is precisely focused. When we are looking at something in the distance, the retinal image of the target is in focus. When we decide to look at a nearby object, the accommodative system

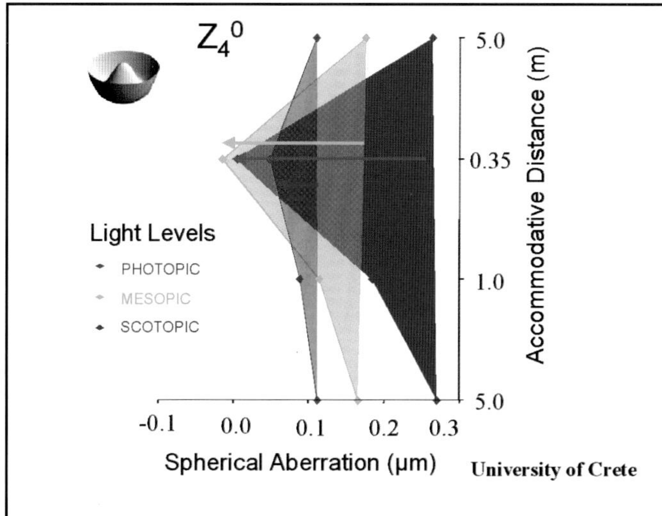

Figure 14-3. Pupil size (mean values and standard deviations) as a function of accommodative distance (5, 1, and 0.35 m) under three light levels (photopic, mesopic, and scotopic). Data were obtained from 60 subjects (age range: 22 to 52).

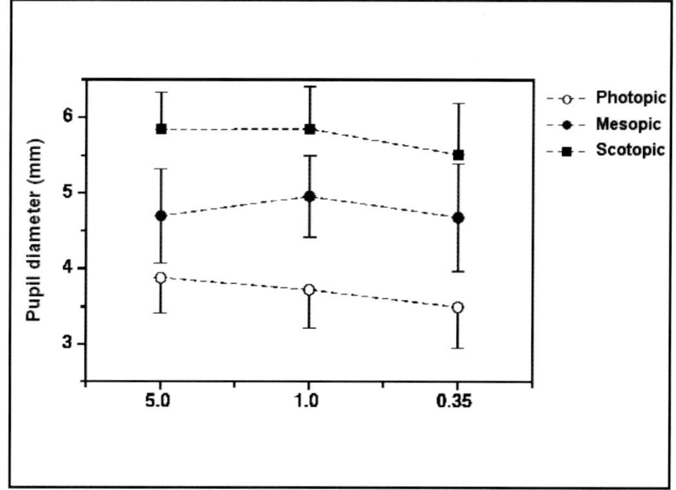

Figure 14-4. Mean values of spherical aberration at different accommodative distances (5, 1, and 0.35 m) under three light levels (photopic, mesopic, and scotopic). Data were obtained from 40 subjects (age range: 22 to 40). Note that the change of spherical aberration toward negative values is more pronounced at scotopic conditions.

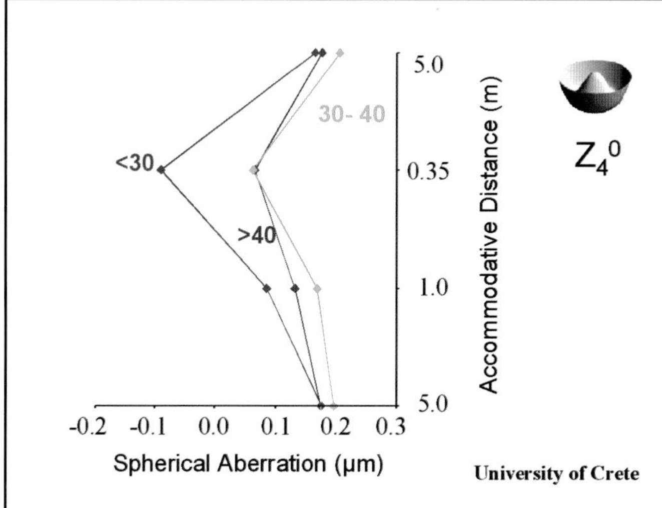

Figure 14-5. Mean values of spherical aberration at different accommodative distances (5, 1, and 0.35 m) for three age groups (<30, 30 to 40, and >40). Photopic conditions were used.

generates signals to minimize the image of blur for the object of interest. In the prepresbyopic eye, two types of focus errors are characteristic of the accommodation system.

First, the system is characterized by overaccommodation for far targets ("leads" of accommodation) and underaccommodation for near targets ("lags" of accommodation).[22] The stability of response is heavily affected at low light levels.[23] Moreover, aberrations change as the eye accommodates[24,25] and are minimum at the resting point of accommodation (about 1.0 to 1.5 diopters [D]),[25] which means that the overall optical quality of the eye will be best at this point. Figure 14-4 presents data collected at the University of Crete with the Wavefront Aberration Supported Corneal Ablation (WASCA) aberrometer (Asclepion-Meditec AG, Jena, Germany) from a group of patients of different ages, highlighting the effect of accommodation on spherical aberration at three light levels. Spherical aberration shows the classical trend toward negative values with the effect being more pronounced at scotopic light levels, confirming results found in previous studies.[26] This could be due to the reduced accommodation stability under scotopic conditions. Moreover, the shift from positive to negative spherical aberration values with accommodation may result in more myopic refraction for small pupils. This is expected to reduce accommodation demand. Figure 14-5 shows the variation in spherical aberration with accommodation for three age groups. The change in spherical aberration to negative values is higher for the young group (< 30 years). This can be attributed to the progressively reduced amplitude of accommodation with age. The wavefront error was measured with the WASCA wavefront analyzer. Second, in normal viewing, the accuracy of accommodation is not perfect; when a target at fixed distance is viewed, the power of the eye changes rapidly and continuously, showing microfluctuations of the order of about 0.2 D.[27] These fluctuations increase at low lighting and as accommodation increases,[27,28] reaching a minimum at its resting point (approximately 1 to 1.5 m). The resulting effect of fluctuations in lens accommodation can cause fluctuations in all of the eye's wave aberrations, not just defocus.[29] Microfluctuations in accommodation, although not considerable enough to produce degradation in high contrast visual acuity, may reduce retinal image quality.

In normal viewing, the accuracy of accommodation is not perfect; when a target at fixed distance is viewed, the power of the eye changes rapidly and continuously, showing microfluctuations of the order of about 0.2 D.

Implications on Wavefront-Guided Refractive Surgery

It is apparent that any changes in accommodation may affect the outcome of wavefront-guided customized refractive surgery. They might, by increasing the effective depth-of-focus of the eye affect the precision of refractive measurement. Furthermore, they may possibly affect the outcome of the wavefront-guided customized ablation, as aberrations of the eye change with the level of accommodation. Hence, the "correction" of the aberrations may only be optimally effective at a range of object distances and may also become less effective as the patient ages. In general, it seems likely that most young individuals who have undergone "aberration correction" will sometimes at best only obtain moderate benefits under natural conditions, where the pupil and accommodation system are active. It may, however, be that a minority of individuals need optimal vision at distance for some specific purpose (such as fighter pilots or marksmen) where higher-order aberration correction is optimized at distance.

The exact trends of different modes of higher-order aberrations when accommodating is not yet fully understood; thus, it is not entirely clear as to how to optimize the visual system at distance and near under a variety of pupil conditions. Therefore, it is important to keep on using the current technology (adaptive optics and wavefront sensing) in order to further understand the dynamics of the visual system.

Editor's note:

Pupil size is one of three critical values that are sometimes confused or mislabeled. The first is ablation optical zone diameter, which determines the effective optical zone depending on tissue reaction and biomechanics. An ablation optical zone diameter of 6 mm for different laser manufacturers may have different effective optical zones, depending on the ablation optical zone and transition zone design and the length of the transition zone.

The second important value is the mesopic pupil size, which should be measured under controlled conditions similar to night driving as mentioned above at 0.1 to 2 lux. Better control of luminance levels with pupillometry will improve our understanding of the role of the mesopic pupil in low light visual performance.

The third value of importance is the wavefront aperture diameter. The wavefront aperture diameter can be varied (either decreased or increased by the user) to a maximum of the pupil diameter when the wavefront was captured. (One of the limitations of wavefront sensors is they are limited to only measuring within the pupil diameter.) As we saw in this chapter, the wavefront aperture diameter should always be noted when giving wavefront error since the aperture diameter plays a profound role in determining the magnitude of the wavefront error. As we saw in Figure 14-2, the wavefront error almost doubled when the wavefront aperture diameter increased from 5 mm to 6 mm and then almost doubled again when going from 6 mm to 7 mm. A better understanding of the relationship between these three values gives us important insights into the subtlety of wavefront correction.

S. MacRae, MD

References

1. Ivanoff A. About the spherical aberration of the eye. *J Opt Soc Am A.* 1956;46:901-903.
2. Jenkins TCA. Aberrations of the human eye and their effects on vision: part I. *British Journal of Physiological Optics.* 1963;20:59-91.
3. Guirao A, Porter J, Williams DR, Cox I. Calculated impact of higher order monochromatic aberrations on retinal image quality in a population of human eyes. *J Opt Soc Am A.* 2002;19:1-9.
4. Charman WN. The retinal image in the human eye. *Prog Retin Eye Res.* 1983;2:1-50.
5. Liang J, Williams DR, Miller DT. Supernormal vision and high-resolution retinal imaging through adaptive optics. *J Opt Soc Am A.* 1997;14:2884-2892.
6. Williams D, Yoon GY, Porter J, Guirao A, Hofer H, Cox I. Visual benefit of correcting higher order aberrations of the eye. *J Refract Surg.* 2000;16:554-559.
7. Charman WN. Will correction of ocular aberration lead to "super acuity"? *CE Optometry.* 2001;4:33-36.
8. Roorda A, Williams DR. The arrangement of the three cone classes in the living human eye. *Nature.* 1999;397:520-522.
9. Roorda A, Romero-Borja F, Donnely WJ, Queener H. Adaptive optics scanning laser ophthalmoscope. *Optics Express.* 2002;10:405-412.
10. MacRae S, Schwiegerling J, Snyder R. Customized corneal ablations and super vision. *J Refract Surg.* 2000;16:230-235.
11. Panagopoulou SI, Pallikaris GI. Wavefront customized ablations with the WASCA Asclepion workstation. *J Refract Surg.* 2001;17:608-612.
12. Mrochen M, Kaemmerer M, Seiler T. Clinical results of wavefront-guided laser in situ keratomileusis 3 months after surgery. *J Cataract Refract Surg.* 2001;27:201-207.
13. McDonald MB. Summit-Autonomous custom cornea laser in situ keratomileusis outcomes. *J Refract Surg.* 2000;16:617-618.
14. Pallikaris, IG, Kymionis GD, Panagopoulou SI, Siganos CS, Theodorakis MA, Pallikaris AI. Induced optical aberrations following formation of a laser in situ keratomileusis flap. *J Cataract Refract Surg.* 2002;28:1737-1741.
15. Moreno-Barriuso E, Lloves JM, Marcos S, Navarro R, Llorente L, Barbero S. Ocular aberrations before and after myopic corneal refractive surgery: LASIK-induced changes measured with laser ray tracing. *Invest Ophthalmol Vis Sci.* 2001;42:1396-1403.
16. Williams DR. Aliasing in human foveal vision. *Vision Res.* 1985; 25:195-205.
17. Curcio CC, Sloan KR, Kalina RE, Hendrickson AE. Human photoreceptor topography. *J Comp Neurol.* 1990;292:497-523.
18. Rovamo J, Mustonen J, Nasanen R. Neural modulation transfer function of the human visual system at various eccentricities. *Vision Res.* 1995;35:767–774.
19. Campbell FW, Gubisch RW. The effect of chromatic aberration on visual acuity. *J Physiol.* 1967;192:345-358.
20. Charman WN, Atchison DA, Scott DH. Theoretical analysis of peripheral imaging after excimer laser corneal refractive surgery for myopia. *J Cataract Refract Surg.* 2002;28:2017-2025.
21. Stiles WS, Crawford BH. The luminous efficiency of rays entering the eye pupil at different points. *Proc Roy Soc B.* 1933;112:428-450.
22. Charman WN. Optics of the eye. In: Bass M, Van Stryland EW, Williams DR, Wolfe WL, eds. *Handbook of Optics.* Vol 1. 2nd ed. New York: McGraw Hill; 1995:24.3-24.54.
23. Johnson CA. Effects of luminance and stimulus distance on accommodation and visual resolution. *J Opt Soc Am A.* 1976;66:138-142.
24. Lopez-Gill N, Iglesias I, Artal P. Retinal image quality in the human eye as a function of the accommodation. *Vision Res.* 1998;38:2897-2907.
25. He JC, Burns SA, Marcos S. Monochromatic aberrations in the accommodated human eye. *Vision Res.* 2000;40:41-48.
26. Atchison DA, Collins MJ, Wildsoet CF, Christensen J, Waterworth MD. Measurement of monochromatic ocular aberrations of human eyes as a function of accommodation by the Howland aberroscope technique. *Vision Res.* 1995;35:313-323.
27. Charman WN, Heron G. Fluctuations in accommodation: a review. *Ophthalmic Physiol Opt.* 1988;8:153-164.
28. Stark LR, Atchison DA. Pupil size, mean accommodation response and the fluctuations of accommodation. *Ophthalmic Physiol Opt.* 1997;17:316-323.
29. Hofer H, Artal P, Singer B, Aragon JL, Williams DR. Dynamics of the eye's wave aberration. *J Opt Soc Am A.* 2001;18:497-506.

Clinical Science Section:

Commercially Available Wavefront Devices

Chapter 15

Shack-Hartmann Aberrometry: Historical Principles and Clinical Applications

Maria Regina Chalita, MD and Ronald R. Krueger, MD, MSE

Some of the concepts in this chapter are repetitive to the concepts presented in Chapter 6. This is done in order to emphasize these principles because of the significance they attribute to the content of each of these two chapters.

Introduction

Customized corneal ablation is a refractive methodology developed to perform a personalized treatment that improves the visual acuity and optical quality of the eye. Measurement of the eye's wavefront aberration is becoming an important goal in clinical ophthalmology and plays a critical role leading toward the optical correction of these ocular aberrations.[1]

There are four different principles by which wavefront aberrations can be acquired and measured: outgoing reflection aberrometry (Shack-Hartmann aberrometry), retinal imaging aberrometry (Tscherning and ray tracing aberrometry), ingoing adjustable refractometry (spatially-resolved refractometry), and double pass aberrometry (slit skiascopy). This chapter describes outgoing optics aberrometry, where the slope of the rays exiting the eye defines the wavefront error pattern. This form of wavefront sensing is uniquely characterized and described by the principles of Shack-Hartmann.

There are four different principles by which wavefront aberrations can be acquired and measured: outgoing reflection aberrometry (Shack-Hartmann aberrometry), retinal imaging aberrometry (Tscherning and ray tracing aberrometry), ingoing adjustable refractometry (spatially-resolved refractometry), and double pass aberrometry (slit skiascopy).

History of the Shack-Hartmann Aberrometer

In 1619, Christopher Scheiner, philosopher and astronomy professor at the University of Ingolstadt, demonstrated the focusing ability of the human eye using a device that is widely known in ophthalmology as the *Scheiner disk*.[2] Scheiner stated that if an optically imperfect eye looks through an opaque disk with two pinholes, a single distant point of light would create two separate retinal images (Figure 15-1). If the eye's optical imperfection is due only to defocus, a simple lens that corrects the ametropia will bring the two retinal images into coincidence. However, for optical aberrations other than defocus, a more general method is needed for quantifying the refractive imperfections of the eye at each pupil location. In 1961, Smirnov described a subjective aberrometer based on Scheiner's disk. He used a fixed light source for the central reference pinhole and a moveable light source for the outer pinhole. By adjusting the moveable source vertically and horizontally, this ray of light is redirected until it intersects the fixed ray at the retina and the patient can visualize a single point of light (Figure 15-2). After the moveable source adjustment, the displacement distances Δ and Δy are a metric of the ray aberration of the eye at the given pupil point.[3] This latter was adopted into ophthalmology as the spatially-resolved refractometer.

In the early 1900s, Hartmann described another method for measuring the ray aberrations of mirrors and lenses based on Scheiner's idea. The direction of light propagation was reversed by placing a spot of light on the retina, thus converting the Scheiner-Smirnov subjective technique into an objective aberrometer. This spot then became a point source that radiated light back out of the eye. Additional holes were created in Scheiner's disk, then called the Hartmann screen (Figure 15-3). Each aperture in the Hartmann screen isolates a narrow pencil of rays emerging from the eye through a different part of the pupil. These emerging rays intersect a video sensor that registers the vertical and horizontal displacement of each ray from the corresponding, nonaberrated reference position.[4,5]

Seventy years later, Shack and Platt used an array of tiny lenses in each individual aperture of the Hartmann screen that subdivided the wavefront into smaller beams of light (or smaller wavefronts), thereby forming multiple images of the same retinal point source. Their technique is known as *Shack-Hartmann aberrometry*, and it is used extensively by astronomers for measuring the optical aberrations of the atmosphere with telescopes (Figure 15-4).[6]

In the mid-1980s, Dr. Josef Bille began working with Shack to use the lens array to measure the corneal profile. Bille was the first to use the sensor in ophthalmology. He used it first to measure the corneal profile and later to measure aberrations in the eye by projecting a point source onto the retina. His first publication was in 1989.[7]

Principles of Shack-Hartmann Aberrometry

In the Shack-Hartmann technique, the outgoing array of spot images are used to determine the wavefront shape. The wavefront is subdivided into a few hundred small beams that are

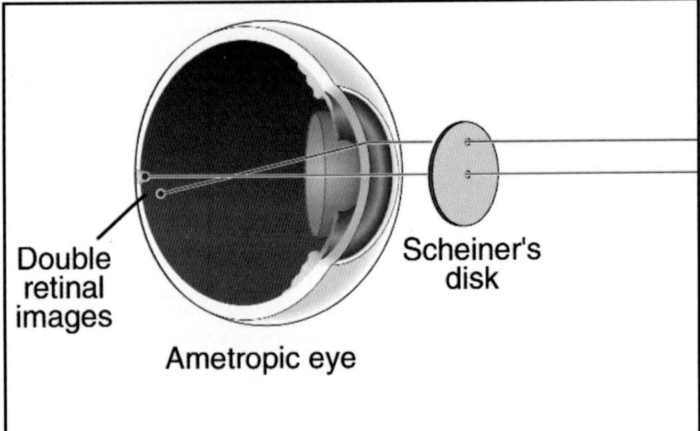

Figure 15-1. Scheiner's disk isolates rays, allowing their aberrated direction of propagation to be traced. An ametropic eye will form two retinal images for each object point when viewing through a Scheiner disk with two apertures. (Adapted from Chapter 6 of MacRae S, Krueger R, Applegate R. *Customized Corneal Ablation: The Quest for Super Vision.* Thorofare, NJ: SLACK Incorporated; 2001.)

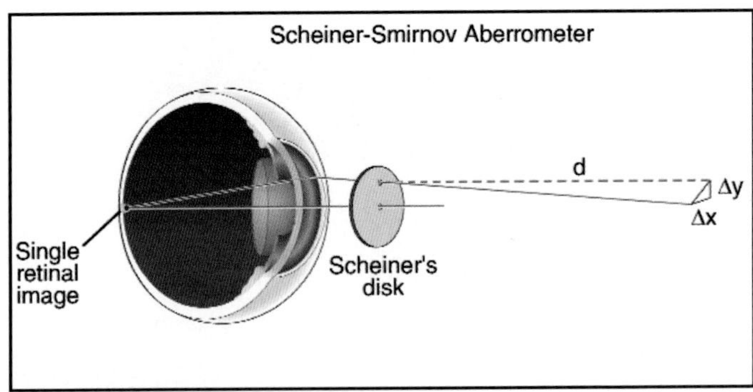

Figure 15-2. Smirnov's aberrometer used the principle of Scheiner's disk to measure the eye's optical imperfections separately at every location in the eye's entrance pupil. (Adapted from Chapter 6 of MacRae S, Krueger R, Applegate R. *Customized Corneal Ablation: The Quest for Super Vision.* Thorofare, NJ: SLACK Incorporated; 2001.)

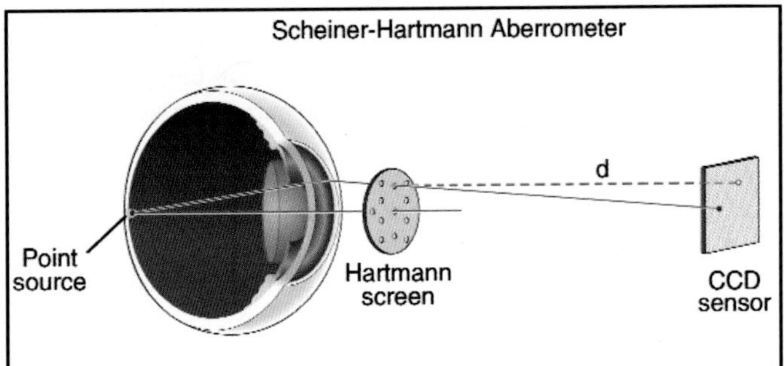

Figure 15-3. The Hartmann screen used to measure aberrations objectively is a Scheiner disk with multiple apertures. (Adapted from Chapter 6 of MacRae S, Krueger R, Applegate R. *Customized Corneal Ablation: The Quest for Super Vision.* Thorofare, NJ: SLACK Incorporated; 2001.)

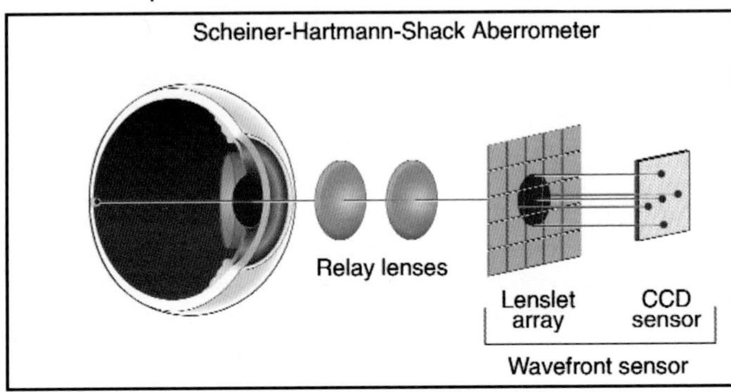

Figure 15-4. The aberrometer built on the Scheiner-Hartmann-Shack principle uses relay lenses to image the lenslet array into the eye's pupil plane. A CCD video sensor captures an image of the array of spots for computer analysis. (Adapted from Chapter 6 of MacRae S, Krueger R, Applegate R. *Customized Corneal Ablation: The Quest for Super Vision.* Thorofare, NJ: SLACK Incorporated; 2001.)

focused onto a charged-coupled device (CCD) video sensor by an array of small lenses or lenslets (see Figure 15-4). For a perfect eye, the reflected plane wave is focused into a perfect lattice of point images, each image falling on the optical axis of the corresponding lenslet (Figure 15-5). In the aberrated eye, the wavefront is distorted. The local slope of the wavefront is now different for each lenslet, thus the wavefront is focused into a disordered collection of spot images (Figure 15-6). The spatial displacement of each spot relative to the optical axis of the corresponding lenslet is a direct measurement of the local slope of the incident wavefront as it passes through the entrance aperture of the lenslet. The integration of these slope measurements reveals the shape of the aberrated wavefront.[8]

> In the Shack-Hartmann technique, the outgoing array of spot images are used to determine the wavefront shape.

> For a perfect eye, the reflected plane wave is focused into a perfect lattice of point images, each image falling on the optical axis of the corresponding lenslet (see Figure 15-5). In the aberrated eye, the wavefront is distorted.

The principles of Shack-Hartmann aberrometry were also applied in 1994 by Liang and colleagues in order to measure aberrations of human eyes.[9] Because the shape of an aberrated wavefront changes as the light propagates, it is important to analyze the reflected wavefront as soon as it passes through the eye's pupil. In order to do this, Liang used a pair of relay lenses that focused the lenslet array onto the eye's entrance pupil. Optically, the lenslet array seemed to reside in the plane of the eye's entrance pupil where it could subdivide the reflected wavefront immediately as it emerged from the eye. The array of spot images formed by the lenslet array was captured by a CCD sensor and then analyzed by computer to estimate the eye's aberration map. The aberrations are expressed as Zernike polynomial derivatives and the fitted coefficients are used to reconstruct the shape of the aberrated wavefront.

Clinical Applications of the Shack-Hartmann Aberrometer

The Shack-Hartmann method of measuring the wave aberration function of the eye is one of today's most promising. This is due to the availability of high-density lenslet arrays as well as the device's speed, objectivity, and high spatial resolution in the pupil plane.[10]

In 1997, Liang and Williams tested the repeatability of the Shack-Hartmann technique by repeatedly measuring the wave-

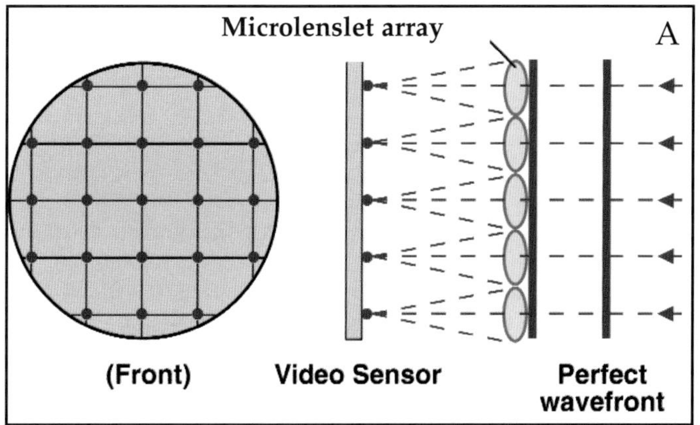

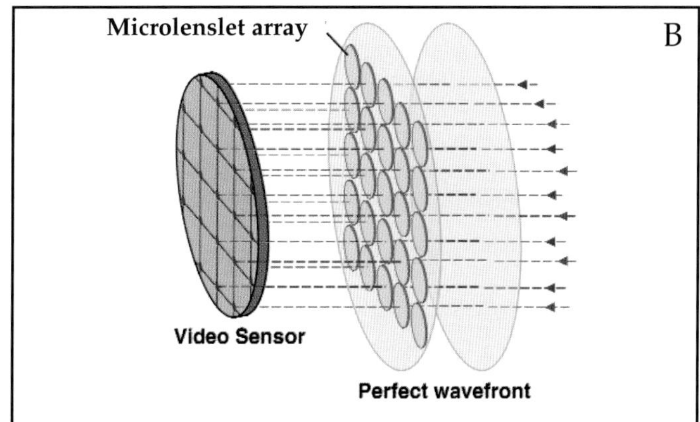

Figure 15-5. The Shack-Hartmann wavefront sensor forms a regular lattice of image points for a perfect plane wave of light. (A) Lateral view of the microlenslet array and front view of the video sensor. (B) Detailed two-dimensional view of the microlenslet array and video sensor. (Adapted from Chapter 6 of MacRae S, Krueger R, Applegate R. *Customized Corneal Ablation: The Quest for Super Vision.* Thorofare, NJ: SLACK Incorporated; 2001.)

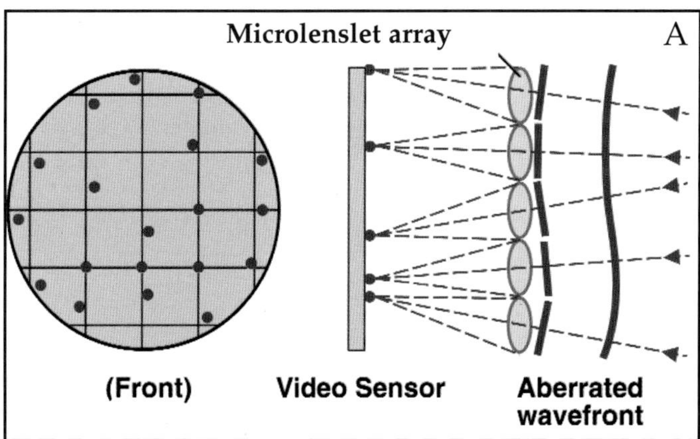

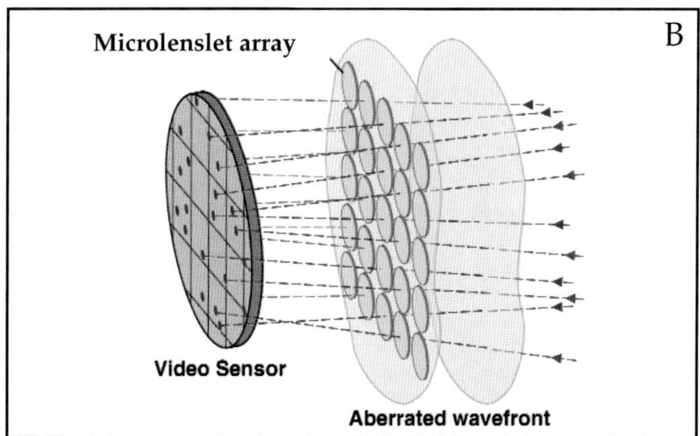

Figure 15-6. The Shack-Hartmann wavefront sensor forms an irregular lattice of image points for an aberrated wave of light. (A) Lateral view of the microlenslet array and front view of the video sensor. (B) Detailed two-dimensional view of the microlenslet array and the video sensor. (Adapted from Chapter 6 of MacRae S, Krueger R, Applegate R. *Customized Corneal Ablation: The Quest for Super Vision.* Thorofare, NJ: SLACK Incorporated; 2001.)

front aberration function along the eye's vertical meridian and accuracy by comparing it with previously measured eyes. They found good repeatability and reasonable agreement with previous measurements.[11] One year later, Salmon and coauthors showed that the Shack-Hartmann sensor could provide accurate and repeatable measurements of the wavefront aberration function in human eyes and that they were in good agreement with independent measurements from the traditional Smirnov psychophysical technique.[12]

In 1999, Thibos and Hong demonstrated that the Shack-Hartmann technique for measuring the optical aberrations of the eye could be applied successfully to a variety of abnormal clinical conditions to provide a comprehensive description of the eye's refractive aberrations. They could measure the aberrations in clinical conditions such as dry eyes, keratoconus, post-laser in-situ keratomileusis (LASIK) surgery, and lenticular cataract.[13]

Limitations of Shack-Hartmann Aberrometry

The Shack-Hartmann data analysis does not take into account the quality of individual spots formed by the lenslet array. Only the spot's displacement is needed for computing local slope of the wavefront over each lenslet aperture. One disadvantage is that in eyes with a large amount of aberrations or extreme irregular corneas, crossover can occur.

Crossover in a Shack-Hartmann aberrometer can take place when light from one lenslet crosses over onto the area where a different spot is expected. Crossover can happen in highly aberrated eyes, such as postcorneal transplant eyes, especially in wavefront sensors with low dynamic range as described in Chapter 16. The crossover creates a false measurement or an inability of the device to calculate the aberration.

Available Commercial Systems That Use Shack-Hartmann Wavefront Sensing

To date, there are six different commercial systems available that utilize a Shack-Hartmann aberrometer: the LADARWave system (Alcon, Fort Worth, Tex), the WaveScan system (VISX, Santa Clara, Calif), the Zywave system (Bausch & Lomb, Rochester, NY), the Topcon Wavefront Analyzer (Topcon America Corp, Paramus, NJ), the Wavefront Aberration Supported Cornea Ablation (WASCA) system (Zeiss Meditec AG, Jena, Germany), and the Complete Ophthalmic Analysis

System (COAS) (WaveFront Sciences, Albuquerque, NM). The systems use different focal lengths, which are positively correlated with the sensitivity of the wavefront sensor and negatively correlated with the dynamic range of the wavefront sensor, as noted in the next chapter. The systems also use different lenslet spacings that also make direct comparisons difficult, since company sponsors generally keep this information proprietary.

> The Shack-Hartmann data analysis does not take into account the quality of individual spots formed by the lenslet array. Only the spot's displacement is needed for computing local slope of the wavefront over each lenslet aperture.

LADARWave System

The LADARWave wavefront device designed by Alcon captures approximately 170 spots within a 6.5 millimeter (mm) pupil aperture (although its maps are typically expressed at 6.5 mm). It can measure up to eighth-order aberrations and has a dynamic range capable of gathering images from spherical errors in the range of -15 to +15 D and cylindrical errors in the range of 0 to -8 D. The device can measure wavefronts with a maximum curvature in any meridian lying between +8 and -14 D (defined for a 8 mm pupil). In order to obtain the patient's true, nonaccommodated refractive profile, the device has an auto-focusing system that automatically fogs the patient until a nonaccommodative refraction is achieved.

WaveScan System

The WaveScan wavefront device from VISX captures about 180 spots within a 6 mm pupil aperture, since the spacing between the lenslet is 0.4 mm. It can measure up to sixth-order aberrations and has a dynamic range capable of measuring from -8 to +6 D. It also has an automated fogging system to avoid undesirable accommodation.

Zywave System

The Zywave wavefront device designed by Bausch & Lomb captures 60 spots within a 6 mm pupil aperture, measuring up to fifth-order aberrations, and is capable of capturing up to seventh order. The system can measure refractive error from +6 to -12 D of sphere and up to -5 D of astigmatism. It can measure wavefront maps with pupil diameters between 2.5 to 8.5 mm in diameter. The system uses a 785 µm infrared light to illuminate the retina and a trombone system to measure the spherical error while maximizing sensitivity.

Topcon Wavefront Analyzer

The Topcon KR9000 PW wavefront analyzer device contains an ordinary refractometer, an 11-ring corneal topographer, and a coaxial Shack-Hartmann aberrometer. It measures up to sixth-order aberrations with 85 spots within a 6 mm pupil diameter and up to fourth order at 4 mm. The system can measure refractive error from +15 to -15 D of sphere with the aberrometer and from +15 to -20 D of sphere with the refractometer, both measuring up to -7 D of astigmatism. The spacing between the lenslet at the entrance pupil plane is 0.6 mm and all measurements are computationally referred to the line of sight. The wavelength is 840 nm, with an exposure time of 300 milliseconds (ms) and the power on the cornea is 18 µW. This device has a rotating d-prism in a common path of an ingoing and an outgoing light to scan the light beam on the focus.

WASCA System

The WASCA system used by Zeiss Meditec incorporates the lenslet array based on the core-patented technology of WaveFront Sciences Inc. The full array consists of lenslets arranged in a rectangular array 44 x 33 (1.452 lenslets). The shape of each lenslet surface is spherical, but each lenslet is a 144 µm square section of this surface. In this way, there is 100% fill of the focusing array, which reduces stray light that could cause interference or background effects that reduce spot localization accuracy. The full array measures 6.5 x 4.8 mm. This array enables approximately 800 lenslets to collect light from a 7 mm entrance pupil, with an effective lateral resolution of 210 µm.

COAS WaveFront Sciences System

The COAS captures 1017 spots within a 6 mm pupil aperture. It can measure up to 16th-order aberrations; however, due to computation time, it is usually set no higher than 10th-order aberrations. This device has a dynamic range capable of measuring from -14 to +7 D, including 5 D of cylinder. It also has a dynamic fogging system that uses a +1.5 D lens.

References

1. Charman W. Wavefront aberration of the eye: a review. *Optom Vis Sci.* 1991;68:574-583.
2. Scheiner C. Oculus, sive fundamentum opticum. *Innspruk.* 1619.
3. Smirnov MS. Measurement of the wave aberration of the human eye. *Biofizica.* 1961;6:687-703.
4. Hartmann J. Bemerkungen uber den bau und die jurstirung von spektrographer. *Zeitschrift fuer Instrumenterkinde.* 1900;20:47.
5. Hartmann J. Objektuventersuchungen. *Zeitschrift fuer Instrumenterkinde.* 1904;24:1.
6. Shack RV, Platt BC. Production and use of a lenticular Hartmann screen. *J Opt Soc Am A.* 1971;61:656.
7. Platt B, Shack R. History and principles of Shack-Hartmann wavefront sensing. *J Refract Surg.* 2001;17:S573-S577.
8. Thibos LN. Principles of Hartmann-Shack aberrometry. *J Refract Surg.* 2000;16:S563-S565.
9. Liang J, Grimm B, Goelz S, Bille J. Objective measurement of the wave aberrations of the human eye using a Hartmann-Shack wavefront sensor. *J Opt Soc Am A.* 1994;11:1949-1957.
10. Munson K, Hong X, Thibos LN. Use of a Shack-Hartmann aberrometer to assess the optical outcome of corneal transplantation in a keratoconic eye. *Optom Vis Sci.* 2001;78:866-871.
11. Liang J, Williams DR. Aberrations and retinal image quality of the normal human eye. *J Opt Soc Am A.* 1997;14:2873-2883.
12. Salmon TO, Thibos LN, Bradley A. Comparison of the eye's wavefront aberration measured by psychophysically and with the Shack-Hartmann wavefront sensor. *J Opt Soc Am A.* 1998;15:2457-2465.
13. Thibos LN, Hong X. Clinical applications of the Shack-Hartmann aberrometer. *Optom Vis Sci.* 1999;76:817-825.

Chapter 16

Optimizing the Shack-Hartmann Wavefront Sensor

Geunyoung Yoon, PhD; Seth Pantanelli, BS; and Scott M. MacRae, MD

A wide range of wavefront sensors have become available for characterization of the eye's aberrations. They have also become a powerful tool for understanding and improving the outcome of conventional and customized laser refractive surgery. Of the designs used in vision science and ophthalmology today, the Shack-Hartmann aberrometer is one of the most popular commercialized sensors used to measure ocular aberrations. While some are specifically designed to achieve high resolution and sensitivity of the wavefront, recent interests are geared more toward being able to measure a large amount of aberration or to have a large dynamic range. A larger dynamic range allows scientists and clinicians to measure a large range of refractive errors and higher-order aberrations as observed in postcorneal transplant and keratoconic eyes. Since each wavefront sensor employs slightly different designs and specifications, it is important to understand the tradeoffs of each parameter for the wavefront sensor. More specifically, the relationship between dynamic range and measurement sensitivity and the factors that affect each will be explored in this chapter.

> A larger dynamic range allows scientists and clinicians to measure a large range of refractive errors and higher-order aberrations as observed in postcorneal transplant and keratoconic eyes.

In the Shack-Hartmann wavefront sensor, a laser beam is sent into the eye so that a spot forms on the retina. The light reflects off of the back of the eye and then continues outward through the lens and cornea. The aberrated wavefront emerging from the eye is relayed onto an array of tiny lenses, called *lenslets*, and transformed into a spot pattern that can be analyzed by a computer program. By measuring the displacement of these spots from a reference, the computer program can reconstruct the original aberrated wavefront.

To accurately measure higher-order aberrations, the number of sampling points (lenslets) must be properly chosen. The measurement performance of the wavefront sensor directly depends on how well the center of each spot can be detected by a centroiding algorithm. If the algorithm fails to correctly detect and assign each spot to its corresponding lenslet for various reasons (to be described later in this chapter), the reconstructed wavefront aberration will be unreliable or completely wrong. Most limitations, such as dynamic range and measurement sensitivity, are related to this task. Now that a basic understanding of the Shack-Hartmann wavefront sensor has been developed, we can look more closely at the relationships between dynamic range and other design parameters that govern its abilities and limitations.

Dynamic Range and Measurement Sensitivity

One of the fundamental limitations in a Shack-Hartmann wavefront sensor is the requirement that each spot generated by an individual lenslet be within the virtual subaperture on a photon detector. This is a problem because the software typically associated with this type of wavefront sensor is not capable of correctly identifying the spot formed by a lenslet once it travels into the space behind an adjacent lenslet (a), closely overlaps with another spot (b), or crosses the path of another spot known as "crossover" (c). These potential problems are illustrated in Figure 16-1.

The dynamic range of a Shack-Hartmann wavefront sensor is defined by the maximum wavefront slope, θ_{max}, that a lenslet is capable of handling without encountering any of the limitations discussed above. This limitation is obviously reached when each spot produces the maximum allowed displacement at a given focal length of the lenslet array, f, as shown in Figure 16-2. Since the wavefront slope can have the opposite sign with the same magnitude, the maximum distance, Δd_{max}, each spot can move is one-half of the lenslet spacing, s. The dynamic range of a wavefront sensor is given by the equation:

$$\theta_{max} = \frac{\Delta d_{max}}{f} = \frac{s/2}{f} \qquad (1)$$

> The dynamic range is, therefore, linearly proportional to the lenslet spacing and inversely proportional to the focal length of the lenslet array. The dynamic range of the wavefront sensor can be increased by increasing the lenslet spacing and/or by reducing the focal length of the lenslet array as expected from equation 1.

Measurement sensitivity is another important factor that should be taken into account when designing this type of wavefront sensor. Although adding dynamic range to the wavefront

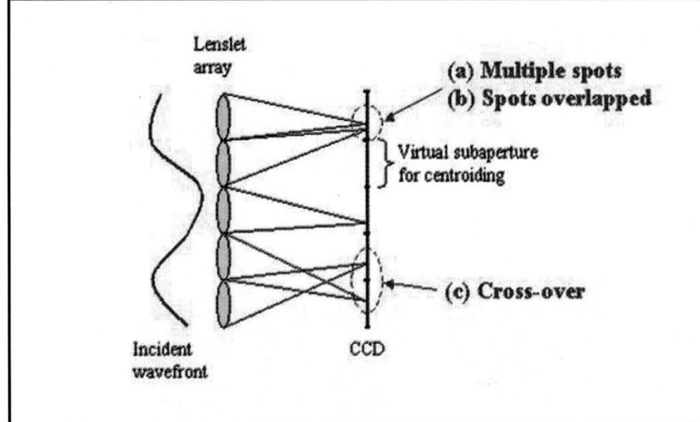

Figure 16-1. Potential problems that may occur in a conventional Shack-Hartmann wavefront sensor (ie, multiple and overlapped spots within the same centroiding area and crossover).

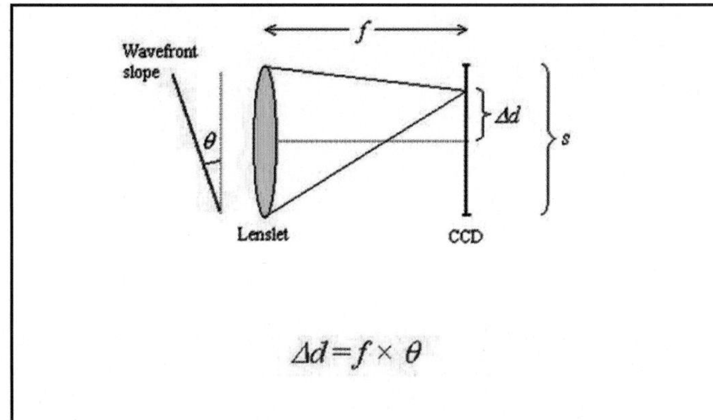

Figure 16-2. A relationship between the spot displacement (Δd), focal length of the lenslet array (f), and averaged wavefront slope (θ) over the lenslet aperture in a Shack-Hartmann wavefront sensor. The dynamic range and measurement sensitivity of a Shack-Hartmann wavefront sensor can be defined using this relationship as shown in equations 1 and 2.

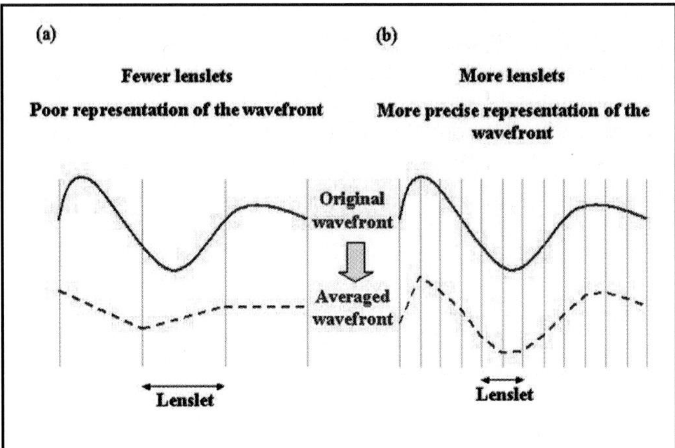

Figure 16-3. Number of lenslets (sampling points) vs accuracy in representation of the wavefront. Using fewer lenslets (A) produces a poorer representation of the wavefront than when the wavefront is sampled with more lenslets (B).

sensor using the above mentioned techniques is possible, the ability to reliably measure a relatively small amount of aberration (measurement sensitivity) is also important in order to achieve better visual outcome from various correction methods. The measurement sensitivity is defined by the smallest wavefront slope, θ_{min}, the sensor can measure. The smaller θ_{min} is, the better the measurement sensitivity. Contrary to the dynamic range, the measurement sensitivity is not limited by the lenslet spacing. As shown in equation 2, it depends directly on the focal length of the lenslet array and the minimum detectable spot displacement, Δd_{min}, determined by the pixel size of the detector and performance of the centroiding algorithm.

$$\text{Measurement Sensitivity} \quad \theta_{min} = \frac{\Delta d_{min}}{f} \qquad (2)$$

If the performance of the centroiding algorithm remains constant, the measurement sensitivity will be directly proportional to the focal length of the lenslet array and inversely proportional to the pixel size of the charged-coupled device (CCD). Increasing the focal length and/or using a smaller pixel size will result in better measurement sensitivity.

> The measurement sensitivity is directly proportional to the focal length of the lenslet array and inversely proportional to the pixel size of the CCD. Increasing the focal length or using a smaller pixel size will result in better measurement sensitivity.

Dynamic Range vs Number of Sampling Points (Lenslets)

The number of lenslets used to image the aberrated wavefront is related to the number of Zernike modes one can accurately calculate. Since each lenslet averages the slope of the local wavefront and displaces a spot from the reference point, more lenslets mean a more accurate representation of the wavefront. This point can be best understood by looking at the diagrams in Figure 16-3. The solid and dotted lines represent the original wavefront and averaged wavefront slope across each lenslet, respectively. Sampling the wavefront with fewer lenslets shown in Figure 16-3A produces a poorer representation of that wavefront than when the wavefront is sampled with more lenslets, as shown in Figure 16-3B. Resolving the more complicated shape of wavefront is exactly what is required to capture the higher-order aberrations in the eye. Thus, the more lenslets you use to sample a wavefront, the more higher-order aberrations you will be able to detect.

> The more lenslets you use to sample a wavefront, the more higher-order aberrations you can detect, but there is a decrease in the dynamic range of the wavefront sensor. This causes greater chance of having crossover with eyes with greater magnitudes of higher-order aberrations.

Unfortunately, there is a tradeoff to increasing the number of lenslets used to sample the wavefront when the pupil size is held constant. Although it does increase the resolution of the wavefront, an increase in the number of lenslets (and a subsequent decrease in their size) causes a decrease in the dynamic range of the system. Therefore, when all other variables are held constant,

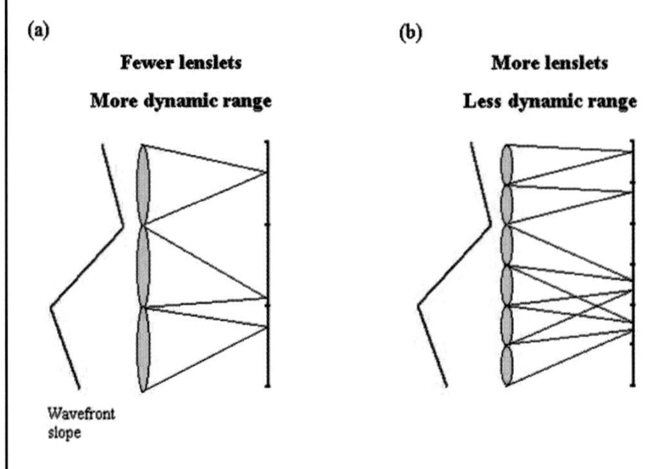

Figure 16-4. Dynamic range vs number of lenslets. With the same wavefront slope incident on the lenslet array, using fewer lenslets (A) or a larger lenslet size provides more dynamic range compared to more lenslets (B) or smaller lenslet sizes, which reduces dynamic range.

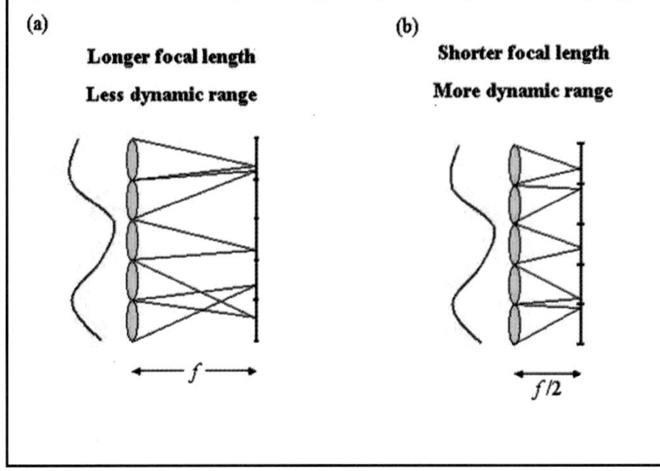

Figure 16-5. Dynamic range vs focal length of the lenslet. Decreasing the focal length of the lenslet array increases the dynamic range of the sensor; however, it also decreases the sensitivity as shown in equation 3. As a result, there is an inverse relationship between sensitivity and dynamic range.

the number of lenslets is inversely proportional to the dynamic range. Doubling the number of lenslets across the diameter of the pupil halves the maximum amount of aberration the system is capable of detecting. As illustrated in Figure 16-4, the potential problems described in the previous section manifest when the number of lenslets is increased.

> There is a tradeoff to increasing the number of lenslets used to sample the wavefront when the pupil size is held constant. Although it does increase the resolution of the wavefront, an increase in the number of lenslets (and a subsequent decrease in their size) causes a decrease in the dynamic range of the system.

Dynamic Range vs Focal Length

Another important constraint that has an effect on the system is the focal length of the lenslet array. Figure 16-5 illustrates the relationship between the dynamic range and focal length. When the wavefront aberration incident upon the lenslet array is held constant, the displacement of each spot is inversely proportional to the focal length of the lenslet as equation 1 indicates. As a result, decreasing the focal length will also decrease the displacement distance of the spots. This causes a subsequent increase in the system's dynamic range. If the lenslet spacing is fixed, using a shorter focal length lenslet array would be the simplest way to compensate for the lack of dynamic range in a Shack-Hartmann wavefront sensor as long as it has proper measurement sensitivity. This tradeoff between dynamic range and measurement sensitivity will be discussed in the next section.

Dynamic Range vs Measurement Sensitivity: The Tradeoff

As we mentioned earlier, the focal length of the lenslet array is linearly proportional to the measurement sensitivity. Reducing the focal length of the lenslet array leads to a decrease in sensitivity, or the ability of the sensor to detect the difference between different amounts of aberration. Increasing the focal length will provide the sensitivity that is clinically acceptable but will limit the system's dynamic range. This concept that the dynamic range of the wavefront sensor has an inverse relationship to the measurement sensitivity is explained by combining equations 1 and 2. The smallest wavefront slope, θ_{min}, redefined using the dynamic range, θ_{max}, from equation 1 is given by:

$$\theta_{min} = \frac{\Delta d_{min}}{f} = \frac{\Delta d_{min}}{(s/2)/\theta_{max}} = \frac{2 * \Delta d_{min} * \theta_{max}}{s} \quad (3)$$

If the lenslet spacing, s, and minimum detectable spot displacement, Δd_{min}, are constant, the measurement sensitivity is decreased (larger θ_{min}) as the dynamic range is increased (larger θ_{max}).

With this example, we have defined the most important limitation of the Shack-Hartmann wavefront sensor. That is, there is an inverse relationship between the sensitivity and dynamic range of the system. Increasing one decreases the other and vice versa.

Table 16-1 shows some practical examples of lenslet array parameters that allow reliable measurement of a range of focusing error for a 7 millimeters (mm) pupil. At a given dynamic range requirement, the maximum focal length of the lenslets is calculated for different lenslet spacings. Since this calculation only takes into account defocus, the actual focal length of the lenslet array may vary when astigmatism and higher-order aberrations are considered. These examples also explain the relationship between dynamic range and lenslet parameters as qualitatively summarized in Table 16-2.

> Reducing the focal length of the lenslet array leads to a decrease in sensitivity or the ability of the sensor to detect the difference between different amounts of aberration. Increasing the focal length will provide the sensitivity that is clinically acceptable but will limit the system's dynamic range.

Table 16-1
Examples of Lenslet Array Parameters to Measure a Required Range of Focusing Error for a 7-mm Pupil

Dynamic Range Required (D)	*Lenslet Spacing (mm)*	*Focal Length of Lenslets (mm)*
±8	0.2	< ~3.9
	0.4	< ~7.8
	0.6	< ~12.5
±16	0.2	< ~1.9
	0.4	< ~3.9
	0.6	< ~6.2

Table 16-2
Qualitative Summary of a Relationship Between Dynamic Range, Measurement Sensitivity, and Lenslet Array Parameters

Wavefront Sensor Parameter	*Result if Increased*
Lenslet spacing	Greater dynamic range Poorer representation of wavefront
Focal length of lenslet array	Increase in measurement sensitivity Decrease in dynamic range
Dynamic range	Decrease in measurement sensitivity

Methods to Increase Dynamic Range Without Losing Measurement Sensitivity

As was discussed previously, resolving the tradeoff between dynamic range and sensitivity will ultimately maximize the ability of the Shack-Hartmann wavefront sensor. Ideally, one would like to increase the dynamic range of the sensor without reducing the focal length of the lenslet array (ie, without sacrificing the measurement sensitivity). In this section, some of the techniques that have been developed to address this tradeoff are discussed below.

Algorithms for Variable Centroiding Area

Using a complex computer algorithm has been suggested as a way of increasing the dynamic range of the Shack-Hartmann sensor. As mentioned earlier, problems arise when spots either leave their respective subapertures, overlap with other spots, or cross paths. The details of the various algorithms that have been developed will not be discussed here; however, we will generalize about their abilities and limitations. Additionally, the algorithms discussed below are not intended to be a full representation of what has been developed but rather a sampling of the research that has been done in this field.

The unwrapping[1] and iterative spline fitting methods[2,3] are the names of two algorithms that have been developed. Generally speaking, these processes assign the spots to their corresponding lenslets even if they are located outside their virtual subaperture on the CCD. The iterative spline fitting methods do this by theoretically predicting the location of the virtual subaperture used to locate the spot centroid. This obviously increases the dynamic range significantly. One limitation of these algorithms, however, is that they are incapable of recognizing conditions in which the spots have either crossed paths or have overlapped (ie, they are only capable of tracking spots that have had no ambiguous interactions with other spots).

Another algorithm[4] that has been suggested in an attempt to compensate for the limitations described above uses a "compare and contrast" technique across multiple exposures. By systematically blocking and unblocking lenslets with a mask and then later comparing the exposures of each configuration, one may determine or match each spot with its corresponding lenslet. This process resolves shortcomings of the unwrapping and iterative spline methods related to crossover. The problem of spot overlap, however, may still reduce measurement reliability. Also, since more than one exposure is required, the total exposure time needed to collect all of the information is increased. The system is, therefore, more sensitive to eye movements and other "noise" contributing factors.

Trombone System (Defocus Corrector)

Statistical analysis of normal population data suggests that over 90% of the total aberration found in eyes (over a 5.7 mm pupil) can be described by second-order Zernike modes (defocus

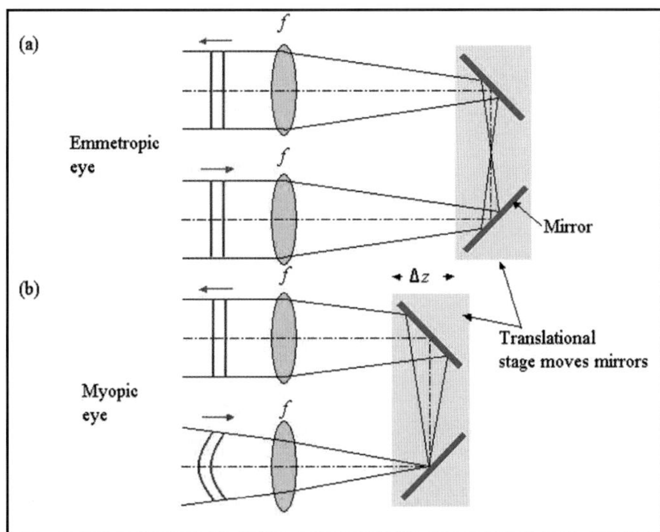

Figure 16-6. Schematic diagram of a trombone system to precompensate for defocus in the eye. (A) Emmetropic eye: The distance between two lenses having the focal length of *f* must be 2 × *f*. (B) Myopic eye: The converged incident wavefront is compensated for by reducing the distance between two lenses. Note that the wavefront coming out of the second lens has no defocus.

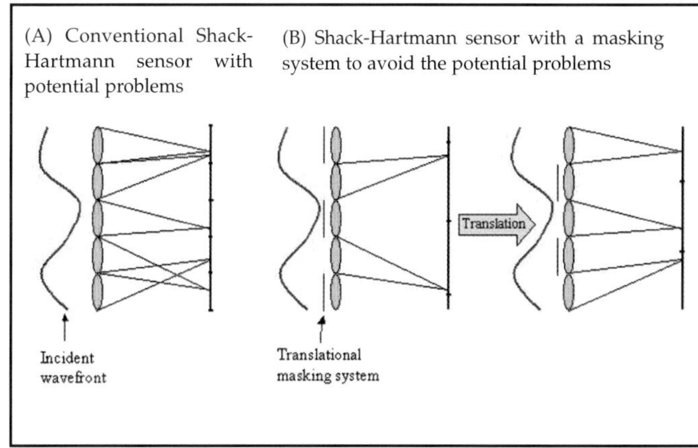

Figure 16-7. Increasing the dynamic range without losing measurement sensitivity. (A) A conventional Shack-Hartmann wavefront sensor showing potential problems described earlier. (B) Masking and unmasking each lenslet using a translational plate with holes can effectively increase the dynamic range without sacrificing measurement sensitivity.

and astigmatism).[5] About 80% of this may be attributed to defocus only. If this defocus is corrected out of the total wavefront aberration before it is measured using a Shack-Hartmann wavefront sensor, the magnitude of the residual aberrations (astigmatisms and higher-order aberrations) to be measured will be significantly decreased. As a result, the chance that the remaining aberration will exceed the dynamic range limitations of the sensor is also decreased. One technique that has been implemented to correct defocus is called a *trombone system*. The trombone works by changing the distance between relay lenses in the Shack-Hartmann wavefront sensor to compensate for positive or negative defocus presented in the eye as shown in Figure 16-6. Later, after measurements have been made, the amount of defocus corrected by the trombone system can be separately added to the measured aberration. A typical trombone system consists of two folding mirrors on a one-axis translational stage. By moving this stage along the optical axis, positive or negative defocus can be added to the wavefront sensor as diagrammed in Figure 16-6. The translational stage should be moved toward the lenses, decreasing the distance between the two lenses (negative Δz), to compensate for defocus error in myopic eyes. For hyperopic eyes, the distance between the lenses should be increased (positive Δz). An amount of refractive power, ΔD, added by changing the distance between the lenses can be calculated by equation 4.

$$\Delta D = \frac{2 \times \Delta z}{f^2} \quad (4)$$

where *f* is the focal length of the relay lenses and Δz is the distance the translational stage is moved. The total change in distance between two lenses is twice as long as Δz. Both Δz and *f* should be in the units of millimeters in this equation.

Since the trombone can be used quite accurately, measuring patients with high myopia or hyperopia becomes a very realistic task for the Shack-Hartmann sensor. This seemingly trivial solution, however, does have its drawbacks. It adds moving mechanical parts, something that the conventional Shack-Hartmann does not have. This can or may introduce undesirable aberrations induced by misalignment. Although the trombone system helps to reduce the requirement for dynamic range for a population of normal eyes, it may not offer a complete solution for eyes with corneal disorders such as keratoconus and penetrating keratoplasty. These eyes typically have a large amount of astigmatism or higher-order aberrations, such as coma and trefoil, which cannot be corrected by using the trombone.

> Trombone systems can increase the dynamic range of the wavefront sensor by measuring the defocus component of the wavefront. This gives the wavefront sensor the ability to measure a large range of myopia and hyperopia.

Masking System to Increase the Centroiding Area

Yet another way of increasing the dynamic range is to increase the spacing between spots generated by the lenslet array by masking certain lenslets so that only a portion of the wavefront aberration data is collected at a time. Figure 16-7 shows a schematic diagram of how the translational masking plate works in the simplified case of a one-dimensional lenslet array. A plate with holes having the same size as a lenslet is placed in front of the lenslet array. Each hole on the plate is spaced every two or more lenslets apart, depending on how much the dynamic range needs to be increased. This plate is translated in the horizontal and vertical directions by a distance equal to the lenslet spacing after taking an image of the spot array pattern at each plate position. Each image is processed separately to measure spot displacement. The spot displacement data from each image are then combined together in the proper order to compute the wave aberration. For example, having holes exposing every other lenslet results in a doubling of the spacing between spots and an increase in the dynamic range by a factor of two. Four images will be required for a single measurement of the aberration.

Although this plate effectively increases spacing between the spots, which results in a larger dynamic range without losing measurement sensitivity, the number of photons per frame taken after each translation of the plate will decrease as the number of translations is increased. If the time needed to complete a single measurement remains constant, the exposure time for each image is reduced by a factor equal to the number of translations required. Shorter exposure times reduce the signal-to-noise ratio of the spot array pattern; this ultimately results in less accurate spot centroiding. In addition, eye movements that occur during measurement or between translations of the mask may result in an increase in error.

> Possible strategies for increasing dynamic range without sacrificing sensitivity include algorithms to allow closer approximations of the light spots and masking techniques that allow covering adjacent lenslets to allow the light spots to be measured sequentially instead of simultaneously.

Summary

In this chapter, we have described the tradeoff that occurs between sensitivity and dynamic range when using a Shack-Hartmann wavefront sensor. Increasing the lenslet size increases the dynamic range of the wavefront sensor but may cause poorer representation of higher-order aberrations. Using a shorter focal length for the lenslet array increases the dynamic range but also reduces the measurement sensitivity.

Various strategies exist for increasing the dynamic range of the sensor while maintaining the measurement sensitivity. These include using special algorithms that can adjust the centroiding area for each spot, a trombone system that precompensates for some amount of defocus before the measurement, and a translational plate with an aperture array that increases spacing between adjacent spots.

References

1. Pfund J, Lindlein N, Schwider J. Dynamic range expansion of a Shack-Hartmann sensor by use of a modified unwrapping algorithm. *Optics Letters*. 1998;23(13):995-997.
2. Groening S, Sick B, Donner K, Pfund J, Lindlein N, Schwider J. Wave-front reconstruction with a Shack-Hartmann sensor with an iterative spline fitting method. *Appl Opt*. 2000;39(4):561-567.
3. Lindlein N, Pfund J, Schwider J. Algorithm for expanding the dynamic range of a Shack-Hartmann sensor by using a spatial light modulator array. *Opt Eng*. 2001;40(5):837-840.
4. Unsbo P, Franzen L, Gustafsson J. Increased dynamic range of a Hartmann Shack Sensor by B-spline extrapolation: measurement of large aberrations in the human eye. ARVO abstract #2021. *Invest Ophthalmol Vis Sci*. 2002;43:E-Abstract #2021.
5. Porter J, Guirao A, Cox I, Williams D. Monochromatic aberrations of the human eye in a large population. *J Opt Soc Am A*. 2001;18(8):1793-1803.

Chapter 17

Retinal Imaging Aberrometry: Principles and Application of the Tscherning Aberrometer

Michael Mrochen, PhD; Mirko Jankov, MD; Hans Peter Iseli, MD; Farhad Hafezi, MD; and Theo Seiler, MD, PhD

The Tscherning Aberrometer

The Tscherning aberrometer is a ray tracing system based on the principles of Tscherning's aberroscope.[1] The commercial device (WaveLight Laser Technologies AG, Erlangen, Germany) was originally designed by Peter Mierdel and associates[2-4] at Technical University of Dresden, Germany. This type of wavefront sensor has been tested for various diagnostic[5-11] and therapeutic[12-15] applications in research, as well as in clinical routine.

System Configuration

The schematic setup of the Tscherning aberrometer is shown in Figure 17-1A. The light source for the measuring rays is a red laser diode (wavelength 670 nanometers [nm]) optically coupled into a monomode fiber and collimated at the end of the fiber tip. The laser beam is enlarged to a diameter of about 25 millimeters (mm) after the collimator to achieve a homogeneous intensity distribution within the central part of the laser beam. The resulting parallel bundle of light is split into a group of parallel rays (diameter 0.30 mm) by means of a mask with a regular matrix of fine holes (Figure 17-1B).

The emerging rays are focused by an adjustable lens system located in front of the eye (in-going optics). Here, the intraocular area of least confusion is located about 2.5 mm in front of the retina to assure a constant retinal image size for different refractions. Therefore, the power of this "aberroscope lens system" depends on the mean ocular spherical refraction. In the case of an emmetropic eye, the dioptric power of this lens system should be in the range of +4 diopters (D); in myopic eyes with a refraction from -6 to -9 D, this lens system can be adjusted to infinity (0.0 D), while for hyperopic eyes of more than +2 D, a refractive power of more than +5 D is needed. In this way, a pattern of light spots is generated on the retina. It should be kept in mind that the purpose of the aberroscope lens system is only to sufficiently enlarge the retinal spot pattern in order to separate and to identify the single light spots. For this reason, the aberroscope lens system changes only the angle of light incidence but not the locations of each single spot in the corneal plane. In this regard, the retinal image size is kept constant in all cases. In an eye with ideal optical performance free of any higher-order optical aberrations, this subjectively, well-recognizable spot pattern has the same regularity as the rays before entering the eye. In a real eye, the retinal light spot pattern is more or less distorted according to the existing ocular optical aberrations. The effect of one's own ocular optical errors (Figure 17-1C) is subjectively visible for the patient and qualitatively describable.

The laser light, controlled by an electromechanical shutter, is opened for 60 milliseconds (msec). This "single shot" retinal spot pattern with a size of 1 x 1 mm^2 is imaged by an optical scheme that is based on the principles of indirect ophthalmoscopy onto the sensor array of a video camera (out-going optics). The optical scheme is adjustable in order to consider the diverse positions of the intermediate image of the retinal spot pattern, depending on the ocular refraction. A small diaphragm (diameter 2 mm) is located in the image plane of the eye's exit pupil, ensuring that only rays through this narrow paraxial space contribute to the image. The coordinates of the geometric centers, x_r, y_r, of all imaged retinal spots are determined by means of image processing software.

The ideal pattern coordinates under aberration-free conditions are calculated from parameters of Gullstrand's simplified eye model,[3] the length of which is assessed by the mean spherical refraction measured with an autorefractometer. Thus, the displacement from its ideal position can be computed for each light spot. This matrix of two-dimensional deviations represents the directional aberrations of the measuring rays from their ideal intraocular course. It is possible to reconstruct the deviation of the wavefront from its ideal desirable spherical shape with the known relationship between the positions of the rays at the cornea, x_c, y_c, and their locations at the retinal plane (L = length of the eye).

$$\frac{\partial W(x, y)}{\partial x} = \frac{x_c - x_r}{L} \qquad \frac{\partial W(x, y)}{\partial y} = \frac{y_c - y_r}{L}$$

The wavefront aberrations were computed by numerical fitting to a Zernike expansion:

$$W(x, y) = \sum_{i=0}^{27} C_i * Z_i(x, y) * R$$

with $x = X/R$, $y = Y/R$, the normalized dimensions of the pupil varying from -1 to 1, R being the pupil radius, X,Y being the coordinates within the pupil plane, and Z_i (x,y) the set of Zernike polynomials.

It should be mentioned that the Zernike coefficients provided by the commercial Tscherning aberrometer must be divided by the appropriate normalization factor, F_n, and multiplied by the

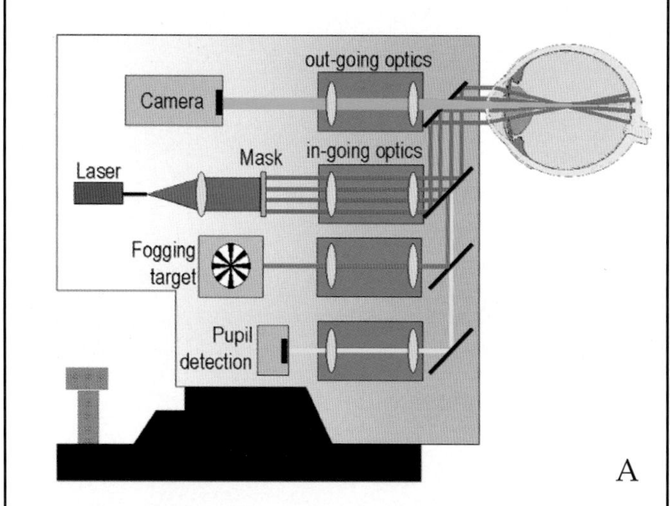

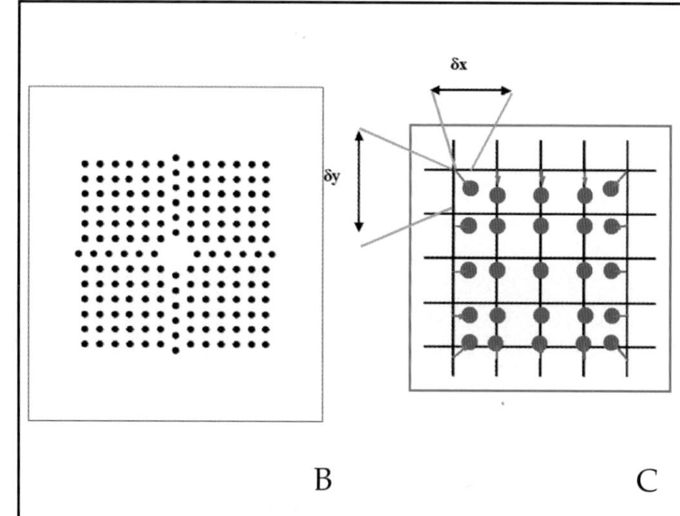

Figure 17-1. (A) Schematic setup of the Tscherning aberrometer mounted on a slit lamp basis. (B) Matrix of regular fine holes used to create a light bundle 168 rays. (C) Determination of the spot displacements, δx, δy, from their ideal positions.

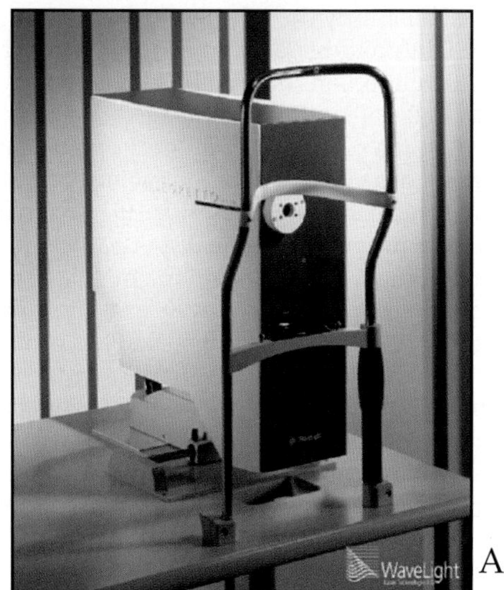

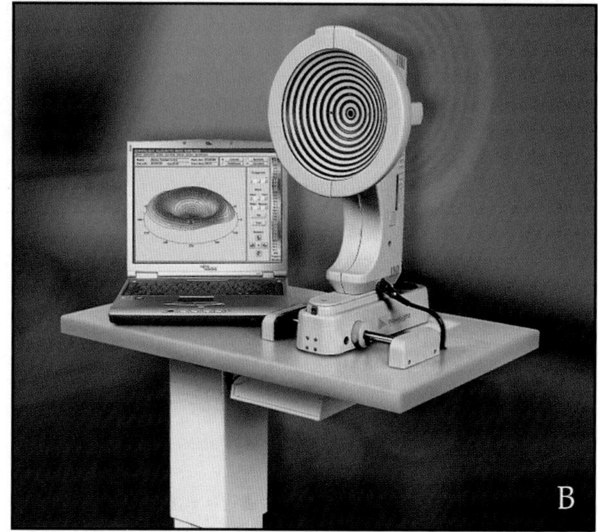

Figure 17-2. (A) Photography of the WaveLight Wavefront Analyzer that is based on the principles of Tscherning's aberrometry. B) Photograph of the Oculus Topographer (Oculus Optikgeräte GmbH, Wetzlar, Germany).

pupil radius to convert them into the Zernike representations proposed by the Vision Science and Its Application (VSIA) taskforce.[16] The normalization factors are determined by:

$$F_{n,m} = \begin{cases} \sqrt{2\,(n+1)} & \text{if } n - 2m \neq 0 \\ \sqrt{(n+1)} & \text{if } n - 2m = 0 \end{cases}$$

where n is the order of the Zernike monomial and m is the angular frequency of the term.

Clinical Experience

The feasibility of the clinical use of the WaveLight Wavefront Analyzer will be demonstrated in a series of interesting cases. In each case, four independent measurements were performed, and the resulting mean wavefront was expressed in terms of Zernike polynomials up to the sixth order. Anterior corneal topography was obtained by means of a placido disk videokeratoscope (Oculus Topographer [Oculus Optikgeräte GmbH, Wetzlar, Germany]) (Figure 17-2). The pupils were dilated to at least 6 mm diameter using tropicamide 1% for both wavefront sensing and topography measurements. The standard protocol for wavefront and topography measurements also includes the control of the centration, head position, pupil size, and the consistency of the tear film during the measurements. Strict rating criteria for the quality of the retinal spot pattern allowed a sure and safe validation of each single measurement.

The "Normal" Case

Case 1 is a 32-year-old female without any ocular treatment or pathological finding in both eyes. She never fully accepted her glasses because sometimes her glasses were subjectively better for near vision and unpleasant for distance, and sometimes the opposite. Under scotopic conditions, the patient complained about "light rays around the street lights." The pupil size was 3.5 mm under photopic conditions and 6.5 mm under scotopic

Table 17-1
Case 1 (32 Years of Age)

	UCVA	Rx	BSCVA
Manifest	20/20-- 20/20-	plano x -0.25 at 80 -0.25	20/20- 20/20-
Phenylephrine	20/25++ 20/20--	plano x -0.25 at 75 plano	20/20-- 20/20--
Cyclopentolate	20/25++ 20/20--	+0.25 x -0.25 at 75 +0.25	20/20-- 20/20-

conditions. The refractive data, as well as her uncorrected (UCVA) and best-spectacle corrected visual acuity (BSCVA), are listed in Table 17-1. Wavefront sensing was possible at a pupil size of 7 mm. All retinal spots within the pupil were detectable with a high predictability. Wavefront refraction was found to be -0.28 D for sphere and -0.51 D at 72 degrees for cylinder at a pupil size of 7 mm. The wavefront sphere, however, shifts slightly from minor myopia to emmetropia (-0.03 D) when calculating the wavefront error for a 4 mm pupil (Figure 17-3). The higher-order wavefront maps display a significant component of coma-like aberration for the 7i mm pupil that is also prominent in the 4 mm pupil. Such a small change can also been seen from the subjective refraction data presented in Table 17-1.

Changing the pupil size in wavefront sensing by means of pharmaceuticals, however, might have an effect on the wavefront refraction data, depending on the amount of higher-order aberrations present in the investigated eye. Usually the defocus, C_4, and astigmatism Zernike terms, C_3, C_5, are the basis to calculate wavefront sphere (*sph*), cylinder (*cyl*), and cylindrical axis[17]:

$$cyl = \frac{4\sqrt{C_3^2 + C_5^2}}{R}$$

$$sph = \frac{4C_4}{R} - \frac{1}{2} Cyl$$

$$\alpha = \frac{1}{2} \arctan \left(\frac{C_3}{C_5}\right)$$

The signs of *sph* and *cyl* are reversed to obtain the ophthalmic correction. The effect of higher-order aberrations on the wavefront refraction was theoretically investigated based on measured wavefront aberration data from 130 normal aberrated eyes. Resulting changes in wavefront sphere due to the change in pupil size from 6 mm to 3 mm were correlated with the initial higher-order aberrations determined for the 6 mm pupil. The wavefront refraction of one eye can change with different pupil sizes, as depicted in Figure 17-4. Consequently, the wavefront determined sphere is strongly influenced by the amount of higher-order aberrations, such as fourth-order spherical aberration. Modification of wavefront sphere with pupil size can be as large as 0.9 D in normal myopic eyes and even larger in highly aberrated eyes.

The wavefront determined sphere is strongly influenced by the amount of higher-order aberrations, such as fourth-order spherical aberration. Modification of wavefront sphere with pupil size can be as large as 0.9 D in normal myopic eyes and even larger in highly aberrated eyes.

The "Lenticular Astigmatism" Case

Case 2 is a 30-year-old male with a manifest refraction of -2 D sphere and with a cylinder of -1.75 D at 90 degrees (against the rule). Similar results were found from wavefront sensing (the wavefront refraction of -2.28 D in sph and -1.53 at 88 degrees cyl). In contrast, corneal topography shows only a slight astigmatism in the order of 0.25 D at 15 degrees. This case demonstrates the different information provided by wavefront sensing and corneal topography (Figure 17-5). While the wavefront sensor determines the optical quality of the total eye, corneal topography can only provide us with data on the anterior front surface. This leads us to the conclusion that corneal topography helps only to analyze the surface quality of the cornea, especially after corneal surgery, but does not provide information on the imaging quality of an individual eye, as done by wavefront sensing. Studies with a larger set of eyes have shown that astigmatism and third-order optical aberrations originate from the cornea in most of the investigated eyes.[18-24] In contrast, fourth-order spherical aberration, as well as all other fourth to sixth orders, do not correlate with the aberrations of the anterior surface of the cornea. This indicates that in most of the normal eyes intraocular structures may, at least to a certain degree, compensate for some of the higher-order aberrations originating at the corneal front surface. In particular, the lack of correlation between corneal and total fourth-order aberration (Figure 17-6) might be due to such an optical compensation mechanism. In normal myopic eyes, the higher-order aberrations are usually limited to the third and fourth Zernike orders, since those of the cornea and total wavefront beyond the fourth order do not contribute much to the total. Thus, the detection of significant corneal aberrations above the fourth order may represent an abnormal condition.

The "Central Island" Case

Case 3 is a 56-year-old male that suffered from poor BSCVA of 20/30 after a laser in-situ keratomileusis (LASIK) procedure with

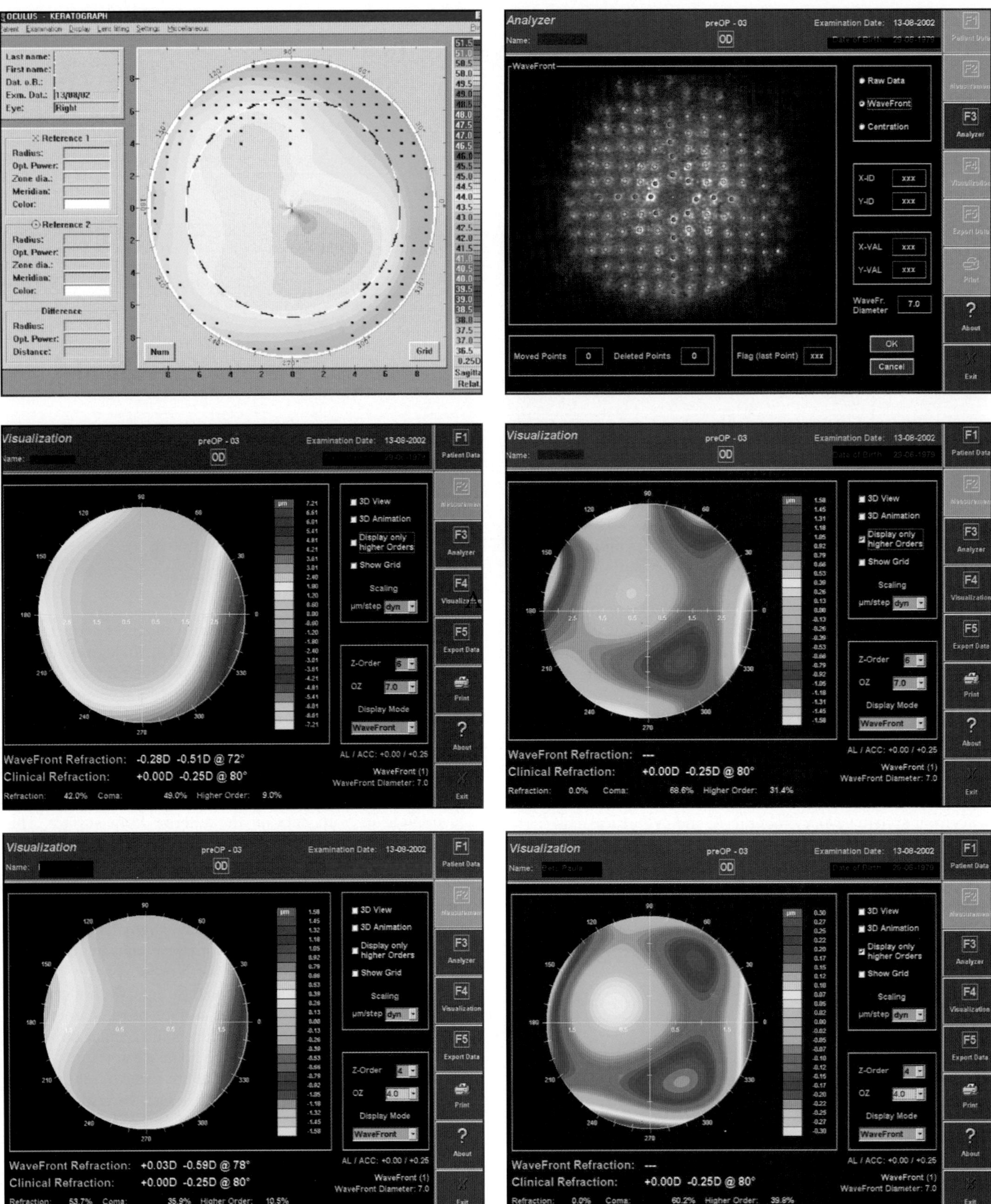

Figure 17-3. The "normal" case. Right eye of case 1 (32-year-old female). (A) Corneal topography. (B) Retinal spot pattern from the Wavefront Analyzer. (C) Total wavefront map for a 7 mm pupil. Here, the wavefront refraction was determined to be sph: -0.28 D and cyl: -0.51 D x 72 degrees. (D) Wavefront map including only third- to sixth-order Zernike aberrations for a 7 mm pupil. (E) Total wavefront map for a 4 mm pupil. Here, the wavefront refraction was determined to be sph: -0.03 D and cyl: -0.59 D x 78 degrees. (F) Wavefront map including only third- to fourth-order Zernike aberrations for a 4 mm pupil. Manifest refraction was determined to be sph: plano and cyl: -0.25 D x 80 degrees.

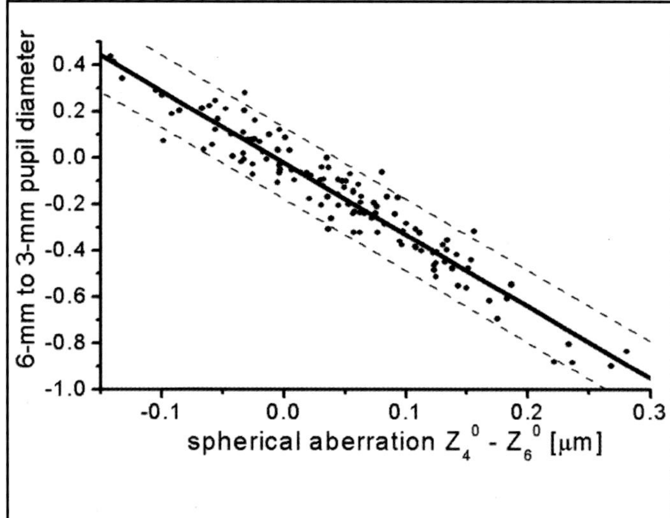

Figure 17-4. Linear correlation ($R^2 = 0.93$) between the change in wavefront sphere (Δsphere) and the amount of fourth- and sixth-order spherical aberration for 130 normal myopic eyes. The maximum amount of sphere change was found to be as large as -0.9 D when varying the pupil size from 3 to 6 mm in some of the investigated eyes.

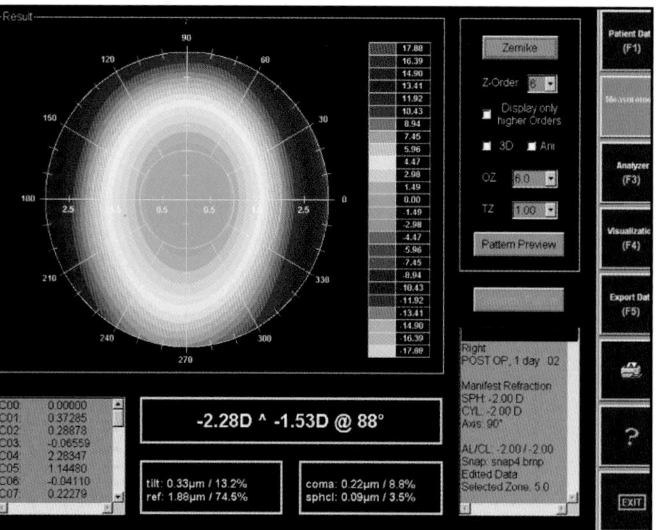

Figure 17-5A. A case of "lenticular astigmatism." Left eye of case 2 (30-year-old male). Total wavefront map for a 6 mm pupil reveals the wavefront refraction to be sph: -2.28 D and cyl: -1.53 D at 88 degrees.

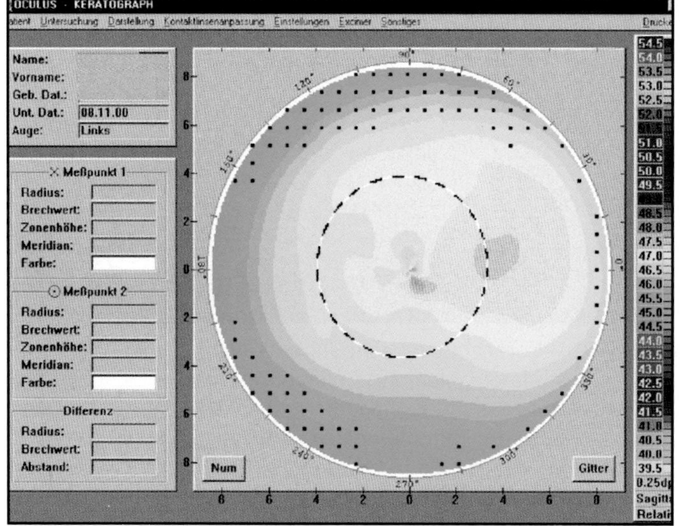

Figure 17-5B. A case of "lenticular astigmatism." Left eye of case 2 (30-year-old male). Corneal topography reveals only cyl: 0.25 at 15 degrees. Manifest refraction was found to be -2 D in sph and -1.75 D at 90 degrees (against the rule) for cylinder.

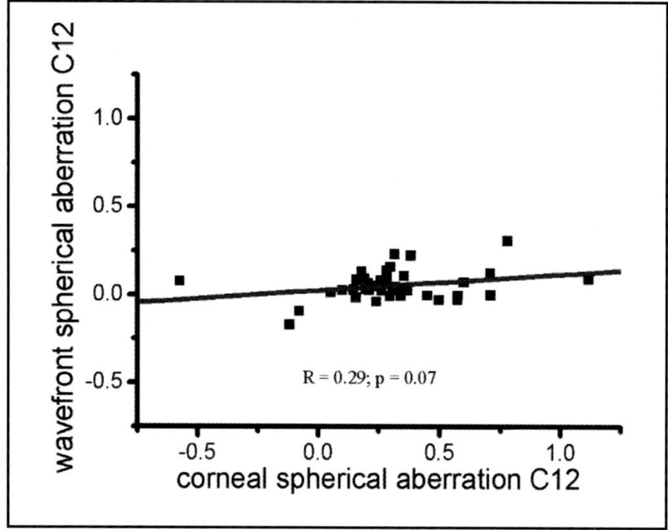

Figure 17-6. Spherical aberration (fourth-order Zernike) measured for the total wavefront as a function of the corneal spherical aberration determined by corneal topography. The correlation was not statistically significant (p = 0.07) with a correlation coefficient of R = 0.29. The data presented was for a 6 mm pupil.

a broad beam laser system. Corneal topography shows a steep area of several diopters centrally within the pupil (Figure 17-7). This small central area, approximately 1 to 2 mm in diameter, was first described as a measuring artifact of the topography system. However, a strong corresponding distortion of the retinal image quality was found during the wavefront measurements. Further analysis demonstrated that the retinal image was completely smeared when the measurement was perfectly centered within a range of less than 50 microns (µm). In contrast, reliable measurements could be achieved when the Wavefront Analyzer was decentered by more than 1 mm from the pupil center during the measurement. This leads to the conclusion that the central irregularity observed in corneal topography can significantly affect the optical path way used to capture the retinal image. Consequently, the irregular central part observed in corneal topography was confirmed to be the source of the visual symptoms of the patient. This eye gained BSCVA to 20/20 1 month after removing the observed irregularity by means of a computer assisted "anticentral island" treatment.

> The central irregularity observed in corneal topography can significantly affect the optical path way used to capture the retinal image.

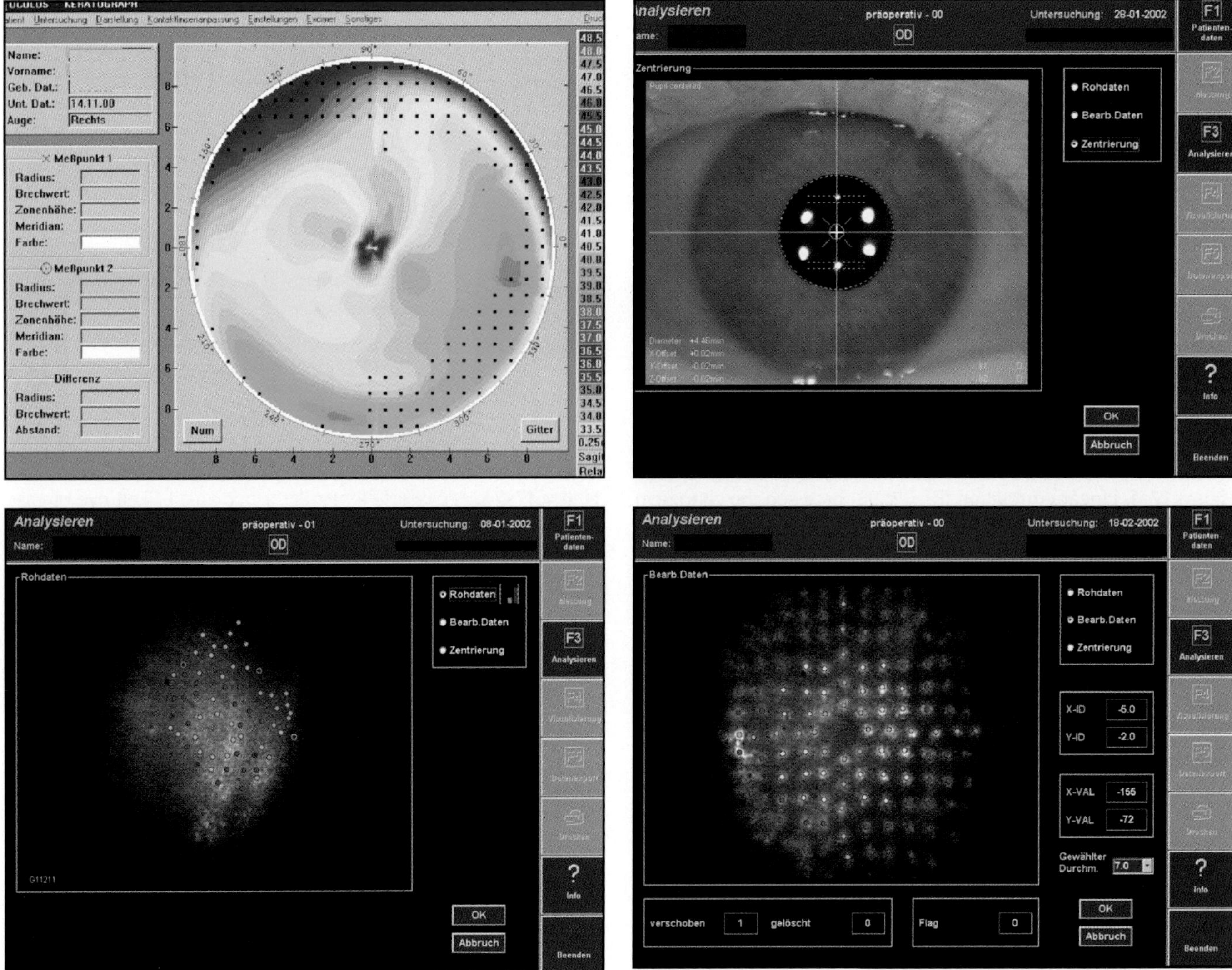

Figure 17-7. The "central island" case. Right eye of case 3 (30-year-old male). (A) Corneal topography shows a steep central irregularity resulting from an initial refractive surgery procedure performed with a broad beam laser system. (B) Centration system of the Wavefront Analyzer including automatic x-y-z alignment onto the line-of-sight. (C) Retinal image of the spot pattern in the case of a well-centered measurement. The retinal image is distorted because the central irregularity is located within the optical pathway of the video camera used to grab the retinal image. (D) Retinal image of the spot pattern in the case of a decentered measurement. The retinal image is sharp because the central irregularity of the cornea is located outside the optical pathway of the video camera.

The "Keratoconus" Case

Case 4 is a 31-year-old female that requested wavefront-guided treatment for vision improvement on her left eye with a UCVA of 20/60. Her manifest refraction oculus sinister (OS) was -2.25 D in sph with -5.5 D at 170 degrees in cyl, reaching BSCVA of 20/25 (-2). Her pupil size was 3 mm under natural light and 5 mm under scotopic conditions. Her corneal topography clearly showed a keratoconus with an inferior paracentral cone (Figure 17-8). She had already undergone a penetrating keratoplasty on her right eye 2 years earlier and wanted to improve her vision in her other eye before it also needed corneal transplantation. The retinal spot pattern, although obtainable with relative difficulty and a moderate repeatability, clearly shows the superior paracentral spot aggregation corresponding to the inferior paracentral corneal cone. Wavefront-guided corneal laser surgery was not intended in this eye because of the diagnosis of advanced keratoconus and the uncertainty of the wavefront measurement.

Summary

Tscherning aberrometry with the WaveLight Wavefront Analyzer represents a clinically useful method for optical aberration diagnosis in human eyes. The measurement principle of retinal imaging helps one to understand and to predict the visual symptoms reported by the patient. The unique method of "photographing" the patient's retinal image, being seen by the patient itself, extends the range of modern wavefront diagnosis and enables clinicians to plan the most advantageous treatment procedure for each individual eye. In addition, the measurement of the wavefront aberration in the image plane makes the WaveLight Wavefront Analyzer a reliable system for clinical wavefront sensing.

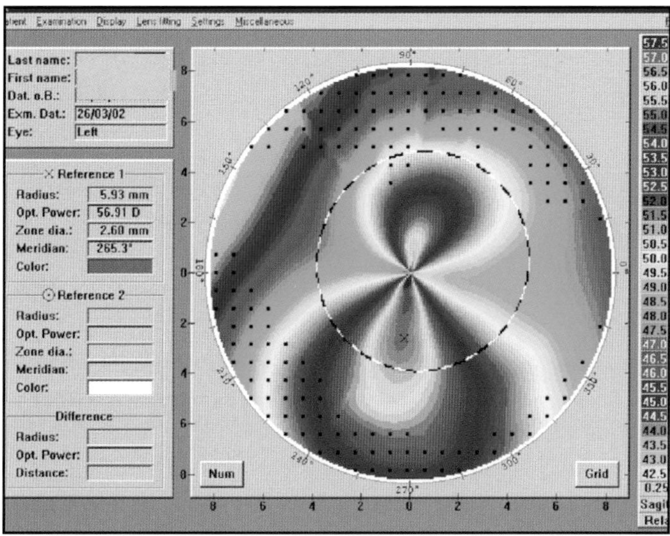

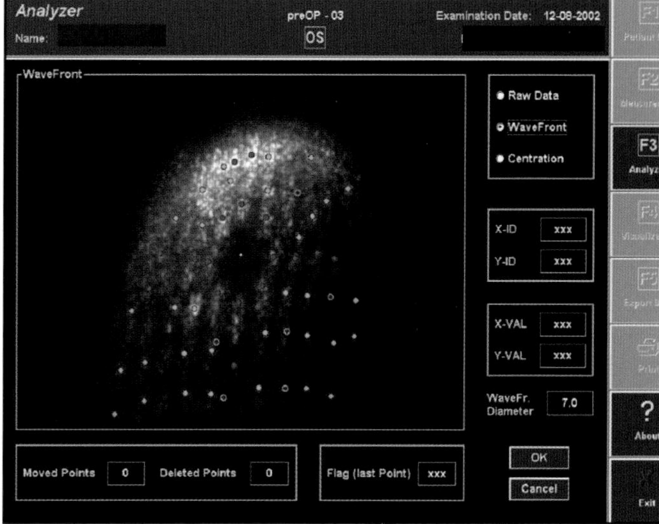

Figure 17-8. The "keratoconus" case. Right eye of case 4 (31-year-old female). (A) Corneal topography shows an irregular astigmatism of more than 6.00 D. (B) The retinal spot pattern clearly shows the superior paracentral spot agglomeration corresponding to the inferior paracentral corneal cone.

References

1. Tscherning M. Die monochromatischen aberrationen des menschlichen auges. *Z Psychol Physiol Sinne.* 1894;6:456-471.
2. Mierdel P, Wiegand W, Krinke HE, Kaemmerer M, Seiler T. Messplatz zur Erfassung der monochromatischen Aberrationen des menschlichen Auges. *Ophthalmologe.* 1997;6:441-445.
3. Mierdel P, Kaemmerer M, Mrochen M, Krinke HE, Seiler T. Ocular optical aberrometer for clinical use. *J Biomed Opt.* 2001;6:200-204.
4. Mrochen M, Kaemmerer M, Mierdel P, Krinke HE, Seiler T. Principles of Tscherning aberrometry. *J Refract Surg.* 2000;16:S570-S571.
5. Mierdel P, Kaemmerer M, Krinke HE, Seiler T. Effects of photorefractive keratectomy and cataract surgery on ocular optical errors of higher order. *Graefe's Arch Clin Exp Ophthalmol.* 1999;237:725-729.
6. Seiler T, Kaemmerer M, Mierdel P, Krinke HE. Ocular optical aberrations after photorefractive keratectomy for myopia and myopic astigmatism. *Arch Ophthalmol.* 2000;118:17-21.
7. Kaemmerer M, Mrochen M, Mierdel P, Krinke HE, Seiler T. Clinical experience with the Tscherning aberrometry. *J Refract Surg.* 2000;16: S584-S587.
8. Mrochen M, Kaemmerer M, Mierdel P, Krinke HE, Seiler T. Is the human eye a perfect optic? *SPIE Proceedings Ophthalmic Technologies XI.* 2001;4245:30-35.
9. Krueger RR, Mrochen M, Kaemmerer M, Seiler T. Understanding refraction and accommodation through retinal imaging aberrometry: a case report. *Ophthalmology.* 2001;108:674-678.
10. Mrochen M, Mostafa Salah Eldine, Kaemmerer M, Seiler T, Hütz W. Improvements of the results after photorefractive corneal laser surgery by using an active eye-tracking system. *J Cataract Refract Surg.* 2001;27:1000-1006.
11. Mrochen M, Kaemmerer M, Mierdel P, Seiler T. Increased higher order optical aberrations after laser refractive surgery—a problem of subclinical decentrations. *J Cataract Refract Surg.* 2001;27:362-369.
12. Mrochen M, Kaemmerer M, Seiler T, Mierdel P. Wavefront-guided in situ keratomileusis: early results in three eyes. *J Refract Surg.* 2000;16:116-121.
13. Seiler T, Mrochen M, Kaemmerer M. Operative corrections of ocular aberrations to improve visual acuity. *J Refract Surg.* 2000;16:S619-S621.
14. Mrochen M, Kaemmerer M, Seiler T. Clinical results of wavefront-guided LASIK at 3 months after surgery. *J Cataract Refract Surg.* 2001;27:201-207.
15. Mrochen M, Krueger RR; Bueeler M, Seiler T. Aberration sensing and wavefront-guided treatment: management of decentered ablations. *J Refract Surg.* 2002;18:418-429.
16. Thibos LN, Applegate RA, Schwingerling JT, Webb R. Report from the VSIA taskforce on standards for reporting optical aberrations of the eye. *J Refract Surg.* 2000;16:S539-S663.
17. Atchinson DA, Scott DH, Cox MJ. Mathematical Treatment of Ocular Aberrations: a User's Guide. OSA Trends in Optics and Photonics Vol 35. Vision Science and its applications. Optical Society of America, Washington, DC, 2000, pp. 110-130.
18. El Hage S, Berny F. Contribution of the crystalline lens to the spherical aberration of the eye. *J Opt Soc Am A.* 1973;63:205-211.
19. Tomlinson A, Hemenger R, Garriott R. Method for estimating the spherical aberration of the human crystalline lens in vitro. *Invest Ophthalmol Vis Sci.* 1993;34:621-629.
20. Millodot M, Sivak J. Contribution of the cornea and lens to the spherical aberration of the eye. *Vision Res.* 1979;19:685-687.
21. Artal P, Guirao A. Contributions of the cornea and the lens to the aberrations of the human eye. *Optics Letters.* 1998;23:1713-1715.
22. Smith G, Cox MJ, Calver R, Garner LF. The spherical aberration of the crystalline lens of the human eye. *Vision Res.* 2001;235-243.
23. Artal P, Guirao A, Berrio E, Williams DR. Compensation of corneal aberrations by the internal optics in the human eye. *Journal of Vision.* 2001;1:1-8.
24. Mrochen M, Jankov M, Bueeler M, Seiler T. Correlation between corneal and total aberrations in myopic eyes. *J Refract Surg.* 2003;19:104-112.

Chapter 18
Retinal Imaging Aberrometry: Principles and Applications of the Tracey (Ray Tracing) Aberrometer

Vasyl Molebny, PhD, DSc; Ioannis Pallikaris, MD, PhD; Sergiy Molebny, MSc; and Harilaos Ginis, PhD

With the advent of modern laser refractive surgery, it has become increasingly important to have instruments that will reliably measure optical aberrations of the human eye's optical system. Consequently, it is also important to understand their impact on retinal image quality and vision. One difficulty in the development of a straightforward methodology for the measurement of ocular aberrations is the anatomy of the eye itself, leading to the "double pass" nature of all measurement techniques. Physiologically, aberrations of human vision are of a single pass nature. In the instruments for measuring the aberrations, many authors undertake countermeasures to minimize the effect of double pass. Moreover, the human optical system is not static but rather time dependent in a complicated manner: age-related changes of the aberration profile have been demonstrated.[1] Short-term changes related to the biomechanical response of the cornea following refractive procedures have been described[2] as have intrameasurement fluctuations of the 1-second time scale, such as accommodation fluctuations.[3] A reliable instrument for the measurement of ocular aberrations should be robust to cover these fluctuations and yet be able to provide accuracy over the broad optical conditions that exist in vision (such as variable pupil diameters, accommodation states) and to allow measurement of the dynamic changes of aberration.

The challenge of objective measurement of ocular aberrations is being attempted with different levels of success by several commercial systems available today.

Ray tracing aberrometry, described earlier,[4] uses measurement of the position of a thin laser beam onto the retina. A beam of light is directed into the eye parallel to the visual axis. Each entrance point provides its own projection on the retina (Figures 18-1 and 18-2). A set of entrance points provides a set of projections.

The Tracey visual function analyzers Tracey-VFA and *i*-Trace (Tracey Technologies, Houston, Tex) are the instruments based on the ray tracing aberrometry principle. In these instruments, a narrow (0.3 millimeter [mm] in diameter) diode laser beam (visible red = 650 nanometers [nm] in Tracey-VFA and invisible infrared 785 nm in *i*-Trace) is being displaced over the entrance pupil of an eye while kept parallel to the visual axis. This procedure is performed with the use of a pair of acousto-optic x-y deflectors and a special collimating lens. The position sensing detectors measure the transverse displacement of the laser spot on the retina. A lens is used to optically conjugate the retina and the detector plane (see Figure 18-2). In the process of beam displacement over the eye aperture, data on the transverse aberration for each point of beam entrance into the eye are collected, these data being the intensity distributions on the linear array photodetectors oriented along x and y axes (Figure 18-3). Registered for a set of entrance points (see Figure 18-1A), they are reconstructed into a two-dimensional distribution: the retinal spot diagram (see Figure 18-1B). The retinal spot diagram corresponds to the actual point spread function of the measured eye. From the retinal spot diagram, wavefront aberrations are reconstructed by means of approximation using either Zernike polynomials or splines. From the reconstructed wavefront, transverse aberrations are calculated using an eye model. Distribution corresponding to the declinations from emmetropia (refraction errors) is called a *refraction map*. The data obtained with the instrument also permit calculation of the suggested ablation map (distribution of the depth of the tissue to be ablated to achieve the required correction of vision).

Additionally, the Tracey ray tracing aberrometer features a charged-coupled device (CCD) video camera and a special target (fixation point) for aligning the eye and the instrument. The alignment method corresponds to the recommendations of the Optical Society of America (OSA) working group.[5] In the process of measurement, an image of the pupil is captured, its size and position are automatically measured in each TV frame. From the size of the pupil, the software calculates optimal locations of all the probing points. The permission on firing the probing radiation is given by the software only when the positions of the pupil and visual axis are within a predetermined correspondence, as well as the predetermined and actual sizes of the pupil. The data, captured with a position sensing detector, are processed and transferred to the computer. The total time of scanning for the entire aperture of the eye is within 50 milliseconds (ms). The duration depends on the number of test points at the eye entrance pupil. The default number of points is 64 and optionally it can be set to 95.

Tracey instruments have a wide range of display possibilities. There are four fields for displaying the diagrams and maps, for which the operator can choose among point spread function (PSF), wavefront, refraction, or simulation of Snellen letter resulting from a total set of aberration components or from its higher-order portion.

Default approximation of the wavefront aberrations is made using Zernike polynomials. Tracey displays Zernike spectrum in its classic form with orthogonal members or in the form of vectors with their amplitudes and orientation angles. In order to better represent high spatial frequency components, spline interpolation is employed as an option in Tracey-VFA. Figure 18-4A demonstrates an example of a refraction map reconstructed using Zernike polynomials, Figure 18-4B using bicubic splines. It

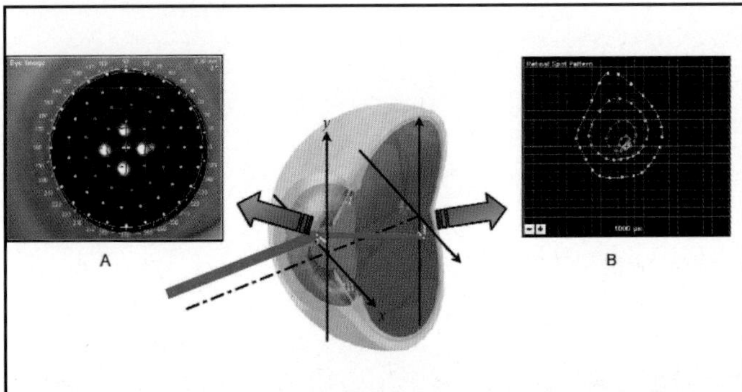

Figure 18-1. Principle of ray tracing aberrometry. A pencil of light entering the eye in the pupil locations (A) intersects the retina at point locations (B), called retina spot diagram.

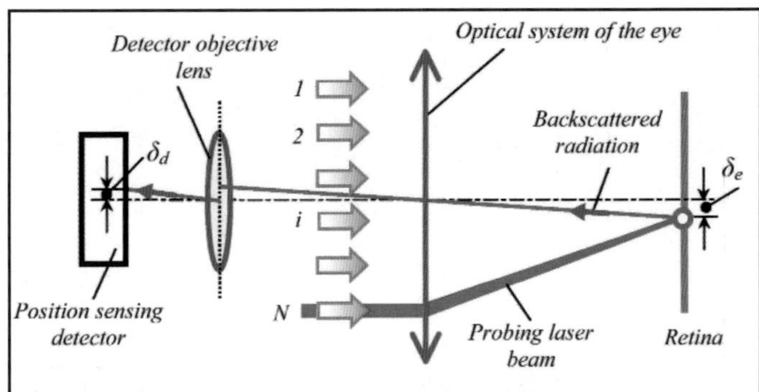

Figure 18-2. Principle of ray tracing aberrometry. Backscattered light from the retina is focused on the detector plane. Retinal spot lateral displacement δ_e is relayed to the plane of the position sensing detector and sensed as δ_d.

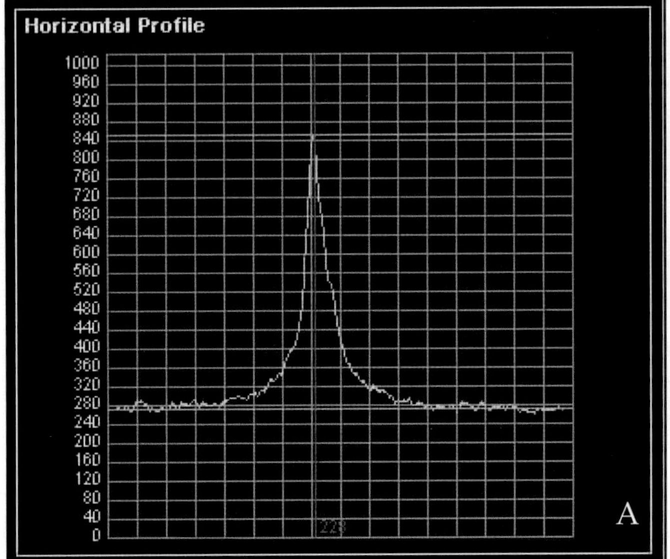

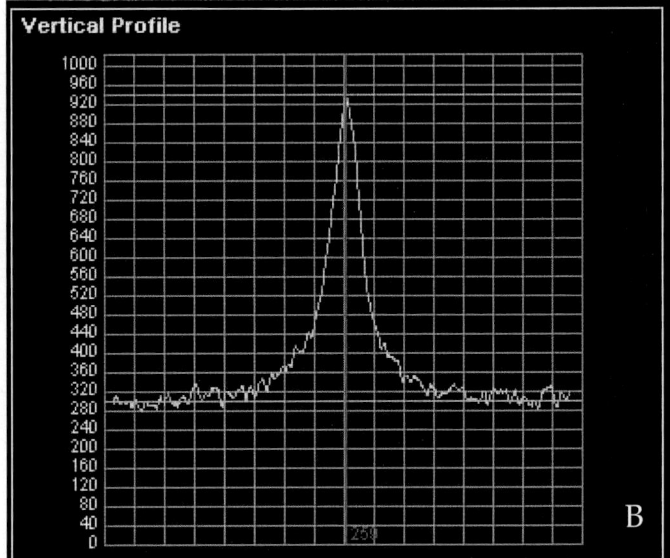

Figure 18-3. Horizontal (A) and vertical (B) profiles of the intensity of the light in the plane of the position sensing detector.

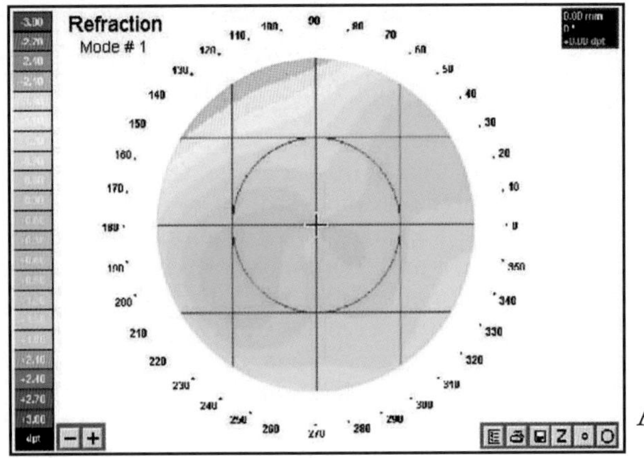

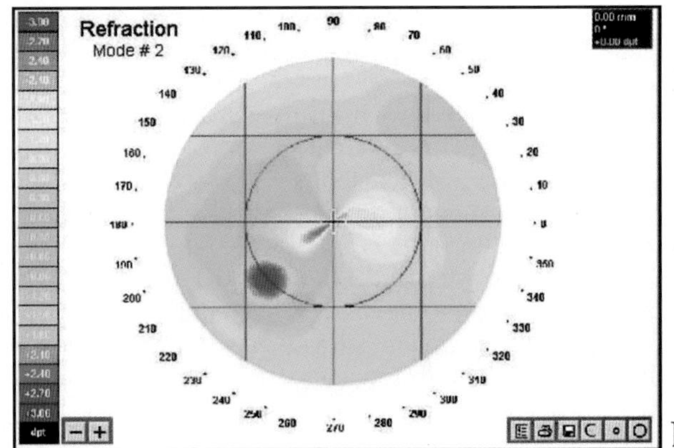

Figure 18-4. Refraction maps reconstructed by means of least mean squares method and approximation using Zernike polynomials (A) and using bicubic spline interpolation (B).

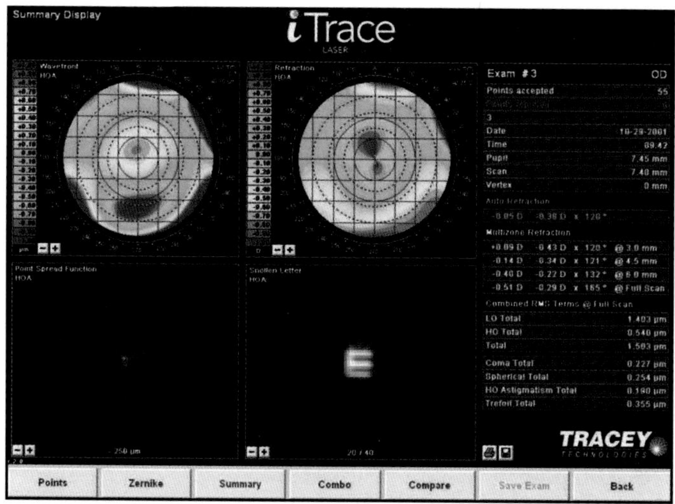

Figure 18-5. Summary display of the *i*-Trace visual function analyzer with the displayed higher-order wavefront aberrations, refraction errors, PSF, simulation of Snellen letter and the table of exam parameters.

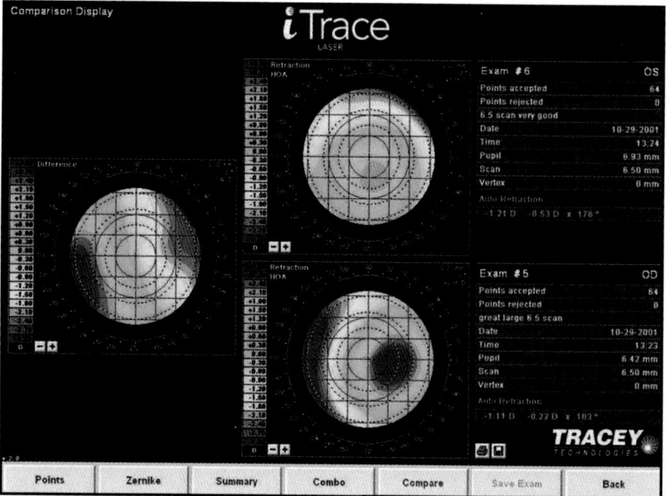

Figure 18-6. Comparison display of the *i*-Trace visual function analyzer with the displayed refraction errors caused by the higher-order aberrations for the left and the right eye of the same patient, their differences, and the table of exam parameters.

can be clearly seen that high spatial frequencies are better represented with spline interpolation. Among the shortcuts of splines, there are artifacts (for their suppression, special algorithms should be applied) and difficulties with classification of aberration types. Combination of these both approximations can be recommended.

In summary display mode, the operator can choose between displaying any possible data, like that shown in Figure 18-5, where four diagrams (wavefront—higher-order aberrations [HOA], refraction—HOA, PSF—total, and Snellen letter—total) and a summary table are displayed. Additionally, intermeasurement comparisons can be made (left-right eyes, pre- and postoperative conditions, etc). An example of a comparison display mode is given in Figure 18-6.

With new photodetector system designs, Tracey can easily measure a large dynamic range of refractive aberrations while maintaining high resolution. This should provide for a significant advantage when measuring a physiologic system, such as the eye, which can easily have a wide dynamic range of refractive errors, as is typically seen in keratoconus or the edge of a laser in-situ keratomileusis (LASIK) flap. Additionally, since each point is sequentially measured, there cannot be a confusion of which entrance pupil location registers with the retinal spot detected, which is often the case in Shack-Hartmann sensor-based systems. In principle, this fact enables the measurement of very aberrated eyes.

With new photodetector system designs, Tracey can easily measure a large dynamic range of refractive aberrations while maintaining high resolution. This should provide for a significant advantage when measuring a physiologic system, such as the eye, which can easily have a wide dynamic range of refractive errors, as is typically seen in keratoconus or the edge of a LASIK flap.

In further comparison to ray tracing aberrometry, the Shack-Hartmann lenslet array method measures the slope changes of the distorted wavefront as it exits the eye. This technology utilizes a bundle of light entering the eye and reflecting from the retina as a secondary light source. It is assumed that this secondary light source is ideal and perfectly centered, which is occasionally not the case and complicates this technique. As the reflected light travels backward through the eye, it is subject to the eye's aberrations and projects out through the exit pupil, striking the Shack-Hartmann sensor. The number of lenslets in the array limits the spatial resolution of this system, and the sensitivity of this system is limited by the focal length of the lenses used in the lenslet array. There is a tradeoff between the greater number of lenses and the greater light-gathering power, or aperture, of each lens.

Although the Shack-Hartmann approach can theoretically avoid the intrameasurement errors related to saccadic movements, it has inherent sensitivity problems arising from the fact that light from a retinal spot has to illuminate all lenslets of the array, whereas each lenslet has a very small surface and therefore small light-gathering power. This effect can become a problem when scattering is present in the eye under measurement, such as when a cataract is developing (Figure 18-7A). In such cases measurement can be made possible with the use of the ray tracing approach in which the retina/detector conjugating lens has substantially higher light-gathering power (Figure 18-7B).

Moreover in Shack-Hartmann–based systems, the focal length of the lenslet array must also be selected and fixed. In other words, this design is limited by the selection of the lenslet array. Once selected, it fixes the resolution and sensitivity of the unit. Shack-Hartmann–based systems tend to have a limited dynamic range in measuring higher-order aberrations. With postrefractive surgery patients or corneal pathologies, this may become a significant limitation.

References

1. Artal P, Berrio E, Guirao A. Contribution of the cornea and internal surfaces to the change of ocular aberrations with age. *J Opt Soc Am A*. 2002;19(1):136-143.
2. Roberts C. Future challenges to aberration-free ablative procedures. *J Refract Surg*. 2000;16:S623-S629.

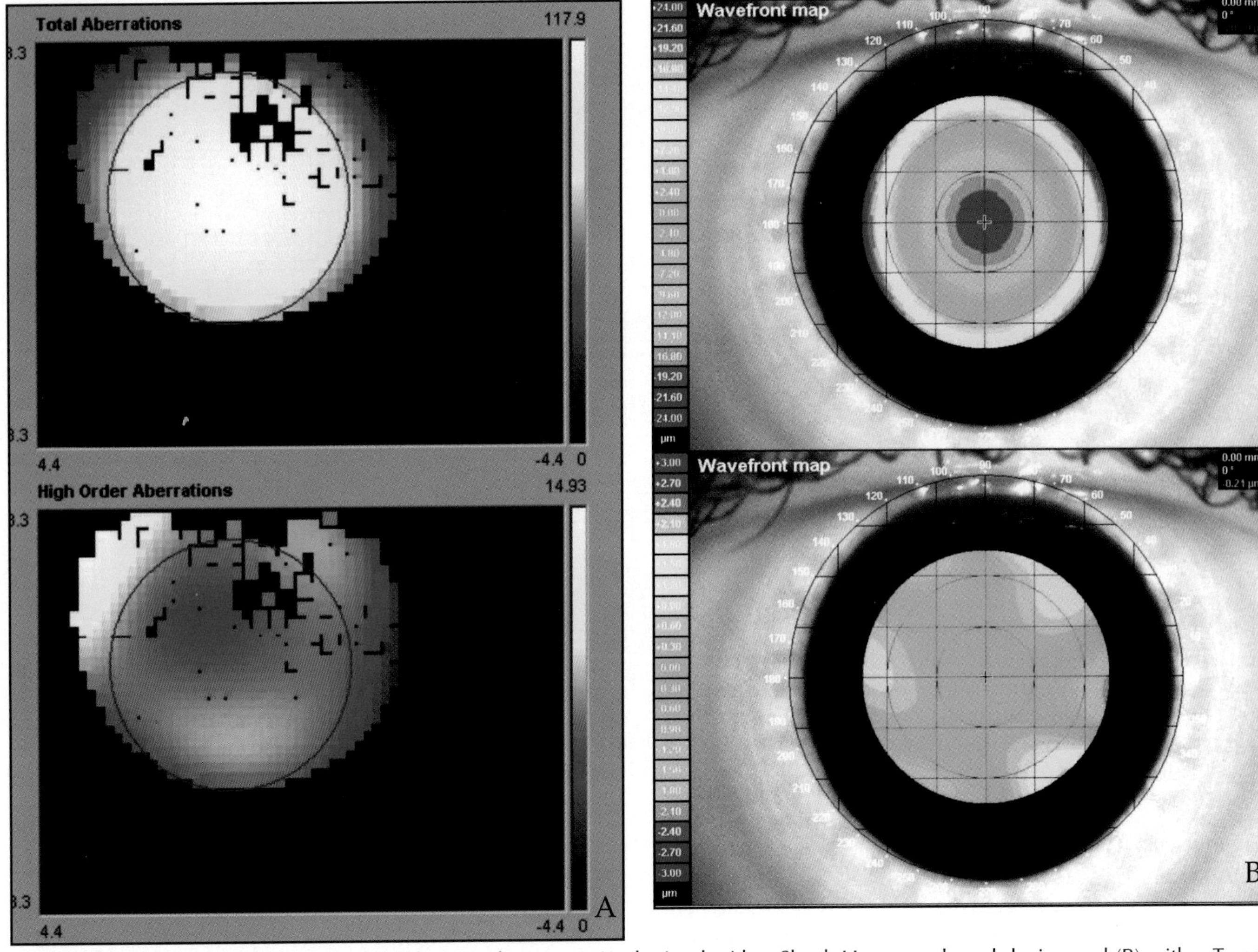

Figure 18-7. Wavefront maps of an eye with cortical cataract (A) obtained with a Shack-Hartmann-based device and (B) with a Tracey ray tracing aberrometer.

3. Charman WN, Heron G. Fluctuations in accommodation: a review. *Ophthal Physiol Opt*. 1988;8:153-163.

4. Molebny VV, Pallikaris IG, Naoumidis LP, Chyzh IH, Molebny SV, Sokurenko VM. Retina ray-tracing technique for eye-refraction mapping. *Proc SPIE*. 1997;2971:175-183.

5. Applegate RA, Thibos LN, Bradley A, et al. Reference axis selection: a subcommittee report of the OSA working group to establish standards for the measurement and reporting of the optical aberration of the eye. *Vision Science and Its Applications. 2000 Technical Digest.* Santa Fe, NM: Optical Society of America; 2000:122-149.

Chapter 19

Retinoscope Double Pass Aberrometry: Principles and Application of the Nidek OPD-Scan

Philip M. Buscemi, OD

The Nidek OPD-Scan (Nidek, Gamagori, Japan) differs from most clinical devices for aberrometry that employ methods to determine the position of a point or points that have passed through the eye's optical system and are projected onto some form of photo detector. The OPD-Scan utilizes an array of photo detectors of known position and measures the time that light takes to reach each detector after reflecting off of the retinal tapetum and passing through the ocular optics. This is the time-based (versus position-based) method to determining the wavefront error of the human eye. Time-based aberrometry allows the instrument to have a broader dynamic range, higher resolution, and increased accuracy. The OPD-Scan can measure patients with -20 to +22 diopters (D) of spherical and up to 12 D of cylindrical refractive error in 1 degree increments. It measures up to 6 millimeters (mm) of the central optical path with 1440 data points in four rings. The measurement time is approximately 0.4 seconds.

> The OPD has a large dynamic range. It can measure patients with -20 to +22 D of spherical and up to 12 D of cylindrical refractive error.

In addition to standard wavefront maps, the OPD-Scan displays a clinically oriented representation of the wavefront error, called the *optical path difference map*. This map represents the spatial distribution of dioptric values of refractive error that are associated with their respective variations from the planar wavefront using color scales similar to those employed in corneal topography.

The OPD-Scan registers the OPD and corneal curvature data using placedo disk-based corneal topography. The corneal topography data consist of 6800 points derived from 19 vertical and 23 horizontal rings using edge detection algorithms.

> The corneal topography system measures corneal curvature with 6800 points derived from 19 vertical and 23 horizontal rings.

The corneal topography map displays include axial, tangential, corneal refractive power (Snell's law), corneal target refractive power (postsurgical estimation using Snell's law), elevation profile, and difference maps. The instrument can measure curvatures from 10 to 100 D. The aberrometry displays include the OPD, total wavefront, and higher-order aberration maps and Zernike graphs with numeric values. The Zernike coefficients can be displayed in groupings of the user's choice or individually and calculated up to eighth-order aberrations.

The OPD-Scan uses three modes of data acquisition: manual, semiautomatic with tracking, or automatic. In manual mode, the user must align and trigger the instrument for data acquisition. Semiautomatic with tracking allows the user to take advantage of the fine tracking mechanism, but allows a manual trigger to initiate the exam. In the automatic mode, the OPD-Scan will automatically trigger when alignment is correct. The unit can perform topography only, aberrometry only, or both in rapid sequence. The instrument has a touch screen display so that a mouse is not necessary. Since many practitioners are more familiar with using a mouse, a mouse port is provided in addition to printer, USB, 10/100 network, and keyboard connections.

All ophthalmic wavefront aberrometers prior to the OPD utilized processed position-based data to determine wavefront error. This started with Dresden- or Tscherning-type aberrometers that project a mosaic of dots onto the retina. These dots are then imaged on a charged-coupled device (CCD), and their positions are determined. The difference between the location of each dot and its expected projected position from a perfect ophthalmic optical system with no refractive error is used to derive the variation in the wavefront.[1]

Although the Dresden and Shack-Hartmann wavefront systems use different methods, in some respects there are similarities. The Shack-Hartmann system uses a different method to derive data points. By projecting a point of coherent light on the retina and imaging the efferent light using a grid of microlenslets, points are once again focused onto a CCD. Each point is associated with a single lenslet in the array, which in turn is conjugate with approximately the plane of the iris to derive each lenslet's exact position in the x,y plane relative to the eye. Once again, the difference in the position of each point on the CCD when compared with that of the perfect optical system is used to calculate the associated wavefront.[2]

A third methodology, the Tracey system, also uses position-based data. The Tracey system differs from the preceding methods in that it projects just one point at a time onto the retina and determines its location with an optical sensor. Sixty-four data

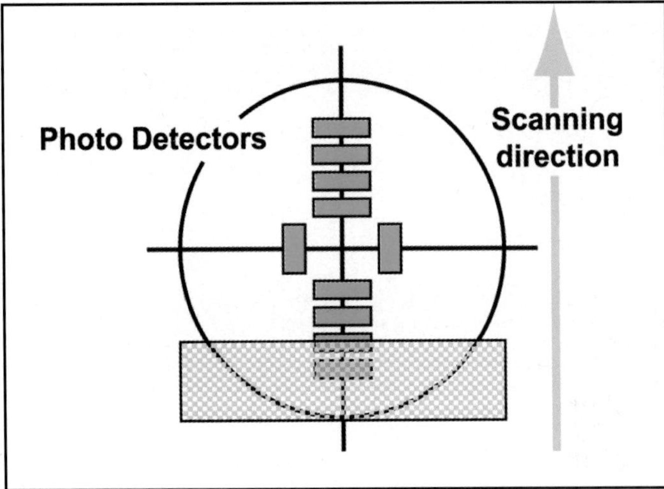

Figure 19-1. The OPD-Scan sensor array employs eight data sensors and two reference sensors to determine relative time differential of the reflected infrared slit in calculating refractive error for each data point.

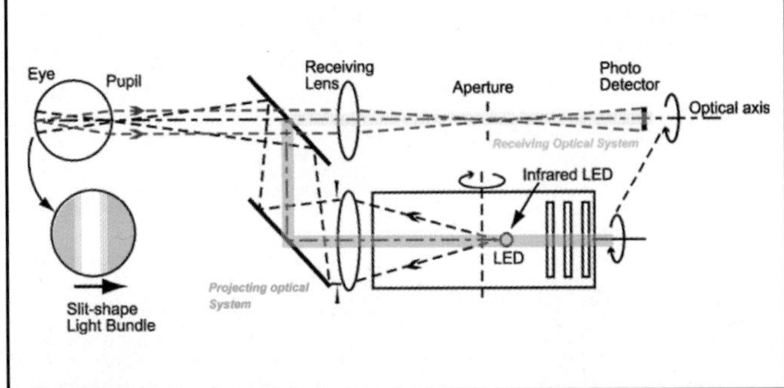

Figure 19-2. The photo detectors and scanning slit rotate in synchrony to produce four rings of data with 360 data points of refractive error per ring. Note the aperture, which is conjugate with the retina in emmetropia.

points are measured five times in 10 milliseconds (ms). Once again, the position of each data point relative to its expected position with a perfect wavefront is used to calculate the aberration.[3]

Position-based systems have certain limitations. The first limitation is actually discerning the dot's image on the CCD and then determining its center to create the data point. In situations of high refractive error and/or higher-order aberration, the dots can be very blurred and irregular in shape. This can lead to lost or misread data points. The second limitation is jumbling of the data points. Higher-order aberrations can make it difficult to determine which measured data point corresponds to its associated ideal theoretical data point. If these are not correctly matched, the derived aberration is incorrect.

There are various techniques that attempt to overcome these inherent deficiencies. Some Shack-Hartmann systems will mask some of the lenslets in the array to prevent jumbling of the data. This reduces the resolution and sensitivity of the device. Others will use multiple steps to gather data by prefocusing the array to eliminate the adverse effects of higher amounts of lower-order aberration. However, as a rule, the higher the resolution of the system, the lower the dynamic range. Conversely, the higher the range, the lower the resolution.

The Tracey system avoids jumbling of data points by projecting just one point at a time, but it may require oversampling of data points for accuracy. This reduces resolution.

The OPD-Scan employs a different approach in determining aberration, using the time it takes reflected light from the retina to reach given points to calculate refractive and wavefront error. Clinicians are familiar with this principle from performing dynamic retinoscopy. As one moves the retinoscope slit across the pupil, the reflected light from the retina will move at a greater speed, either with or against the motion of the slit depending on the refractive error. In emmetropia, all you see is a flash.

The OPD-Scan employs a different approach in determining aberration, using the time it takes reflected light from the retina to reach given points to calculate refractive and wavefront error.

In the OPD-Scan technology, the positions of the data points are predefined. The time for the intensity of reflected light from the retina to peak at a given data point compared to the theoretical time it would take light to maximally illuminate the point in an eye with perfect emmetropia is used to calculate the refractive error at that location in x and y on the reference plane, which is near the iris. The time differential is calculated in four rings of data containing 360 data points in each ring that comprises the data set of 1440 data points. This array of data is then converted into a color map representing the dioptric refractive error values of each component called an *optical path difference* or *OPD map*.

To achieve this, the OPD-Scan uses a rotating set of photo detectors (Figure 19-1). There are eight data sensors and two reference sensors, with four data photo detectors above and below the reference photo detectors, which are on the optical axis. These are illuminated by the reflection off of the retinal tapetum of a moving slit of light, which is created by an infrared light source, a chopper wheel, and a projecting lens (Figure 19-2). The slit bundle is perpendicular to the line of data sensors and scanning along the same axis. Because the chopper wheel rotates rapidly, a constant high-speed scan of the retina is reflecting back through a receiving lens and aperture stop to the sensors, which synchronously rotate around their axis with the scanning slit of infrared light through 180 degrees in 0.4 seconds. This yields 360 degrees of data in four rings.

The emitting infrared light-emitting diode (LED) and the photo detectors are conjugate with the cornea, while the aperture is conjugate with the retina in the emmetropic eye. In myopia, the aperture stop is in front of the retina. In hyperopia, it is behind the retina (Figure 19-3). As in retinoscopy, this causes the reflected light to flash all at once across the pupil in emmetropia, but to lead or reverse when compared to the movement of the projected slit of light in ametropic conditions. This causes time differences in the peak illumination between the reference and data photo detectors (Figures 19-4A, 19-4B, and 19-4C). The time difference at any location within the 6 mm examination zone is due to differences in the optical path distance between the retina and the aperture. By comparing the peak of light intensity of each data sensor with respect to the peak of intensity in the reference sensor, the refractive error for each of the 1440 data points is determined and an OPD map is generated (Figure 19-5).[4]

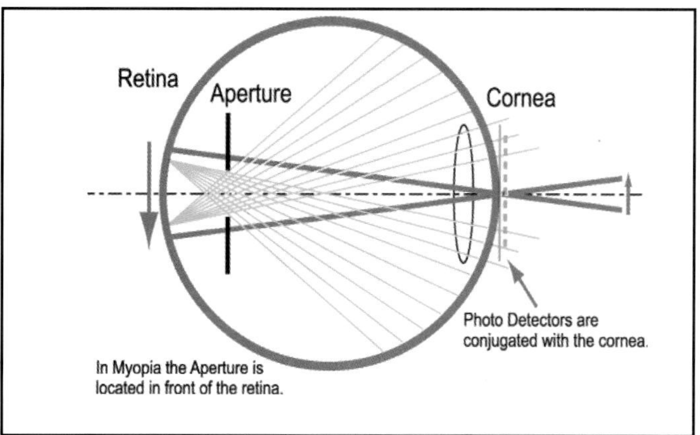

Figure 19-3. The aperture is conjugate with the retina in emmetropia, conjugate in front of the retina in myopia (shown), and behind in hyperopia.

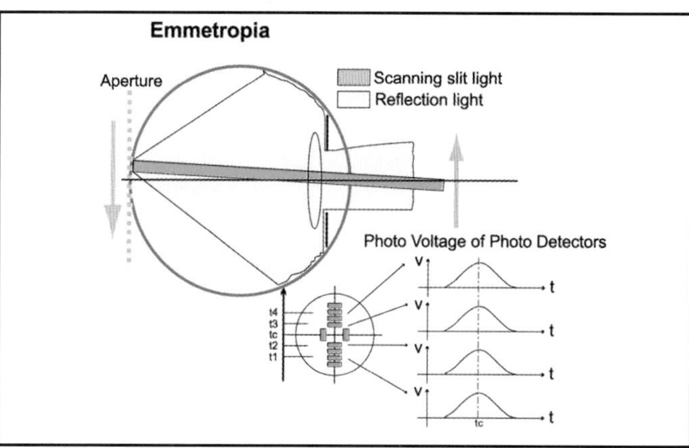

Figure 19-4A. In emmetropia, the aperture at the retinal plane causes the slit reflex to flash across all photo detectors at once.

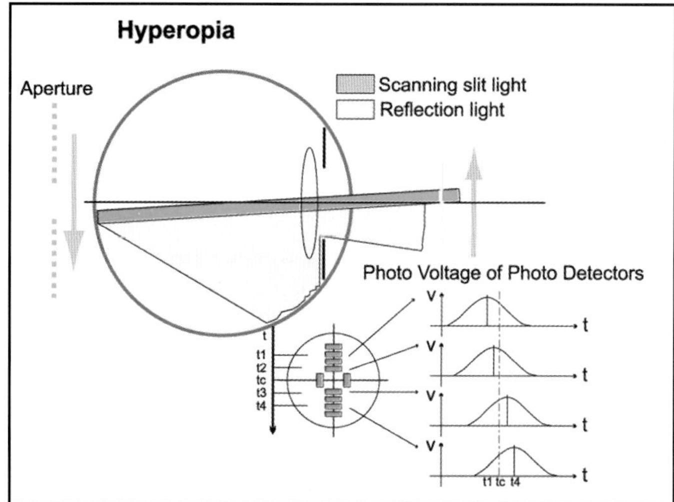

Figure 19-4B. In hyperopia, the aperture is behind the retinal plane, causing the slit reflex to move in the opposite direction of the projected slit. The rate of movement is measured by the time difference between the peak voltage of the reference and sensor photodetectors and converted to refractive error.

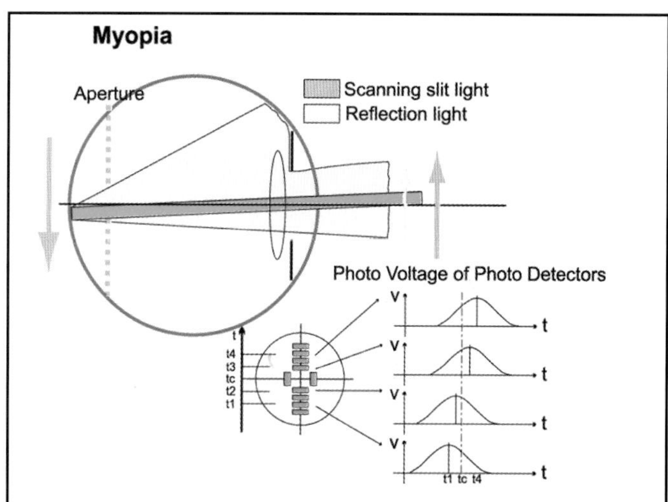

Figure 19-4C. In myopia, the aperture is in front of the retinal plane, causing the slit reflex to move more rapidly in the same direction as the projected slit. The rate of movement is measured by the time difference between the peak voltage of the reference and sensor photodetectors and converted to refractive error.

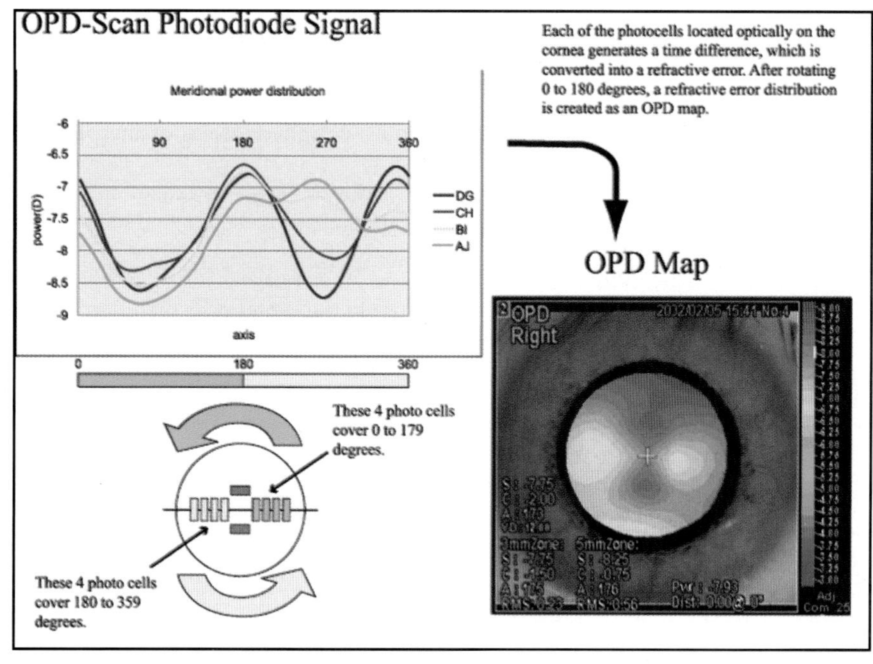

Figure 19-5. The OPD map is a spatial representation of the refractive error across the reference plane.

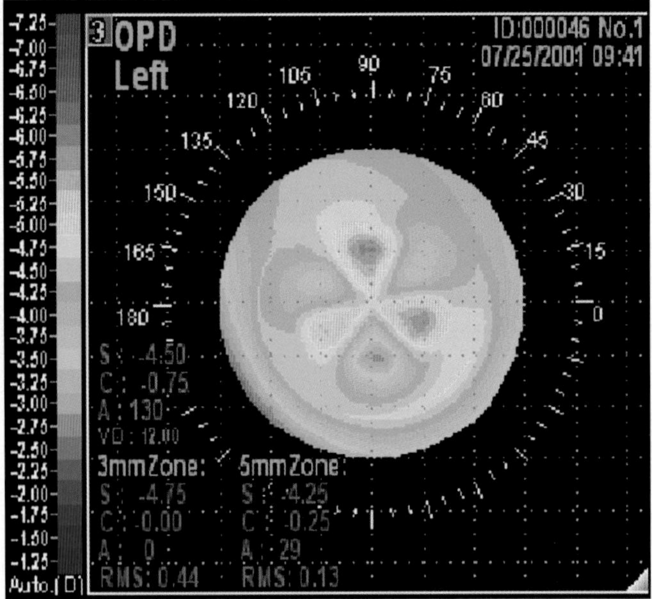

Figure 19-6. The OPD map displays the spatial distribution of refractive error in trefoil. It is very easy for the practitioner to associate this with the patient's symptoms of monocular triple images.

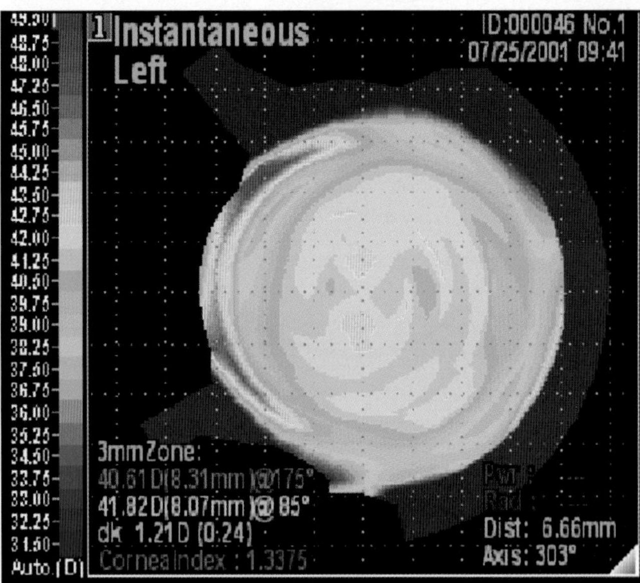

Figure 19-7. Corneal topography of the same patient in Figure 19-6 does not show the trefoil. The OPD-Scan can differentiate the onternal OPD/wavefront data from corneal surface data because both data sets are registered on the same instrument.

> Editor's note:
>
> The OPD system fires a rapid sequence of slits into the eye in 0.4 sec. The photodetectors measure the time that the light takes to hit each photodetector to determine if there is myopia, hyperopia, or higher-order aberrations.
>
> S. MacRae, MD

This dioptric data is easy for the clinician to understand and frequently will illuminate optical aberrations not intuitively ascertained through the corneal topography. An OPD map of a patient with trefoil (Figure 19-6) when compared to the corneal topography (Figure 19-7) makes it obvious why the patient was seeing three images monocularly. When viewing the OPD map, it is easy to understand that each of the three red lobes acts optically like a small lens; hence, the three images from one eye. The topography does not give any hint of the trefoil or explain the etiology of the patient's chief subjective complaint—monocular triplopia. In addition, the patient's lower-order aberration—basically sphere, cylinder, and axis—can be easily differentiated from the higher-order aberration in the OPD map because the data is displayed in diopters.

> The OPD map makes it easier to see higher-order aberrations, like trefoil, that are difficult to visualize with corneal topography.

The OPD map is converted to a traditional, more scientifically- and, in some ways, less clinically-oriented, wavefront error map with variations from the plane wave denoted in microns by reverse ray tracing (Figure 19-8). Each data point on the reference plane is a dioptric value. A point is plotted on a line tangential to the reference plane that is equal to the distance of the focal length of the data point. Note that this measurement is made from the intersection of the line and reference plane. A reference line connecting the point on the tangential line and the original data point is then determined.

A small plane that is associated with the data point and is tangential to the reference line is then moved along the line so that its edges approximate the edges of the planes associated with the surrounding data points. Combining all of these small planes yields the shape of the wavefront. The distance from the wavefront to the reference plane is calculated in microns and displayed on a color wavefront map. This data is used to calculate the Zernike polynomials that comprise the mathematical model of the wavefront.

It is clinically important to compare the OPD map (see Figure 19-5) with the higher-order aberration wavefront map (Figure 19-9) that is derived from the same data set. Note that the OPD map displays the actual optical effect within the central areas of the cornea. The higher-order wavefront map could lead the unsuspecting practitioner to believe that the effect on the patient's vision is actually in the more peripheral areas of the patient's optical system.

The reason for this may be due to the leveraging of the peripheral wavefront by central anomalies. To better understand this effect, imagine a straight line with one end anchored in the center of the wavefront and the other floating in the periphery. A small push in the z-axis close to the center near the fulcrum will cause the periphery of the line to move a lot. The same may happen with wavefront errors (ie, smaller changes centrally compound their effect peripherally in the wavefront, leading to higher gross errors there). This is not the case with the OPD map because it is displaying refractive error and not microns of deviation from a plane wave.

Dr. Stephen Klyce has proposed an easy way to remember these differences by using the acronym MD: microns (produced by wavefront maps) is for machines, diopters (displayed in OPD maps) is for doctors. The point being that wavefront maps may

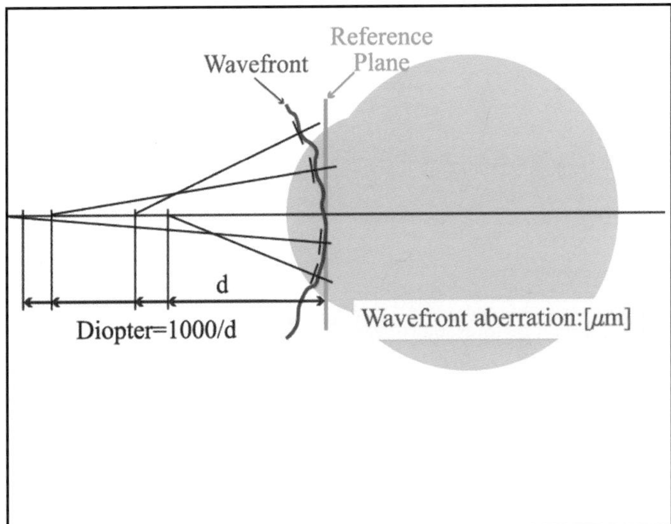

Figure 19-8. Reverse ray tracing of the OPD data yields a wavefront map that can then be differentiated into its various components by Zernike deconvolution.

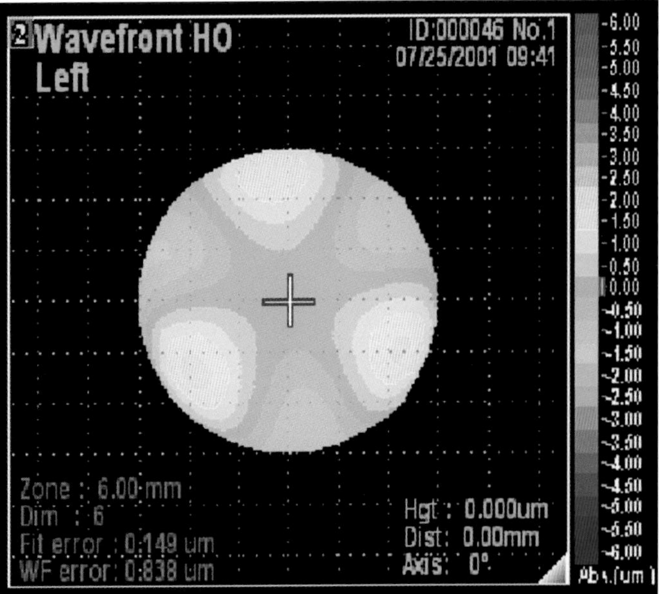

Figure 19-9. The wavefront map derived from the OPD map in Figure 19-6. Note that the wavefront data can mislead the practitioner in thinking that the optical effect occurs peripherally when the effects in fact are in the central area of the reference plane.

be best employed when calculating shot data in performing ablations, while the OPD map may be the most intuitive for diagnostics by physicians.

The OPD-Scan is an aberrometer that is unique among its peers in its fundamental principles of operation, acquisition technology, methodology, and data generated. It can provide comprehensive wavefront data, Zernike polynomials, OPD maps, and corneal topography. When combined with Nidek's Final Fit Software and EC-5000 in their NAVEX system, its output is used to drive customized ablation to repair both lower- and higher-order aberrations. It is also an extremely useful tool for contact lens practitioners and in determining whether the etiology of vision loss is of optical origins. Its high range, resolution, and registered corneal topography will likely find more clinical applications in the future.

References

1. Mierdel P, Kaemmerer M, Mrochen M, Krinke HE, Seiler T. Ocular optical aberrometer for clinical use. *J Biomed Opt*. 2001;6(2):200-204.
2. Platt BC, Shack R. History and principles of Shack-Hartmann wavefront sensing. *J Refract Surg*. 2001;17(5):S573-S577.
3. Molebny VV, Panagopoulou SI, Molebny SV, Wakil YS, Pallikaris IG. Principles of ray tracing aberrometry. *J Refract Surg*. 2000;16(5):S572-S575.
4. MacRae S, Fujieda M. Slit skiascopic-guided ablation using the Nidek laser. *J Refract Surg*. 2000;16(5):S576-S580.

Chapter 20

Spatially Resolved Refractometry: Principles and Application of the Emory Vision InterWave Aberrometer

Jonathan D. Carr, MD, MA, FRCOphth; Henia Lichter, MD; Jose Garcia, BS; R. Doyle Stulting, MD, PhD; Keith P. Thompson, MD; and P. Randall Staver, MS

The 21st century has seen excimer lasers become increasingly sophisticated, with laser beam delivery size becoming smaller (slits or spots of laser light), treating the cornea at greater frequencies. This has created a need for eye trackers to monitor the delivery of the treatment during laser ablation. The commercialization of wavefront aberrometers, long the province of optical scientists, has allowed refractive surgeons the opportunity to move beyond the correction of spherocylindrical refractive errors. The potential exists for patients to enjoy a quality of vision that is superior to that provided by spectacles and contact lenses and to have new treatment options for presbyopia.

The Emory Vision InterWave (interactive wavefront) scanner (Emory Vision, Atlanta, Ga) is one example of an aberrometer that is currently being used in refractive surgery practice. It is a patient-interactive aberrometer that measures visual aberrations across the entire entrance pupil and throughout the entire visual system, from the cornea to the visual cortex. It is based upon the Scheiner principle, first described by Scheiner in the 17th century[1] and subsequently modified by Smirnov.[2] The InterWave scanner is a solid-state version of a spatially resolved refractometer, developed by Webb and colleagues at Schepens Eye Research Institute and described by He.[3]

There are four types of aberrometers in use today. The Shack-Hartmann wavefront sensor is an example of reflection aberrometry, whereby light exiting the eye is acquired at the entrance pupil and the wavefront error reconstructed after passing through a lenslet array.[4] Retinal imaging aberrometry was first described by Tscherning and later modified by Howland and Howland.[5,6] More recently Mierdel, Seiler, and colleagues have employed this technique to study the aberrations of the human eye.[7] Double pass retinoscopic aberrometry looks at both ingoing and outgoing passage of light, and has been adapted for clinical use in Nidek's OPD-Scan system (Gamagori, Japan). The InterWave scanner is an example of spatially resolved refractometry[3,8-15] and it is different from other methods in that it allows subjects to interact during the testing process, a strategy that may prove to be an advantage in the arena of customized laser treatment.

We report herein the principles behind spatially resolved refractometry and the Emory Vision InterWave scanner and the practical uses of this exciting technology.

THE INTERWAVE SCANNER

In the 17th century, Scheiner described a simple optometer that consisted of a disk with two holes.[1] A patient then viewed a distant point light source through the disk. Each of the two holes allowed a ray of light to pass through a discrete region of the pupil. If the eye were emmetropic, both rays of light would be brought to a focus at the fovea and the patient perceived ONE light source. In the presence of a refractive error or other visual aberration, the light source formed TWO images on the retina and the patient perceived two spots (Figure 20-1).

The Emory Vision InterWave scanner incorporates the Scheiner principle with modern solid-state computer controls and optical interfaces into a unit that integrates well into the busy clinical practice at our institution (Figure 20-2). Data acquisition is rapid, generally requiring 3 minutes per eye. InterWave measurements have become the standard of care for preoperative, operative, and postoperative decision making at Emory Vision.

The InterWave scanner records the wavefront error at approximately 70 individual positions across the dilated pupil. The instrument possesses a Badal optometer that allows for neutralization of the eye's spherical equivalent refractive error, allowing the bandwidth of the instrument (-15 to +7 diopters [D]) to measure the higher-order aberrations. This allows test subjects to easily visualize the test spot and background alignment reticule. Each of the 70 measurements requires the patient to use a computer joystick to center a movable test spot to the center of a fixed cross hair reticule. The test spot and the alignment reticule are delivered through two independent optical channels (test channel and reference channel) in the instrument. A charged-coupled device (CCD) camera occupies the third optical channel; it allows for passive pupil monitoring during data acquisition. These optical channels are shown in Figure 20-3.

The InterWave scanner records the wavefront error at approximately 70 individual positions across the dilated pupil. The instrument possesses a Badal optometer that allows for neutralization of the eye's spherical equivalent refractive error, allowing the bandwidth of the instrument (-15 to +7 D) to measure the higher-order aberrations.

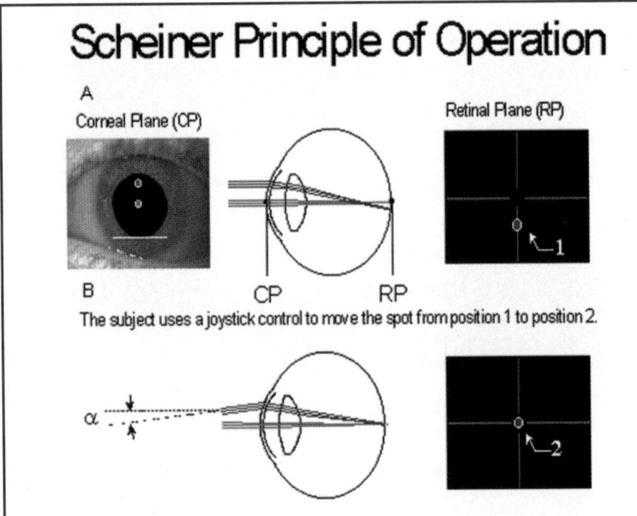

Figure 20-1. The Scheiner principle of operation. Two lights are projected onto the cornea. A reference light and a test light, the latter used to measure the local refraction at all points within the pupil. In an emmetropic, aberration-free eye, ONE light will be perceived by the test subject. In the presence of a refractive error, two spots will be perceived, a central one and one that is separated from the center of the cross hairs ("1" in the figure). The subject uses a joystick to move the spot from position "1" to position "2." The angle required to move the light from position "1" to position "2" represents the slope of the wavefront at that location.

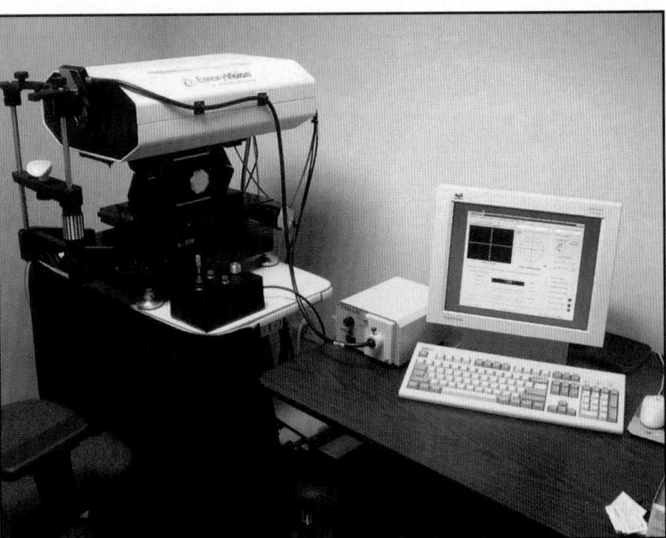

Figure 20-2. The InterWave is a compact solid-state device that integrates easily into our busy refractive surgery practice.

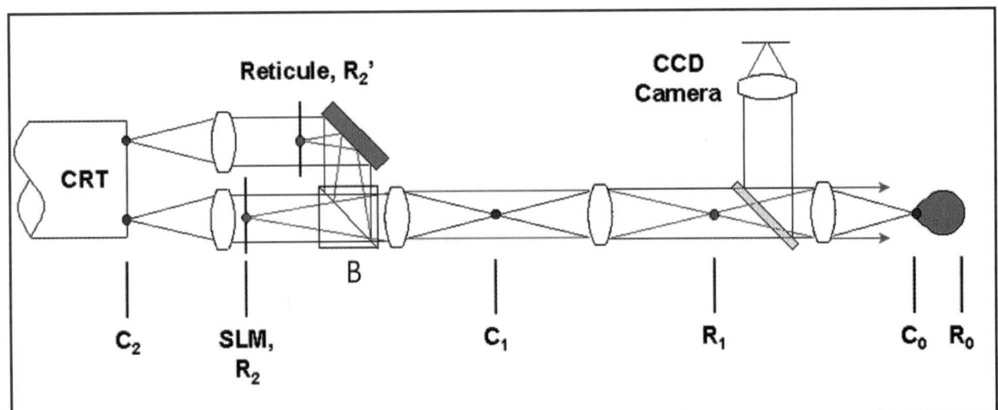

Figure 20-3. Optical configuration of the InterWave scanner. The planes defined by C_0, C_1, and C_2 represent the corneal plane and its two conjugate planes, respectively. The planes defined by R_0, R_1, and R_2 are the retinal plane and its two conjugate planes, respectively. The cathode ray tube (CRT) is conjugate to the corneal plane; the spatial light modulator (SLM) is conjugate to the retinal plane. A CCD camera focused at infinity observes the corneal plane through a beam splitter. A beam splitter acts as a beam-combining device that superimposes the reference and test channel images into one image. In the reference channel, a fixed reticule is used in place of the SLM to create the image of an alignment cross hair.

The channel projecting the test spot generates the image by illumination of a spatial light modulator (SLM) with a small spot from a cathode ray tube (CRT). The size and location of the test spot on the CRT determines the size and location of the test spot at the entrance pupil of the eye. The CRT is located at a plane conjugate to the patient's entrance pupil, while the SLM is located at a plane conjugate to the patient's retina.

The second channel projects the alignment reticule, illuminated by a second spot on the CRT. A beam splitter acts as a beam-combining device that combines test and reference channels into one image. Because the SLM and the reticule are conjugate to the patient's retinal plane, the test subject sees a replica of the pattern on the SLM, typically a small spot. The location of this test spot on the SLM is used to determine the local derivative of the wavefront error at a discrete region within the entrance pupil of the eye.

The CCD camera has two main functions in the system. First, it acquires the image of the eye and tracks its location with

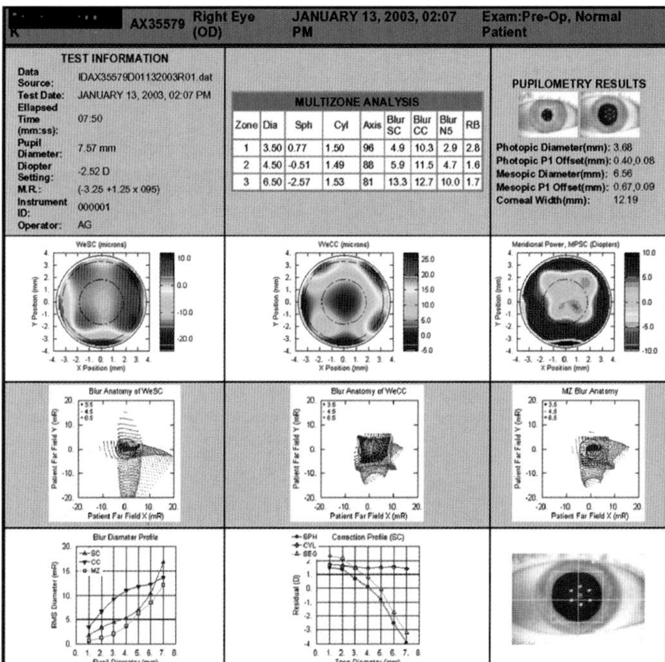

Zone	Dia	Sph	Cyl	Axis	Blur SC	Blur CC	Blur N5	RB
1	3.50	0.77	1.50	96	4.9	10.3	2.9	2.8
2	4.50	-0.51	1.49	88	5.9	11.5	4.7	1.6
3	6.50	-2.57	1.53	81	13.3	12.7	10.0	1.7

Figure 20-4. The standard InterWave report shows infrared pupillometry data, wavefront maps with and without spherocylindrical correction, retinal blur anatomy maps, and measures of spherical aberration as the pupil becomes larger for the eye tested. This report shows a highly aberrated eye of a patient that had previously undergone refractive keratotomy.

respect to the instrument's optical axis during the acquisition procedure. This information is then used to adaptively maintain the alignment of the test and reference spots as the subject's eye moves during the test. Secondly, it measures the pupil diameter and the position of the pupil centroid and Purkinje image reflection under different illumination conditions. The tracking system has the flexibility to provide registration based upon the dilated pupil or the Purkinje axis, an option that provides flexibility for registering InterWave data with the excimer lasers that perform customized laser ablation. This may have particular importance in hyperopic customized treatments, since the center of the pupil might not be the optimal location to center laser treatment in lieu of the visual axis.

InterWave testing requires cycloplegia, achieved by instillation of one drop of 1% cyclopentolate 20 minutes prior to testing. Once correctly positioned, the test subject is presented with a test spot that is projected through a specific region of the entrance pupil. In the presence of a local refractive error (or higher-order aberrations), the spot lies away from the center of the cross hair. The subject uses a joystick to move the test spot to the center of the cross hair. The joystick drives optics in the system that move the angle at which the test beam impinges on the pupil without moving its position. The subject presses a button to indicate that the alignment of test spot and cross hair is satisfactory. A new test spot is presented to the test subject and the alignment task is repeated, and so on until the end of the test.

In the presence of a local refractive error (or higher-order aberrations), the spot lies away from the center of the cross hair. The subject uses a joystick to move the test spot to the center of the cross hair. The joystick drives optics in the system that move the angle at which the test beam impinges on the pupil without moving its position.

Data Analysis

For each position tested within the pupil, an angle pair is produced. The angle measurement at each location is proportional to the slope of the local wavefront error at the particular position within the entrance pupil. A least-square procedure is used to fit the slope measurements at each location to the derivatives of the Zernike polynomials as described by Webb.[16] The derived coefficients are used to reconstruct the overall wavefront aberration of the eye. He and colleagues have previously reported the method for data acquisition and analysis.[3]

Having obtained aberration data for a widely dilated pupil, it is now possible to determine the optical performance of the eye with different pupil sizes. This has clinical significance, since some patients have larger pupils than others under mesopic and scotopic conditions.

Data Output

The InterWave scanner produces a detailed output of the eye's aberration structure (Figure 20-4). Infrared pupillometry is recorded for photopic and mesopic conditions and shown at the top of the InterWave report. The wavefront error contour map is generated and shown for the uncorrected eye and for the eye with a spherocylindrical spectacle correction. These wavefront error maps show the difference in microns between the measured wavefront and a perfect reference wavefront. They are a representation of how a wavefront of light is distorted as it travels through the ocular media. A meridional power map is also generated and is comparable to maps generated on corneal videokeratography instruments; InterWave-derived power maps reflect optical power throughout the entire optical system, not just the cornea as is the case for corneal topographic maps.

Three blur anatomy maps are also generated (see Figure 20-4). These maps are a graphical representation of the predicted blur pattern that is perceived by patients when the eye views a point source of light at infinity. Ten thousand rays, traced from a point light source through the pupil to the retina, are used to generate the blur anatomy maps. The resulting figure is measured in milliradians (mR) of blur. For reference purposes, the image size of the moon high in the sky is shown, which is known to subtend 8.7 mR for an observer on earth. The resulting image on the blur anatomy map is color-coded according to the region of the pupil through which the light rays passed that are responsible for the particular parts of the image. The central pupil zone reports information from the central 3.5 millimeters (mm), the next zone, the area from 3.5 mm to 4.5 mm, and the outer zone from 4.5 mm to 6.5 mm. These zones are color-coded, so that the papillary

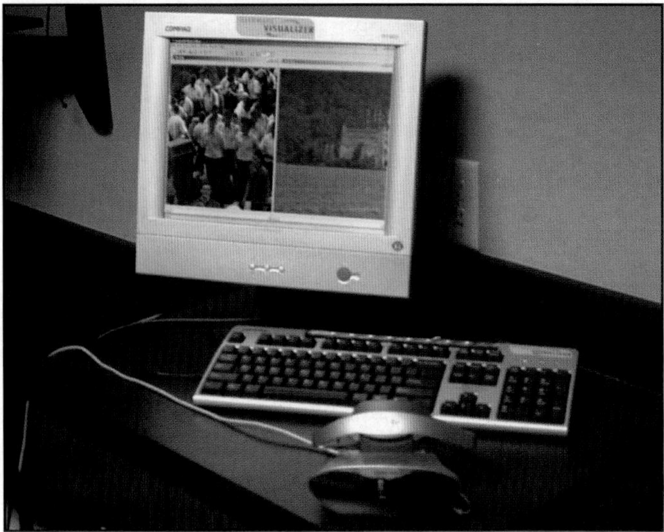

Figure 20-5. The InterWave Visualizer is a clinic-based tool that allows prospective patients to see (either on screen, or with heads-up display goggles) the type of result that might be expected from laser eye surgery in comparison to their spectacle correction.

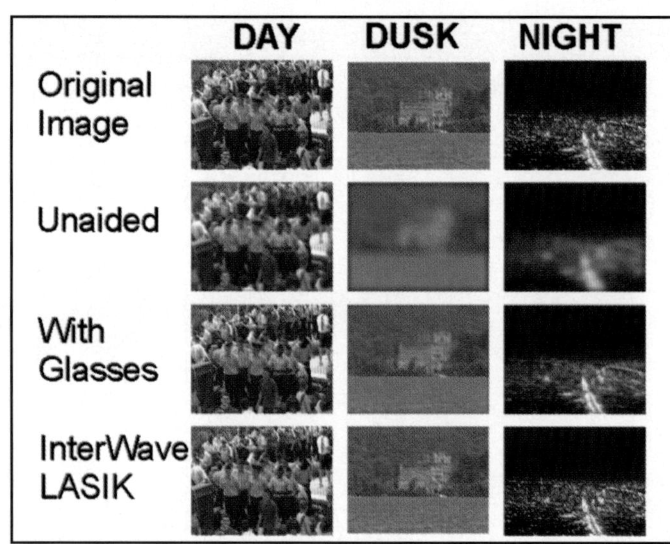

Figure 20-6. The InterWave Visualizer can provide patient-specific renditions of standard photographs that best show vision quality in daylight, at dusk, or at night.

regions (inner-blue, middle-green, outer-red) can be identified with the corresponding blurs that they cause. The blur anatomy is shown for the uncorrected eye and for the eye with spectacle correction. A third map shows the residual blur anatomy that would follow multiple pass, multizone laser ablation with the Nidek EC-5000 (Gamagori, Japan), using InterWave-derived sequential spherocylindrical treatments that are optimized for each papillary zone. This has allowed surgeons to customize treatments to minimize axisymmetric aberrations.

> The resulting image on the blur anatomy map is color-coded according to the region of the pupil through which the light rays passed that are responsible for the particular parts of the image. The central pupil zone reports information from the central 3.5 mm, the next zone, the area from 3.5 mm to 4.5 mm, and the outer zone from 4.5 mm to 6.5 mm. These zones are color-coded, so that the papillary regions (inner-blue, middle-green, outer-red) can be identified with the corresponding blurs that they cause.

In addition to the zonal blur anatomy maps, a zonal refraction can be derived by using an optimization algorithm to minimize the blur in each of the three zones. This algorithm selects the best combination of sphere, cylinder, and axis that minimizes the patient's resultant retinal blur anatomy within each zone independently. This process of calculating zonal refraction is highly accurate and precise. Staver and colleagues reported the standard deviation of measurements on sphere, cylinder, and axis to be 0.04 D, 0.07 D, and 2.8 degrees, respectively, for zone 1 (the central 3.5 mm), and 0.07 D, 0.04 D, and 0.5 degrees for zone 3.[17] Staver also reported that the zonal refraction for zone 1 was highly correlated with the manifest refraction ($r^2 = 0.915$).[17] This accuracy and precision has allowed the use of the excimer laser to perform multiple pass, multiple zone laser ablation to treat axisymmetric higher-order aberrations, such as spherical aberration. A recent retrospective analysis of laser in-situ keratomileusis (LASIK), to correct myopia and astigmatism with the Nidek EC-5000 excimer laser platform, compared multiple pass/multiple zone ablation based on InterWave zonal refraction data to standard spherocylindrical treatment based on manifest refraction. The multipass, multi-zone InterWave-based ablations reduced the retinal blur area by 48% compared to matched eyes treated with the standard sphero-cylindrical algorithm. In addition, the percentage of patients reporting night time halo symptoms was significantly reduced from 12.9% in the standard spherocylindrical treatment group to 1.3% in the multi-pass, multi-zone InterWave group.[18] This study demonstrated that InterWave-guided laser treatment significantly improved the quality of vision in patients undergoing LASIK surgery compared to patients treated with standard spherocylindrical laser treatment.

> The multipass, multizone InterWave-based ablations reduced the retinal blur area by 48% compared to matched eyes treated with the standard spherocylindrical algorithm.

InterWave Visualizer

The data generated from the InterWave is put to good use for prospective refractive surgery patients. The InterWave Visualizer allows patients to view the quality of vision that they might achieve after laser treatment in comparison to conventional correction that does not correct for higher-order aberrations (Figure 20-5). The pupil function is computed from the wavefront error and pupil diameter information and then Fourier transformed to obtain the point spread function (PSF). The reference color image is then resolved into its component red, green, and blue images. The PSF data undergo convolution with the red, green, and blue images. The red, green, and blue images are now blurred, or aberrated, as a result of the InterWave data. Reconstruction of the color image from the component red, green, and blue images allows the image to reflect the aberration structure of the eye. Patients are presented with images that best illustrate the quality of their vision when viewing daytime, dusk, and night time scenes on a high resolution/definition computer screen. These images can be modified to show the quality of vision achieved for the test eye with no refractive correction, with spherocylindrical spectacle correction, or after neutralization of higher-order aberrations with laser surgery (Figure 20-6).

> Editor's note:
>
> With increasing attention to neural processing as an important component in visual perception, the InterWave scanner provides the unique advantage of eliciting a patient response while capturing wavefront error. In this regard, assessment of visual perception is more complete because it measures the status of the visual system from the cornea to the occipital cortex, rather than just the retinal image plane used with reflection-based aberrometers. The disadvantage of this system, however, is that it requires a longer testing time of 3 minutes for each eye, and a more skilled device operator in capturing the wavefront error.
>
> R. Krueger, MD, MSE

Future Uses of InterWave Technology

InterWave technology is now providing the refractive information that surgeons at Emory Vision use to perform laser ablations for elimination of refractive errors, including higher-order aberrations. InterWave has a number of potential advantages over other aberrometers. The patient-interactive process for data acquisition allows the InterWave to measure the status of the visual system from cornea to occipital cortex. This may be an advantage compared to reflection-based aberrometers that have no patient input, because the location of the retinal image plane preferred by the patient is crucial to obtaining optimal measurements. For example, autorefractometers have been used for several decades to measure the spherocylindrical error of the eye, but prescription of glasses and contact lenses has required a patient-interactive step—the manifest refraction—in which the patient fine tunes the measurement to his or her preference. In a method similar to a manifest refraction, the InterWave scanner allows the patient to optimize the image to his or her preference.

The InterWave scanner allows sampling of the entrance pupil with a variable number of spots and variable spot sizes if regions of the cornea require an increased resolution. In addition, registration of data acquired with wavefront aberrometers is vital if subtle imperfections are to be corrected with excimer lasers. The InterWave scanner can track and register the wavefront error to either the center of the dilated pupil or the Purkinje images; this flexibility may become important in customized laser ablation, particularly when involving hyperopic corrections. The image minification that results from hyperopic laser correction, together with the fact that the optical zone of the hyperopic ablation zone is small, makes it vital that laser treatment be delivered as close to the "visual axis" as possible. The center of the pupil, though a reproducible landmark, may not be the optimal place to center hyperopic ablations. All of these features make the InterWave an ideal instrument to study highly aberrated eyes such as those with irregular astigmatism following previous corneal surgery. Measurement of highly aberrated eyes with reflection-based aberrometers can be complicated by image crossover during data acquisition.

> The InterWave scanner can track and register the wavefront error to either the center of the dilated pupil or the Purkinje image

InterWave aberrometry has some disadvantages. The testing method, like a visual field test, requires an alert cooperative subject. The testing time is longer (3 minutes per eye) than that required for reflection-based methods (a few seconds). The present generation of the InterWave system requires an operator with greater skill than that required to operate a less sophisticated system.

InterWave technology is also being used to conduct studies on customizing the refractive correction in contact lenses. The InterWave scanner is fully capable of acquiring data from the eye when a contact lens is in place on the cornea, an advantage that would facilitate a study of contact lenses that were customized to correct higher-order aberrations. Prospective evaluation of the ability of InterWave to guide a flying spot excimer laser with high repetition rate for the correction of aberrations will be underway shortly.

References

1. Scheiner C. Oculus, sive fundamentum opticum. *Innspruk.* 1619.
2. Smirnov H. Measurement of the wave aberration in the human eye. *Biophys.* 1961;6:52-66.
3. He JC, Marcos S, Webb RH, Burns SA. Measurement of the wavefront aberration of the eye by a fast psychophysical procedure. *J Opt Soc Am A.* 1998;15:2449-2456.
4. Liang J, Grimm B, Goelz S, Bille JF. Objective measurement of wave aberrations of the human eye with the use of a Shack-Hartmann wavefront sensor. *J Opt Soc Am A.* 1994;11(7):1949-1957.
5. Howland HC, Howland B. A subjective method for the measurement of monochromatic aberrations of the eye. *J Opt Soc Am A.* 1977; 67:1508-1518.
6. Walsh G, Charman WN, Howland HC. Objective technique for the determination of monochromatic aberrations of the human eye. *J Opt Soc Am A.* 1984;1:987-992.
7. Mierdel P, Krinke HE, Wiegand W, Kaemmerer M, Seiler T. [Measuring device for determining monochromatic aberration of the human eye]. *Ophthalmologe.* 1997;94(6):441-445.
8. Webb RH, Penney CM, Thompson KP. Measurement of ocular wavefront distortion with a spatially resolved refractometer. *Appl Opt.* 1992;31:3678-3686.
9. He JC, Burns SA, Marcos S. Monochromatic aberrations in the accommodated human eye. *Vision Res.* 2000;40(1):41-48.
10. Penney CM, Webb RH, Tieman JT, Thompson KP. Spatially resolved objective refractometer. USA patent 5. 1993.
11. Webb RH, Burns SA, Penney CM, inventors. Coaxial spatially resolved refractometer. USA patent 6,000,800. 1999.
12. Marcos S, Burns SA. On the symmetry between eyes of wavefront aberration and cone directionality. *Vision Res.* 2000;40(18):2437-2447.
13. Marcos S, Barbero S, Llorente L, Merayo-Lloves J. Optical response to LASIK surgery for myopia from total and corneal aberration measurements. *Invest Ophthalmol Vis Sci.* 2001;42(13):3349-3356.
14. Webb RH, Penney CM, Staver PR, Burns SA, Sobiech J. The SRR: an aberrometer with null endpoint. *OSA Technical Digest Series.* 2001: 114-117.
15. Burns SA. The spatially resolved refractometer. *J Refract Surg.* 2000; 16(5):S566-S569.

16. Webb R. Zernike polynomial description of ophthalmic surfaces. *OSA Technical Digest Series*. 1992;3:38-41.
17. Staver PR, et al. Accuracy and reproducibility of the InterWave scanner in clinical practice. Paper presented at: American Society of Cataract and Refractive Surgery Annual Meeting; June 1-4, 2002; Philadelphia, Pa.
18. Thompson KP, Staver PR, Garcia JR, Burns SA, Webb RH, Stulting RD. Using InterWave aberrometry to measure and improve the quality of vision in LASIK surgery. *Ophthalmology*. In press.

Chapter 21

Comparing Wavefront Devices

Daniel S. Durrie, MD and Erin D. Stahl

Introduction

In January of 2001, we began investing significant time and resources into the emerging field of wavefront diagnostics. As time passed, one aspect of our research began to focus on clinical uses of wavefront analysis and on the advancement of clinical diagnostics. Over the past 2 years, we have been fortunate to acquire multiple wavefront devices in our clinic. As a result of having many different devices, we have been challenged to undertake preliminary studies in comparing these instruments. The goal of our research was to identify the strengths and weaknesses that these different techniques and technologies bring to this field.

In this chapter, we will identify many of the challenges and obstacles that we faced in attempting to compare these devices. We will also highlight data we have collected to compare the parameters of repeatability, raw Zernike output, and wavefront surface description between devices. In addition to direct comparison, we have also included some preliminary analysis correlating performance of the individual devices with number of data points available in a 6 millimeter (mm) acquisition zone. Finally, data from a test eye study will be discussed.

Initial Comparison Challenges

Standards

Early in ophthalmic wavefront study it was recognized by the medical and optics communities that in order for wavefront reporting to be consistent and repeatable standards must be set. These standards were published by the Vision Science and Its Application (VSIA) standards taskforce in 2001.[1] Although these standards have been available for some time, many of the devices utilize output formats and analysis techniques that are not consistent with the recommendations. The main discrepancy we identified in this study was the issue of Zernike identification and numbering. Manipulating the data from the different devices to fit into the Optical Society of America (OSA) standards often required reordering of terms as well as magnitude and sign changes. Inevitably, this ensures a great difficulty in the comparison between devices. It is very important that before undertaking any type of wavefront data comparison, one must be clear that the measurements are being reported and analyzed under the same parameters.

The main discrepancy we identified in this study was the issue of Zernike identification and numbering. Manipulating the data from the different devices to fit into the OSA standards often required reordering of terms as well as magnitude and sign changes.

Measurement and Analysis Diameter

One of the most influential variables in wavefront data collection is the diameter of the analysis zone. It is important to keep in mind that wavefront measurements can only be made through the pupil area. If the pupil is 4 mm when the measurement is taken, the maximum analysis diameter is only 4 mm. As Zernike measurements are highly correlated with increasing pupil size, it is imperative that any measurements to be compared are done so at the same analysis diameter. On some devices, there is an option to set the analysis diameter to a certain size. On others, there is no clinician choice, so all measurements are calculated based on the maximum pupil size. For example, Figures 21-1 and 21-2 show an eye measured and analyzed at 3 mm on the left and the same eye measured at 7 mm on the right. The three-dimensional (3-D) map and the histogram clearly show the increase in aberration with the increase in pupil size when all other variables are held constant.

Accommodation Challenges

As with many other diagnostic devices, device-induced accommodation is also a challenge with wavefront measurement. The Topcon (Paramus, NJ), Alcon (Fort Worth, Tex), Nidek (Gamagori, Japan), WaveFront Sciences (Albuquerque, NM), and Bausch & Lomb (Rochester, NY) devices use an auto-fogging technique to adjust for accommodation. The Tracey device (Kiev, Ukraine) utilizes a system in which the subject focuses at a distant point while looking through the measurement device. We believe that each of these devices may reduce the effect of accommodation at differing levels, and in so doing it introduces further challenges in the attempt to compare devices. We would like to see more study into reducing the influence of accommodation in all devices.

Instrument Goals

A final challenge in our study to compare devices is in the fact that these devices were not all designed with the same purpose.

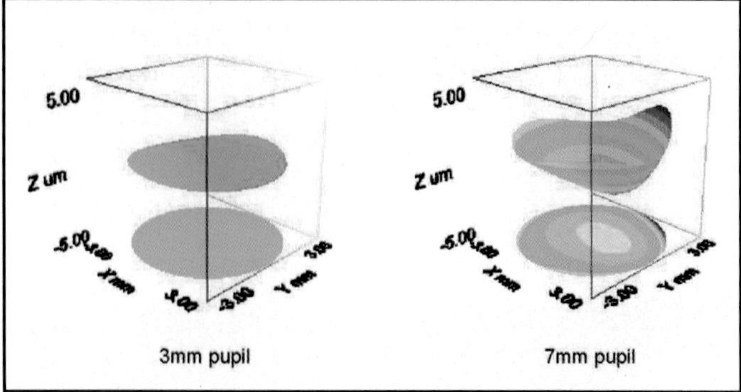

Figure 21-1. 3-D wavefront profile of an eye at 3 mm (left) and 7 mm (right) pupil aperture, demonstrating a more aberrated shape in the latter.

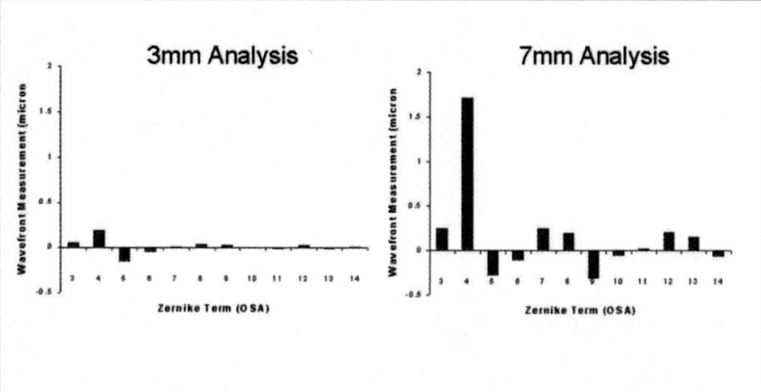

Figure 21-2. Wavefront histogram of an eye at 3 mm (left) and 7 mm (right) pupil aperture, demonstrating an increase in aberrations with the larger pupil size.

Manufacturer	Device	Data Points (6mm)	Technology	Additional Capabilities
Alcon	LADARwave	170	Hartmann-Shack	communicates with the Alcon LADARwave laser for customized treatments
Bausch and Lomb	Zywave	60	Hartmann-Shack	communicates with the B&L 217z laser for customized treatments
Nidek	OPD-Scan	1440	Dynamic Skiascopy	simultaneous topography and autorefraction, communicates with the Nidek excimer laser system for customized treatments
Topcon	Wave-Front Analyzer	85	Hartmann-Shack	simultaneous topography and autorefraction
Tracey	VFA	64	Ray-tracing	
Wavefront Sciences	COAS	1017	Hartmann-Shack	

Figure 21-3. Comparison of technology type, number of data points, and additional capabilities for the wavefront devices utilized in this study.

Some were designed to perform as robust diagnostic devices for use in a wide range of ophthalmic applications. Others were designed to achieve the most accuracy when measuring eyes of refractive surgery candidates with the intent of driving excimer lasers. The impact of these design goals can be clearly seen in the outcomes of the comparison data as presented in the sections on pp. 165 and 166

Study Devices

A total of six wavefront devices were utilized in this study. They include the following (Figure 21-3).

Alcon LADARwave

The LADARwave is a Shack-Hartmann device with a maximum of 170 data points across a 6 mm pupil. The Alcon device includes software to determine customized treatment algorithms for its LADARVision excimer laser system.

Bausch & Lomb Zywave

The Zywave is a Shack-Hartmann device with a maximum of 60 data points across a 6 mm pupil. This device contains the Zyoptics software to combine an Orbscan measurement with the Zywave reading to export a customized treatment pattern to the Bausch & Lomb 217z excimer laser system.

Nidek OPD-Scan

This device utilizes a dynamic skiascopy technique to calculate optical path difference with maximum data sampling of 1440 points at a 6 mm pupil. The unit also takes simultaneous placido disk topography and an autorefraction reading. It is capable of exporting this data for customized treatment into the Nidek excimer laser system.

Topcon Wavefront Analyzer

The Topcon unit is a Shack-Hartmann system with a maximum of 85 data points at a 6 mm pupil. This device also takes a simultaneous placido disk topography image and calculates the topography into Zernike terms.

Tracey VFA

The Tracey unit uses a single ray tracing technology with 64 points. The rays are emitted sequentially in a "gatling gun" fashion and are detected individually.

WaveFront Sciences COAS

The COAS is a Shack-Hartmann device with a maximum of 1017 data points across a 6 mm pupil.

Comparison Study Design

The basis of this study was to evaluate the six devices on both individual performance (repeatability) and on performance against the group with raw Zernike data and wavefront mapping comparisons. Additionally, the devices were also identified by the number of data points in a 6 mm pupil, which allowed us to examine trends with respect to data density.

To accomplish this task we recruited patients in four groups (Figure 21-4). The groups were defined as:

- Group 1: Normal, nonoperative, low higher-order aberrations
- Group 2: Nonoperative, significant higher-order aberrations
- Group 3: Postrefractive surgery, low higher-order aberrations
- Group 4: Postrefractive surgery, significant higher-order aberrations

Group 1	Group 2	Group 3	Group 4
Non-operative		Operative	
Low higher order aberrations	Significant higher order aberrations	Low higher order aberrations	Significant higher order aberrations
e.g. normal preop	e.g. keratoconus	e.g. good outcome LASIK	e.g. symptomatic LASIK

Figure 21-4. Four analysis groups utilized in this study categorized by nonoperative vs operative and low vs significant higher-order aberrations.

n	m	OSA #	Name	Shape
2	-2	3	Astigmatism	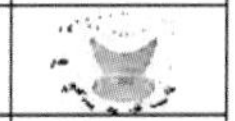
2	0	4	Defocus	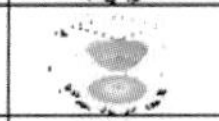
2	2	5	Astigmatism	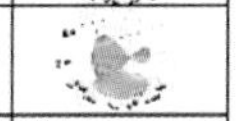
3	-3	6	Trefoil	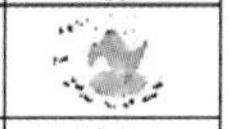
3	-1	7	Coma	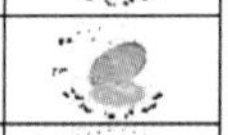
3	1	8	Coma	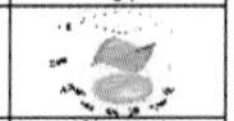
3	3	9	Trefoil	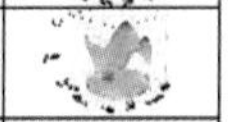
4	-4	10	Tetrafoil	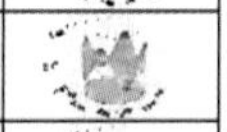
4	-2	11	Astigmatism	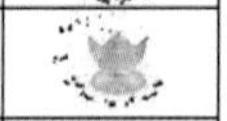
4	0	12	Spherical Aberration	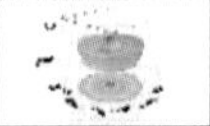
4	2	13	Astigmatism	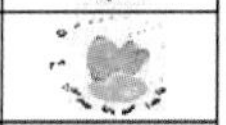
4	4	14	Tetrafoil	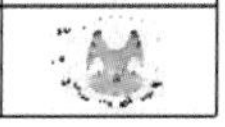

Figure 21-5. OSA standards of wavefront reporting published by the VSIA taskforce.

Five eyes were selected for each of the groups with a total of 20 eyes.

Measurements were collected over 2 months (October to December, 2002). Each eye was dilated with 1.0% tropicamide HCl and 2.5% phenylephrine HCl to a minimum of 6 mm. Three consecutive measurements were taken on each of the six devices. All analysis was performed over a 6 mm pupil regardless of maximum pupil size. Zernike data was entered in to CTView software[2] for graphical comparison analysis.

Repeatability

To study repeatability with the six different instruments, each eye underwent three consecutive measurements on each of these devices. The raw Zernike data were compiled in a spreadsheet and standard deviation was calculated for each term from OSA 3 to 14 (second through fourth orders) (Figure 21-5). These individual term deviations were averaged to determine the "average deviation" or "repeatability" for each eye on each device. The repeatability data were then averaged by group. Group average, standard deviation, and range are shown in Figure 21-6. In Figures 21-7 to 21-10, the group data are displayed graphically with the devices arranged on the graph by increasing number of data points. We were interested to determine if repeatability data varied according to data density. These data show that for Group 1, the group with the lowest aberrations, the Wavefront Sciences, Topcon, Bausch & Lomb, Alcon, and Nidek instruments performed consistently well with an average deviation of less than ±0.05 microns (µm). It is evident in this group and in the following three that the Tracey unit has a consistently larger deviation than the other instruments. It must be noted that due to some of the variables in how different devices calculate Zernike values, the measurements made by the Tracey unit are of a greater magnitude than the other devices. Due to this general trend toward greater values with the Tracey unit, the deviation values are also slightly larger. Further study needs to be made into the cause of this discrepancy. For the other devices, there is not a significant trend between repeatability and number of data points in this group.

In Group 2, the eyes have a higher level of natural aberrations, which is reflected in the larger average deviation values. The Alcon unit was the only device with an average deviation below ±0.05 µm. There is also no evidence of a trend between number of data points and repeatability in this group. Group 3 patients represent satisfied refractive surgery patients with low aberrations. The average deviations of the WaveFront Sciences, Bausch & Lomb, and Alcon units all remained below ±0.05 µm. Again, there was no significant trend between repeatability and number of data points. The final group, Group 4, represents the most highly aberrated postrefractive surgery eyes. This group would be similar to those patients seeking retreatment customized with wavefront-guided algorithms. The data shows that the Alcon and Nidek devices have an average deviation below ±0.05 µm. Although not statistically significant, there appears to be some trend that the instruments with greater than 170 data points perform better in this analysis.

> Although not statistically significant, there appears to be some trend that the instruments with greater than 170 data points perform better in this analysis.

It should be noted that the WaveFront Sciences and Bausch & Lomb data are not included in this portion of the study. The Wavefront Sciences unit is unable to measure postmyopic refractive surgery patients at a 6 mm pupil. The device is capable of taking consistent readings on these patients but due to the design of the instrument, corrected myopes measure at a smaller pupil. With this data reported at a smaller pupil than 6 mm, the values are smaller than the other instruments and consequently would reflect a smaller repeatability deviation than the other devices. The Bausch & Lomb unit failed to acquire measurements on two of the five eyes in this group.

Figure 21-6. Repeatability data averaged by group for each of the G wavefront devices utilized in this study. In Group 4, WaveFront Sciences' data could not be analyzed at 6.0 mm, while the Bausch & Lomb device could not capture two of the five eyes in this group (N/A).

Instrument	Group 1		SD	Range	Group 2		SD	Range
Wavefront Sciences	0.0346	+/-	0.02	(0.019-0.067)	0.0515	+/-	0.02	(0.025-0.085)
Topcon	0.0278	+/-	0.02	(0.010-0.050)	0.1290	+/-	0.10	(0.025-0.240)
Tracey	0.1582	+/-	0.09	(0.080-0.301)	0.1653	+/-	0.03	(0.129-0.199)
Bausch & Lomb	0.0320	+/-	0.02	(0.026-0.058)	0.0960	+/-	0.04	(0.053-0.154)
Alcon	0.0220	+/-	0.01	(0.012-0.030)	0.0259	+/-	0.01	(0.011-0.049)
Nidek	0.0293	+/-	0.01	(0.015-0.044)	0.0858	+/-	0.03	(0.036-0.117)

Instrument	Group 3		SD	Range	Group 4		SD	Range
Wavefront Sciences	0.0275	+/-	0.01	(0.021-0.037)	N/A			
Topcon	0.1037	+/-	0.16	(0.014-0.381)	0.1721	+/-	0.16	(0.015-0.408)
Tracey	0.2144	+/-	0.19	(0.078-0.553)	0.2756	+/-	0.15	(0.097-0.489)
Bausch & Lomb	0.0387	+/-	0.03	(0.034-0.063)	N/A			
Alcon	0.0227	+/-	0.01	(0.012-0.040)	0.0332	+/-	0.01	(0.014-0.050)
Nidek	0.1122	+/-	0.19	(0.020-0.444)	0.0468	+/-	0.02	(0.020-0.079)

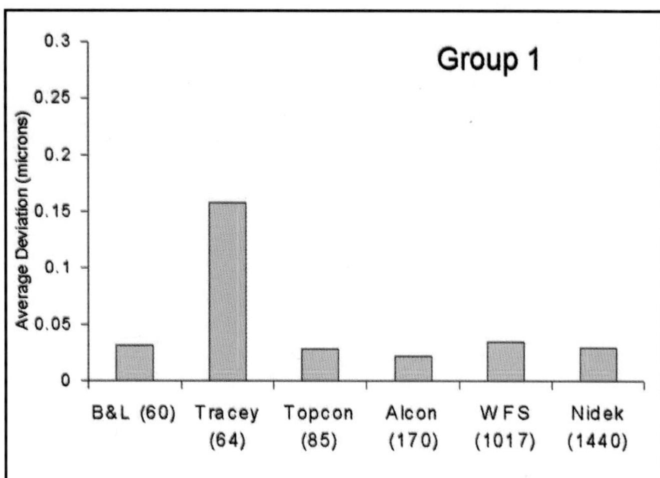

Figure 21-7. Repeatability (average deviation) of group 1 (ie, normal) eyes, revealing less than ±0.05 μm variability in all devices except the Tracey.

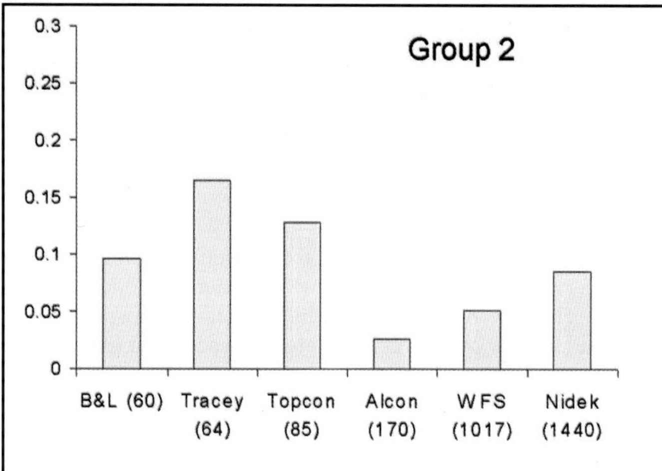

Figure 21-8. Repeatability (average deviation) of group 2 (ie, keratoconus) eyes, revealing less than ±0.05 μm variability in only the Alcon device.

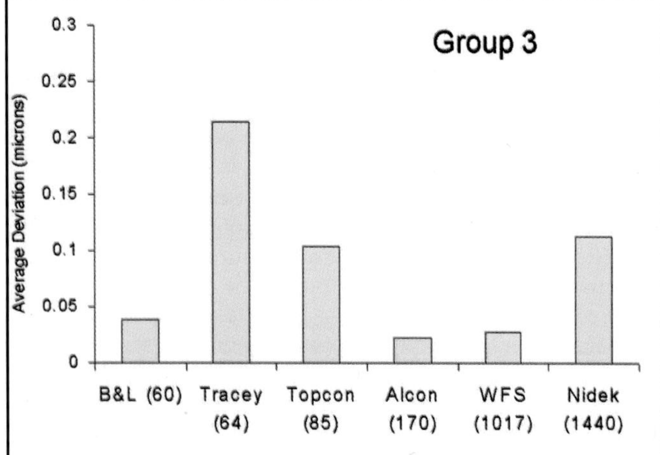

Figure 21-9. Repeatability (average deviation) of group 3 (ie, good outcome laser in-situ keratomileusis [LASIK]) eyes, revealing less than ±0.05 μm of variability in the WaveFront Sciences, Bausch & Lomb, and the Alcon devices.

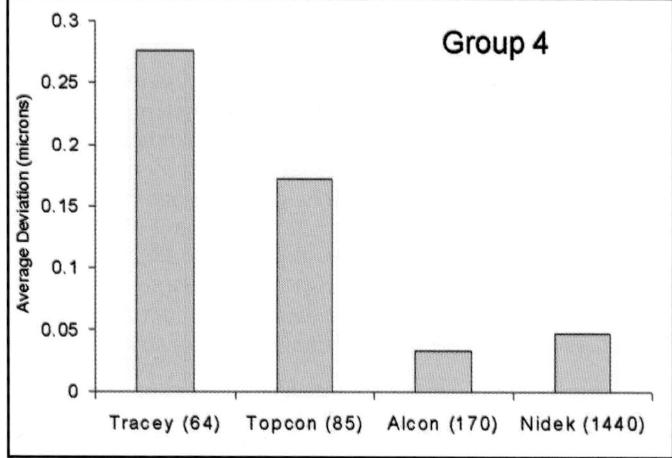

Figure 21-10. Repeatability (average deviation) of group 4 (ie, symptomatic LASIK) eyes, revealing less than ±0.05 μm of variability in Nidek and Alcon devices (the WaveFront Sciences and Bausch & Lomb devices were excluded).

Instrument	Group 1		SD	Range	Group 2		SD	Range
Wavefront Sciences	0.0798	+/-	0.03	(0.055-0.125)	0.2345	+/-	0.14	(0.051-0.406)
Topcon	0.0640	+/-	0.03	(0.043-0.116)	0.2706	+/-	0.19	(0.075-0.495)
Tracey	0.3428	+/-	0.05	(0.267-0.411)	1.1397	+/-	0.54	(0.371-1.690)
Bausch & Lomb	0.1224	+/-	0.07	(0.140-0.166)	0.4229	+/-	0.22	(0.188-0.671)
Alcon	0.0911	+/-	0.02	(0.067-0.121)	0.2861	+/-	0.20	(0.079-0.507)
Nidek	0.1118	+/-	0.12	(0.041-0.333)	0.2500	+/-	0.16	(0.062-0.462)

Instrument	Group 3		SD	Range	Group 4		SD	Range
Wavefront Sciences	0.0776	+/-	0.02	(0.047-0.095)	N/A			
Topcon	0.0798	+/-	0.11	(0.024-0.038)	0.1383	+/-	0.05	(0.072-0.210)
Tracey	0.4061	+/-	0.24	(0.226-0.818)	0.7614	+/-	0.38	(0.575-1.447)
Bausch & Lomb	0.1206	+/-	0.11	(0.084-0.303)	N/A			
Alcon	0.0775	+/-	0.06	(0.027-0.176)	0.1169	+/-	0.02	(0.098-0.144)
Nidek	0.0915	+/-	0.07	(0.050-0.217)	0.0889	+/-	0.02	(0.052-0.107)

Figure 21-11. Average deviation of the raw Zernike data for each deviation relative to the mean Zernike values averaged from all of the devices (except Tracey). Tracey measurements are analyzed but not included in the average from all devices due to their significantly larger values.

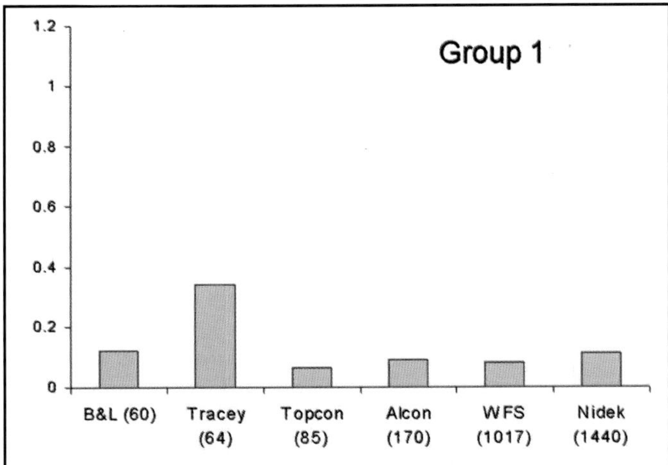

Figure 21-12. Raw Zernike data comparison of each device relative to the mean value of all devices (except Tracey) for Group 1 eyes. All devices show less than ±0.20 μm deviation, except Tracey.

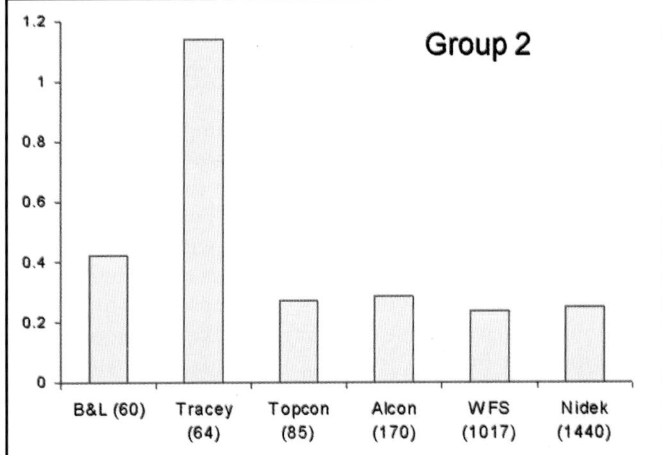

Figure 21-13. Raw Zernike data comparison of each device relative to the mean value of all devices (except Tracey) for Group 2 eyes, revealing a similar ration of values to group 1, but with none less than ±0.20 μm.

Raw Zernike Data Comparison

When comparing wavefront data between devices, it is necessary to consider that at this point there is no standard against which measurements can be judged. In order to perform a comparison, we calculated the mean Zernike values for each individual term between the five devices—Alcon, Bausch & Lomb, Topcon, WaveFront Sciences, and Nidek—on each eye. Due to the issue of consistently greater values with the Tracey unit, we elected to not include the Tracey measurements in this average. We then used the mean from the five instruments to calculate the deviation from the mean for terms 3 through 14 on each individual instrument. This mean was determined for each eye and then averaged by group. Group average, standard deviation, and range are shown in Figure 21-11. The outcomes from this analysis are shown in Figures 21-12 to 21-15 and are stratified by group number and instrument. Noted along with the instrument type is the number of data points in a 6 mm pupil.

In Group 1, the deviation from the group average was below ±0.20 μm for the Bausch & Lomb, Topcon, Alcon, WaveFront Sciences, and Nidek devices. As expected, the Tracey values are much larger because they were not included in average determination. It will be shown in the wavefront comparison section that although the Tracey values are greater, the shapes of the wavefronts are consistent with the other instruments. In looking for a trend between Zernike deviation and number of data points, there is no trend to suggest that more data points may provide a more consistent wavefront with this group.

The data from Group 2 show a larger deviation for all terms in comparison with Group 1, although the shapes of the graphs are similar. The four instruments with higher data densities—Topcon, Alcon, WaveFront Sciences, and Nidek—all had consistent results in measuring this group of highly aberrated eyes. The eyes in Group 3 show a very similar trend to Group 1 with the majority of devices measuring the Zernike terms within ±0.20 μm of the average. Group 4 shows only small deviations for the Alcon, Nidek, and Topcon units. Bausch & Lomb and WaveFront Sciences have been excluded from this analysis because of the aforementioned issues with Group 4 eyes. Again, there is not a statistically significant relationship, but a trend does exist between an increase in number of data points and a decrease in deviation from average Zernike values.

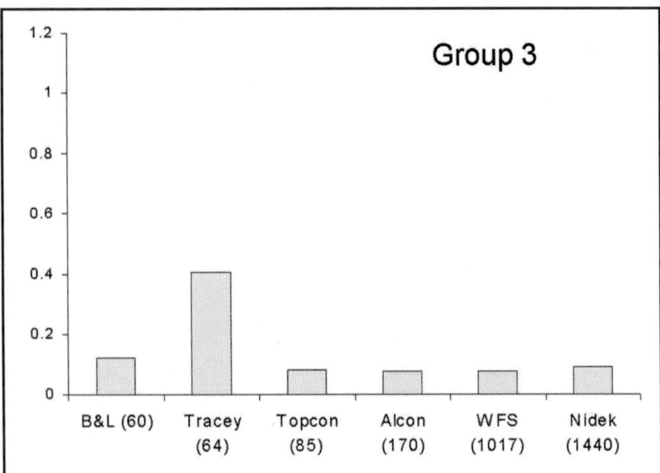

Figure 21-14. Raw Zernike data comparison of each device relative to the mean value of all devices (except Tracey) for Group 3 eyes. All devices show less than ±0.20 µm, except Tracey.

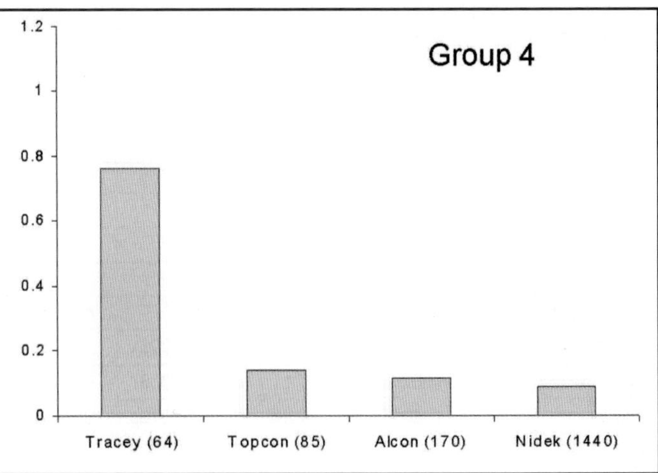

Figure 21-15. Raw Zernike data comparison of each device relative to the mean value of all devices (except Tracey) for Group 4 eyes. Again, Tracey only device with a deviation not less than ±0.20 µm (WaveFront Sciences and Bausch & Lomb devices excluded).

Wavefront Comparison

Due to some of the difficulties in comparing raw Zernike values, we also found it useful to display the wavefront maps generated by mapping the second-, third-, and fourth-order terms. Looking at the data in this manner allows for some compensation for a difference in magnitude as shown with the Tracey unit. Although the magnitudes may differ between the various instruments, it can be seen that the wavefront maps are in most cases very similar. To create these maps, raw Zernike data were manipulated to reflect the OSA reporting standards and then entered into CTView V4.0 software. 3-D maps were created on standard axes with scales from 5 to -5 µm. In each example, the color steps are divided by 0.50 µm. A two-dimensional (2-D) map is projected beneath the 3-D map to clarify the location of the aberrations. One patient from each of the four groups is displayed in this manner (Figures 21-16 to 21-19)

> Editor's note:
>
> To facilitate a more direct comparison of wavefront maps generated by each device according to a set standard, the raw Zernike data of wavefront error was reconstructed using CTView software into new standard maps, reflecting the OSA reporting standards. The new maps for each device are displayed side-by-side for comparison.
>
> R. Krueger, MD, MSE

> Although the magnitudes may differ between the various instruments, it can be seen that the wavefront maps are in most cases very similar.

The patient from Group 1 has a very low profile with slight hyperopia and astigmatism. It is evident from the maps that although the different instruments detect a similar wavefront pattern, the outputs are not identical.

The patient from Group 2 has mild keratoconus with significant astigmatism and higher-order aberrations. Each instrument in this study mapped a very similar wavefront surface for this highly aberrated eye. The patient from Group 3 underwent laser subepithelial keratomileusis (LASEK) surgery 18 months before measurement and was 20/15 OU at the time of measurement. In this case, each device detects some mild residual astigmatism and higher-order aberrations. The patient from Group 4 underwent LASIK surgery for monovision 3 years ago. Although this patient can read J1, there is significant coma (OSA 7 and OSA 8) detected by all devices.

Test Object Comparison

The difficulties we have faced in trying to compare these very diverse systems are evident at this point in the wavefront study. Many of the individual companies have designed test objects that are used to measure and calibrate their devices. Unfortunately, many of the test objects mount to the instruments in a specific way that does not enable their use on other devices. We were able to use an Alcon test object to successfully make measurements on the Alcon, WaveFront Sciences, and Tracey units. Although there was no mounting system on the WaveFront Sciences and Tracey units, we were able to acquire measurements that suggested a promising future for the use of test objects across different devices. The outcome of this test is shown in Figure 21-20 with 2-D maps from CTView software. Figure 21-21 shows the histogram representation of the raw Zernike values on each device. These maps show only the higher-order terms of OSA 6 to 14. Although there are some subtle differences between devices, some of this may be accounted for with alignment problems. Overall, this test was a promising step for further study.

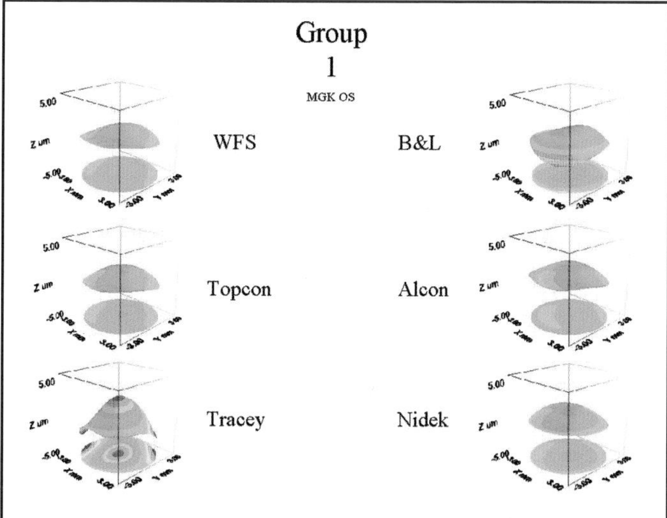

Figure 21-16. Wavefront profile comparison of a normal eye with slight hyperopia and astigmatism (Group 1).

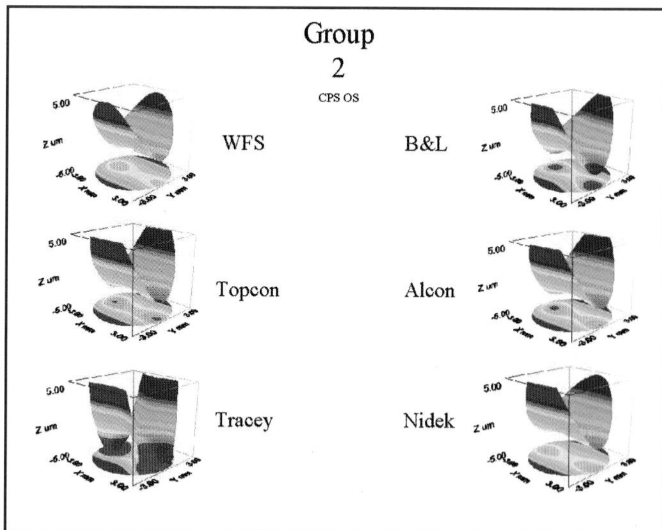

Figure 21-17. Wavefront profile comparison of a keratoconus eye with significant astigmatism and higher-order aberrations (Group 2).

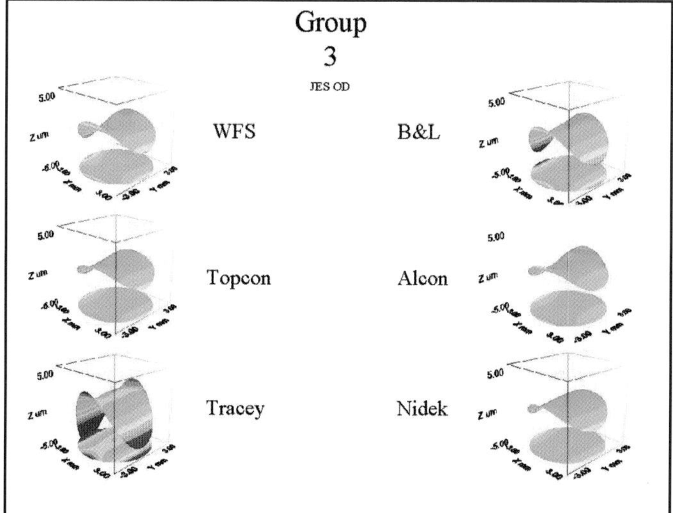

Figure 21-18. Wavefront profile comparison of a post-LASEK eye (20/15) with mild astigmatism and subtle higher-order aberrations (Group 3).

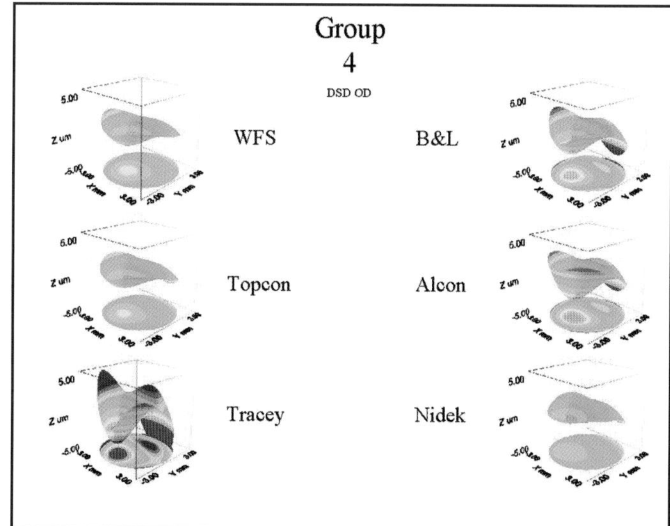

Figure 21-19. Wavefront profile comparison of a monovision LASIK eye with significant coma (Group 4).

Conclusion

As of a result of this preliminary device comparative study, there are two significant outcomes. The first is that wavefront devices cannot be used or easily studied interchangeably. The reasons for the differences are varied and complex and are a topic for further analysis. The important result is that the study of wavefront diagnostics is aimed at determining therapeutic treatments; therefore, it is most evident that a diagnostic device must be used only with specific therapeutic systems. The idea that raw Zernike data could be fed into any system is not a reality at this time.

The second main outcome of this study shows that in both repeatability and raw Zernike comparison, no significant relationship exists between number of data points and performance at this time. It does appear as a trend, however, that the devices with a greater number of points do perform slightly better with more highly aberrated eyes than those with fewer data points. It appears that the devices with very few data points (<70 points in a 6 mm pupil) may be less robust in their diagnostic capabilities. Interestingly, there does not seem to be a great difference in the diagnostic capabilities between those instruments with a moderate number of data points (greater than 85 and less than 200) and those with a very large number of points (>200 points). Future study may show further correlation between device technology, number of data points, and performance in different groups of eyes.

> It appears that the devices with very few data points (<70 points in a 6 mm pupil) may be less robust in their diagnostic capabilities.

In attempting to bring together six complex and highly diverse devices for study, we faced many evident challenges and obstacles. It is our hope that initiating an effort to solve just a few of these issues will lead the device companies and other users to further this effort. It is our strong recommendation that each of

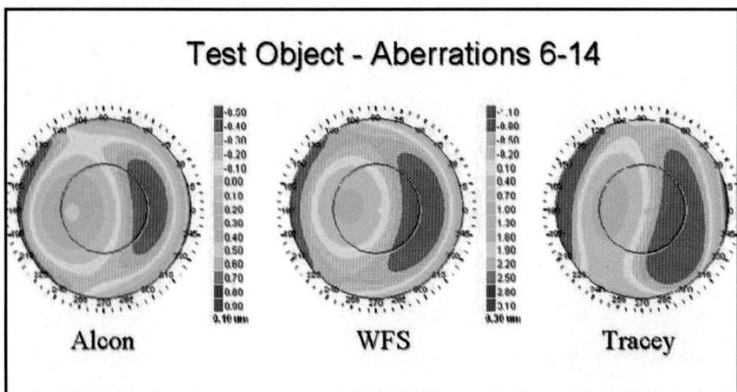

Figure 21-20. 2-D wavefront profile of an Alcon test object as successfully captured by the Alcon, WaveFront Sciences, and Tracey devices.

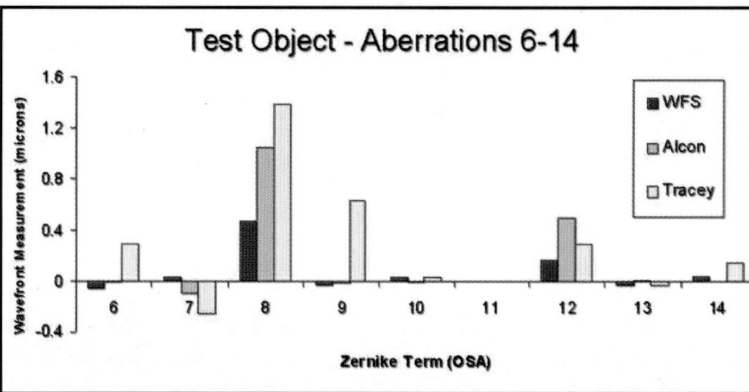

Figure 21-21. Wavefront histogram revealing the relative differences between devices in measuring the known aberrations of a test object (ie, horizontal coma and spherical aberration).

the participating companies and the others in the field implement the standards for reporting of wavefront data outlined by OSA. A movement in our field toward uniform reporting standards will ultimately lead to a more complete understanding of wavefront diagnostics and treatment.

References

1. Thibos LN, Applegate RA, Schwiegerling JT, Webb R. Standards for reporting the optical aberrations of eyes. In: Lakshminarayanan V, ed. *Trends in Optics and Photonics*. 2000;35:232-44.
2. CTView Software V4.0. Sarver and Associates, Inc. Available at: http://www.sarverandassociates.com. Accessed November 13, 2003.

Section III

Wavefront Customized Corneal Ablation

Basic Science Section

Chapter 22

Physics of Customized Corneal Ablation

David Huang, MD, PhD

INTRODUCTION

In a broad sense, refractive surgeons are already performing customized corneal ablation today. After all, the same laser ablation is not applied to every eye. Each ablation in laser in-situ keratomileusis (LASIK) and photorefractive keratectomy (PRK) is tailored to the eye's subjective spherocylindrical refraction. The current usage of the term *custom cornea*, however, refers specifically to laser ablation of the cornea customized to each eye's higher-order as well as spherocylindrical aberrations. Eliminating higher-order aberrations may allow us to achieve a supranormal vision (20/10 perfect vision). Reduction of higher-order aberrations is also useful in restoring vision to a normal level in pathologic condition such as corneal scar and complicated keratorefractive surgery (steep central island, decentered or small optical zone). Customized corneal ablation requires new technology and more precision in all aspects of the surgery. Novel wavefront sensors are used to map the aberrations of the eye. Small-spot scanning lasers are used for more precise corneal ablation. Accurate alignment of laser ablation with wavefront and/or corneal topographic maps is critical.

> Eliminating higher-order aberrations may allow us to achieve a supranormal vision ("20/10 perfect vision").

In order to use, evaluate, and improve "customized corneal ablation," the ophthalmic surgeon needs to understand the physical principles behind the technology. This chapter introduces these principles.

WAVEFRONT OPTICS

Why Wavefront?

Wavefront-guided correction reduces the aberration of the entire optical system of the eye. If one only corrects corneal topographic aberration, vision would still be limited by aberrations in the posterior corneal surface, the crystalline lens, and other optical elements of the eye.

What is a Wavefront?

Wavefront optics is not a familiar subject to most people outside of the field of optical engineering and physics. This introductory chapter starts with a graphical explanation of wavefront.

Light is a traveling electromagnetic wave. A wavefront is a continuous iso-phase surface. To simplify our mental picture, let's first consider waves on the surface of water. Imagine throwing a stone into still water and observing the expanding circles of waves.

If we take a snap shot of this wave at one point in time (Figure 22-1), we can draw circular wavefronts along the crests (phase 0) of the waves. We can also draw the wavefronts at any arbitrary reference phase such as the troughs (phase π) or the midpoint of descent (phase $\pi/2$). Note that the wavefronts are perpendicular to the directions of wave propagation, which are represented by rays (see Figure 22-1). Water waves are confined to a two-dimensional surface and therefore the wavefronts are lines. Optical waves propagate in three dimensions and optical wavefronts are surfaces.

> Wavefront-guided correction reduces the aberration of the entire optical system of the eye. If one only corrects corneal topographic aberration, vision would still be limited by aberrations in the posterior corneal surface, the crystalline lens, and other optical elements of the eye.

Both wavefronts and rays can be used to describe wave propagation (eg, an optical wavefront from a point source propagates through a lens) (Figure 22-2). As the wave travels through the lens, the speed of propagation is slowed because the lens material has a higher index of refraction than air. The center of the lens is thicker and therefore retards the center of the wavefront relative to the periphery. The differential slowing imparted by the shape of the convex lens in air converts the incoming diverging wavefront with a center of curvature at the object point into a converging wavefront on exit with a center of curvature at the focal point (see Figure 22-2). In the absence of aberration, wavefront converges to a diffraction-limited spot at the focus. Wavefront aberration is defined by the deviation of the actual wavefront from an ideal reference wavefront as a function of

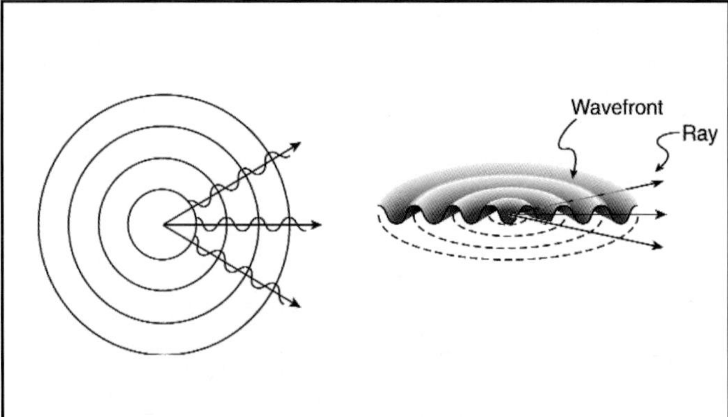

Figure 22-1. The relationship between wavefront and rays in a surface wave example.

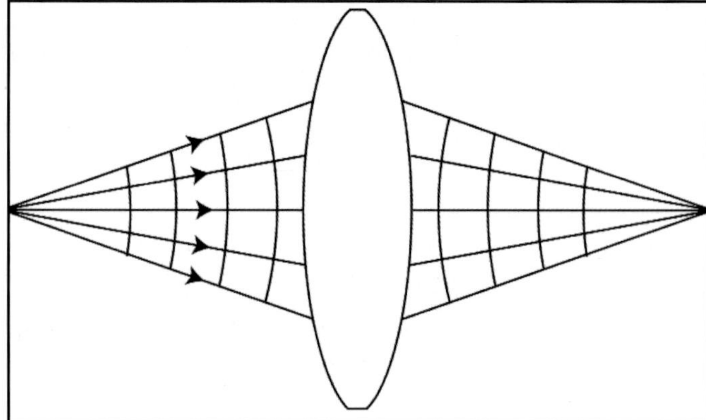

Figure 22-2. An ideal optical system. Light from the object plane is focused by the lens and converges at the image plane. Deviation from the ideal wavefront defines aberration.

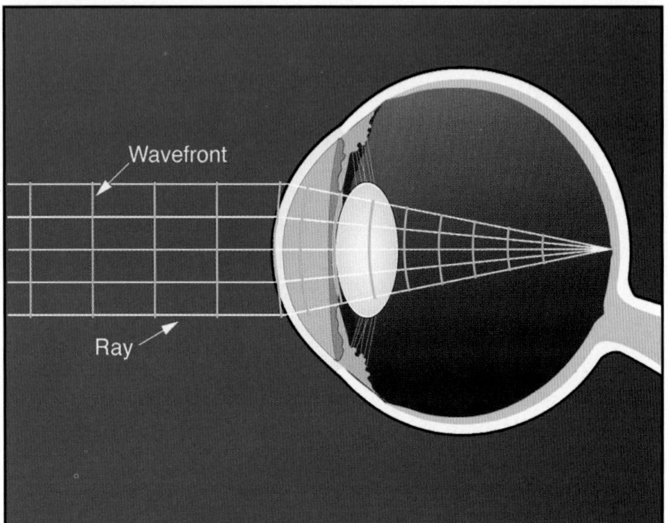

Figure 22-3. An ideal eye. Deviation from the ideal wavefront defines aberration.

location within the exit pupil of the system. We can describe the same focusing system using a bundle of rays (ray tracing). At the lens surfaces, the incoming diverging rays are refracted according to Snell's law at each lens location and, again, converge toward the focus (see Figure 22-2). The deviations of the rays from the ideal ray path contain information that is equivalent to the wavefront aberration. The advantage of the wavefront formulation is that the wavefront deviation at the corneal surface can be directly translated into the depth of customized corneal ablation.

> The advantage of the wavefront formulation is that the wavefront deviation at the corneal surface can be directly translated into the depth of customized corneal ablation.

How Wavefront Aberration is Used to Guide Corneal Ablation

Wavefront aberration of the eye is defined as the deviation of the actual wavefront from an ideal reference wavefront emanating from a foveal point source (Figure 22-3). For an eye focused at infinity, the ideal wavefront exiting the aberration-free eye is a flat plane (see Figure 22-3). In a real eye, there are optical aberrations, and the exit wavefront deviate from that of the plane wave (Figure 22-4). This wavefront aberration is $W(x,y)$, where x and y are the horizontal and vertical axes. $W(x,y)$ is conventionally measured in microns. To see how $W(x,y)$ translates into ablation depth, imagine it reversing direction and propagate into the eye (Figure 22-5). Because light propagation is symmetric in both forward and backward directions, we know that the aberrated wavefront $W(x,y)$ will exactly cancel out the ocular aberration and focus to a point (strictly speaking, a diffraction-limited* spot) at the fovea. On the other hand, a plane wave entering the eye will form an aberrated pattern on the retina due to the imperfect optics of the eye. In order for the plane wave to achieve perfect focus in this aberrated eye, we need a lens at the corneal surface that converts the flat wavefront to $W(x,y)$. This lens can be etched onto the corneal surface by customized ablation. Removal of 1 micron (μm) of corneal tissue reduce wavefront retardation by $n_{cornea} - n_{air}$ μm. Therefore, the equation for the customized corneal ablation depth $A(x,y)$ needed to correct ocular wavefront aberration W(x,y) is:

$$A(x,y) \times (n_{cornea} - n_{air}) = C - W(x,y) \qquad (1)$$

where n_{cornea} = corneal index of refraction, n_{air} = refractive index of air, and C is the smallest constant depth needed to keep $A(x,y)$ from becoming negative anywhere. Ablation depth $A(x,y)$ cannot take on a negative value because ablation cannot add tissue to the cornea.

Equation 1 is a basic starting point for designing wavefront-guided ablation. As with the Munnerlyn formula for spherocylindrical ablation, equation 1 ignores the eye's response to laser ablation. In the context of PRK, Munnerlyn described this

*Diffraction of light limits the size of the focused spot even in the absence of optical aberration. The diffraction limit depends on the wavelength and numerical aperture of the optical system. The smaller the aperture, the larger the diffraction effects.

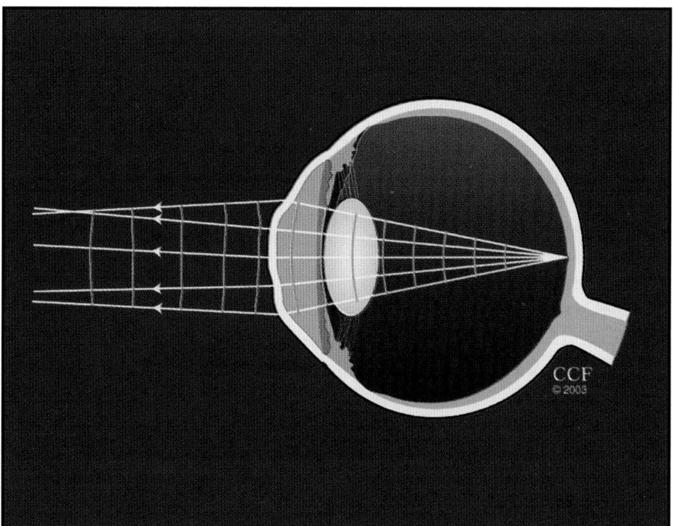

Figure 22-4. Wavefront aberration exiting the eye from a foveal point source.

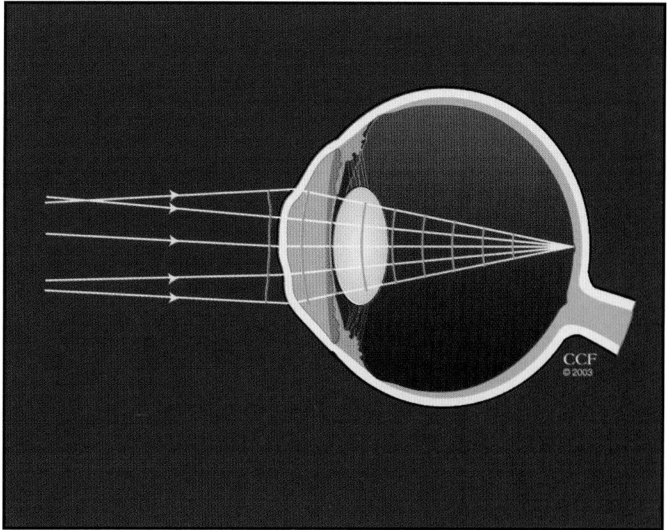

Figure 22-5. Entrance wavefront needed to nullify ocular aberrations.

simplifying assumption very well in his classic paper[1]: "The following analysis assumes that if an area of the epithelium is removed and a portion of the stroma is ablated, the epithelium will regrow with a uniform thickness and produce a new corneal curvature determined by the new curvature of the stroma." Reality differs from this assumption and modification of the corneal surface does occur after both PRK and LASIK.[2,3] To realize the full potential of customized corneal ablation, we will eventually need to understand and deal with the corneal biological response. With lamellar keratotomy and laser ablation, tension is released in the anterior lamellae and shifted to the posterior lamellae, resulting in corneal biomechanical changes. Biomechanical changes include shifts in hydration and posterior curvature and are discussed in more detail in a latter chapter. Epithelial smoothing is another important healing response that, if it could be understood and predicted, may be compensated for in the design of the laser ablation pattern.[4]

> To realize the full potential of customized corneal ablation, we will eventually need to understand and deal with the corneal biological response.

How Wavefront Aberration is Mapped

Mapping devices for ocular aberrations have proliferated recently due to commercial interest. The multitude of new devices leaves many of us struggling to understand the physical principles behind each of them. I hope the following classification schemes will provide a conceptual scaffold for understanding. Wavefront devices are described elsewhere in the book. We will adopt the name *wavefront sensor* to describe all of these devices because the wavefront aberration map is their final output.

Wavefront sensors can be divided into subjective and objective types. Subjective methods require response from the subject and usually take more time. Subject motion and cooperation are limitations. Objective methods use imaging systems to analyze reflections from the ocular fundus. Since fundus reflection can arise from multiple chorioretinal layers, the reference focal plane is not as well defined as that for subjective methods, which are based on light perception at photoreceptor layer. This focal plane uncertainty is relatively small and should be important only for the defocus (spherical equivalent) term.*

Besides the subjective/objective division, wavefront sensors can also be divided into three categories based on the optical information that is directly measured.

Exit Wavefront From an Illuminated Foveal Spot

In this class of instruments, the fovea is illuminated by a narrow, focused beam and the backscattered wavefront is measured (see Figure 22-4). In the Shack-Hartmann wavefront sensor, the slope of the exit wavefront $W(x,y)$ is mapped with a Shack lenslet array. The wavefront can also be mapped with an interferogram.[5]This class of instruments can provide rapid single-shot wavefront measurement. These devices work best when backscattering from the fovea closely approximates a point sources. Challenges to this ideal include multiple scattering from choroidal structures, interference speckle from coherent light sources (eg, lasers), and limits to the brightness and quality of foveal illumination.

Entrance Wavefront Needed to Cancel Ocular Aberration

In this class of instruments, patches of the corneal surface are probed with incoming light beams to determine the ray directions needed to overcome aberrations and focus at the fovea (see Figure 22-5). The map of ray directions is used to derive the entrance wavefront $W(x,y)$ needed to cancel ocular aberration (see Figure 22-5). In the spatially resolved refractometer, the subject provides

---

*Chorioretinal structures that backscatter into objective wavefront sensors are generally within 200 μm of the photoreceptor plane. The axial length of the eye is approximately 23 millimeters (mm). Therefore the uncertainty is roughly 1% (200 μm/23 mm). The eye's focusing power is about 60 diopters (D). Therefore, objective wavefront sensors can be wrong by up to 0.6 D in defocus. For astigmatism and even higher-order terms, 1% error should be insignificant.

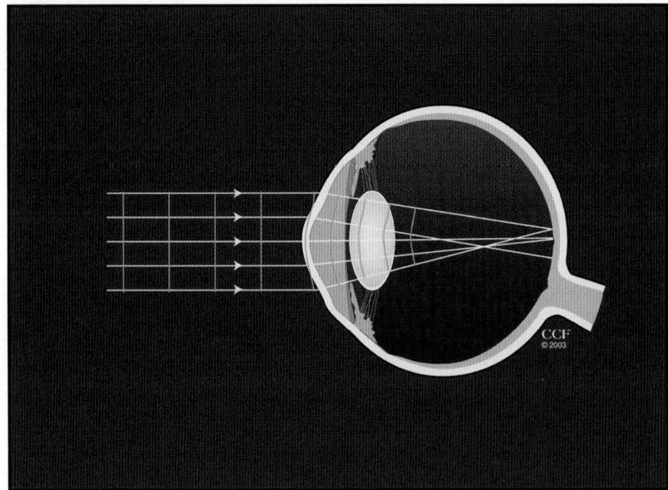

Figure 22-6. Aberration of retinal image.

feedback by manually steering the probe beam. The Nidek slit skioloscope (Gamagori, Japan) is an objective variant in which the direction of a slit beam entering the eye is rapidly scanned and the fundus reflection is measured by a detector array. The slit axis is then successively rotated to map the wavefront aberration over the entire cornea. These instruments are intrinsically sequential and may take more time to acquire data. However, objective measurements can be acquired in a rapid sequence.

Aberration of Retinal Image

In these instruments, an image is projected on the retina through a large pupil aperture over which the wavefront is to be mapped. (This is to be contrasted with the narrow beam used to illuminate the fovea in the first type of wavefront sensors.) The retinal image is a grid or point pattern that is distorted on the inbound pass by the aberration of the eye (Figure 22-6). The retinal image is captured by a camera that typically has a small conjugate aperture on the pupil plane so that ocular aberration minimally affects the image on the outbound pass. The deviation of the retinal image from the ideal is used to compute the ocular aberration by a ray tracing algorithm. The Howland crosscylinder aberroscope (both subjective and objective) projects a grid line pattern.[6] The Tscherning-type aberroscope projects a grid pattern of points simultaneously. The Tracey system projects a point grid pattern sequentially. The double-pass ophthalmoscope projects a single point and uses the retinal point spread function to compute ocular aberration.[7] These instruments must assume an idealized eye model in order to perform the ray tracing computation that derives the wavefront aberration at the corneal or pupil plane.

Topography-Guided Ablation

Corneal topography can only measure the aberration of the corneal surface. Therefore, on its own, it cannot measure or guide the elimination of all ocular aberrations. However, there may be situations in which corneal topography may be superior to wavefront sensors. Placido-ring–based corneal topography is a mature technology. It maps the surface of the cornea based on several thousand sampled points on the reflected ring pattern. By comparison, wavefront sensors typically sample only a few hundred points.[8,9] In cases in which corneal aberration is predominant and contain small-scale irregularities (scar, dystrophy, and surgical complications such as steep central island), corneal topography may be able to map aberrations with higher resolution than current wavefront sensors.

The basic formula for topography-guided ablation is simple in form:

$$A(x,y) = C - \{T(x,y) - T_{target}(x,y)\} \qquad (2)$$

where $A(x,y)$ is the ablation pattern, $T(x,y)$ is the actual corneal elevation topography, $T_{target}(x,y)$ is the target corneal topography one which to achieve, and C is the smallest constant depth needed to keep A(x,y) from becoming negative anywhere. Ablation depth A(x,y) cannot take negative value because ablation cannot add tissue to the cornea. C = the maximum value of $\{T(x,y) - T_{target}(x,y)\}$ over the optical zone.

There are several limitations to the accuracy and completeness of corneal topography in practice. Placido-ring–based devices measure the local radial slope of the cornea at discrete sampling points. Slope data are converted to height topography by an integration algorithm starting from the center outward. Integration introduces error in a cumulative fashion, and the height topography becomes less reliable further from the center. The coverage of the ring projections on the cornea can be obscured by the nose and brow. The tear film is variable over time and often there are also poorly wet areas on the cornea where measurement cannot be made. These patches of missing slope data can introduce large errors into height calculations. With all these limitations, Placido-ring technology is still the most successful corneal topographic method so far.

A tricky step in topography-guided ablation is the determination of the target topography $T_{target}(x,y)$. If one ignores lenticular aberration, then $T_{target}(x,y)$ should be a parabolic surface with the right refractive power to achieve emmetropia or other postoperative refractive target. This can be derived from the spherical-equivalent power of the preoperative cornea and the spherical-equivalent refraction of the preoperative eye. However, these measurements are difficult to determine in cases with severe aberration and poor best-corrected visual acuity. One may need to use rigid contact lens over-refraction to estimate these quantities.

Eventually, we may learn to use both wavefront and topographic data in a complementary fashion. For example, we may wish to completely remove corneal aberration but limit the correction of lenticular aberration in anticipation of age-related lenticular changes and the possibility of future cataract surgery.

Laser Physics

Photons: Particles of Light

While the propagation of light is described very well by electromagnetic wave theory, many aspects of the interaction between light and matter can only be understood through quantum mechanics. A basic tenet of quantum mechanics is that physical systems such as atoms and molecules can be found, upon measurement, in discrete energy states. Light interacts with these physical systems by the absorption or emission of photons. When an atom transitions from a higher energy state E_2 to a lower energy state E_1, a photon of energy $E = E_2 - E_1$ is emitted. When an atom transitions from the lower to higher state, a pho-

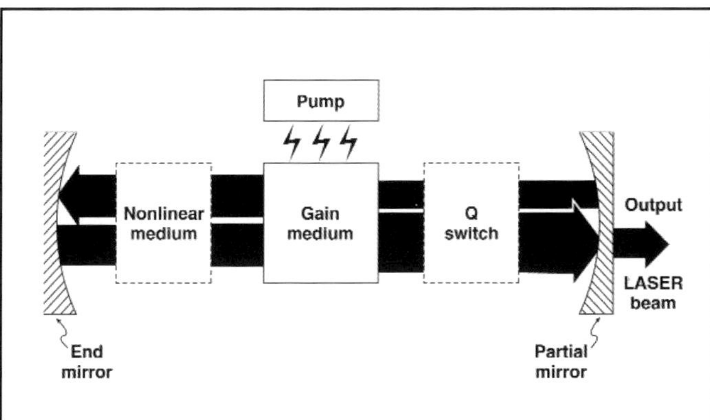

Figure 22-7. Laser oscillator.

ton is absorbed. The energy of the photon is related to its frequency υ by $E = h\upsilon$, where h is Plank's constant.[10] The wavelength λ of the photon is related to its frequency by the relation $\lambda = c/\upsilon$, where c is the speed of light in a vacuum.

LASE: Light Amplification by Stimulated Emission

When a photon of energy E travels through a medium, it can induce atomic transitions by either absorption or emission. When there are more atoms or molecules in a higher energy state E_2 than in the lower energy state E_1 (population inversion), the probability of a stimulated emission is higher than absorption. Thus light is amplified by gaining more photons as it passes through the gain medium. This action defines light amplification by stimulated emission (LASE).[10]

A laser is most often constructed as an oscillator (Figure 22-7), where light bounces back and forth between two end mirrors. The two mirrors form the laser cavity. Each time light completes a round-trip between the mirrors, energy is gained by passage through the gain medium and lost by transmission through the output end mirror. Oscillation is maintained by population inversion in the gain medium. To obtain population inversion, energy is replenished by a pump source, which can be electrical, optical, or chemical. The laser output is shaped by the gain medium, the resonant modes of the laser cavity, and other cavity elements. Since light circulates through a typical laser cavity about a billion times per second, extremely powerful control of the laser output can be obtained. The laser output can be very constant (continuous wave) or concentrated in extremely short (nanoseconds to femtoseconds) pulses. Continuous-wave lasers typically emit over a very narrow wavelength band (monochromatic), while a femtosecond laser outputs a broad range of wavelengths. The spatial coherence imposed by cavity resonance conditions (repeated shaping by mirrors and apertures) means that lasers can often be focused to near diffraction-limited spots.

Since light circulates through a typical laser cavity about a billion times per second, extremely powerful control of the laser output can be obtained. The laser output can be very constant (continuous wave) or concentrated in extremely short (nanoseconds to femtoseconds) pulses.

A method of producing a powerful short pulse from a laser is Q-switching.[10] The quality factor Q is proportional to the ratio of the optical energy in laser cavity over the power dissipated by the cavity. Thus, a high Q cavity leaks energy very slowly while a low Q cavity loses energy quickly. In Q-switching, the Q of the laser cavity is lowered by some means during the pumping phase (see Figure 22-7). Low Q in the cavity prevents amplification of cavity oscillation so the gain in the laser medium can be built up to a very high level. Once the population inversion in the medium reaches its peak, the Q is suddenly switched to a high value. This causes a very rapid buildup of the oscillation that quickly drains energy in the laser medium by the output of a giant laser pulse. The duration of the pulse is a few nanoseconds to hundreds of nanoseconds (a few to a few hundred round-trips in the cavity). Q-switching has been used to obtain the high peak power needed to convert the neodymium:yttrium-aluminum-garnet (Nd:YAG) laser's infrared (IR) output into ultraviolet (UV) wavelength needed for corneal ablation.

Another method for obtaining short pulses and high peak power is "modelocking." In this technique, nonlinear or time dependent medium (see Figure 22-7) is placed inside the laser cavity to select for a circulating pulse inside the laser cavity. A fraction of the circulating pulse exits the laser cavity each time it meets the output mirror, generating a train of pulses at the output. These pulses can be extremely short, typically lasting picoseconds to femtoseconds. By concentrating the laser energy in such short pulses, the peak power is greatly enhanced. High peak power allows the laser output to be efficiently converted to a different wavelength by second harmonic generation or optical parametric oscillation.[10]

Harmonic generation combines several photons of a longer wavelength laser light into a single photon of shorter wavelength and greater energy. Optical parametric oscillation converts one photon into two photons of longer wavelength.

Laser Ablation Rate

Removal or ablation of tissue requires that the amount of laser energy absorbed per tissue volume is sufficient to break up the tissue through chemical decomposition, mechanical stress, and/or heating. As laser light travels deeper into tissue, absorption decreases the fluence (energy per area) until it falls below the threshold for ablation. Below threshold, tissue remains in place, but thermal coagulation may still occur. Ablation is a dynamic and complex event[11] that is only described approximately by the following equation that assumes fluence decreases with depth in an exponential fashion described by the Lambert-Beer's Law. Empirically, the depth of ablation is approximately related to the incident fluence by[12]:

$$d = m \times \ln(F/F_{th}) \text{ for } F > F_{th} > 0 \quad (3)$$

where d is the ablation depth per pulse, m is the slope efficiency of ablation*, F is the incident fluence of the laser pulse, and F_{th} is the threshold fluence for ablation.

*The ablation efficiency m is usually close to but not identical to the absorption length measured under nonablative conditions.

Lambert-Beer's law states that, as light travels trough a medium (tissue) that absorbs it, its energy decreases exponentially with depth.

The ablation efficiency *m* is measured in units of microns (μm) and corresponds to the ablation depth per pulse at a pulse fluence 2.7 times that of threshold.* For efficient tissue ablation, one should operate at a fluence level that removes approximately *m* μm per pulse. Thus, *m* is of an important measure of the precision of ablation when comparing the various laser available for laser vision correction. Smaller *m* corresponds to less ablation depth per pulse and finer precision.

Laser ablation parameters are determined primarily by the wavelength and pulse duration. For precise corneal ablation, it is desirable to have the laser radiation absorbed over a superficial depth of few microns or less. This is possible in the far ultraviolet (ie, 193 to 213 nanometers [nm]) where there is strong absorption by peptide bonds,[13] and at the water absorption peak in the mid-IR (3.0 μm). It is also desirable to have a short pulse duration that does not permit heat to diffuse into deeper layers. On a micron scale, laser pulse duration of less than 1 microsecond (ms) is needed to avoid thermal diffusion.

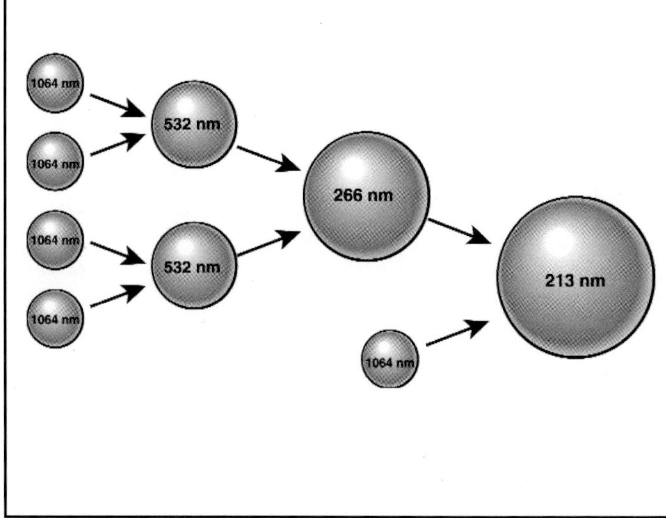

Figure 22-8. Fifth harmonic generation from a 1064 nm Nd:YAG laser. Five 1064 nm photons are combined in a cascade up-conversion to obtain a more energetic 213 nm photon.

Ultraviolet Lasers and Photodecomposition

In order to directly breakup an organic molecule, the photon energy must surpass that of the intramolecular bonding energy. Photons in the far UV range are capable of ablating tissue through this "photodecomposition" mechanism.[14] The photochemical interaction also powers the expansion and ejection of tissue material. This differs from photothermal ablation in which tissue heating and subsequent vaporization or plasma formation provide the energy for expansion and ejection. When photodecomposition is the predominant mechanism, tissue ablation occurs at a lower fluence and tissue heating is greatly reduced. This is why the UV excimer lasers are often tauted as being "cool" lasers. At the 193 nm argon-fluoride (ArF) excimer wavelength, thermal effect is small and thermal coagulation of adjacent tissue become negligible. This clean ablation characteristic is one reason why the 193 nm laser dominates vision correction.

The dynamic event of tissue ejection during excimer laser ablation has been studied using high-speed photography.[15,16] Immediately after the ablation, hot gaseous product leaves the ablation site and rapidly expands outward. The expansion and cooling forms a low pressure zone that draws in surrounding air, which constricts the base of the ejection plume and forms a mushroom cloud appearance. Subsequent recirculation of ablation product toward the low pressure zone forms ring vortices. Eventually, most of the ejected material dissipates with air flow while part of it falls back into the tissue surface. With larger ablation diameter, the plume evolves more slowly and more ablated material redeposits on the center of the ablation zone. Both the airborne and redeposited material can block subsequent laser pulses. This has been implicated as a mechanism that contributes to the formation of steep central islands with broad beam laser ablation.[16]

The practical methods of generating far UV pulses at this time include the excimer lasers and harmonic generation from lasers of longer wavelengths.

The active gain medium of the excimer lasers are transient rare gas-halogen molecular states that emit a photon on dissociation. Different molecular combinations emit different wavelengths ranging from 157 to 10,600 nm. The ArF excimer laser at 193 nm has been found to be optimal for optimal tissue ablation in the context of vision correction.[14] At shorter wavelengths, beam delivery systems are very difficult to build because of lack of optical material that can transmit and withstand the radiation. At longer wavelengths, thermal effects become increasingly dominant over the photodecomposition mechanism and thermal coagulation of adjacent tissue becomes significant.[17] At 193 nm, the ablation efficiency *m* is approximately 0.30 μm and collateral thermal damage to adjacent tissue is negligible.[18,19] This is the most precise laser currently being used for corneal ablation.

Harmonic generation using output from the Nd:YAG laser is an alternative method for generating UV radiation. The Q-switched Nd:YAG laser is a very efficient basis for generating nanosecond laser pulses at 1064 nm wavelength. Passage of the 1064 nm radiation through a nonlinear medium allows the up conversion of two 1064 nm photons into a more energetic 532 nm photon. A cascade of this up conversion process can be used to generate 213 nm laser pulses (Figure 22-8). The 213 nm laser has an absorption length[13] twice that of the ArF excimer laser. However, the ablation efficiency appears to be only slightly deeper (0.40 μm)[20] and collateral thermal damage is less than 1 μm deep.[21] Thus, the 213 nm laser is a viable alternative to the excimer laser for corneal ablation. A potential disadvantage of fifth harmonic generation is that pulse-to-pulse energy fluctuation is increased roughly five-fold by the harmonic generation process, which can reduce the accuracy of laser ablation.† Potential advantages of the 213 nm laser compared to the 193 nm

*e = 2.718 is the basis of the natural logarithm.

†The intensity of the fifth harmonic output is proportional to the fifth power of the input power at the fundamental frequency. Thus, for example, a 1% pulse-to-pulse energy variation translates to a 5% pulse-to-pulse variation in the fifth harmonic output (1.01^5 = " 1.05).

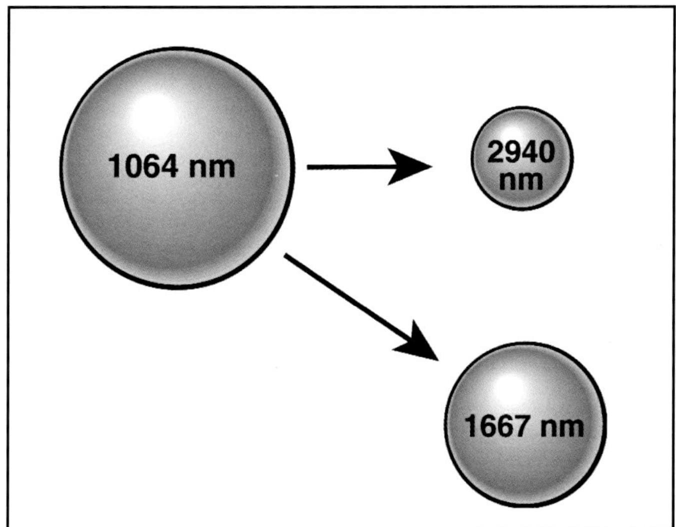

Figure 22-9. Down conversion in an OPO divides the energy in a 1064 nm photon between two photons of longer wavelengths.

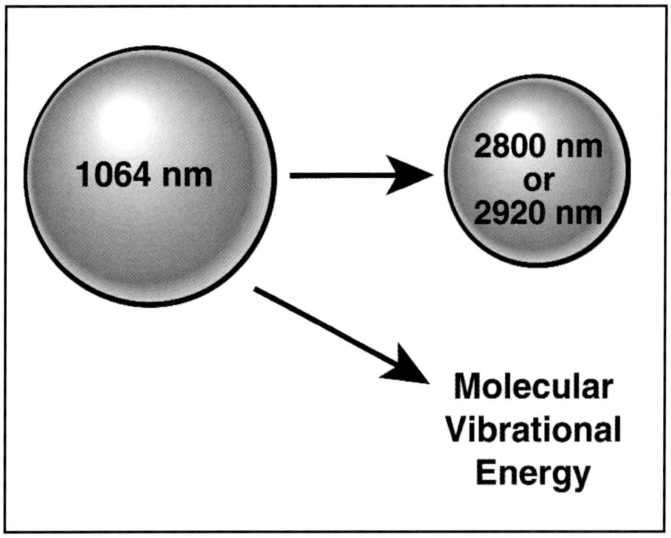

Figure 22-10. Down conversion by Raman shift. A 1064 nm photon is absorbed and a less energetic photon at a longer wavelength is emitted. The balance of energy is left behind as vibration energy in the Raman medium.

excimer are the reliability of the Nd:YAG laser, reduced wear on optical elements, and ablation rate that is less influenced by tissue hydration level.[22]

Infrared Lasers

Laser output at a mid-IR wavelength of around 3 µm is strongly absorbed by tissue water. Several mid-IR sources have been tested for corneal ablation. In general, because there is no photochemical decomposition, mid-IR lasers have larger ablation depth per pulse and produce more thermal coagulation of adjacent tissue. The Q-switched erbium:yttrium-aluminun-garnet (Er:YAG) laser at 2.94 µm and 100 nanosecond (ns) has an ablation efficiency of 4 µm.[12] Down conversion of the Q-switched Nd:YAG laser with the optical parametric oscillator (OPO) (Figure 22-9)[23] or the Raman shift (Figure 22-10)[24] can produce mid-IR pulses of less than 10 ns. One report[23] showed that the OPO can produce ablation depth per pulse under 1 µm and a thermal coagulation zone of 0.1 to 0.2 µm, which are comparable to the 193-nm excimer laser. The lack of thermal damage is explained by an ablation mechanism called *photospallation,* in which tissue is removed by a fast expanding bipolar pressure wave that induces a strong mechanical tension at the surface of the tissue. Further studies are needed to determine whether photospallation by nanosecond mid-IR pulses can be practically used for refractive surgery.

> Raman shift converts photons to a longer wavelength and lower energy as part of the energy of the photons are converted to molecular vibrational energy in the Raman medium.

Accuracy of Aberration Correction

The goal of eliminating higher-order aberrations from the eye demands more accuracy in both measurement and ablation. The required resolution increases with increasing Zernike order. To understand these issues, we will review the representation of optical aberrations (Zernike polynomials), establish the relevant criteria for optimal optical and visual performance, and compare these criteria to the performance of current lasers and wavefront sensors.

Zernike Polynomials

Wavefront aberrations can be represented by an infinite series of terms called *Zernike circle polynomials*[25] or *Zernike expansion.* Zernike polynomials can also be used to represent an optical surface such as corneal elevation topography.[26] Zernike polynomials are ideal for describing the optics of the eye because they are defined based on a circular geometry (the cornea and pupil have circular geometry), can be interpreted in terms of common optical elements (defocus, astigmatism, and higher-order aberrations), and are mathematically well-behaved.

Zernike terms Z_n^m are defined by a radial order n and a azimuthal frequency m, which is never larger than n and m-n must be an even integer (see Appendix 1 for standards for expressing the Zernike polynomial for ocular optics). They are defined inside a unit circle. For our application, we would normalize the radial dimension against the radius of the optical zone (radius = 3 mm for a 6 mm diameter circular optical zone). The lowest order Zernike polynomials are familiar quantities. Z_0^0 is a flat piston, such as a flat circular phototherapeutic keratectomy (PTK) ablation. Z_1^1 and Z_1^{-1} represent tilts (prismatic displacements) along the vertical and horizontal meridians. Z_2^0 represents defocus or spherical equivalent refractive error. Z_2^2 and Z_2^{-2} are cardinal (against and with-the-rule) and oblique (45/135 degrees) astigmatisms.* Higher-order terms have more complex

*Cardinal and oblique cylinders are Jackson crosscylinders[27] oriented along cardinal and oblique axes.[28] They have spherical equivalents of zero and therefore are orthogonal from the defocus (spherical) term.

variation and finer features over the radial and azimuthal dimensions. Zernike polynomials provide us with a tool to separate these spherocylindrical aberration terms from higher-order aberration.

> Zernike polynomials are ideal for describing the optics of the eye because they are defined based on a circular geometry (the cornea and pupil have circular geometry), can be interpreted in terms of common optical elements (defocus, astigmatism, and higher-order aberrations), and are mathematically well-behaved.

Zernike polynomials have useful mathematical properties such as orthogonality, normality, and completeness. Completeness means that any aberration over a circular aperture can be completely represented by a series of Zernike polynomial terms. Orthogonality means that each Zernike term can be arithmetically manipulated and recombined separately. For example, lenticular and corneal components of Z_2^2 (cardinal astigmatism) can be simply added arithmetically to give the Z_2^2 for the eye. Orthogonality is lacking in our traditional system of refraction in either positive or negative cylinder notations.* Normality means that the unit measures of Zernike terms are adjusted so that they contribute equally to the root mean square (RMS) wavefront aberration. For example, 1 μm RMS of Z_2^0 plus 1 μm RMS of Z^2_2 equals $\sqrt{2}$ μm of combined RMS aberration. The RMS aberration value does not have a simple relationship to the visual acuity potential of an eye. For a highly aberrated eye, different Zernike terms with the same magnitude can have unequal effects on optical and visual performance. However, for small aberrations, the RMS wavefront aberration of an optical system is directly related to its Strehl ratio,† a measure of optical performance.[29] This allows us to use the RMS aberration value to set a criteria for near-ideal optical performance in the next section. The Strehl ratio is the ratio between the actual and ideal values of maximum light intensity at the focus. A perfectly aberration-free optical system has a Strehl ratio of 1.

Wavefront Elevation

Criteria for Optical and Visual Performance

The Marechal and Rayleigh criteria are often used to assess whether an optical system can be termed *near diffraction-limited*. They are simple approximate guidelines that relate wavefront aberration to optical performance (Strehl ratio).

The Marechal criteria[25] states that an optical system can be regarded as well-corrected when the Strehl ratio is greater than or equal to 0.80 and that this condition is equivalent to the requirement that the RMS departure of the wavefront from a reference sphere that is centered on the diffraction focus shall not exceed the value $\lambda/14$, where λ is the wavelength of light.

Rayleigh's quarter wavelength rule[25] is based on the amplitude of maximum wavefront departure rather than the RMS departure. Rayleigh showed that when a system suffers from primary spherical aberration of such an amount that the wavefront in the exit pupil departs from the Gaussian reference sphere by less than a quarter wavelength, the intensity at the Gaussian focus is diminished by less than 20%. Other types of aberration also roughly follow this $\lambda/4$ rule.

In the human eye, how many orders of Zernike terms must we eliminate in order to achieve diffraction limit? By applying the Marechal criterion, Liang and Williams showed that correction of up to fourth-order (up to $Z_4^{\pm 4}$) Zernike terms is sufficient for a 3.40 mm pupil and correction of up to eighth-order terms is needed for a 7.30 mm pupil.[1]

Beside monochromatic optical aberration, human vision is also limited by chromatic aberration and photoreceptor spacing. Thus the more relevant criteria relates to visual performance as a whole rather than optical performance in isolation. Experience with adaptive optics correction of the eye's monochromatic aberrations suggest that correction of up to fourth-order Zernike terms is sufficient for reaching the photoreceptor resolution limit in some subjects.

Precision of Laser Ablation

In order to bring the eye to near diffraction-limited performance, the laser system must be able to sculpt the cornea with sufficient precision to meet the Rayleigh and Marechal criteria we just discussed.

Where the ablation depth is small, the precision of laser ablation is limited by the ablation depth per pulse. Current ArF excimer lasers used in vision correction operate at an ablation depth per pulse of roughly 0.30 μm. This corresponds to a change in wavefront retardation of 0.11 μm (equation 1). When applied to the average visible wavelengths (green light at 0.51 μm), the Rayleigh quarter wavelength rule requires that the wavefront departure be less than 0.13 μm. Therefore, the 193 nm excimer laser satisfies the Rayleigh rule. The 213 nm fifth harmonic of the Nd:YAG laser has also demonstrated this level of precision.

The RMS accuracy of laser ablation is influenced by many factors. Pulse-to-pulse energy fluctuation affects all lasers. For broad-beam lasers, beam profile inhomogeneity, plume dynamics,[16] and aperture steps can all introduce errors. Small spot scanning lasers are limited by eye-tracking accuracy. Whether these lasers satisfy the Marechal criterion can only be determined empirically. Because broad-beam lasers can produce steep central islands and other types of ablation irregularity, small spot scanning laser with accurate eye tracking is likely to be essential to customized corneal ablation.

Precision and Accuracy of Wavefront Sensors

According to the Marechal criterion, wavefront sensors for custom cornea need to measure wavefront elevation with a RMS precision and accuracy of better than $\lambda/14$. For green light, $\lambda/14$ is 0.04 μm.

---

*For example, 1 D of positive corneal cylinder at axis 180 degrees plus 1 D of positive lenticular cylinder at axis 30 degrees do not add to 2 D of positive cylinder along any axis. In order to add them by simple arithmetic, they need to be broken down into orthogonal terms. One diopter of positive cylinder at axis 180 degrees is broken down into 0.50 D of Z_2^0 (defocus or spherical equivalent) and 1 D of Z_2^2 (cardinal astigmatism).

†Excluding Z_0^0, a flat piston surface which has no effect on optical performance.

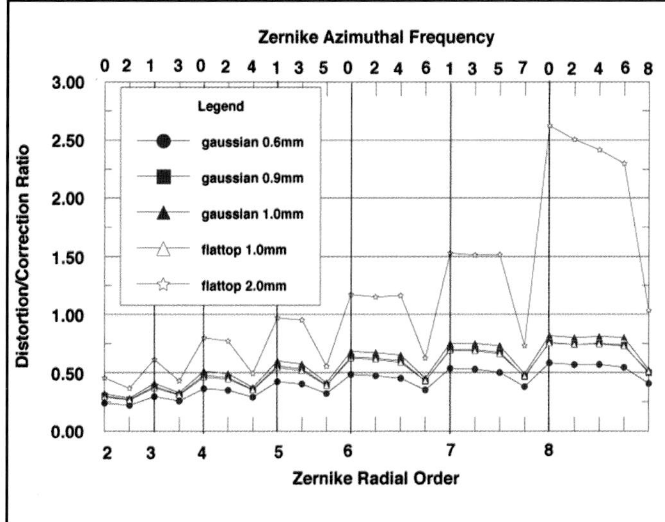

Figure 22-11. Distortion/correction ratio (DCR) for aberrations correction with various beam diameters and shapes. (Reprinted with permission from Huang D, Arif M. Spot size and quality of scanning laser correction of higher order wavefront aberrations. *J Cataract Refract Surg.* 2002;28(3):407-416.)

The precision of a wavefront sensor can be easily gauged by the variability of repeat measurements. This performance figure should be routinely reported for any study using a wavefront sensor. The repeatability of ocular wavefront mapping appears to be limited at about λ/14 by the variability of the eye.[1] A Shack-Hartmann wavefront sensor can have an intrinsic repeatability of λ/487,[1] which is more than precise enough for the measurement of the human eye.

> Shack-Hartmann wavefront sensors can have an intrinsic repeatability of λ/487,[1] which is more than precise enough for the measurement of the human eye.

The accuracy of wavefront sensors needs to be measured against a reference optical system with well-characterized optical aberrations. A trefoil phase plate has been proposed as a reliable standard that is relatively insensitive to displacement and tilt in a test setup.[30]

Transverse Resolution

Resolution of Wavefront Measurement

The transverse (x-y) resolution requirement for wavefront sensors proves to be relatively easy to satisfy. Wang et al showed that uniform sampling of 80 points is sufficient for the computation of eighth-order Zernike coefficients.[29] This is easily satisfied by most commercial Shack-Hartmann wavefront sensors.

Spot Size for a Scanning Laser

The transverse resolution requirement for aberration correction with a scanning laser depends on the order of aberration one wishes to correct. The finer details of higher-order aberrations require smaller beam size to correct, just as a finely detailed painting requires smaller brushes. To assess the relationship between spot size and the quality of scanning laser correction of ocular aberrations, we performed computer simulations of ablations with Gaussian and top-hat beams of 0.6 to 2 mm full-width-half-maximum diameters.[31] The fractional correction and secondary aberration (distortion) were evaluated. Using a DCR of less than 0.5 as a cutoff for adequate performance (Figure 22-11),* we found that a 2 mm or smaller beam is adequate for spherocylindrical correction (Zernike second order), a 1 mm or smaller beam is adequate for correction of up to fourth-order Zernike modes, and a 0.6 mm or smaller beam is adequate for correction of up to sixth-order Zernike modes. Since ocular aberrations above Zernike fourth order are relatively insignificant in normal eyes, current scanning lasers with a beam diameter of 1.0 mm or less are theoretically capable of eliminating the majority of higher-order ocular aberration.

> A 2 mm or smaller beam is adequate for spherocylindrical correction (Zernike second order), a 1 mm or smaller beam is adequate for correction of up to fourth-order Zernike modes, and a 0.6 mm or smaller beam is adequate for correction of up to sixth-order Zernike modes.

Are Current Systems Accurate Enough for Customized Corneal Ablation?

The above review indicates that at least some of the current wavefront sensors and small-beam scanning laser systems are precise and accurate enough to correct a significant fraction of the eye's higher-order aberrations. There is no fundamental physical reason why we should not succeed. The main stumbling blocks to success are likely to come from the variability of the eye itself. During surgery, the variability of corneal hydration may limit the accuracy of tissue removal even with a perfectly accurate laser. The cornea responds to the surgery with epithelial thickness modulation, hydration shifts, structural changes, and stromal remodeling. These changes may be difficult to predict. The cornea and lens undergo aging changes that may degrade the aberration correction over time. Only long-term clinical experience will tell us how much real-life benefit we will derive from custom cornea.

References

1. Munnerlyn CR, Koons SJ, Marshall J. Photorefractive keratectomy: a technique for laser refractive surgery. *J Cataract Refract Surg.* 1988; 14(1):46-52.
2. Gauthier CA, Fagerholm P, Epstein D, Holden BA, Tengroth B, Hamberg-Nystrom H. Failure of mechanical epithelial removal to reverse persistent hyperopia after photorefractive keratectomy. *J Refract Surg.* 1996;12(5):601-606.
3. Gauthier CA, Holden BA, Epstein D, Tengroth B, Fagerholm P, Hamberg-Nystrom H. Factors affecting epithelial hyperplasia after photorefractive keratectomy. *J Cataract Refract Surg.* 1997;23(7):1042-1050.

*A DCR of 0.50 means that after the simulated ablation, the overall aberration (RMS) is reduced by half.

4. Huang D, Tang M, Shekhar R. Mathematical model of corneal surface smoothing after laser refractive surgery. *Am J Ophthalmol*. 2003; 135(3):267-278.
5. Malacara D, DeVore SL. Interferogram evaluation and wavefront fitting. In: Malacara D, ed. *Optical Shop Testing*. 2nd ed. New York, NY: John Wiley & Sons; 1992:455-499.
6. Howland HC, Howland B. A subjective method for the measurement of monochromatic aberrations of the eye. *J Opt Soc Am A*. 1977; 67(11):1508-1518.
7. Artal P, Santamaria J, Bescos J. Retrieval of wave aberration of human eyes from actual point-spread-function data. *J Opt Soc Am A*. 1988;A5:1201-1206.
8. Liang J, Williams DR. Aberrations and retinal image quality of the normal human eye. *J Opt Soc Am A*. 1997;14(11):2873-2883.
9. Liang J, Grimm B, Goelz S, Bille JF. Objective measurement of wave aberrations of the human eye with the use of a Hartmann-Shack wave-front sensor. *J Opt Soc Am A*. 1994;11(7):1949-1957.
10. Yariv A. *Optical Electronics*. 3rd ed. New York, NY: Holt, Rinehart and Winston; 1985.
11. Sauerbrey R, Pettit GH. Theory for the etching of organic materials by ultraviolet laser pulses. *Applied Physics Letters*. 1989;55(5):421-423.
12. Mrochen M, Semshichen V, Funk RH, Seiler T. Limitations of erbium:YAG laser photorefractive keratectomy. *J Refract Surg*. 2000; 16(1):51-59.
13. Pettit GH, Ediger MN. Corneal-tissue absorption coefficients for 193- and 213-nm ultraviolet radiation. *Appl Opt*. 1996; 35(19):3386-3391.
14. Trokel SL, Srinivasan R, Braren B. Excimer laser surgery of the cornea. *Am J Ophthalmol*. 1983;96(6):710-715.
15. Puliafito CA, Stern D, Krueger RR, Mandel ER. High-speed photography of excimer laser ablation of the cornea. *Arch Ophthalmol*. 1987; 105(9):1255-1259.
16. Noack J, Tonnies R, Hohla K, Birngruber R, Vogel A. Influence of ablation plume dynamics on the formation of central islands in excimer laser photorefractive keratectomy. *Ophthalmology*. 1997; 104(5):823-830.
17. Krueger RR, Trokel SL, Schubert HD. Interaction of ultraviolet laser light with the cornea. *Invest Ophthalmol Vis Sci*. 1985;26(11):1455-1464.
18. Kitai MS, Popkov VL, Semchishen VA, Kharizov AA. The physics of UV laser cornea ablation. *IEEE J Quant Electron*. 1991;27:302-307.
19. Krueger RR, Trokel SL. Quantitation of corneal ablation by ultraviolet laser light. *Arch Ophthalmol*. 1985;103(11):1741-1742.
20. Dair GT, Pelouch WS, van Saarloos PP, Lloyd DJ, Linares SM, Reinholz F. Investigation of corneal ablation efficiency using ultraviolet 213-nm solid state laser pulses. *Invest Ophthalmol Vis Sci*. 1999; 40(11):2752-2756.
21. Gailitis RP, Ren QS, Thompson KP, Lin JT, Waring GOd. Solid state ultraviolet laser (213 nm) ablation of the cornea and synthetic collagen lenticules. *Lasers Surg Med*. 1991;11(6):556-562.
22. Dair GT, Ashman RA, Eikelboom RH, Reinholz F, van Saarloos PP. Absorption of 193- and 213-nm laser wavelengths in sodium chloride solution and balanced salt solution. *Arch Ophthalmol*. 2001; 119(4):533-537.
23. Telfair WB, Bekker C, Hoffman HJ, et al. Histological comparison of corneal ablation with Er:YAG laser, Nd:YAG optical parametric oscillator, and excimer laser. *J Refract Surg*. 2000;16(1):40-50.
24. Stern D, Puliafito CA, Dobi ET, Reidy WT. Infrared laser surgery of the cornea. Studies with a Raman-shifted neodymium:YAG laser at 2.80 and 2.92 micron. *Ophthalmology*. 1988;95(10):1434-1441.
25. Born M, Wolf E. *Principles of Optics*. 7th ed. Cambridge, United Kingdom: Cambridge University Press; 1999.
26. Schwiegerling J, Greivenkamp JE, Miller JM. Representation of videokeratoscopic height data with Zernike polynomials. *J Opt Soc Am A*. 1995;12(10):2105-2113.
27. Thibos LN, Wheeler W, Horner D. Power vectors: an application of Fourier analysis to the description and statistical analysis of refractive error. *Optom Vis Sci*. 1997;74(6):367-375.
28. Huang D, Stulting RD, Carr JD, Thompson KP, Waring GO, 3rd. Multiple regression and vector analyses of laser in situ keratomileusis for myopia and astigmatism. *J Refract Surg*. 1999;15(5):538-549.
29. Wang JY, Silva DE. Wave-front interpretation with Zernike polynomials. *Appl Opt*. 1980;19(9):1510-1518.
30. Thibos LN, Applegate RA, Schwiegerling JT, Webb R, Members VST. Standards for reporting the optical aberrations of eyes. In: Lakshminarayanan V, ed. *Vision Science and its Applications*. Vol 35. Washington, DC: Optical Society of America; 2000.
31. Huang D, Arif M. Spot size and quality of scanning laser correction of higher order wavefront aberrations. *J Cataract Refract Surg*. 2002; 28(3):407-416.

Chapter 23

Technology Requirements for Customized Corneal Ablation

Ronald R. Krueger, MD, MSE

Introduction

The introduction of wavefront sensing technology and customized corneal ablation has revolutionized the field of refractive surgery. With last year's United States Food and Drug Administration (FDA) approval of CustomCornea (Alcon, Fort Worth, Tex) for the correction of myopia, customized corneal ablation made its debut into the mainstream of refractive surgery, and together with other similar platform approvals, will likely revolutionize our field in the months and years to come.

In order for the successfulness of customized laser vision correction to reach its full potential, a number of technology requirements must be addressed and implemented by the specific laser vision correction platform offering this customized procedure. The aberrations that are induced by conventional laser vision correction have the potential for being minimized and eliminated with customized corneal ablation.[1,2] In addition, pre-existing aberrations may be minimized or eliminated by this same technology.[3]

The technology required to achieve aberration-free laser vision correction is still under development. At present, several different technology platforms exist. Each of these have a different methodology for providing custom ablation, and a more thorough understanding of these technology platforms will help in evaluating which system is best at eliminating aberrations. Although the following technology requirements may be considered biased, they provide an accurate representation of what is considered optimal within the current state of technology and knowledge in this field. The following four requirements—scanning spot laser delivery, robust eye tracking, accurate wavefront device, and the wavefront-laser interface—are considered essential components that need to be considered when designing a customized corneal ablation system.[4]

Scanning Spot Laser Delivery

Scanning Spot Size

Although many of today's commercially available excimer lasers have begun to offer scanning and flying spot delivery patterns, it is the size of the spot that has more recently been looked at with greater scrutiny. This is especially so with the advent of wavefront customized corneal ablation because of the higher-order aberrations that the laser vision correction platform is now attempting to correct. Two independent mathematical analysis have been recently published to substantiate the importance of the small scanning spot in correcting these aberrations and defining the optimal sizes for adequate correction of higher-order aberrations.

> Two independent mathematical analyses have been recently published to substantiate the importance of the small scanning spot in correcting these aberrations and defining the optimal sizes for adequate correction of higher-order aberrations.

In the first study by Huang et al, a polynomial analysis reveals that treating up to fourth-order aberrations (N = 4) with a total optical zone diameter of 6 millimeter (mm) (D = 6) requires a scanning spot beam diameter of 1 mm or less.[5] Correcting further detail, up to sixth-order aberrations, with a 6 mm zone requires less than or equal to a 0.6 mm diameter scanning spot. Numerical simulation of the percentage correction (correction factor) with beam diameter varying between 0.6 and 2.0 mm confirms the relationship that higher-order Zernike modes require a smaller ablation spot for efficient correction (Figure 23-1).

In an independent analysis by Guirao et al, a scanning spot beam diameter of 1 mm was again determined to be the maximum desirable spot size for correcting fifth-order aberrations by viewing the power spectrum of the wave aberration.[6] The need for a small spot was further confirmed by a third, separate analysis of performance degradation of both low and high spatial frequency during custom ablation using a 2 mm top hat beam profile. This is in contrast to <1.0 mm Gaussian beam, which shows good performance when treating both high and low spatial frequency aberrations.[7]

Table 23-1 lists seven excimer laser systems that attempt to provide a small scanning spot beam size. The first five listed correct refractive error with a less than 1 mm spot during the entire treatment. The fifth excimer laser system, the Zeiss Meditec MEL 80 (Jena, Germany), was recently updated from the MEL 70, which previously had a larger spot of 1.90 mm. The MEL 80 became the new updated excimer laser system of Meditec following the merger with Zeiss Humphrey (Dublin, Calif). The latter two laser systems in this table, the Bausch & Lomb Technolas 217Z (Rochester, NY) and the VISX STAR S4 smooth scan (Santa Clara, Calif), both use a larger, 2 mm diameter beam for the

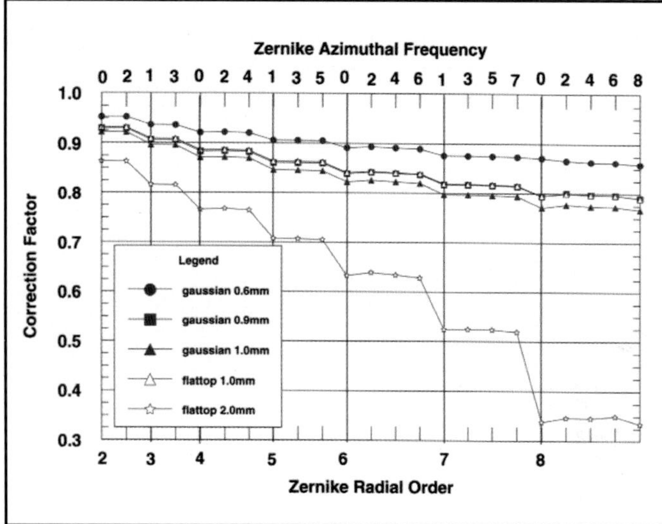

Figure 23-1. The simulated percentage correction (correction factor) of higher-order aberrations is dependent on the ablation spot size, shap, and the order of aberration to be corrected. Higher-order aberrations require increasingly smaller ablation spots for efficient correction. (Reprinted with permission from Huang D, et al. Spot size and quality of scanning laser correction of higher order wavefront aberrations. *J Cataract Refract Surg.* 2002;28:407-416.)

majority of their correction, and then attempt to correct any fine, higher-order aberrations with a 1-mm masked or truncated spot.

Scanning Spot Shape

In Table 23-1, the spot beam profile is listed for each of the laser systems and once again, among the first five listed systems, a Gaussian beam shape is implemented whereas in the latter two, the Bausch & Lomb Technolas uses what they refer to as a truncated Gaussian beam, and the VISX STAR S4 uses a top hat beam profile. The Gaussian beam profile is considered the most desirable scanning spot shape because it allows for a very uniform overlap in the creation of the ablation zone profile. This is important because small spatial errors in beam placement could result in spikes and valleys in the ablation profile with a top hat beam, whereas the Gaussian beam avoids abrupt edges, resulting in an overall, smooth beam profile. This can be illustrated in the profilometry of a -3 diopter (D) correction using a gaussian versus a top hat spot profile (Figure 23-2). Although the difference between these may be considered small, it is during the treatment of the highly aberrated eye that the beam profile and size have the greatest importance.

A modification of the Gaussian beam is utilized by the Bausch & Lomb laser system, which truncates a 2 mm diameter Gaussian spot along the edges to allow for a smaller 1 mm beam, but without the gradual taper of the Gaussian profile. With the VISX STAR S4 laser, a broad excimer beam is masked to the desired spot sizes, ranging from 0.65 to 6 mm, but purely in a top hat fashion. Ultimately, the masking process allows for the beam to be placed with the same kind of spatial variation as a scanning spot delivery system, yet with a different beam profile.

Scanning Spot Rate

Table 23-1 also identifies the spot frequency of each of the seven lasers listed. The majority of the small spot Gaussian profile lasers use a spot scanning rate of approximately 200 Hz. The Alcon LADARVision laser (Fort Worth, Texas), however, uses a slightly lower rate of 60 Hz. Although the slower rate is thought to extend the time of treatment, the volume ablated per shot is also an important factor and with the LADARVision system, the actual ablation time is shorter (8 seconds/D with standard myopic treatment) than when using the Laser Sight LSX system (Orlando, Fla). The higher fluence with the LADARVision system results in a greater volume ablated per shot, which helps to reduce treatment time.

Table 23-1
Laser Spot Size and Scanning Rate Among Scanning Spot Excimer Lasers

LASER	SPOT SIZE	SCANNING RATE
LADARVision	0.8 mm	60 hertz (Hz)
LaserSight	0.6 mm	200 Hz
Wavelight	0.95 mm	200 Hz
Schwind	1.0 mm	200 Hz
Zeiss Meditec	0.7 mm	250 Hz
Technolas	2 + 1 mm TG	50 Hz
VISX STAR S4	2 + 1 mm TH	>10 Hz

The frequency of spot placement is important with regard to hydration changes that occur over time, as treatments that take too long can adversely affect hydration. The scanning spot rate, noted in Table 23-1, however, must not be more rapid than the sampling and response rate that can be adequately followed by the tracking system (Table 23-2). A large saccadic eye movement can experience delays in mirror realignment with the slower tracking systems and consequently result in a greater number of pulses being misplaced on the cornea with a rapid spot scanning rate.

The frequency of spot placement is important with regard to hydration changes that occur over time, as treatments that take too long can adversely affect hydration.

Finally, the placement of the scanning spot is best when non-sequential, or pointillistic, such that one spot is not directly placed next to the preceding spot. This helps to avoid thermal buildup of energy at any given location or improper shielding of the ablation plume during treatment (Figure 23-3).

The Three S's of Scanning Spot Delivery

Steep Central Islands

Although most of the laser systems we are discussing no longer use a broad beam form of delivery, it is worth mentioning here, that scanning small spot delivery does add intrinsic benefits beside custom ablation potential over and beyond the broad beam profile.

The formation of steep central islands has been documented with the early use of broad beam lasers in more than 80% of eyes treated with photorefractive keratectomy (PRK).[8] Although this phenomena was felt to be due, in part, to localized pooling of fluid

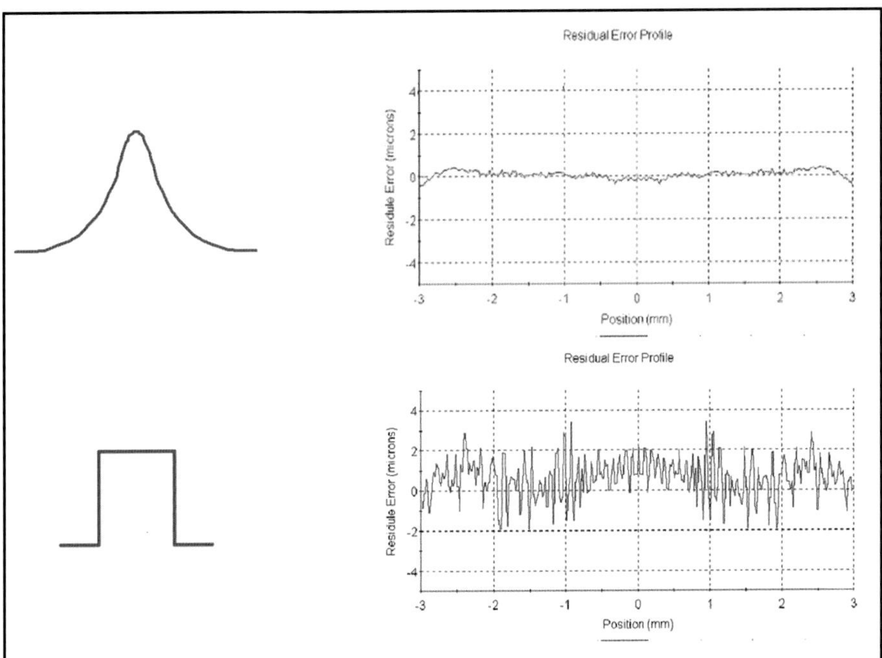

Figure 23-2. Profilometry of a three-dimensional (3-D) myopic ablation performed with a Gaussian vs top hat small spot beam shape. The top hat beam results in greater nonuniformity, due to overlapping edges, than the Gaussian beam.

Table 23-2
Comparative Features of Eye Tracking in Scanning Excimer Lasers

	LADARVision	*Video Camera*
Laser system	Autonomous	Technolas (120) Nidek, VISX (60) LaserSight (60) WaveLight (250) Zeiss Meditec (250)
Method	Laser radar	Charged-coupled device (CCD)/infrared
Transmitted signal	905 nanometers (nm) diode laser	None
Detection frequency	4000 Hz	60, 120, and 250 Hz
Response time	3.00 millisecond (ms) rise time (100 Hz bandwidth)	50 ms rise time (6 Hz bandwidth)

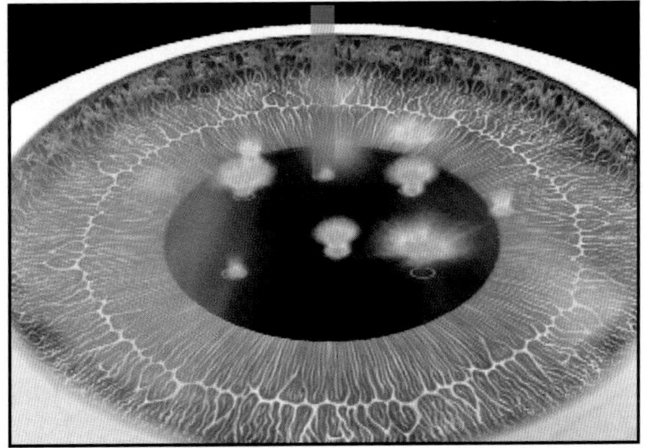

Figure 23-3. Nonsequential (pointillistic) scanning spot placement, as noted with the LADARVision platform.

in the center of the myopic ablation zone treatment, a profilometry of broad beam ablation in plastics demonstrates this same phenomena due to broad beam ablation physics. This can be seen as a peripheral overablation and central underablation (Figure 23-4).[9] Since this profilometry was performed in plastic, the total explanation of central islands being due to an accumulation of central stromal fluid would be unsubstantiated. With the development of special ablation software to compensate for central island formation, the incidence of steep central islands has decreased over the years. Nevertheless, they still occur with broad beam lasers, making the outcome less predictable and ultimately preferable with the small, scanning spot. Consequently, broad beam laser treatment may result in corneal macroirregularities, which are not present when using a scanning spot delivery system.

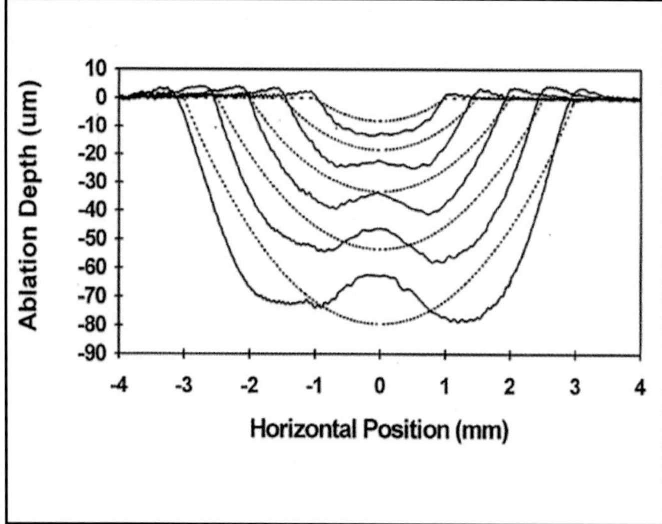

Figure 23-4. Profilometry of broad beam ablation in plastic polymethylmethacrylate (PMMA) resulting in steep central island formation with peripheral over-ablation and central undercorrection. (Reprinted with permission from Shimmick JK, et al. Corneal ablation profilometry and steep central islands. *J Refract Surg.* 1997;13:235-45.)

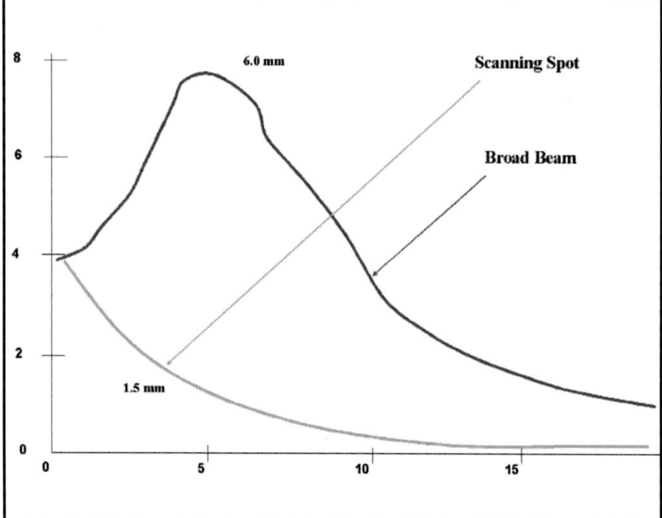

Figure 23-6. Excimer laser induced stress waves as a function of spot diameter and distance within a porcine eye. With the 1.5 mm beam, the stress wave amplitude quickly dissipates as it travels through the eye, while the 6 mm beam develops a pressure focus. In human eyes, the pressure focus is 7 to 8 mm posterior to the cornea.

Surface Smoothness

In addition to the macroirregularities of a steep central island, broad beam laser delivery can also result in inhomogeneities or hot spots within the beam. In contrast, scanning spot ablation with perfect overlap at spot placement demonstrates no inhomogeneities or hot spots. This results in greater smoothness of the surface as determined by laser profilometry of ablated plastic with the four most popular laser vision correction platforms. In the study published by Richard Yee and colleagues, the LADARVision laser platform, possessing the smallest Gaussian scanning spot, demonstrates the smoothest profile from among the four (Figure 23-5).[10]

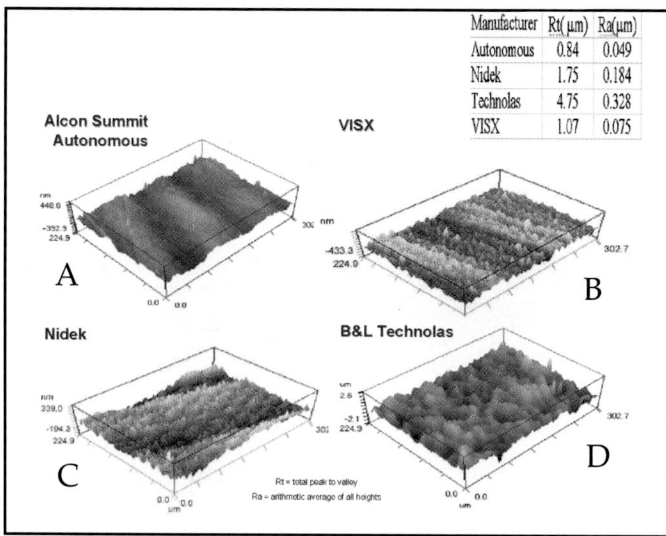

Figure 23-5. Ablation profilometry of the major, commercially available laser platforms. (A) Alcon LADARVision, (B) VISX STAR S2, (C) Nidek ED-5000 d, and (D) Bausch & Lomb Planoscan.

Stress Waves

The impact of the excimer laser photoablation process of the cornea produces a stress wave that propagates through the eye as well as an ablation plume projected away from the eye. The magnitude of this excimer laser induced stress wave is approximately 40 atmospheres on the plane of the cornea. With small spot ablation (less than or equal to 1.5 mm), this energy quickly dissipates beyond the corneal endothelium and is negligible at the level of the vitreous and retinal structures. However, for larger spots (greater than/or equal to 3 mm), a pressure focus is found at approximately 7 to 8 mm behind the corneal endothelium, which is at the level of the posterior lens or anterior vitreous (Figure 23-6). For a 6 mm diameter beam, the magnitude of the pressure focus is approximately 80 atmospheres or twice that seen at the level of the corneal surface.[11] This additional acoustic stress at the level of the anterior vitreous and lens may pose a risk for vitreoretinal or lens abnormalities with broad beam ablation. Although the incidence of retinal detachments after PRK or laser in-situ keratomileusis (LASIK) is no greater than the general population,[12] isolated cases, such as a report of bilateral giant retinal tears with detachment,[13] bring this acoustic effect and the pressure induced by the suction ring into question.

Robust Eye Tracking

Fixation-Related Eye Movements

During patient fixation, frequent saccadic eye movements have been recorded. They are 1) random, 2) about 5 times per second, and 3) at a rapid rate proportional to the distance traversed.[14] These characteristics of fixation-related saccadic eye movements make careful treatment of patients requiring laser vision correction less effective without the aid of a sophisticated eye tracking system. Typical fixation related saccades can traverse the distance of 1 to 10 degrees (0.2 to 2 mm) at a rate varying from 100 to 800 degrees per second (22 to 170 mm/second).[14-16] Figure 23-7 demonstrates the movement of fixation-related saccades dur-

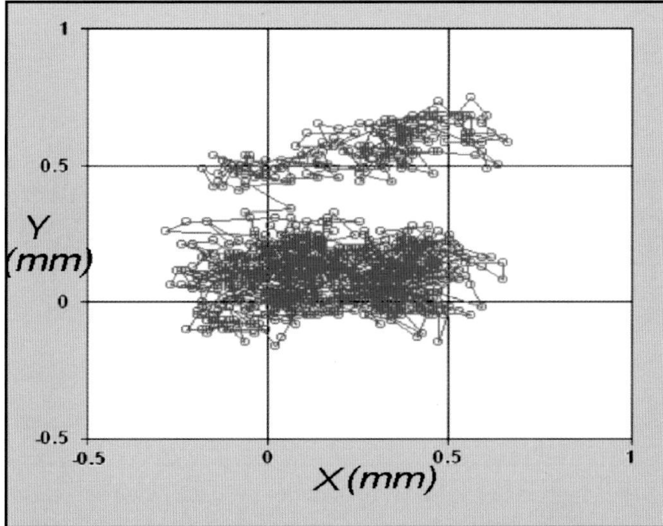

Figure 23-7. Recorded tracing of fixation-related saccades as captured by the LADARVision tracker during a myopic treatment. The saccadic movement extends >0.7 mm both horizontally and vertically from the point of fixation.

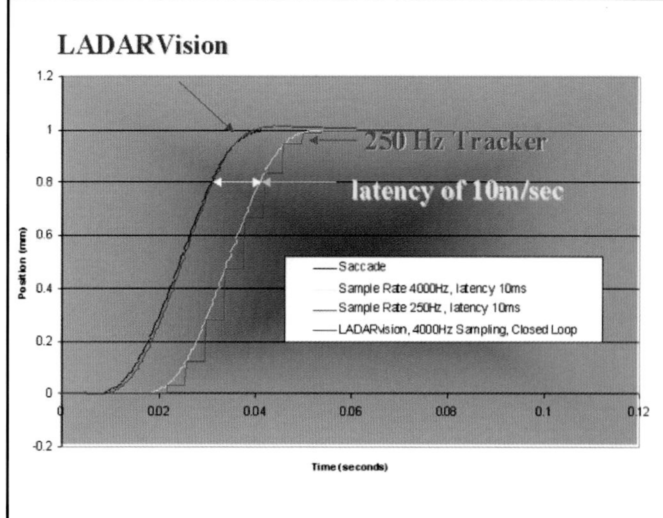

Figure 23-8A. Tracking response of a 1 mm saccadic eye movement (black), demonstrating the time latency of laser radar (blue) vs video camera tracking (red).

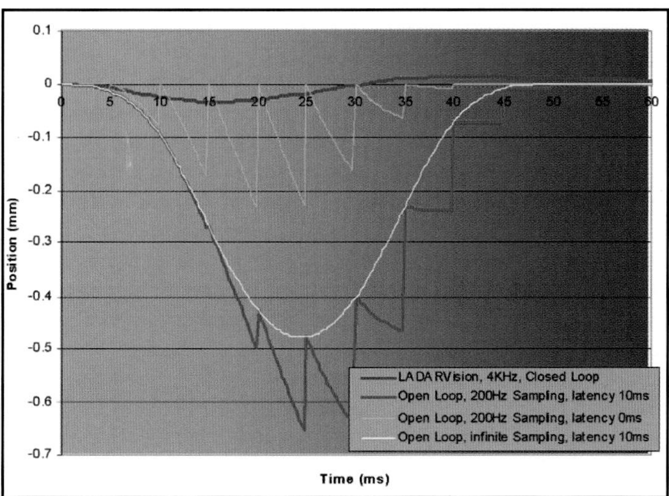

Figure 23-8B. Tracking response of a 1 mm saccadic eye movement (black), demonstrating the corresponding peak position error of pulse placement for laser radar (blue) vs 200 Hz video camera tracking (red) vs 200 Hz sampling, no latency (green) vs infinite sampling, 10 ms latency (yellow).

ing laser vision correction as recorded by the LADARVision tracking system. The figure shows translational movement extending greater than 0.7 mm in both the x and y directions from the point of original fixation. Only the most robust eye tracking system can follow these rapid saccadic eye movements during laser vision correction. For larger excursions, passive eye tracking is often used to avoid gross misalignment, but this is also subject to a latency in the laser shutoff.

Tracking Nomenclature

In order to understand the eye tracking systems, a number of terms need to be defined. These include sampling rate, latency, tracker type, and closed vs open loop tracking.

Sampling Rate

Sampling rate describes how often the tracker measures the eye's location. Tracking frequencies vary from 60 Hz, based on the frame rate of certain video camera trackers, to up to 4000 Hz, seen with laser-radar tracking.

Latency

Latency is the time required to determine the eye's location, calculate the required response, and move the laser tracker mirrors to compensate for the new location. The latency period is therefore due to both the processing delay and the mirror readjustment delay. Typical infrared video camera-based tracking systems have a processing delay due to the time for the image to be integrated onto the image sensor and for the sensor image to be transferred from the camera to an image processing unit. Both of these steps each require a period of 16.67 ms (NTSC) or 20.0 ms (PAL) with a typical video camera-based tracker.[17] This amounts to a total processing delay of 33 ms (NTSC) or 40 milliseconds (PAL). Custom high-speed video processing systems are touted to reduce the delay to 4 to 8 ms; however, this may still be for only one component step rather than both processing and mirror realignment.[17] The exact latencies in most of the commercial video camera tracking systems used in laser vision correction are unknown by the author and cannot be compared at this time. Nevertheless, even an 8 ms processing delay can result in beam spot malposition errors of up to 700 microns (μm). Figure 23-8A demonstrates the tracking of a 1 mm saccadic eye movement (black line) by the <1 ms latency LADARVision tracker at 4000 Hz sampling rate (blue line), as well as the highest sampling video-based tracker at 250 Hz with the high speed latency of 10 ms(red line). The peaked position error corresponding to these two tracking examples can be seen in Figure 23-8B as only 30 μm with the laser radar tracker (blue line) and as much as 650 μm with the high speed video camera tracker (red line). The green line and yellow lines in Figure 10-8B correspond to a zero latency tracking at 200 Hz and a 10 ms latency tracking with an infinite sampling rate, respectively. Based on these figures, one can

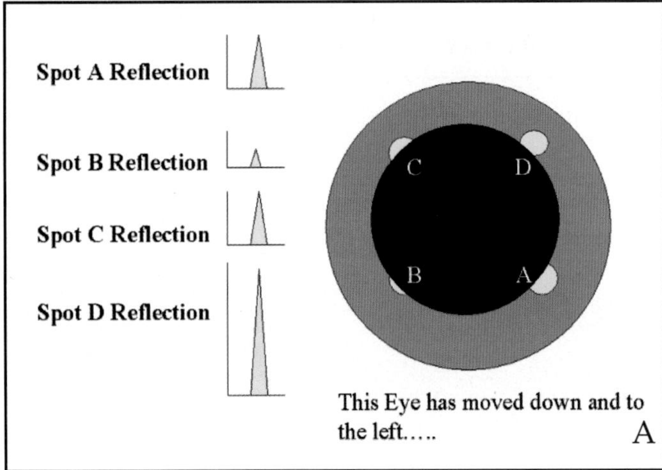

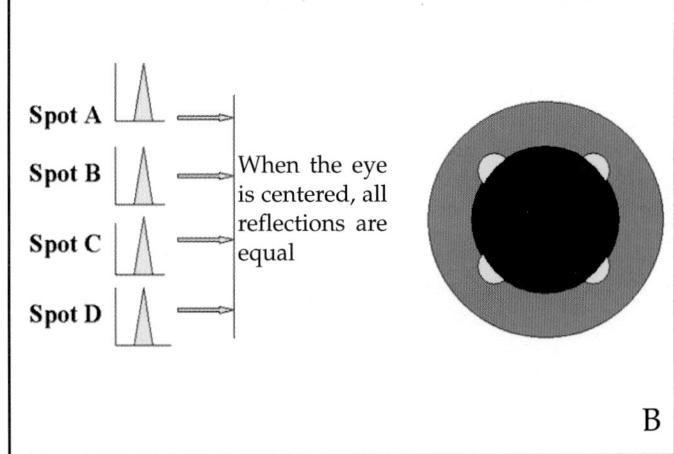

Figure 23-9. Closed loop eye tracking of the LADARVision system, demonstrating the four contrast boundaries (A, B, C, D) which reflect the laser signal. The reflected spot amplitude of the laser radar signal is recorded. Movement down and left results in a non-uniform spot pattern (A), which instantaneously corrects itself by mirror realignment based on feedback from the eyes position prior to movement (B).

deduce that latency due to processing delay and mirror realignment contributes a notable limitation to adequate tracking during laser vision correction. Even passive eye tracking, which typically shuts off the laser for >1.50 mm excursions in some laser systems, does not protect for fixation-related saccades.

Latency is the time required to determine the eye's location, calculate the required response, and move the laser tracker mirrors to compensate for the new location. The latency period is therefore due to both the processing delay and the mirror readjustment delay.

Tracker Type

Table 23-2 illustrates the comparative features of eye tracking among small spot scanning excimer lasers. The table lists only two columns, referring to LADARVision tracking using laser radar and video camera-based tracking using an infrared video image. The difference in sampling rates are included in this table and even though latency periods are not listed, the previously illustrated figures illustrate the important contributions of latency for video camera vs laser radar trackers. Typical video camera eye tracking uses infrared light illumination of the iris against a dark pupil in most refractive surgical systems. This video-based tracking captures a new image without maintaining a reference of the eye's position previously so that no feedback of the eye's current position exists. It simply sees a deviation from the intended position and moves to respond to that deviation.

Closed vs Open Loop Tracking

In open loop (video) tracking, once a new image is taken, the change from the previous image location is calculated and an error signal is sent to then move the mirrors. This is in contrast to closed loop tracking, represented by the laser-radar–based system (LADAR) where the rapid sampling rate together with this system's closed loop servo response feeds back information on the eye's new position continually, thus maintaining a space stabilized image and accurate tracking without latency.

When initiating tracking, the LADARVision system scans the eye to find four contrast boundaries (A, B, C, D) that reflect the 905 nm laser signal back to the detector device in the eye tracking system. When the detected spots vary in size, the eye position is immediately readjusted so that all reflections are of equal magnitude. An equal reflected spot magnitude is essentially maintained, providing a space-stabilized image throughout the engagement of the tracker. Figure 23-9A demonstrates the spot reflection magnitude when the eye has moved down and to the left. This is adjusted instantaneously to allow an equal spot reflection magnitude to be maintained, as in Figure 23-9B. This maintenance of a space-stabilized image is the essence of closed loop eye tracking, such that the controlled variable (eye movement) can be fed back and compared to the reference input (eye position) in order to minimize the position error. In contrast, open loop eye tracking has no comparison of the controlled variable with the desired input. For closed loop eye tracking to be maintained, the sampling rate needs to be at least 10 times the tracker bandwidth, which for eye tracking is approximately 100 Hz.[18] Hence, a tracker sampling rate of at least 1000 Hz is sufficient for maintaining a space-stabilized image with closed loop eye tracking.

For closed loop eye tracking to be maintained, the sampling rate needs to be at least 10 times the tracker bandwidth, which for eye tracking is approximately 100 Hz.[18] Hence, a tracker sampling rate of at least 1000 Hz is sufficient for maintaining a space-stabilized image with closed loop eye tracking.

Clinical Significance of Eye Tracking

When discussing the important components of eye tracking, such as sampling rate, latency time, tracker type, and open loop vs closed loop, the clinical significance of these components are demonstrated by comparative studies of laser vision correction when the eye tracker is on, compared to the same when the eye tracker is off. In a presentation at the American Academy of Ophthalmology Meeting in 2001, Hardten et al used the VISX ActiveTrac, which is a 60 Hz video camera tracker with open loop tracking, to treat a cohort of 202 eyes in comparison to 110 eyes in which the tracker was not engaged. Statistically significant improvement in vision was noted with the active tracker engaged (mean SCVA = 20/19.3) in comparison to no tracker (mean SCVA = 20/20.2) ($p = 0.020$). This study is in comparison to that reported by Mrochen et al,[19] in which a faster, 250 Hz, video camera tracker employed by the Wavelight Allegretto (Erlangen, Germany) laser demonstrated a statistically significant improvement in vision (mean SCVA = 20/17.7) when tracking 20 eyes in comparison to 20 eyes with no tracker (mean SCVA = 20/20.8) ($p = 0.013$). Both studies showed clinical improvement with eye tracking, yet the latter study required a smaller number of eyes to achieve statistical significance. Performing a similar comparison with the LADARVision eye tracker system at 4000 Hz cannot be done because the laser will not fire with the tracker turned off. Nevertheless, one can infer that significant clinical improvement would also be achieved when using the LADARVision tracker. In conclusion, we recommend the use of a high sampling rate tracker with minimal or no latency and closed loop servo response to achieve the maximum benefit.

Accurate Wavefront Device

Wavefront vs Corneal Topography

Although customized corneal ablation and especially customized visual correction, as specified by this book, refer predominantly to information gathered from a wavefront measurement device, computerized corneal topography can also be used in customizing corneal ablation by breaking down the corneal topographic map into the same aberrations and irregularity terms presented in ocular wavefront analysis. The concept of topographic customized corneal ablation was first proposed by Gibralter and Trokel in the mid-1990s.[20] Although a number of companies have attempted to make a successful clinical link between corneal topography and laser ablation, wide spread adaptation has been limited due to difficulties in the registry of the topographic information with the laser. Nevertheless, highly irregular corneas after previous laser vision correction, or other corneal surgery, can be in part corrected with several different customized topographic platforms presented later in the book. With many of these platforms, however, although the cornea can be more successfully regularized, a precise refractive outcome is yet difficult to achieve as clinical topography gives no information about the patient's refraction and this must be implemented as a separate step.

The more popular focus of customized corneal ablation, as well as customized visual correction, utilizes ocular wavefront sensing as the refractive information being used in wavefront-guided customized ablation. The wavefront measurement device gives a two-dimensional (2-D) profile of refractive error much in the same way as computerized corneal topography gives a 2-D mapping profile of keratometry. Therefore, wavefront-guided customized corneal ablation should be more precise than topography-guided ablation, as the wavefront not only attempts to smooth the cornea, but provides a sharp focus of all corneal points on the retinal fovea.

> The wavefront measurement device gives a two dimensional profile of refractive error much in the same way as computerized corneal topography gives a two-dimensional mapping profile of keratometry.

Principles of Wavefront Measurement Devices

Much in the same way that computerized corneal topography devices became available during the past decade, there are now a number of different types of wavefront measurement devices being made available on the market. Although it is often difficult to adequately categorize new products in an understandable fashion, there appears to be four different principles by which wavefront aberration information is collected and measured. A summary of the principles of measurement and their devices are included in Table 23-3.

Outgoing Refractive Aberrometry (Shack-Hartmann)

At the turn of the past century, Hartmann first described the principles by which optical aberrations in lenses could be characterized.[21] This was later modified by Shack and found practical application in adaptive optics telescopes to eliminate the aberrations of the earth's atmospheres for the past 20 years. It was finally introduced into ophthalmology by Liang and Bille in 1994.[22] The Shack-Hartmann wavefront sensor was used to objectively measure the wave aberrations of the human eye. Further application of adaptive optics in ophthalmology found use in viewing retinal structures with greater detail than ever before. In 1996, images of the cone photoreceptors were viewed in the living human eye by adaptive optics defined by a Shack-Hartmann wavefront sensor.[23] This first attempt at customizing the optics of the eye to increase the resolution of structures within it defined the need for the measurement specificity provided by wavefront technology in achieving better resolution when viewing structures outside the eye.

The typical Shack-Hartmann wavefront sensor utilizes approximately 100 spots or more, created by approximately 100 lenslets that focus the aberrated light exiting the eye onto a CCD detection array. Figure 23-10 demonstrates the principles of Shack-Hartmann wavefront sensing, in which a low energy laser light reflects off the retinal fovea, passing through the optical structures of the eye and creating an outgoing wavefront. After the light passes through the array of lenslets, each small segment of the wavefront is then focused to a small spot on the detection array, and the distance of displacement of the focused spot from the ideal very accurately defines the degree of ocular aberration. Figure 23-11 shows a segment of the wavefront going through a single lenslet and focusing at a distance (dx) from an ideal perpendicular point of focus. To the left of this figure, the entire aberrated wavefront spot profile in red is slightly more peripheral than the ideal wavefront spot profile in blue. This particular wavefront spot profile is representative of a patient with myopia.

Although the Shack-Hartmann method of wavefront aberrometry is a very accurate method, the level of accuracy is

Table 23-3
Categorical Listing of Commercial Wavefront Devices

OUTGOING REFLECTION ABERROMETRY (SHACK-HARTMANN)

- Alcon LADARWave
- VISX Wavescan
- Schwind Aberrometer
- Bausch & Lomb Zywave
- Meditec WASCA

RETINAL IMAGING ABERROMETRY (TSCHERNING)

- WaveLight Analyzer
- Tracey Ray Tracing

INCOMING ADJUSTABLE REFRACTOMETRY (SCHEINER)

- InterWave SRR

DOUBLE PASS ABERROMETRY (SLIT SKIASCOPY)

- Nidek OPD-Scan

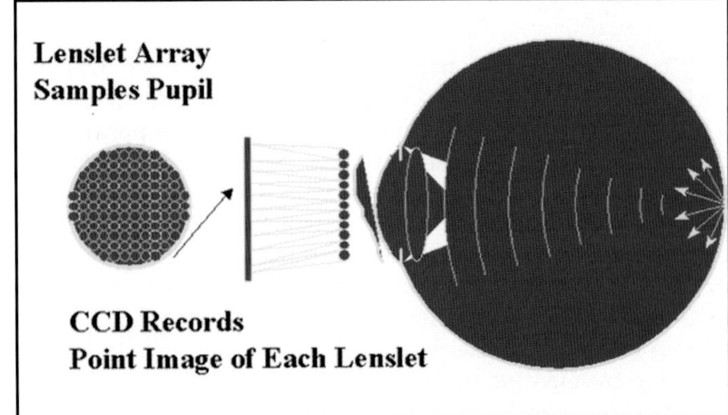

Figure 23-10. Principle of Shack-Hartmann wavefront sensing in which a low energy laser light reflects off the retinal fovea, passing through the optical structures of the eye to create the outgoing wavefront. The wavefront passes through a lenslet array to define the deviation of focused spots from their ideal. (Courtesy of Raymond Applegate, PhD.)

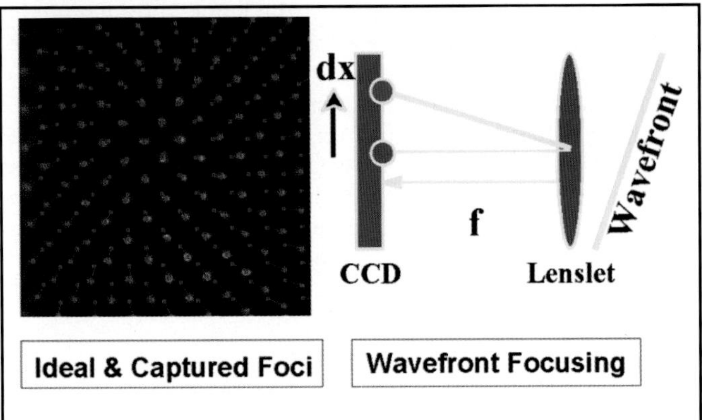

Figure 23-11. A small segment of the wavefront passing through a single lenslet demonstrating the deviation (dx) of the focused spot (red) from its ideal location (blue). When presented as an array of spots, the more peripheral location of the focused spots (red) from the ideal spots (blue) represents a myopic wavefront spot pattern.

dependent on the number of spots that are collected within a 7 mm pupil area. Commercially, Shack-Hartmann wavefront devices vary from as little as 70 spots (Bausch & Lomb Zywave) to as many as 800 spots (WaveFront Sciences COAS). In general, it appears that approximately 200 spots within a 7 mm pupil area appears to be sufficient for accurately measuring up to eighth-order aberrations (see Chapter 21). The potential limitations of Shack-Hartmann wavefront sensing may include multiple scattering from choroidal structures beneath the fovea, but this is likely to be insignificant in comparison the axial length. Also, highly aberrated eyes may find a crossover of the focused spots. Although potentially a concern with some devices,[24] this has not been found to be of concern with other devices, even in capturing the most complex wavefronts (see Chapters 26 and 29).

> Although the Shack-Hartmann method of wavefront aberrometry is a very accurate method, the level of accuracy is dependent on the number of spots that are collected within a 7 mm pupil area.

Retinal Imaging Aberrometry (Tscherning and Ray Tracing)

The next type of wavefront sensing was characterized by Tscherning in 1894, when he described the monochromatic aberrations of the human eye.[25] Tscherning's description, however, was not supported by the leaders of ophthalmic optics, including Gullstrand, and was not favorably accepted. It was not until 1977 that Howland & Howland used Tscherning's aberroscope design together with a crosscylinder lens to subjectively measure the monochromatic aberrations of the eye.[26] This same concept was more recently modified by Seiler using a spherical lens to project a 1 mm grid pattern unto the retina.[27] This, together with a paraxial aperture system, could visualize and photographically record the aberrated pattern of up to 168 spots as a wavefront map. This 13 x 13 spot grid of laser light is projected through a 10 mm corneal area and represents an analysis of approximately 100 spots within a 7 mm pupillary area. Figure 23-12 illustrates the optical principals of the modified Tscherning aberrometer, demonstrating the optics of retinal imaging (A) and image capture (B).

The potential limitation of this type of wavefront sensing is the use of an idealized eye model (Gullstrand Model I) to perform the ray tracing computation. The Gullstrand model, which varies with refractive error, however, is modified within the commercial device according to the patient's refractive error to maintain an accurate assessment of the axial length.

An alternative form of retinal imaging has been introduced over the past several years by a Ukrainian scientist, Vasyl Molebny.[28] Tracey retinal ray tracing is a slightly different form of retinal imaging in that it uses a sequential projection of spots onto the retina, in a "gatling gun" fashion, that are captured and traced to find the wavefront pattern. A total of 64 sequential retinal spots (recently increased to nearly 100) can be traced within 12 ms, and converted to a wavefront pattern on the pupillary plane. The number of spots with this method of analysis is nearly the same as that of the Tscherning aberrometer within a

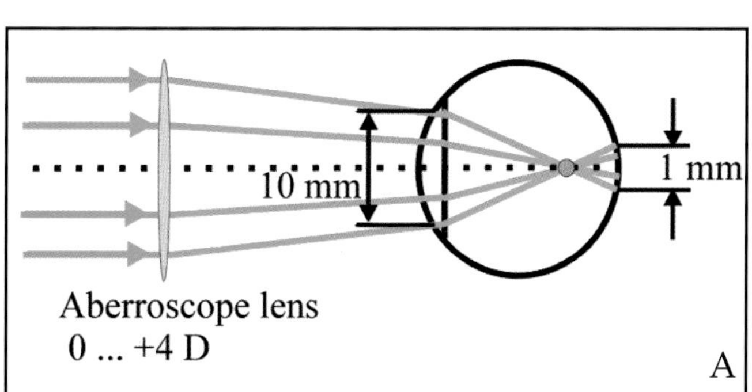

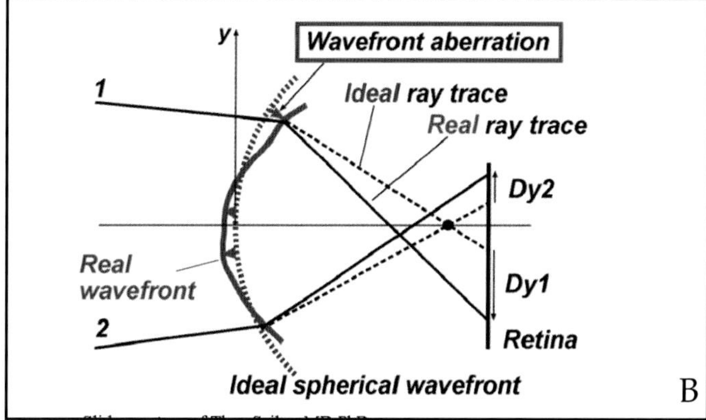

Figure 23-12. Principles of Tscherning aberrometry with (A) low energy laser light as a 13 x 13 spot grid, passing through 10 mm of the cornea and defocusing to an aberrated grid of 1 mm on the retina, and (B) aberrated retinal spot position is compared to the ideal retinal spot pattern to determine the wavefront error at the level of the entrance pupil. (Courtesy of Theo Seiler, MD, PhD.)

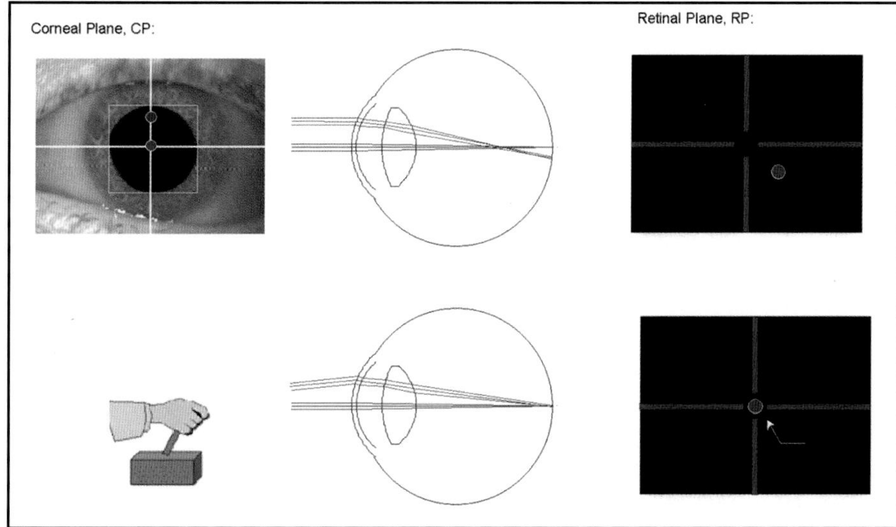

Figure 23-13. Principles of spatially resolved refractometry: a peripheral light source projected through a wheel (mask) can be subjectively redirected by a joystick to overlap a reference point in the center of the pupil. The movement varies the angle of incidence of the peripheral ray and can be used to mathematically characterize the wavefront error at that point. Multiple peripheral rays are tested to construct the wavefront profile. (Courtesy of Stephen Burns, PhD.)

7 mm pupillary area, but the Tracey technology has the flexibility of analyzing a greater number of spots within a critical area, expanding the specificity of resolution, especially in more aberrated eyes.

Ingoing Adjustable Refractometry (Spatially-Resolved Refractometer)

The third method of wavefront sensing is based on the 17th century principle of Sheiner and described by Smirnov in 1961 as a form of subjectively adjustable refractometry.[29] Peripheral beams of incoming light are subjectively redirected toward a central target to cancel the ocular aberrations from that peripheral point. This was modified by Webb, Penny, and Thompson in 1992 as a subjective form of wavefront refractometry of the human eye.[30] Figure 23-13 demonstrates the optical schematic of the spatial resolved refractometer (SRR), which measures the wavefront pattern according to these principles. The InterWave (Emory Vision, Atlanta, Ga) device commercializes the SRR technology utilizing approximately 37 testing spots that are manually directed by the observer to overlap the central target in defining the wavefront aberration pattern. Although this technology is unique and potentially beneficial by subjectively verifying the aberration seen by the patient, the limitation of this technique is a lengthy time required for subjective alignment of the aberrated spots.

Double Pass Aberrometry (Slit Skiascopy)

The final method of wavefront sensing is based on methods of double pass aberrometry or retinoscopic aberrometry which considers both the passage of light into the eye and reflection of light out of the eye in defining the wavefront pattern. Slit retinoscopy (skiascopy) rapidly scans a slit of light along a specific axis and orientation. The fundus reflection is then captured to define the wavefront aberration pattern onto a parallel array of photodetectors and one set of perpendicular photodetectors to define the orientation.[31] A total of four spots can be defined at each meridian of scanning with 360 meridia being scanned (at each degree of 360 degrees) for a total of 1440 data points. Figure 23-14 shows the retinoscopic scanning slit of light into the eye and reflected light out of the eye. The temporal delay of photo voltage peaks from the photodetector signify the points of wavefront information. Although this technique, utilized by the Nidek OPD-Scan (Gamagori, Japan), is also sequential at various axes, the objective capture of the reflex makes it possible to acquire the information in a rapid sequence. The potential limitation of this technology includes the small amount of information collected axially within a given meridian (four spots) and the sequential nature of the capture.

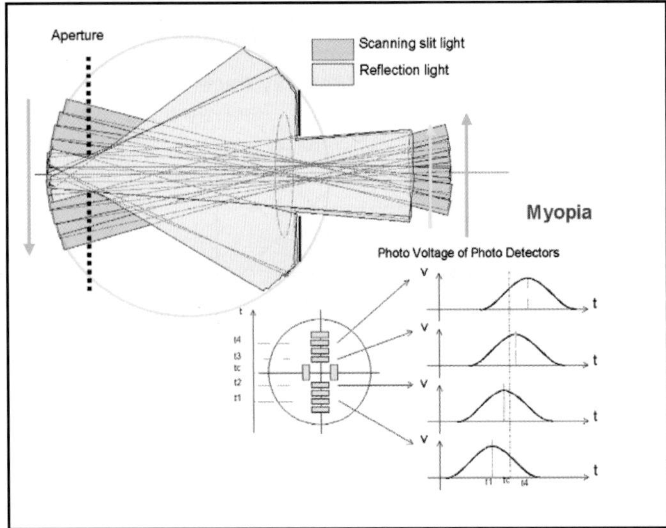

Figure 23-14. Principles of slit skiascopy used in the Nidek OPD-Scan. A scanning slit of light (aqua blue) enters the eye and is reflected out (yellow) with a temporal delay. An array of photo detectors capture the temporal delay, which defines the refractive or aberration error specific to that meridian. Multiple meridia characterize the total ocular wavefront profile.

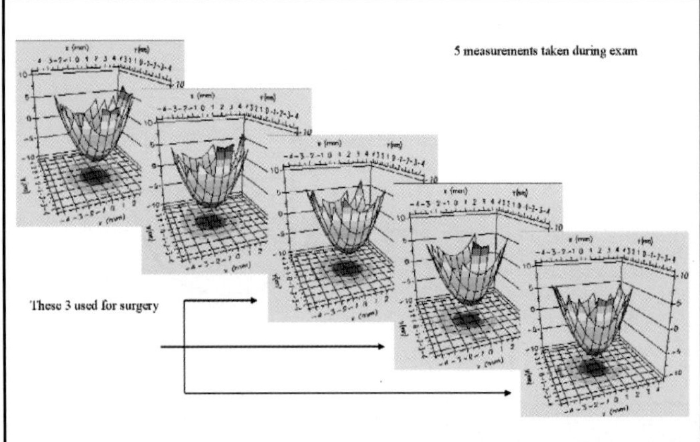

Figure 23-15. Capture and comparison of five consecutive wavefront maps in a myopic eye before custom cornea LASIK surgery. The three closest in agreement were used to generate a composite profile map to be used in creating the wavefront-guided laser ablation profile.

Practical Aspects of Wavefront Measurement Devices

Table 23-3 outlines the categorical listing of commercially available wavefront devices. Each has a representation by at least one or several companies. Each company has made its own proprietary modifications to provide a practical device for clinical use. Careful comparison of these various wavefront measuring principles and their specific devices are only beginning to be performed clinically, and this is represented in Chapter 21. The practical utility of one device vs another will continue to be the subject of future investigation. A more detailed description of these various principles of wavefront sensing is discussed in Chapters 15 to 20.

Laser/Wavefront Interface

Wavefront Capture and Comparison

The first step to properly linking up the wavefront device and measurement with the actual laser treatment is to ensure the most accurate and reproducible wavefront has been captured and implemented. Many commercial wavefront devices have steps to assure an accurate wavefront capture. For example, with the Alcon LADARWave aberrometer, each patient exam requires five consecutive wavefront measurements, each of which is saved, with the three closest in agreement being compared and used to generate a composite profile (Figure 23-15). This new composite wavefront map can be used diagnostically or used to create a wavefront-guided laser ablation profile and spot pattern for treatment. Whether other wavefront/laser link-ups require the creation of a composite map is unknown, but a very reproducible and accurate map can best be achieved with multiple captures, comparisons, and the generation of a composite map.

Just prior to the wavefront capture, small ink marks may be placed along the limbus at two locations using an eye marking pen. This step is specifically done with the LADARVision platform for custom cornea, where the eye geometry of the markings is captured together with the wavefront information. At this point, the wavefront and geometry information is electronically transferred to the treatment laser. This link-up is achieved by a computer disc that downloads the information from the wavefront device to the treatment laser. This transfer includes not only the wavefront error information, but also the orientation data gathered during the wavefront measurement and defined by the position of the ink marks and the limbus.

Conversion to Ablation Profile

The next step in the wavefront to laser link-up is the conversion of the wavefront measurement to an actual ablation profile. The tissue that needs to be removed from the cornea to correct the refractive error and higher-order aberrations is determined from an ablation profile that is fundamentally the inverse of the wavefront error map. When implementing this step, it is important to have a wavefront measurement that has been captured through a diameter at least 0.50 mm larger than the scotopic pupil size. To achieve a pupil diameter of this size, pharmacological dilation is necessary. Although subtle variations in the wavefront pattern have been demonstrated with the use of pharmacologic agents,[32] a customized laser vision correction requires a large ablation profile in excess of the typical scotopic pupil, hence necessitating pharmacologic dilation. The actual conversion process of the wavefront into the ablation profile is a complex mathematical inversion of the three dimensional maps that often factors in other variables, such as corneal curvature[33] and biomechanics (Figure 23-16A).[34] The actual ablation profile diameter used in customized laser vision correction may vary somewhat for different custom laser platforms. For instance, with the Alcon LADARVision platform, the CustomCornea ablation profile is defined by a 6.5 mm optical zone together with a 1.25 mm blend zone for a total ablation diameter of 9 mm.

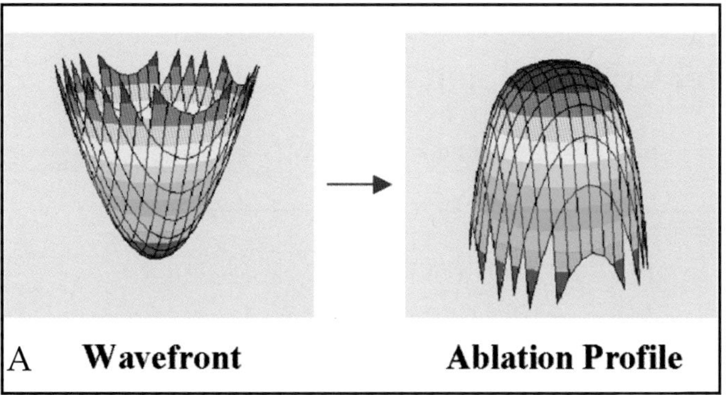

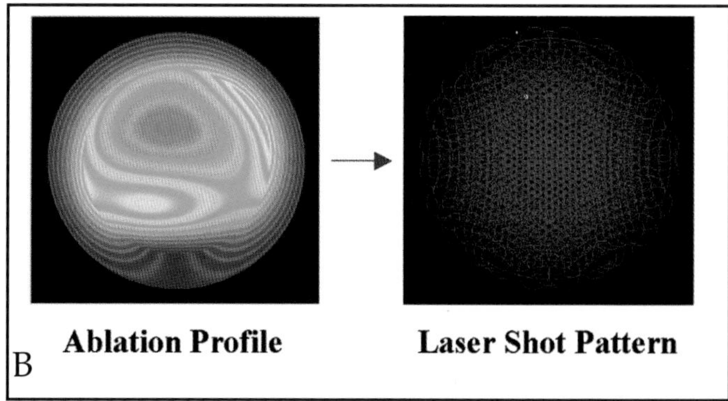

Figure 23-16. (A) Conversion of the wavefront map into an ablation profile by a complex mathematical inversion that factors in other variables (corneal curvature, biomechanics, etc). (B) Calculation of the excimer laser shot pattern to achieve the desired ablation profile. This depends on the laser fluence during the calibration process and other environmental and surgeon factors, which can be compensated for by a spherical offset.

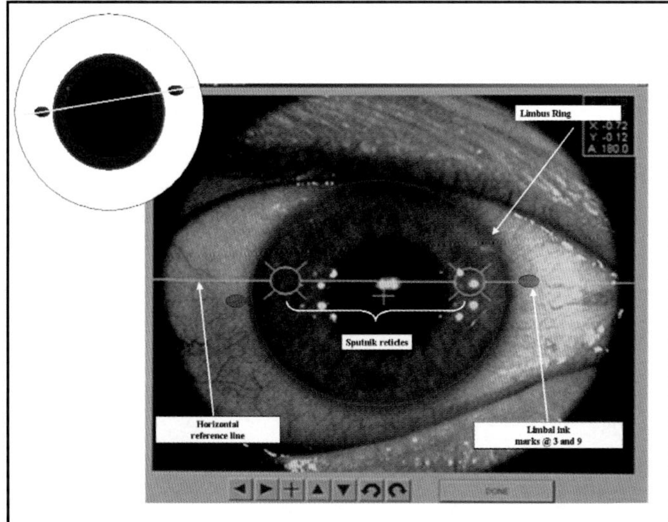

Figure 23-17. Registration process, which includes a limbus ring for xy alignment and orientation marks for cyclorotation. The latter can be overlapped by virtual sputniks to register the wavefront data to the actual eye and laser tracker.

A customized laser vision correction requires a large ablation profile in excess of the typical scotopic pupil, hence necessitating pharmacologic dilation.

In every instance of customized ablation, a blend zone is necessary to produce a smooth transition between the correction of higher-order aberrations at the edge of optical zone and the residual unablated cornea. With the Tscherning aberrometer link-up to the Wavelight Allegretto laser, a blend zone of at least 0.5 mm is added to the calculated ablation zone. In cases where the residual stromal thickness after LASIK makes it unsafe to meet a full 7 mm optical zone, a slightly smaller optical zone diameter is implemented.

The final step in the conversion process is determining the excimer laser shot pattern (Figure 23-16B). This step is generally an automatic process in which the typical ablation depth per pulse is used, corresponding to the measured fluence of the laser during the calibration process. Subtle variations of laser ablation technique and environmental conditions, including temperature and humidity, can affect the ablation depth per pulse. For the most part, the currently approved customized ablation platforms have a spherical offset to compensate for individual surgeon variability, while maintaining the same shot pattern for cylinder and higher-order aberrations.

For the most part, the currently approved customized ablation platforms have a spherical offset to compensate for individual surgeon variability, while maintaining the same shot pattern for cylinder and higher-order aberrations.

Dynamic Registration

Once the ablation profile and laser shot pattern is in place, the patient is ready for customized laser vision correction. For most laser vision correction platforms, this means aligning the geometric center of the laser vision ablation profile with the center of the undilated pupil. For many of these systems, infrared video camera eye tracking can also be engaged to maintain this position in the midst of low grade eye movements.

For CustomCornea and the LADARVision platform, this goes one step further. Dynamic registration can be achieved by engaging the laser radar eye tracker, which registers the wavefront-determined laser shot pattern to its corresponding position on the cornea by overlaying the identification reticles. The first reticle is the limbus ring which provides the xy alignment, and dynamically maintains that alignment throughout the tracking of the dilated pupil margin. The second reticle is the cyclorotation alignment which is implemented by rotating the image of the limbus ring in such a way that virtual "sputniks", taken from the orientation marks recorded during the wavefront capture, are overlapped with the actual ink marks that still remain on the eye. In this way, true registration can be achieved dynamically, not only in XY orientation, but also statically with regard to cyclorotation. The graphic user interface on the LADARVision 4000 laser demonstrates the alignment of the limbus and overlap of the orientation marks for verification prior to treatment (Figure 23-17). In the future, registration and tracking based on iris detail will provide a possible alternative for dynamic capture of cyclorotation, as well.

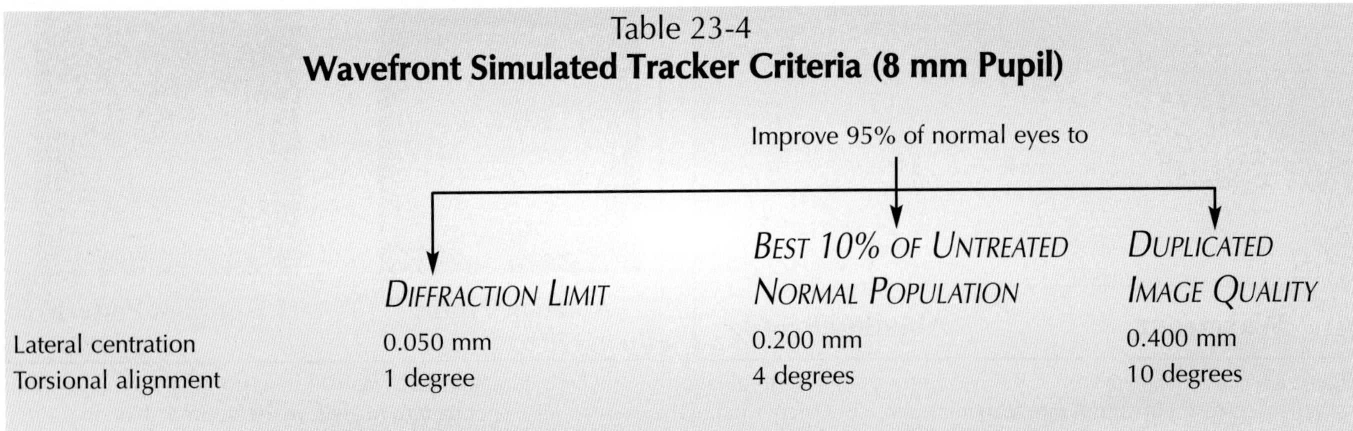

Table 23-4
Wavefront Simulated Tracker Criteria (8 mm Pupil)

Improve 95% of normal eyes to

	Diffraction Limit	Best 10% of Untreated Normal Population	Duplicated Image Quality
Lateral centration	0.050 mm	0.200 mm	0.400 mm
Torsional alignment	1 degree	4 degrees	10 degrees

The process of registration is actually the most important technology requirement for accurate customized ablation of higher-order aberrations. The importance of registration regarding lateral movement and cyclorotation can be seen in Table 23-4. Here the criteria for registration and tracking requires: 1) less than 50 μm of decentration to maintain an ideal wavefront ablation; 2) less than 200 μm of decentration to achieve results consistent with the best 10% of the untreated, normal population; and 3) approximately 400 μm of decentration to only duplicate the mean preoperative image quality. These same lateral decentrations can be noted with tortional misalignment of 1 degree, 4 degrees, and 10 degrees, respectively, for the aforementioned criteria.

The process of registration is actually the most important technology requirement for accurate customized ablation of higher-order aberrations

Algorithm Development

A final consideration in the wavefront/laser interface requires an understanding of the variable of the ablation process. With many of the existing customized laser vision correction platforms, a complex algorithm needs to be implemented to insure the effectiveness of the custom treatment. Fortunately, the software received by the user already has the appropriate algorithm in place. This makes it even easier for the surgeon, who merely has to download the wavefront information rather than develop a nomogram based on refraction data. Subtle adjustment can be implemented depending on the surgeon factor and environmental conditions. However, this offset is not intended to be an actual nomogram adjustment, but rather a preset spherical refinement that considers variables based on an individual surgeon and location. Both the actual laser algorithm and the offset are to be carefully established.

With a proper algorithm and "nomogram" offset, together with the technology requirements of a small, scanning spot, very fast eye tracking system, accurate wavefront device and state of the art wavefront/laser interface, it is truly possible achieve the optimum results with customized corneal ablation. These technology requirements serve as a foundational basis in our current attempts to provide state of the art wavefront-guided customized corneal ablation.

References

1. Seiler T, Kaemmerer M, Mierdel P, Krinke HE. Ocular optical aberrations after photorefractive keratectomy for myopia and myopic astigmatism. *Arch Ophthalmol.* 2000;118:17-21
2. Marco S. Aberrations and visual performance following standard laser vision correction. *J Refract Surg.* 2001;17:S596-S601.
3. Mrochen, M, Krueger R, Bueeler M, Seiler T. Aberration sensing and wavefront-guided treatment: management of decentered ablations. *J Refract Surg.* 2002;18:418-429.
4. Krueger R. Technology requirements for customized corneal ablation. In: MacRae S, Krueger R, Applegate R, eds. *Customized Corneal Ablation: The Quest For Super Vision.* Thorofare, NJ: SLACK Incorporated; 2001:133-147.
5. Huang D, Arif M. Spot size and quality of scanning laser correction of higher-order wavefront aberrations. *J Cataract Refract Surg.* 2002; 28:407-416.
6. Guirao A, Williams DR, MacRae SM. Effect of beam size on the expected benefit of customized laser refractive surgery. *J Refract Surg.* 2003;19:15-23.
7. Campin JA, Pettit GH, Gray GP. Required laser beam resolution and PRK system configuration for custom high fidelity corneal shaping. *Invest Ophthalmol Vis Sci.* 1999;38:S538.
8. Krueger RR, Saedy NF, McDonnell PJ. Clinical analysis of steep central islands after excimer laser photorefractive keratectomy. *Arch Ophthal.* 1996; 114:377-381.
9. Shimmick JK, Telfair WB, Munnerlyn CR, Bartlett JD, Trokel SL. Corneal ablation profilometry and steep central islands. *J Refract Surg.* 1997;13:235-245.
10. Thomas JW, Mitras S, Chuang AZ, Yee RW. Comparison of surface smoothness of porcine cornea and acrylic calibration plastic by electron microscopy after laser ablation. *J Refract Surg.* 2003.
11. Krueger RR, Seiler T, Gruchman T, Mrochen M, Berlin MS. Stress wave amplitudes during laser surgery of the cornea. *Ophthalmology.* 2001;27:1018-1024.
12. Arevalo JF, Ramirez E, Suarez E, et al. Incidence of vitreoretinal pathologic conditions within 24 months after laser in-situ keratomileusis. *Ophthalmology.* 2000;107:258-262.
13. Ozdemar A, Aras C, Sener B, et al. Bilateral retinal detachment associated with giant retinal tear after laser-assisted keratomileusis. *Retina.* 1998;18:176-177.
14. Bollen E, Bax J, Van Dijk JG. Variability of the main sequence. *Invest Ophthalmol Vis Sci.* 1993;34:3700-3704.
15. Boghea D, Troost BT, Daroff RB, Dell'osso LF, Birkett JE. Characteristics of normal human saccades. *Invest Ophthalmol Vis Sci.* 1974;13:619-623.

16. Bahill AT, Clark MR, Stark K. Glissades eye movements generated by mismatched components of the saccadic motorneural control signal. *Mathematical Biosciences*. 1975;26:303-318.

17. Huppertz M, Schmidt E, Teiwes W. Eye tracking and refractive surgery. In: MacRae SM, Krueger RR, Applegate RA, eds. *Customized Corneal Ablation: The Quest for Super Vision*. Thorofare, NJ: SLACK Incorporated; 2001:149-160.

18. Krueger RR. In perspective: eye tracking and Autonomous laser radar. *J Refract Surg*. 1999;15:145-149.

19. Mrochen M, Eldine MS, Kaemerrer M, Seiler T, Hutz W. Improvement in photorefactive corneal laser surgery results using an active eye-tracking system. *J Cataract Refract Surg*. 2001;27:1000-1006.

20. Gibralter R, Trokel S. Correction of irregular astigmatism with the excimer laser. *Ophthalmology*. 1994;101:1310-1315.

21. Hartmann . Bemerkurgen uber den bau und die jurstirung von spektographer. *Zeitschrift fuer Instrumenter Kinde*. 1900;20:47.

22. Liang J, Grimm B, Goelz S, Bille JF. Objective measurement of wave aberrations of the human eye with the use of a Hartmann-Shack wavefront sensor. *J Opt Soc Am A*. 1994;11:1949-1957.

23. Miller D, Williams DR, Morris GM, Liang J. Images of cone photoreceptors in the living human eye. *Vision Res*. 1996;36:1067-1079.

24. Wang L, Wang N, Koch DD. Evaluation of refractive error measurements of the WaveScan Wavefront system and Tracey Wavefront aberrometer. *J Cataract Refract Surg*. 2003.

25. Tscherning M. Die monochromatischen aberrationen des merschlichen auges. *Z Psychol Physiol Sinne*. 1894;6:456-471.

26. Howland HC, Howland B. A subjective method for the measurement of monochromatic aberrations of the eye. *J Opt Soc Am A*. 1977; 67:1805-1818.

27. Mierdel P, Wiegard W, Krinke HE, et al. Measuring device for determining monochromatic aberrations of the human eye. *Ophthalmologe*. 1997;6:441-445.

28. Molebny VV, Pallikaris IG, Naoumidis LP, et al. Retinal ray tracing technique for eye refraction mapping. *Proc SPIE*. 1997;1971:175-183.

29. Smirnov HS. Measurement of the wave aberration in the human eye. *Biophys*. 1961;6:52-66.

30. Webb RH, Penney CM, Thompson KP. Measurement of ocular wavefront distortion with a spatially resolved refractometer. *Appl Opt*. 1992;31:3678-3686.

31. MacRae S, Fujieda M. Slit skiascopic-guided ablation using the Nidek laser. *J Refract Surg*. 2000;16:S576-S580.

32. Fankhauser F, Kaemmerer M, Mrochen M, Seiler T. The effect of accommodation, mydriasis and cycloplegia on aberrometry. *Invest Ophthalmol Vis Sci*. 2000;41(4):S461.

33. Mrochen M, Seiler T. Influence of corneal curvature on calculation of ablation patterns used in photorefractive laser surgery. *J Refract Surg*. 2001;17:S584-S587.

34. Dupps WJ, Roberts C. Effect of acute biomechanical changes on corneal curvature after photokeratectomy. *J Refract Surg*. 2001;17: 658-659.

Chapter 24

Eye Tracking and Alignment in Refractive Surgery: Requirements for Customized Ablation

Natalie Taylor, PhD and Winfried Teiwes, Dr Ing

Introduction

With the increasing demands of customized corneal ablation—smaller beam sizes, faster repetition rate, and greater precision of correction—exact positioning of each laser shot onto the eye becomes increasingly more important. This need for greater positioning accuracy has provided the impetus for several refractive laser companies to implement eye tracking as the "target acquisition system," to position the ablation beam accurately onto the corneal surface and compensate for patient head and eye movements during the surgery procedure. As the sophistication of the laser delivery systems and the whole treatment process increases, so do the requirements of this eye tracking system.

This chapter will outline the overall accuracy requirements of beam placement for accurate and repeatable customized ablation; how the physiological parameters of eye movements can affect the accuracy of beam placement, and hence the overall outcome; and the requirements and design of the overall eye tracking system to be considered to achieve accurate, repeatable customized surgery.

Overall Accuracy Requirements

How accurate does beam placement need to be for the quest for ideal refractive corrections? Several studies[1,2] have used computers to calculate the effect of displacement of the correction on the cornea or cyclotorsion on a simulated refractive outcome. Results indicated that a maximum constant decentration during surgery of 0.45 millimeters (mm) ensured that the optical quality of the model eye was not decreased by the simulated surgery. This requirement was reduced to a mere 0.05 mm when the aim is to achieve a diffraction-limited eye (ie, optically perfect). The results for cyclotorsion or rotatory displacement of the correction on the cornea were 15 degrees to ensure the optical quality was not further reduced and 1 degree to ensure a diffraction limited outcome.

> Editor's note:
> Work by Guirao and coworkers demonstrated that 50% of the visual benefit of higher-order aberration is lost with a 250 microns (μm) decentration or a 10 degree eye rotation.[1]
> S. MacRae

This requirement of 0.45 mm may seem coarse and simple to achieve, in comparison to the micron resolution of the diagnosis and tissue ablation per shot. However, this offset to the perfectly aligned procedure may have many causes: either systematic errors such as misalignment in the axis of the laser beam or incorrect initial alignment of the patient's eye; or random or dynamic errors such as the eye movements of the eye. Each of these factors must be carefully controlled to ensure that the desired refractive correction is aligned correctly to the eye accurately enough to ensure a successful and repeatable visual outcome.

It is the purpose of the eye tracking system to measure the eye position at the beginning of the surgery; measure movements throughout the surgery; to send the offset data to the laser system; and to ensure that the position of the laser beam is compensated for changes in eye position. It is a requirement of the eye tracking system that it can have an overall accuracy that ensures an improved visual outcome, that is giving an overall offset of less than 0.45 mm in translation (ideally 0.05 mm), and a rotary offset of less than 15 degrees (ideally 1 degree).

Effect of Eye Movements

This section will first describe eye movements in general situations, and then describe eye movements as they occur during the laser surgery and to some extent also during the diagnostic procedure. For correct measurement of eye movements, it is essential to understand the principles of the static and dynamic behavior of the eye's high performance actuator system—the muscular structure that holds and controls the eye and its movements— and the neurological and vestibular control system that controls the actuator system.

Kinematics of Eye Movements

The eye can be modeled as a ball and socket mounted, rigid spherical body and eye movements can be described as a series of infinitesimal rotations around three orthogonal axes that intersect in the center of the sphere. Three pairs of extraocular muscles, acting according to the push-pull principle, rotate the eye around these three axes, therefore performing eye movements in three dimensions of rotation: horizontal rotation around the vertical axis, vertical rotation around the horizontal axis, and torsional rotation around the line of sight (Figure 24-1). Eye move-

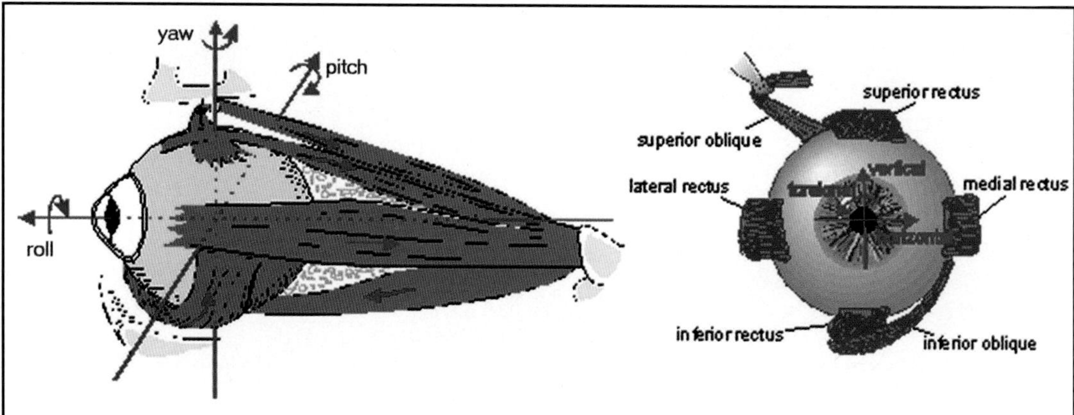

Figure 24-1. Eye movement coordinates and their generation from extraocular muscles.

ment coordinates are normally described in an eye-fixed coordinate system (Euler angles).

The necessity to also control torsional eye position becomes clear if we consider that the same horizontal and vertical rotation of the eye but in different sequence results in a different torsional eye position in space (rotations are not commutative). For example, rotation of first 45 degrees up, then 45 degrees right results in a counterclockwise rotated retinal image; rotation first 45 degrees to the right, then 45 degrees up results in a clockwise rotation of the retinal image. A corrective torsional movement of the eye is therefore required to provide the same orientation of the image on the retina independent from the sequence. As identified more than a hundred years ago by Donders and Listing[3,4] all eye positions during a fixation may be described as a rotation around a single axis from a primary eye position (approximately straight ahead). All rotation axes are lying in a single plane perpendicular to the primary position of the eye (Listing's law) (Figure 24-2).

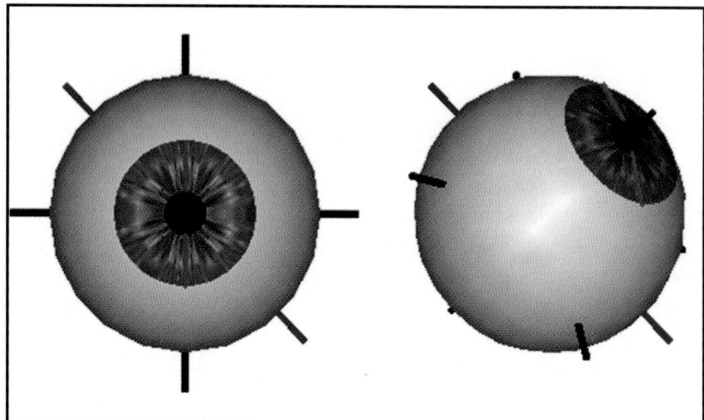

Figure 24-2. Eye rotations according to Listing's law.

Dynamics of Eye Movements

Eye movements are needed for five main purposes and hence are performed at different velocities and angular ranges (Table 24-1)*:

a. Saccades: The eye normally performs fast eye movements (saccades) to jump from one target position to the other (fixation). Peak velocities of saccades are somewhat proportional to the amplitude of the saccade ranging from 10 degrees per second (deg/s) (2 mm/s) to 800 deg/s (170 mm/s).[3] The duration of saccades depends on the amplitude, ranging from 30 milliseconds (ms) for small saccades of 5 degrees to 100 ms or even more for 20 degrees and above
b. Vestibular eye movement stabilizes the retinal image to avoid blurring due to head movements. Linear (translatory) and rotational acceleration of the head are measured by the vestibular system in the inner ear and lead to slow compensatory eye movements up to approximately. 100 deg/s, (21 mm/s), which are often compensated by faster saccades in the range of 100 deg/s to 400 deg/s, (84 mm/s) in the opposite direction if the amplitude of the movement reaches a certain limit (nystagmus). Also static rotations are introduced. Different orientation of the head toward gravity results in a different torsional eye position (ocular counter-roll) in the order of ±7 degrees[14]
c. Pursuit and optokinetic movement stabilize the retinal image due to moving objects relative to the eye. A retinal image slip creates again a pursuit eye movement of up to 40 deg/s (8 mm/s) to follow the target and minimize retinal slip.[8] Movements with larger amplitudes create also fast saccades in the opposite direction, resulting in an optokinetic nystagmus
d. Vergence eye movement removes retinal disparity introduced by looking at objects at different distances and by accommodation (retinal blur).[9] In humans, these are slow eye movements in the order of 10 deg/s (2 mm/s) and are mainly horizontal with amplitudes up to 15 degrees; however, vertical and torsional vergence can be observed by introducing prisms[10]
e. Miniature movements occur while the subject is trying to maintain fixation on a stationary target. These movements consists of three components: 1) tremor, a high frequency movement with a bandwidth up to 90 hertz (Hz),[11] which introduces retinal image movement with velocities in the range of 10 min/s[12] in the range 10 to 40 seconds of arc and comparable in size to the smallest cones on the retina (some 24 seconds of arc); 2) comparatively large but slow drift movement with amplitudes in the range of 5 min and velocities in the region of 4 min/s[13]; and 3) microsaccades in the range of 10 feet and peak velocity in the order of 300 min/s.[12] Therefore, even during a perfect fixation, humans perform eye movements at least within a range of approx-

*Note: Degrees of eye rotation can be calculated as microns at the corneal surface using an assumed center of rotation. There is no one center of rotation, as it differs depending on which direction the eye rotates, but it can be approximated as 15 mm behind the corneal apex (along the optical axis).[5] Therefore, where x is the rotation in degrees, the translational displacement is equal to 15 tan (x degrees).

Table 24-1
Type of Eye Movements and Corresponding Dynamics

TYPE OF MOVEMENT	VELOCITY RANGE	ANGULAR RANGE
Saccades	10 to 800 deg/s; (2 to 170 mm/s)	0.1 to 100 degrees
Vestibular eye movements	<100 deg/s; (21 mm/s); or 100 to 400 deg/s; (21 to 84 mm/s)	1 to 12 degrees
Pursuit and optokinetic movement	<40 deg/s; (8 mm/s)	>1 degree
Vergence eye movements	10 deg/s; (2 mm/s)	Approximately 15 degrees
Miniature movements	10′ to 300′/s; (0.03 to 1 mm/s)	10′′ to 10′; (0.003 to 0.2 degrees)

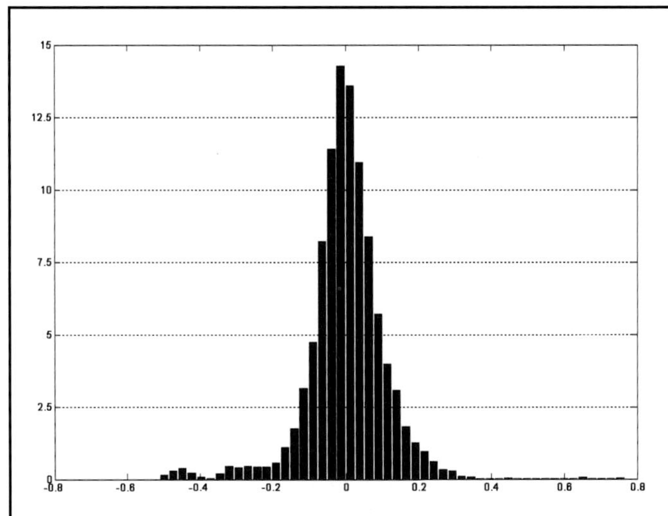

Figure 24-3. Distribution of pupil size changes during laser in-situ keratomileusis (LASIK) surgery for one patient.

imately 0.2 degrees (corresponding to 45 μm on the cornea) and peak velocities of around 5 deg/s (corresponding to 1000 μm/s on the cornea)

Eye Movement Specific to Laser Refractive Surgery

Laser refractive surgery may induce different amounts of eye movements to the amount of eye movement measured during laboratory examination. For example, the patient fixates on a target, which may be difficult to see due to the removal of the flap, or the pharmaceutical dilation of the pupil. The surgeon may also introduce head movements while trying to correct the patient's drifting eye movements. In addition, the mental state of the patient together with auditory cues of the laser during the procedure create distractions from the fixation task.

Schwiegerling and Snyder[14] measured eye movement during LASIK performed with a VISX STAR S2 laser system (Santa Clara, Calif). Videotapes of five surgeries were recorded and the results were analyzed off-line. Eye movement was measured by measuring the displacement of the pupil image in the videotapes. Two of these eyes were decentered by approximately 0.25 mm relative to the axis of treatment, and the standard deviation of eye movement overall was 0.10 mm.

Other aspects of the eye, apart from pure rotation of the globe, also affect the accuracy of beam position on the eye. These factors include the movement of certain features within the globe, such as the pupil. Most alignment and tracking techniques rely on the pupil center as the reference point for alignment. The doctor is recommended to manually align the patient on the line of sight, defined as the broken line passing through the entrance pupil and exit pupil, connecting the point of regard to the foveola.[15] Most automatic tracking systems take advantage of the high contrast between pupil and iris to track on this feature. However, the pupil is not a fixed point relative to the corneal tissue being ablated.

The pupil center does not dilate evenly and the change of pupil center with pupil diameter cannot be predicted.[16,17] A study at SMI measuring 11 patients comparing pupil center relative to fixed markers on the eye between a dilated state (as is common during wavefront measurement) and a natural state (as is common during surgery) showed an average pupil center shift of 0.20 mm and a maximum of 0.60 mm. The change in pupil size between diagnosis and surgery can vary from 8 mm to 3 mm. The natural pupil size during surgery varies significantly less. Figure 24-3 shows the pupil size changes during a typical surgery. Therefore, it can be assumed that the pupil center shift during surgery is also significantly less. Hence, to achieve accurate alignment it is more important to control the axis of alignment between the diagnostic device and the eye-tracking device (ie, pupil center shift between diagnosis and surgery).

Requirements of Eye Tracker to Compensate for Eye Movements

Given that there is an overall requirement for accuracy of beam placement on the cornea (eg, 0.05 mm) and a known expected amount of eye movement, the design requirements for a system that measures and compensates for eye movements can also be derived. Overall accuracy is a combination of the dynamic accuracy of the system and the static accuracy.

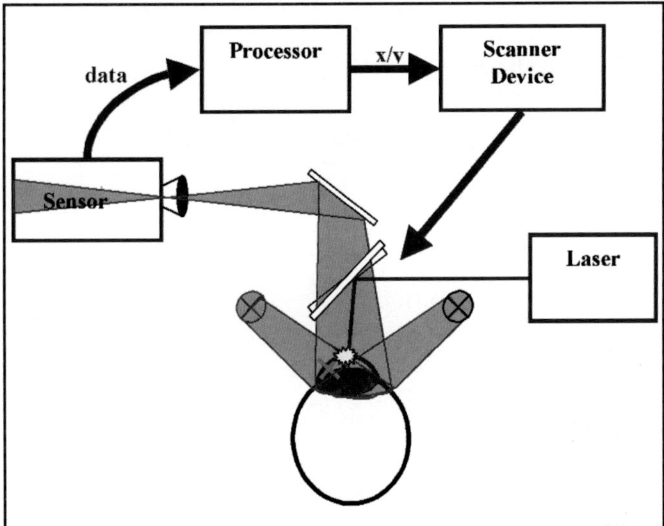

Figure 24-4. Open loop image-based eye tracking system

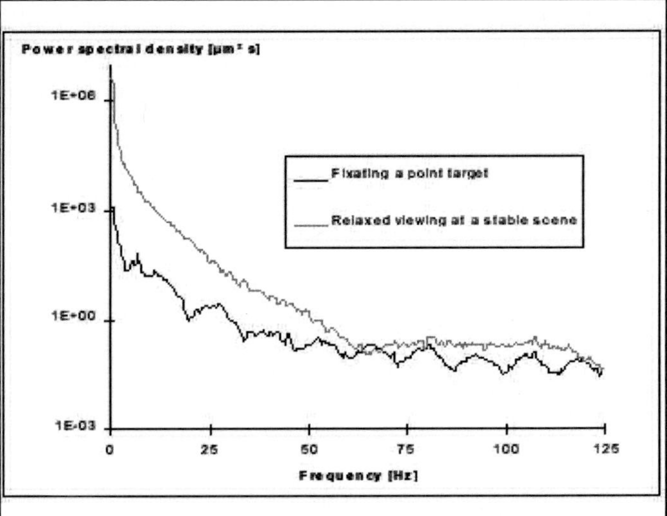

Figure 24-5. Power spectral density of 60 second recordings of horizontal eye-movements fixating a point target (black) and observing a fixed scene image similar to the scene during refractive surgery (gray) (sampling-frequency 250 Hz; binwidth 0.49 Hz, 256 bins; using Parzen-windowing). Standard deviation of horizontal eye movement was 66 µm during fixation and 2.7 mm viewing the visual scene.

Dynamic Accuracy

Dynamic accuracy can be defined as the errors induced by the fact that the target is moving. For example, if the eye position is measured completely accurately, but it takes a certain latency period to move the laser beam to the measured eye position, any eye movement during this latency period will contribute to the overall inaccuracy.

Figure 24-4 shows an open loop image-based eye tracking system. Each step illustrated in this diagram contributes to the overall latency between the eye position and the laser beam compensation.

a. The eye is illuminated and the light imaged on a sensor device
b. This image is transferred from the sensor to a processing device
c. The processor calculates the x,y position from the image and sends it to a scanner
d. The scanner sends a signal to rotate a mirror to redirect the laser beam
e. The laser beam fires and hits the cornea

Knowing the type of eye movements to take into account, now the question is what are the necessary requirements—sampling rate and delay—for measuring them in the context of refractive surgery. One technique is to use the power spectral density* of eye movements (Figure 24-5)—converted already into movement of the cornea—while a subject fixates for 60 seconds either on a single target or viewing relaxed at a fixed picture similar to the scene observed during surgery, which reflects the extreme situation for eye movements during refractive surgery.

This figure shows that if a fixation cannot be performed accurately, then the main energy of eye movements is found below 60 Hz. The above power spectrum also demonstrates that for being able to perform accurate reconstruction of eye movements and avoid aliasing† sampling rates of 200 Hz and above (at least 4 to 5 times higher than the significant power spectrum bandwidth) should be used.

These results were confirmed by a second study, in which 250 Hz eye tracking data was used to simulate the amount of error that that would occur for a given overall delay between eye position measurement and laser shot. Figure 24-6 shows the different scenarios for the same eye movement pattern given a varying amount of latency or delay. For an overall latency of 48 ms, 80% of the shots were within 0.065 mm of the target. This error was reduced to 80% better than 0.007 mm, when latency was reduced to 4 ms. To put this data into context, state-of-the-art video–based tracking systems may have an overall delay of less than 8 ms. A system based on a standard NTSC (60 Hz) camera may have a latency of more than 50 ms.

Static Accuracy

The accuracy of the eye position measurement, independent of eye movement, must also be given due consideration. Static inaccuracy can come from either errors in the feature detection (eg, errors in the image or signal processing required to detect the pupil center or edge) or due to the assumptions used in measuring eye movement. As errors in feature detection depend heavily on the individual system, this section will discuss only errors

*The power spectral density quantifies the size and amount of eye movements within a certain frequency range, calculated via a transformation from time to frequency domain of the recorded eye position data. The unit of the power spectral density is in our case $\mu m^2 s$ or $\mu m^2/Hz$, thus giving a measure for the uncertainty (hence variance) of the eye position related to a given frequency range.

†Aliasing is the effect of measuring power components of higher frequency components in lower frequencies. This occurs due to the limitation of measurement frequencies. In order to avoid aliasing all significant power spectrum components of the signal (eye position data) should be at frequencies significantly below the measurement frequency.

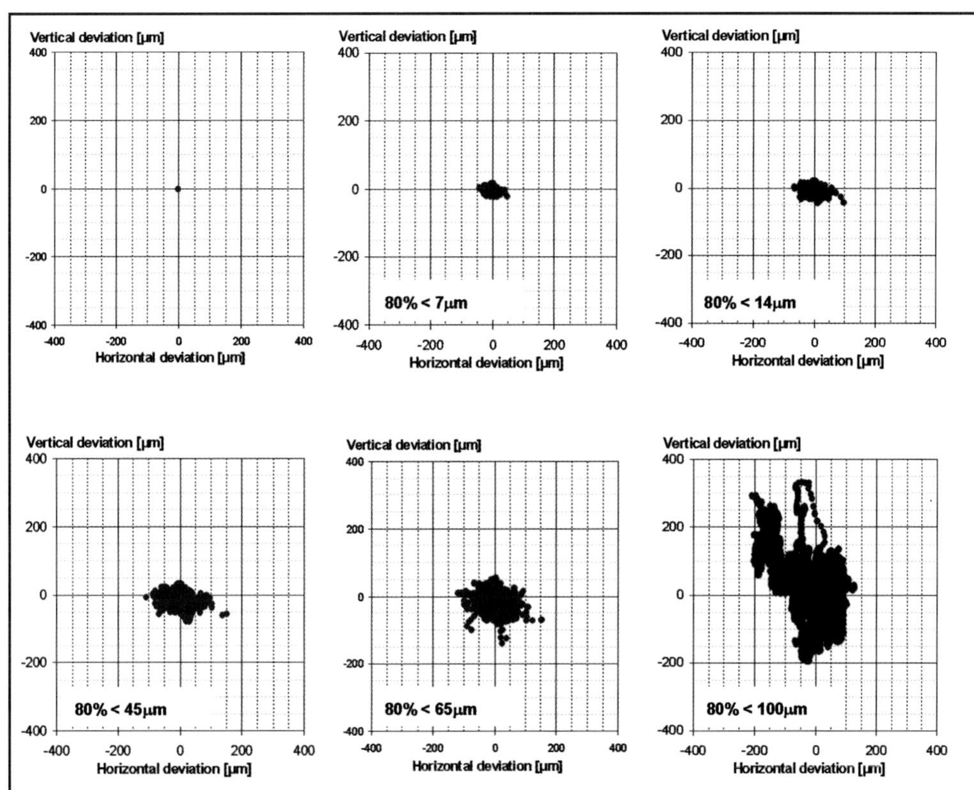

Figure 24-6. Errors for different latency scenarios.

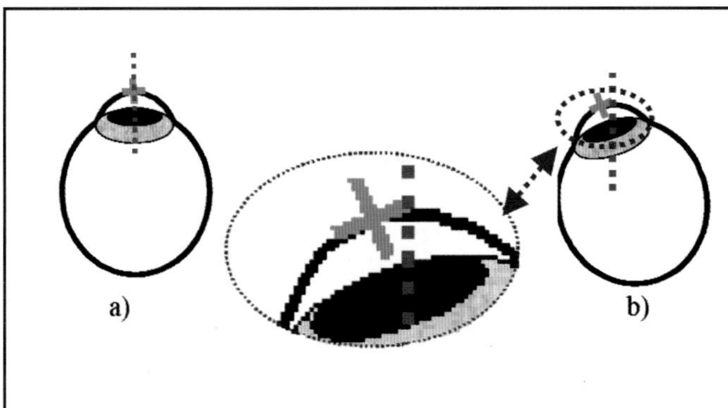

Figure 24-7. Rotation vs translation of the eye.

For an overall latency of 48 ms, 80% of the shots were within 0.065mm of the target. This error was reduced to 80% better than 0.007 mm, when latency was reduced to 4 ms.

There is no eye tracking system that currently actively differentiates between translation and rotation of the eye. Decentration can be minimized by reducing the active or hot zone of the tracking system and switching the laser off when the eye extends beyond this zone, as is done with passive tracking.

due to the assumptions common to most eye tracking systems—assumptions made in tracking a particular feature, such as the pupil.

The eye can move in six different dimensions—translation in x, y, and z; and rotation around x, y, and z, known as pitch, yaw, and roll, respectively—but it is a common assumption to only consider x and y translation movement. Rotation around the x- and y-axis can be approximated as translation, when projected onto a two-dimensional (2-D) image plane. It is a common trait of all refractive surgery eye trackers to track the pupil or to be exact, the projection of the pupil image onto an image plane. Figure 24-7 illustrates the errors caused by this assumption.

In Figure 24-7A, the eye is perfectly aligned and the center of the pupil is aligned to the corneal center (green cross = target for the laser beam). When the whole eye translates (eg, during a translation of the chair), the center of the pupil will remain aligned with the corneal center. Figure 24-7B shows the same eye, rotated around the y-axis. When viewed by the surgeon through the microscope, this rotation will appear like a translation of the pupil center and the corneal center in x. This is the assumption made by all present refractive eye-tracking systems—that eye movement can be approximated by this projected translation. It can be seen in the zoomed view in the middle, that the pupil center underestimates the movement of the corneal surface, as it is a different distance from the center of rotation of the eye. For a rotation of 0.20 degrees or translation of 0.05 mm, this error is only 0.011 mm (calculated assuming a distance of x between pupil and corneal surface). However, for a rotation of 0.80 degrees or 0.20 mm, this error is 0.046 mm and hence significant.

At present, no eye tracking system actively differentiates between rotation and translation of the eye. However, the error

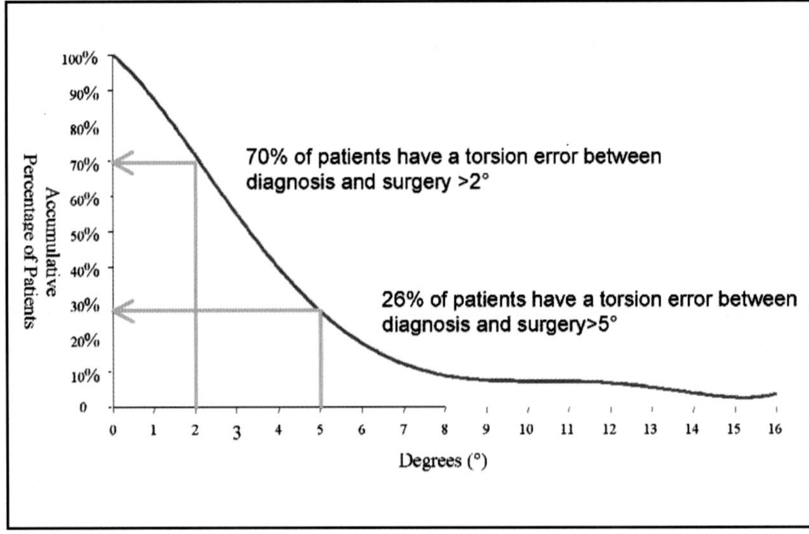

Figure 24-8. Torsion between diagnosis and surgery (n = 46 subjects).

due to this assumption can be minimized by minimizing the active or hot zone of the tracking system. When the eye moves beyond a given threshold, the laser is switched off and the eye realigned (passive tracking).

Errors in measuring eye position may also be caused by ignoring translations in z, or changes in height of the eye. This depends on the focal depth of the imaging system and is worsened when the tracking system is not coaxial.

Rotation around z, or torsion of the eye during fixation, is relatively small within ±1 degree. However, torsion during surgery is also caused by events such as the flap cut, wiping or marking the eye, or small changes in head position. As there is a large change in head position between surgery and diagnosis, the majority of torsion error is caused as a constant offset between the sitting up position during diagnosis and the prone position under the laser. Figure 24-8 shows an accumulative graph of the amount of torsion measured using the iris registration between an auto-refractor and a refractive laser.

> Editor's note:
>
> "Locking on" in the proper position is the most important step in laser surgery registration. You can have an excellent tracker, but if it isn't "locked on" properly, it will be ineffective. To get excellent static accuracy in any system, it is critical that the surgeon "lock on" with the eye centered and fixated.
>
> S. MacRae, MD

Present Eye Tracking Technology

Eye tracking has been used in a variety of applications but the requirements for laser refractive surgery are quite particular. The eye tracker must be fast, reliable, nonintrusive, work on all iris colors, and be insensitive to alignment lights and to the removal of tissue from the cornea. The main techniques applied in refractive surgery can be classified as either open loop or closed loop tracking systems and as either image-based eye tracking systems or photoelectric-based systems.

Open Loop vs Closed Loop Tracking System

A closed loop system uses the output from the previous measurement as input for the new measurement; hence, it closes the loop. An open loop system does not use information from the previous measurement in the new measurement. These two different control techniques have different affects on both the dynamic requirement of the eye tracking system and the robustness of the eye tracking system.

Strictly speaking, an open loop system does not track or follow the eye. Instead, an open loop system aims to take a snapshot of the eye position as close as possible in time to the laser shot. It is not necessary for an open loop system to follow every eye movement, but instead to have a very small delay between eye position measurement and laser shot. Saccades that occur between laser shots may be safely ignored. Therefore, for an open loop eye tracking system, the most important "speed" factor is delay or latency. A closed loop system must capture every movement of the eye to keep locked onto the eye; therefore, for a closed loop system, the most important factor is frequency. The required frequency to capture the eye movements can be derived from the power spectrum shown in Figure 24-5.

> Therefore, for an open loop eye tracking system the most important "speed" factor is delay or latency. A closed loop system must capture every movement of the eye to keep locked onto the eye; therefore, for a closed loop system, the most important factor is frequency. An objective performance comparison should be based on the resulting dynamic accuracy.

As these requirements for the two systems are different, the best way to compare the "speed" of the systems is to compare the resulting dynamic accuracy. The dynamic accuracy of a synchronized 250 hertz (Hz) open-loop system with a delay of 8 ms is shown in Figure 24-6—80% of shots better than 14 µm. The dynamic accuracy of a 4 kilahertz (kHz) closed-loop system is approximately 1 µm, with a peak position error of 30 mm during fast saccades.[18]

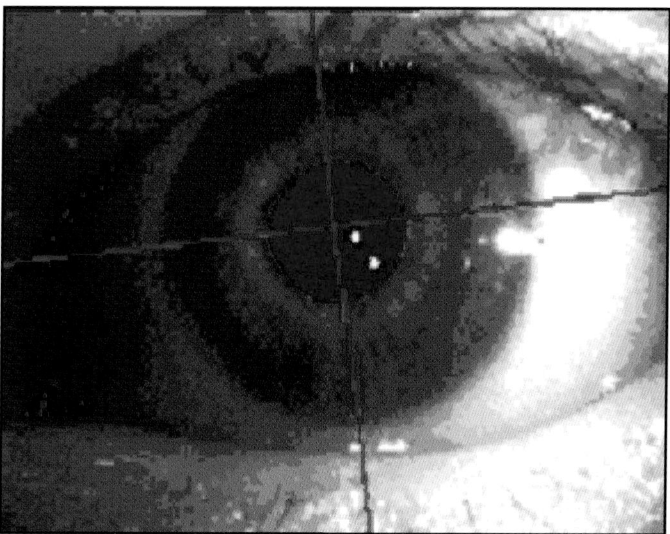

Figure 24-9. Tracked eye with dark pupil tracker for x, y coordinates and ocular torsion using the three-dimensional (3-D) VOG system by SensoMotoric Instruments (Boston, Mass).

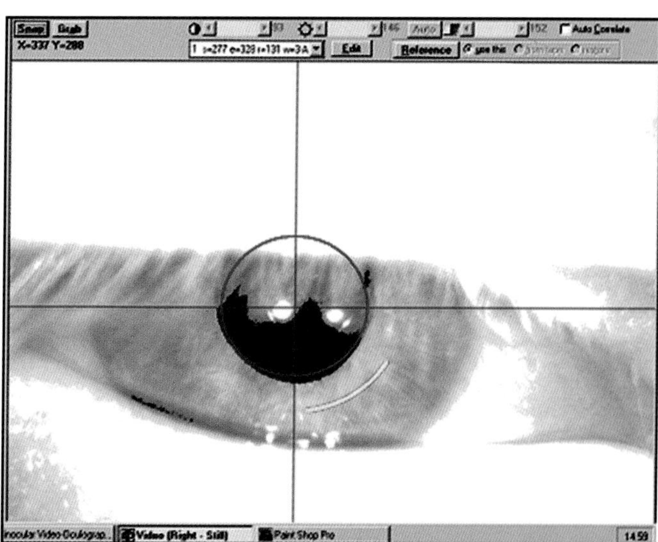

Figure 24-10. Detection of partly occluded eye with image processing using the 3-D VOG system by SensoMotoric Instruments.

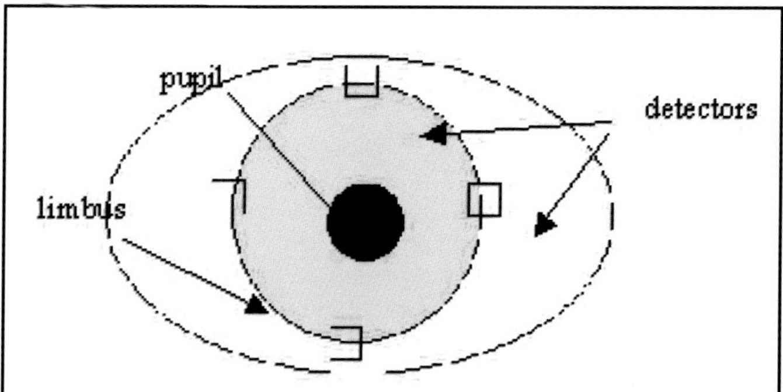

Figure 24-11. Detector array for limbus tracking used in IRVision AccuScan 2000 (San Jose, Calif).

The decision whether to use open loop or closed loop tracking also affects the stability or robustness of the eye tracking system. As an open loop system does not use information from the previous measurement, it is unlikely to "lose track" when a doctor's hand or instrument is placed between the eye and the tracking system.

Image-Based (Digital) Systems

In image-based eye tracking, infrared (IR) light illuminates the eye and IR sensitive cameras acquire the eye image. If the axis of the illumination and the camera differ significantly, the pupil is a sink for IR light and appears dark on the image. (If the IR illumination and camera are close to or on the same optical axis, the IR light is reflected by the retina and the pupil appears light on the image.) The dark pupil approach is more commonly used in refractive surgery, since it is more robust in illumination set-up. Figure 24-9 shows a typical dark pupil-tracking situation with cross hair overlay for pupil center and tilt of cross hair for torsion of the eye around the visual axis.

With more powerful imaging sensors and processing units and more sophisticated algorithms for determining the pupil center and the limbus, video eye tracking is getting increasingly robust and insensitive to a broad range of disturbances, changes of the illumination, and image quality during refractive surgery.

The following image (Figure 24-10) shows an example of a partly occluded eye, in which the pupil is still detected.

Image-based tracking also has the advantage of improved static accuracy using enhanced image processing. Measuring both pupil and limbus in the same image can compensate errors caused by pupil center shift. Misalignment caused by ocular cyclotorsion between diagnosis and surgery can also be compensated using iris registration.

Although it is technically feasible to use image-based systems as a closed loop system, most are open loop tracking systems.

Photoelectric-Based (Analog) Systems

Photoelectric analog techniques detect eye movement from changes in reflected light. Either focused spots, slits, or rings of light are projected onto the cornea, and the response from multiple light detectors is analyzed using analog signal processing techniques. Figure 24-11 shows the configuration of one such tracker detector array. Either the pupil/iris border or the limbus is monitored. If the pupil is tracked, it is generally back-lit to maximize contrast and dilated to minimize interference from the procedure itself. The limbus does not suffer these limitations, as it is located further away from the surgical zone.

Because analog methods are used, the frequency response can be very high (eg, 4 kHZ), which lends these techniques to closed loop tracking systems. On the other side, these techniques tend to measure only a limited number of points on the eye, such as the four spots to define the pupil shown in Figure 24-11, compared to the approximately 75,000 points measured by a high- speed video system. This may result in a lower measurement resolution, and limits these systems to 2 diopter (D) translation tracking.

Conclusion

Eye trackers are a basic requirement of laser refractive surgery and essential for optimal correction. In the quest—not only for ideal corrections but also for reliable repeatable results for all patients—more accurate centration is required. To be certain that the alignment of the patient's eye is sufficiently accurate, several factors need to be considered:

- Accurate registration between diagnosis and surgery, including compensation for pupil center shift and cyclotorsion (mean values 0.20 mm and 3.40 degrees measured from clinical trials)
- Pupil size changes and hence pupil center shift during surgery
- Eye movement measured as the translation of the projected image of the pupil (mean 0.25 mm)
- Rotation versus translation (0.00 to 0.25 mm for eye movement between 0 to 1 mm)
- Rotation around z (torsion) during surgery (0 to 1 degree based on a fixating eye in laboratory conditions)
- Height (z translation)
- Dynamic accuracy of the system (80% < 0.014 mm based on high-speed video-based system)

When the typical values for each of these factors (shown in brackets above) are summed together, the goal of 0.45 mm to ensure at least a consistent optical quality after refractive surgery does not seem so modest! Each of these factors must be carefully controlled to ensure that the desired refractive correction is aligned correctly to the eye, accurately enough to ensure a successful and repeatable visual outcome. Present eye tracking systems control some dimensions of alignment and tracking automatically, repeatably, and objectively and have been demonstrated to improve optical outcome.[21] Until eye tracking systems can control all of these factors, the clinician should be aware of how each of these considerations can affect the alignment and hence the visual outcome, and actively work to monitor and control the alignment of the patient's eye. The fully automatic six dimensional high-speed eye alignment system integrated into both the diagnostic and surgical device, however, is the ultimate goal for controlled consistent customized surgery.

> Most patients move their eye only minimally during surgery. Therefore, it is important that the laser "locks on" and gets excellent correspondence between the axis and the orientation of the eye measured by wavefront sensor and the axis and orientation of the eye identified by the eye tracker during ablation.

As the science and technology behind refractive surgery and customized ablation improves so too will the eye tracking and alignment systems. The goal of not only an "ideal correction," but reliable repeatable results for all patients will be reached not just by faster eye trackers, but also by smart imaging technology eye trackers.

Acknowledgements

We would like to acknowledge the cooperative work of our clients, especially within the eye movement research field, who made this work possible, as well as all our colleagues at SensoMotoric Instruments.

References

1. Guirao A, Williams DR, Cox IG. Effect of rotation and translation on the expected benefit of an ideal method to correct the eye's higher-order aberrations. *Opt Soc Am A*. 2001;18(5).
2. Bueeler M, Mrochen M, Seiler T. Required accuracy of lateral and torsional alignment in aberration sensing and wavefront guided treatments. Proceedings of SPIE. Vol. 4611: 185-196, In: Manns F, Soederberg PG, Ho A, eds. *Ophthalmic Technologies XII*. 2002:185-196.
3. Donders FC. Beitrag zur Lehre von Bewegungen des menschlichen Auges, Holländische Beiträge zu den anatomischen und psychologischen. *Wissenschafte*. 1847;1:101-145, 384-386.
4. Listing, JB. *Beitrag zu Physiologischen Optik*. Vandenhoeck & Ruprecht: Göttingen; 1845.
5. Atchison DA, Smith G. *Optics of the Human Eye*. Oxford, United Kingdom: Butterworth-Heinemann; 2000.
6. Bahill AT, Clark, MR, Stark L. Glissades-eye movements generated by mismatched components of the saccadic motoneuronal control signal. *Mathematical Biosciences*. 1975;26:303-318.
7. Miller EF. Counterrolling of the human eyes produced by head tilt with respect to gravity. *Acta Otolaryngol*. 1962;54:479-501.
8. Honrubia V, Scott BJ, Ward PH. Experimental studies on optokinetic nystagmus. I. Normal cats. *Acta Otolaryngol*. 1967;65:441-448.
9. Müller J. *Zur vergleichenden Physiologie des Gesichtssinnes*. Leipzig, Germany: C. Cnobloch; 1826.
10. Helmholtz H. *Handbuch der Physiologischen Optik*. 1st ed. Voss, Hamburg; 1867. [3rd edition translated by Southall JPC for the Optical Society of America (1924)].
11. Findlay JM. Frequency analysis of human involuntary eye movement. *Kybernetik*. 1971;8:207-214.
12. Ditchburn RW. The functions of small saccades. *Vision Res*. 1980;20:271-272.
13. Ditchburn, RW. *Eye-movements and Visual Perception*. Oxford, United Kingdom: Clarendon Press; 1973.
14. Schwiegerling J, Snyder RW. Eye movement during laser in situ keratomileusis. *J Cataract Refract Surg*. 2000;26(3):345-351.
15. Applegate RA, Thibos LN, Bradley A, et al. Reference axis selection: subcommittee report of the OSA working group to establish standards for measurement and reporting of optical aberrations of the eye. *J Refract Surg*. 2000;16:S656-S658.
16. Loewenfeld IE, Newsome DA. Iris mechanics I. Influence of pupil size on dynamics of pupillary movements. *Am J Ophthalmol*. 1971; 71:347-362.
17. Wilson MA, Campbell MCW, Simonet P. Change of pupil centration with change of illumination and pupil size. *Technical Digest on Ophthalmic and Visual Optics*. 1991;220-223.
18. Krueger RR. In perspective: eye tracking and Autonomous LADAR radar. *J Refract Surg*. 1999;15:145-149.
19. Mrochen M, Eldine MS, Kaemmerer M, Seiler T, Hutz W. Improvement in photorefractive corneal laser surgery results using an active eye-tracking system. *J Cataract Refract Surg*. 2001;27(7): 1000-1006.

Chapter 25
Wound Healing in Customized Corneal Ablation: Effect on Predictability, Fidelity, and Stability of Refractive Outcomes

Joel A.D. Javier, MD; Puwat Charukamnoetkanok, MD; and Dimitri T. Azar, MD

Introduction: Basic Aspects of Corneal Wound Healing

Customized Corneal Ablation

Innovations in an evolving field of refractive surgery have made possible the customization of laser vision correction based on the ability to detect and correct higher-order optical abnormalities (wavefront errors) beyond simple sphere and cylinder. The goal of refractive surgery can now include enhancement of visual performance beyond Snellen acuity of 20/20 by improving retinal image resolution and contrast. This potential for better than the natural best corrected visual acuity has been termed *super vision*.[1] Customized ablation may also improve our ability to treat the patients who are disappointed with the outcomes of their refractive surgeries despite excellent visual acuity because of complaints related to decrease in quality of vision such as glare, halo, and reduced contrast sensitivity. Furthermore, customized corneal ablation will benefit patients whose eyes have irregular or atypical aberrations as the results of postkeratoplasty astigmatism, corneal scarring, decentered ablations, central islands, or lenticular abnormalities.

Wound Healing Responses After Photorefractive Keratectomy, Laser In-Situ Keratomileusis, and Laser Epithelial Keratomileusis

Currently, there are three potential refractive surgical procedures that may be used for customized corneal ablation: photorefractive keratectomy (PRK), laser assisted in-situ keratomileusis (LASIK), and laser assisted subepithelial keratomileusis (LASEK) (Figure 25-1). It is not known which procedure will deliver the best fidelity of transmitting the intended correction to the anterior corneal surface (tear film, epithelium, and anterior stroma). This is, in part, due to the qualitative and quantitative differences in three major aspects of wound healing following these procedures: scarring (fibroblast proliferation), epithelial hyperplasia, and collagen deposition.

In PRK, the corneal epithelium is mechanically or photoablatively removed and the anterior cornea is ablated to correct the refractive error.[2] This results in the greatest degree of scarring and epithelial hyperplasia. Furthermore, interindividual variability of wound healing is greatest after PRK. In LASIK, a corneal flap is first raised, the underlying stroma is ablated, and the flap is repositioned.[3,4] Despite the relatively small degree of scarring and epithelial hyperplasia after LASIK, the thickness and irregularity of the flap may mitigate the benefits of customized ablation.[5] In LASEK, the corneal epithelial adhesion to the underlying Bowman's layer is chemically reduced by the application of diluted ethanol, the underlying stroma is exposed and ablated, and the epithelial sheet is returned to cover the ablated corneal surface.[6-8] It is not known, at the time of this writing, whether the degree of scarring and epithelial hyperplasia are reduced after LASEK as compared to PRK.

> Interindividual variability of wound healing is greatest after PRK.

Although the wound healing response after refractive surgery may sometimes be undesirable, it aims to restore the structural integrity of the injured tissues. An important determinant of the visual outcome of patients undergoing refractive surgery is our ability to predict and compensate for the eye's biologic response to laser surgery. While better understanding of wound healing response is crucial for first generation refractive surgeries, it is indispensable for customized corneal ablation. Biological variability of wound healing confounds and modifies intended results of corneal topography-coupled or wavefront-guided excimer laser ablation.

Clinical Implication of Corneal Wound Healing

Scarring (fibroblast proliferation), cellular hyperplasia, and collagen deposition coexist during the eye's response to laser; however, they confer distinct effects on refraction and aberration profiles. The scarring or haze leads to a decrease of contrast sensitivity. The irregular deposition of cells or collagen is responsible for treatment regression or generation of higher-order optical aberrations.

> The irregular deposition of cells or collagen is responsible for treatment regression or generation of higher-order optical aberrations.

A pharmacologic approach to modifying the complex corneal wound healing cascade has been tried to suppress subepithelial haze and regression after ablation. While available wound heal-

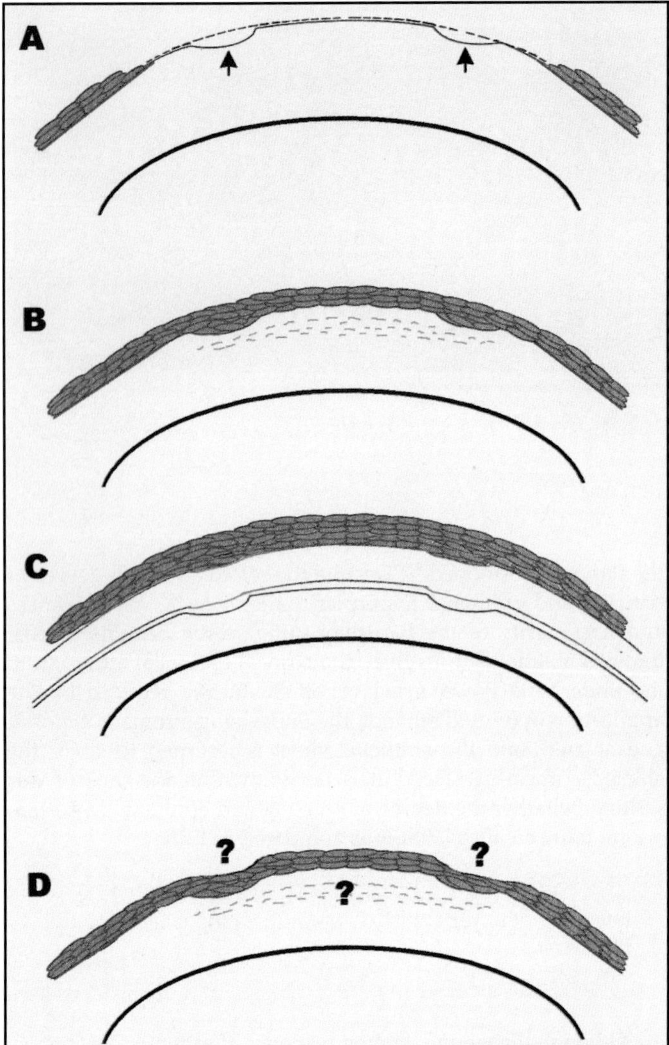

Figure 25-1. Potential effect of corneal wound healing on customized corneal ablation. (A) Customized vs noncustomized ablation: the simulation of PRK includes hypothetical additional ablative pattern (arrows) designed to correct higher-order aberrations. The corresponding noncustomized ablation is indicated by the dotted line. (B) Post-PRK healing: there is epithelial hyperplasia at the site of the custom alterations that tends to mask the custom effect. Stromal remodeling (green broken lines) may also influence these alterations. (C) Post-LASIK healing: In LASIK, the flap may diminish the benefit of customized ablation and contribute to higher-order aberrations. (D) Post-LASEK healing: it is not known whether the degrees of scarring and epithelial hyperplasia are reduced after LASEK as compared to PRK. (Adapted from Wilson SE, Mohan RR, Hong JW, Lee JS, Choi R. The wound healing response after laser in situ keratomileusis and photorefractive keratectomy: elusive control of biological variability and effect on custom laser vision correction. *Arch Ophthalmol.* 2001;119(6): 889-896.)

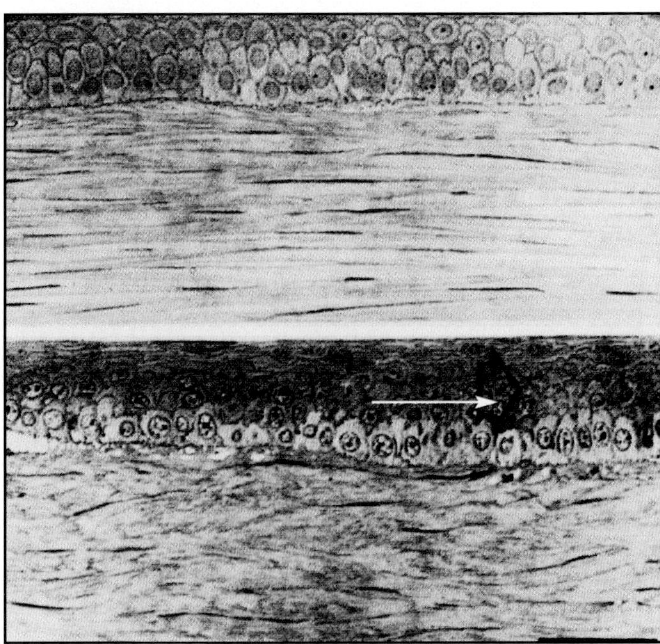

Figure 25-2. Light micrographs of the interface between corneal epithelium and stroma (monkey) in areas of excimer laser ablation 6 months after exposure. Top: central area of ablation. Bottom: peripheral area of ablation. Top: Notice the regularity of the basal organization in the central areas as well as a near normal number of cells in the overlying epithelium. Bottom: An increase in the number of layers of cells within the epithelium is seen at the edge of the ablation. The arrow indicates the direction of the lesion center. Bars = 50 microns (µm). (Courtesy of Marshall J, Trokel SL, Rothery S, Krueger RR. Long-term healing of the central cornea after photorefractive keratectomy using an excimer laser. *Ophthalmology.* 1988;95(10):1411-1421.)

ing modulating agents such as corticosteroid and antimetabolites (Mitomycin C) are effective,[9-13] they are nonspecific and have many potentially dangerous side effects. Surgical techniques can also be modified to modulate wound healing to clinical advantage. A detailed understanding of various cellular and molecular processes that regulate the wound healing responses to laser will lead to adjunct therapeutic strategies that may mitigate the adverse effects and more precisely modulate refractive outcomes. With these insights, surgeons can confidently plan a laser ablation profile, knowing that the results will be more predictable and reproducible. We can then truly realize the worthy goal of "super vision" in the unaided eyes.

Epithelial Wound Healing

Following 6 millimeter (mm) excimer ablation of the human cornea, epithelial cells migrate over the wound within 1 to 3 days.[14-16] Data from studies of animal and human corneal wound healing following excimer laser keratectomy have shown that there is a tendency for the epithelium to undergo hyperplasia over the ablation bed, which is more pronounced in nontapered ablations (Figure 25-2).[14,17-24] Additionally, the epithelial surface does not totally reflect surface irregularities of the stromal ablation bed.[20-23]

> There is a tendency for the epithelium to undergo hyperplasia over the ablation bed, which is more pronounced in nontapered ablations.

In epithelial defects that do not involve the basement membrane, reformation of corneal epithelial adhesion promptly follows epithelial resurfacing.[24,25] Adhesion structure reformation, however, is delayed for up to 2 to 3 months following keratectomy wounds that go below the basement membrane.[25,26] Electron microscopy (EM) and immunolocalization of hemidesmosomes, basement membrane, and anchoring fibril components provide evidence of synchronous reappearance of the adhesion structures following keratectomy wounds.[26-35] Postexcimer EM analyses of corneal epithelial basement membrane zones in monkey eyes have shown discontinuities, duplication, and thickening of the basement membrane as late as 18 months postoperatively.[2,14,17,18,36,37] Normalization of the basement membrane and hemidesmosomal attachments were seen only at 9 months after wounding.

Data from keratoplasty specimens[38] showed that, after excimer laser, 29% of cells had normal basement membrane at 6 months, compared with 86% at 15 months. Multilamellar basement membrane was seen in one cornea. Anchoring fibrils were initially decreased but increased gradually after 6 months. Irregular collagen peaked at 9 months, which coincided with the reduction of keratocytes adjacent to the wound. These data corroborate the findings of previous studies and suggest that significant alterations of corneal epithelial adhesion and basement membrane persist after 6 months and do not normalize until 1 year.

Laminin, present in normal corneas in and below the basement membrane, was immunolocalized to the anterior stroma as early as 1 week after wounding.[14] It concentrated in the basement membrane zone by 3 months and continued to show discontinuities as late as 18 months after excimer wounding. Type III collagen, ordinarily seen in corneal scars but not in normal cornea, began to appear below the epithelium 3 weeks postoperatively and persist in the anterior stroma.

Bowman's layer, a cellular, fibrotic collagen layer, does not regenerate once it's ablated, and its edges retain their tapered appearance after a graded ablation. The exact physiologic role of Bowman's layer is not clear. A long-standing, but experimentally unproven, hypothesis has been that this layer provides an important contribution to the biomechanical stability of the cornea. Histologically, this point of view was easily accepted because the collagen fibers in Bowman's layer are omnidirectionally oriented and strongly interwoven. However, experiments of uniaxial stress-strain analysis performed on the human cadaver eyes showed that Bowman's layer does not contribute significantly to corneal stability.[39]

Stromal Wound Healing

Phases of Stromal Wound Healing

Concomitant with the epithelial wound healing, the process of stromal wound healing commences but often lasts for a longer time period. Stromal wound healing occurs in four phases (Figure 25-3). In the first phase, the keratocytes adjacent to the area of epithelial debridement undergo apoptosis, leaving a zone devoid of cells. This cell death has been suggested to initiate the healing response.[40,41]

In the second phase, the keratocytes immediately adjacent to the area of cell death proliferate to repopulate the wound area. In rat corneas, proliferation occurs 24 to 48 hours after wounding. As part of the second phase of stromal wound healing, the keratocytes transform into fibroblasts and migrate into the wound area. This migration may take up to a week. Transformation of keratocytes to fibroblasts can be visualized at the molecular level as reorganization of the actin cytoskeleton (with development of stress fibers and focal adhesion structures) and activation of new genes encoding extracellular matrix (ECM) components such as fibronectin, ECM adhesion molecule, α5 integrin, ECM-degrading metalloproteins (MMPs), and cytokines.

This same transition occurs when keratocytes are isolated from the corneal stroma and cultured in serum-containing medium; by the time these cells are subcultured, they have acquired the fibroblast phenotype. The migratory repair fibroblasts (filamentous-actin positive) are elongated, spindle shaped, highly reflective and are present in the wound edge and within the wound. Repair fibroblasts turn on the synthesis of the α5 integrin chain that results in formation of the α5b1 integrin heterodimer, the classic fibronectin receptor. This occurs concomitant with deposition of fibronectin in the wound area. Synthesis of dermatan sulfate proteoglycan increases whereas lumican synthesis decreases. In addition to depositing extracellular matrix, repair fibroblasts synthesize several matrix MMPs including MMP-1, -2, -3, and -9, and -14 (MT1-MMP).

> In addition to depositing extracellular matrix, repair fibroblasts synthesize several MMPs.

Freshly isolated keratocytes differ from subcultured cells, or from migratory repair fibroblasts, in their incompetence to synthesize collagenase in response to treatment with agents that stimulate remodeling of the actin cytoskeleton, such as phorbol myristate acetate (PMA) or cytochalasin B (CB).[42] Collagenase expression requires activation of an autocrine interleukin (IL) 1α feedback loop, which in turn requires two different stimuli. Agents such as CB or PMA provide an initial stimulus. However, in order for the positive feedback amplification to occur, cells must subsequently be responsive to the stimulation from their self-generated IL-1 (autocrine pathway). The incompetence for expression of IL-1α by fresh corneal stromal cells is the result of failure to activate the transcription factor NF-kB. Interestingly, NF-kB regulates many cell functions with potential to disturb corneal structure, including expression of inflammatory, stress, degradative proteinase genes, apoptosis, and cell replication. Therefore, NF-kB regulatory pathway likely represents an important mechanism for maintaining corneal homeostasis and preserving functions.[43]

In the third phase of stromal wound healing, fibroblasts may be transformed into myofibroblasts (evidenced by α smooth muscle actin staining). This occurs primarily after incisional wounds. Myofibroblasts appear as stellate cells, are highly reflective, but are limited to within the wound area. The extent of transformation into myofibroblasts seems to be dependent on the type of wound. In general, gaping wounds and wounds that remove Bowman's membrane result in greater myofibroblast generation than wounds that do not penetrate Bowman's layer. Myofibroblast transformation may take up to a month to become apparent.

> In general, gaping wounds and wounds that remove Bowman's membrane result in greater myofibroblast generation than wounds that do not penetrate Bowman's layer.

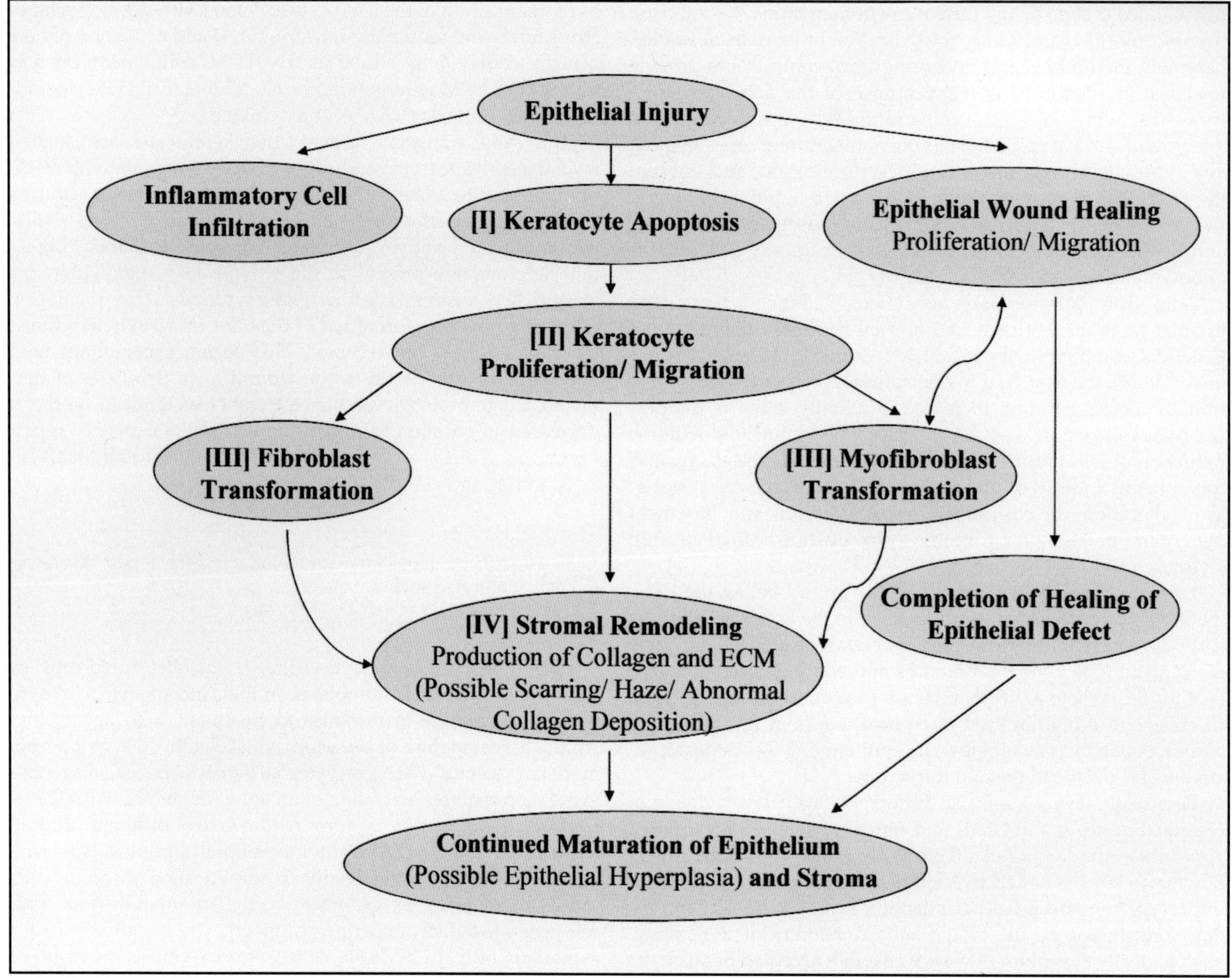

Figure 25-3. Schematic of wound healing after excimer ablation. To simplify the diagram, only important events are illustrated. The four phrases of stromal wound healing are: [I] Keratocytes adjacent to epithelial debridement undergo apoptosis. [II] Keratocytes (fibroblasts) repopulate area adjacent to the apoptosis site. [III] Keratocytes transform into fibroblasts or myofibroblasts. [IV] Stromal remodeling occurs. Although exact details remain to be studied, the inflammatory cells likely play important roles throughout the healing process (not shown).

The final (fourth) phase of stromal healing involves stromal remodeling and is greatly dependent on the original wound. Wounds that have completely healed contain few if any myofibroblasts, presumably because they revert to the fibroblast phenotype or undergo apoptosis during wound healing.[44] This may take a year or more.

Factors Involved in Wound Healing After Excimer Laser Surgery

Cytokines communication between corneal epithelial cells and stromal fibroblasts is complex but can be grouped into four general patterns (Table 25-1).[45,46] Although these patterns are based on in vitro studies and represent simplified and incomplete model of epithelium-stromal interaction, they provide useful conceptual framework for understanding the complex cellular regulation by cytokines during wound healing. In Type I pattern of signaling, the corneal epithelium exclusively produces cytokines that act predominantly on stromal fibroblasts (TGFα, IL-1β, and PDGF-β). In Type II pattern, there is a reciprocal communication between the epithelium and stromal fibroblasts in which both cell types produce cytokines and their receptors (IGF-1, TGF-β1, TGF-β2, LIF, and bFGF). In Type III pattern, stromal fibroblasts produce cytokines that affect the corneal epithelium (KGF and HGF). Finally, in Type IV pattern, the epithelium and stromal fibroblasts produce and release cytokines whose receptors are expressed only by inflammatory or immune cells (M-CSF and IL-8). Lacrimal gland cells also synthesize and secrete cytokines such as EGF and TGF-α< which influence corneal wound healing.

Transforming growth factor (TGF)-β and basic fibroblast growth factor (bFGF, FGF-2) have opposing effects on the stromal cell phenotype during wound healing and in culture conditions. TGF-β1 (and activin A) stimulates myofibroblast differentiation.[47-49] Cytokines such as FGF-2 and platelet-derived growth factor (PDGF) inhibit such transformation.[44,50] In addition, FGF-2 has been shown to induce conversion of myofibroblasts to the fibroblast phenotype.[51] The opposing effects of FGF-2 and TGF-

Table 25-1
Patterns of Epithelial-Fibroblast Interaction Mediated by Cytokines

Type I	*Epithelium secretes:* TGF-a IL-1ß PDGF-ß	*Receptors in fibroblasts for:* EGFR IL-1R PDGFR-ß
Type II	*Epithelium and fibroblasts secrete and have receptors for:* IGF-1, TGF-β1, TGF-β2, LIF, bFGF	
Type III	*Fibroblasts secrete:* KGF HGF	*Receptors in epithelium for:* KGFR HGFR (c-met)
Type IV	*Epithelium or fibroblasts secrete:* M-CSF IL-8	*Receptors in immune cells for:* M-CSFR IL-8R

TGF = transforming growth factor; EGFR = epidermal growth factor receptor; IL = interleukin; IL-1ß = interleukin-1 receptor; PDGR = platelet-derived growth factor; PDGF-ß = platelet-derived growth factor receptor; IGF = insulin-like growth factor; LIF = leukemia inhibitory factor; bFGF (FGF-2) = basic fibroblast growth factor; KGF = keratinocyte growth factor; HGF = hepatocyte growth factor; HGFR (c-met) = hepatocyte growth factor receptor; M-CSF = macrophage colony-stimulating factor; M-CSFR = macrophage colony-stimulating factor receptor; IL-8R = interleukin-8-receptor.

Adapted from Li DQ, Tseng SC. Three patterns of cytokine expression potentially involved in epithelial-fibroblast interactions of human ocular surface. *J Cell Physiol.* 1995;163:61-79.

ß are consistent with the findings that these two growth factors participate in different signaling pathways and that these pathways converge on the regulation of Smad proteins downstream to the TGF-β receptors (TβRI and TβRII).[51-54]

> TGF-β and bFGF, FGF-2 have opposing effects on the stromal cell phenotype during wound healing and in culture conditions. TGF-β1 stimulates myofibroblast differentiation. Cytokines such as FGF-2 and PDGF inhibit such transformation.

In culture, if the fibroblasts are confluent, addition of TGF-β does not induce myofibroblast differentiation.[55] This density-dependent differentiation correlates with the finding that high-density cells express fewer receptors (Tβ RI and Tβ RII) than low-density cells.[56]

Matrix Metalloproteins in Corneal Wound Healing

Corneal wound healing is a complex process that relies on the interplay of proteinases and their inhibitors for proper ECM remodeling. MMPs are thought to play a major role in ECM remodeling during corneal development and wound healing. Several MMPs have been identified in the cornea, and their expression has been characterized during wound healing. We have previously published our work on MMPs that are present in rat corneal cells: MMP-14, MMP-13, and MMP-12.[57-59]

Under our experimental conditions, the corneal re-epithelialization usually occurred 0 to 4 days after wounding. We have demonstrated that MMP-13 was localized to basal epithelial cells in the leading edge of wounded corneas at 6 hours and in the wound area at 1 and 3 days after surgery, but not in normal rat corneas. Using reverse transcription polymerase chain reaction (RT-PCR), we confirmed that MMP-13 is expressed in the regenerating rat corneal epithelium 18 hours and 3 days after wounding but not in normal epithelium. The temporal and spatial correlation between MMP-13 and corneal re-epithelialization suggests that MMP-13 plays a role in re-epithelialization after corneal wounding.

> The temporal and spatial correlation between MMP-13 and corneal re-epithelialization suggests that MMP-13 plays a role in re-epithelialization after corneal wounding.

In contrast, MMP-14 was expressed in both normal and wounded corneas. In situ hybridization has localized MMP-13 mRNA to migrating basal epithelial cells and MMP-14 predominantly to superficial stromal keratocytes in the wound area. Similar findings have been reported during rat skin wound healing. Rat MMP-13 (collagenase III), originally named rat collagenase,[60,61] shares 86% identity with human MMP-13 at the amino acid level but not with human collagenase I (MMP-1).[62] Collagenase I expression has been shown in fibroblasts, macrophages, chondrocytes, and certain tumor cells.[63] On the contrary, we found that collagenase III (MMP-13) is expressed in the corneal epithelium but not in the stroma.

Collagenase I (MMP-1) is expressed in human and rabbit mesenchymal and epithelial cell types.[60,64,65] Fini and colleagues, however, have found data to the contrary in that there was no evidence indicating the presence or synthesis of MMP-1 in injured rat corneas.[64]

Human gelatinase B (MMP-9) is activated by MMP-13 in vitro.[66] Our previous experiments[58,67] showed MMP-9 localization to the basal epithelial cells in corneas after wounding. We demonstrated the colocalization of MMP-9 and MMP-13 in a time dependent fashion and provided the first line of evidence that MMP-13 may play a part in MMP-9 activation in vivo.

MMP-14 plays a role in MMP-2 activation.[68,69] In a previous study,[58,67] we demonstrated the low level expression of MMP-2 wounded and unwounded epithelia and also in normal stroma. MMP-2 was shown to be predominantly expressed by superficial stromal keratocytes after excimer keratectomy. Interestingly, we were able to demonstrate MMP-14 to have a similar stromal expression pattern. This suggests that MMP-14 is a possible pro-MMP-2 activator at the stromal cell surface. We can also hypothesize that MMP-14 may play a role in the maintenance of the normal balance between ECM synthesis and degradation during normal ECM turnover and during connective tissue restoration in wound healing.

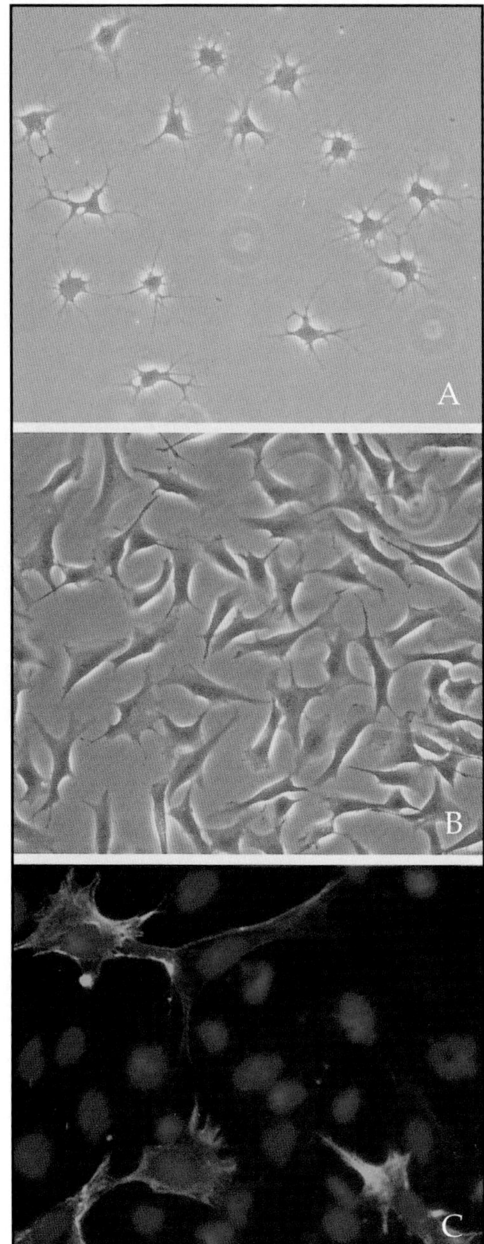

Figure 25-4. (A) Examples of keratocytes grown in serum free medium. (B) Keratocytes that have been transformed into a fibroblastic phenotype. (C) Myofibroblast phenotype is demonstrated by alpha smooth muscle actin staining (green). The nuclei are stained by propidium iodine (red).

Biological Differences Between Wound Healing in LASIK and PRK/LASEK

Several complex cytokine-mediated interactions exist between epithelial cells and active and inactive keratocytes during the wound healing process after refractive surgery. Injured epithelial cells, sustained in the creation of a LASIK flap and during epithelial debridement and removal in PRK and LASEK, release cytokines such as IL-1/IL-1 receptor and Fas/Fas ligand.[70-72] Evidence from Wilson and associates[72] have suggested that IL-1 mediated production of Fas/Fas ligand can result in keratocyte apoptosis.

> Injured epithelial cells release cytokines such as IL-1/IL-1 receptor and Fas/Fas ligand. Evidence from Wilson and associates[72] have suggested that IL-1 mediated production of Fas/Fas ligand can result in keratocyte apoptosis.

Keratocyte apoptosis occurs immediately after epithelial insult. Keratocytes that do not undergo the apoptotic cascade are transformed into fibroblasts or myofibroblasts (Figure 25-4) that move into the injured zone and release factors that induce epithelial recovery and proliferation.[73] Myofibroblast migration and action may be regulated by epithelial cells. These interactions between the epithelium and stroma, which modulate the reactionary response to injury, are responsible for the return to the normal corneal milieu.

There are differences in the wound healing patterns between LASIK and PRK/LASEK. The apoptotic patterns may offer some hypotheses as to the variation in clinical outcomes between the different techniques seen, especially in the treatment of higher-order aberrations.

In PRK, the apoptotic response is in the immediate vicinity of the epithelial injury. Myofibroblast migration and proliferation accompany its release of factors favoring epithelial cell proliferation which, may in turn result in an over-proliferation of epithelial cells.[40] It has been published that regression in PRK is in part due to epithelial hyperplasia and is caused by an abrupt change in the contour of the ablated area.[74-76] Epithelial proliferation and migration are mediated by epidermal growth factor (EGF), transforming growth factor-α (TGF-α), fibroblast growth factor (FGF), keratocyte growth factor (KGF), and hepatocyte growth

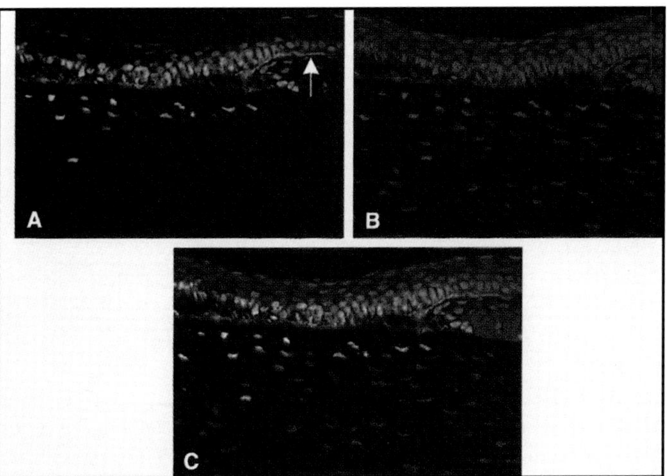

Figure 25-5. Apoptosis in LASEK. (A) Tunnel assay performed on chicken cornea 4 hours after LASEK (basement membrane arrow). (B) Nuclear staining (propidium iodine) is in red. (C) Combined tunnel and nuclear staining.

factor (HGF).[46] The replacement of the basement membrane and its associated attachment complexes—hemidesmosomes, fibronectin, collagen type IV, and anchoring fibrils—have been demonstrated by immunolocalization 3 months after surgery.[77,78] These are all necessary for the maintenance of a normal regenerated epithelium.

> In PRK, the apoptotic response is in the immediate vicinity of the epithelial injury, favoring epithelial cell proliferation that may, in turn, result in an overproliferation of epithelial cells.

The epithelium is disrupted in LASIK only at the area where the microkeratome cuts through to create the flap. The over-proliferation of epithelial cells then is less likely to be observed in LASIK. This may then be the substantiating evidence for the observation of less regression in patients who undergo LASIK vs those who are managed with PRK with the same order of myopic aberration.[40] However, an epithelial ingrowth may sometimes result from hyperplastic epithelial plugs at the site of the microkeratome incision, causing haze in the interface.[78] Type IV collagen has been localized at this region suggesting that basement membrane components may be responsible.[79] The proliferation of myofibroblasts after LASIK occurs further away from the epithelial layers separated by normal stroma. It has been recently described that there is an apparent loss of keratocytes in the most anterior portion of the cornea 6 months after LASIK. The consequences of this finding, however, have not been elucidated.[80]

> The epithelium is disrupted in LASIK only at the area where the microkeratome cuts through to create the flap. The overproliferation of epithelial cells then is less likely to be observed in LASIK.

In our laboratory, we have demonstrated the phenomenon of apoptosis occurring in the anterior portion of the treated stromal bed post-LASEK in the avian model (Figure 25-5). The alcohol-assisted removal of the epithelial flap separated at the basement membrane is then reapproximated to its original position. Questions pertaining to the aforementioned arise: 1) would there be more apoptosis induced by repositioning a viable epithelial flap[81,82] onto a newly treated stromal bed; and 2) would the existence of viable tissue serve as a barrier to attenuate epithelial hyperplasia mediated by myofibroblastic activity?[82]

> We have demonstrated the phenomenon of apoptosis occurring in the anterior portion of the treated stromal bed post-LASEK in the avian model.

Effect of Wound Healing on Clinical Outcomes After Excimer Laser Surgery

Effect on Predictability of Refractive Outcomes

Achievement of intended refractive correction depends on the delicate balance that occurs during tissue response to laser. While robust wound healing response results in myopic regression, inadequate healing leads to hyperopic shift. Durrie and associates studied clinical response after PRK and classified patients in to three groups according to the degree of wound healing.[83] Normal (Type I) responders are patients who had refraction within +1 diopter (D) of attempted correction at 6 months (84.5%). Inadequate (Type II) responders are patients who had greater than 1 D of overcorrection at 6 months (11.2%). Aggressive (Type III) responders are patients who had greater than 1 D of undercorrection at 6 months (4.3%).

These observations underscore the variability of wound healing responses in refractive surgery patients. To date, there are no reliable methods to preoperatively classify patients according to their wound healing response. The ideal evaluation of patients for the customized ablation may need to include not only detailed wavefront profiles but also wound healing patterns. We need a greater understanding of events involved in the tissue remodeling process in order to devise objective tests to characterize and classify patients according to their potential healing response.

> To date, there are no reliable methods to preoperatively classify patients according to their wound healing response. The ideal evaluation of patients for the customized ablation may need to include not only detailed wavefront profiles but also wound healing patterns.

Effect on Fidelity of Custom Ablation Pattern to the Corneal Surface

Customized ablation to correct for wavefront errors requires precise sculpting of the cornea. The ablation pattern can be so subtle that even slight changes of cell thickness may interfere with desirable outcome. Wound healing-related alterations such as epithelial hyperplasia or stromal remodeling may readily mask many features incorporated into customized ablation. The flap thickness and irregularity in LASIK may also cover intended wavefront correction or generate new higher-order aberration. In addition, remodeling changes in the cornea after the ablation may contribute to postoperative wavefront errors.

Many factors have been found to influence epithelial thickness, including eyelid pressure, lid shearing causing exfoliation, rate of cell metabolism, surface area requiring epithelialization,[84] and rate of cell sliding.[76] Using very high-frequency (VHF) ultrasound corneal analysis, Reinstein and colleagues[85] suggested an intriguing concept that after lamellar refractive surgery the epithelium appears to possess the ability to remodel itself to compensate for stromal surface abnormalities caused by either flap irregularity or irregular stromal resection. While the origin of this epithelial behavior is not known, it was postulated that the tarsus of the eyelid provides a semirigid, concave template that rubs and polishes the epithelial surface during blinking. Because the observed epithelial compensation masks asymmetry of the stromal surface relative to the visual axis, the authors suggested that ideal laser ablation should symmetrize the stromal surface. In the customized ablation, the use of an accurate layer-by-layer analysis (confocal microscopy or high resolution ultrasound biomicroscopy) to unmask the true shape of the stromal surface may enable more accurate preoperative assessment and surgical planning.

> After lamellar refractive surgery, the epithelium appears to possess the ability to remodel itself to compensate for stromal surface abnormalities caused by either flap irregularity or irregular stromal resection.

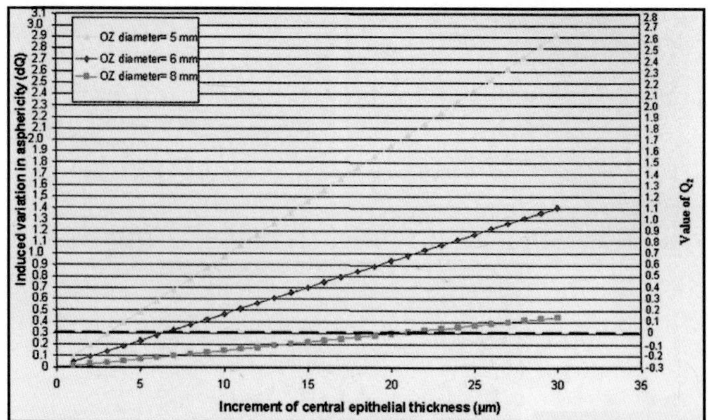

Figure 25-6. The theoretical induced variation in asphericity consecutive to different maximal central epithelial thickening with no paraxial refractive change after excimer laser correction of myopia is shown for different optical zone (OZ) diameters. The y-axis shows the value of the modified asphericity (Q2) for an initial asphericity of -0.3. For an optical zone of 6 mm, 7 µm of central epithelial hyperplasia is sufficient to induce an oblate final corneal contour (Q2 >0). The corresponding magnitudes of epithelial hyperplasia for optical zones of 5 and 8 mm are 3 and 21 µm, respectively. (Courtesy of Gatinel D, Malet J, Hoang-Xuan T, Azar DT. Analysis of customized corneal ablations: theoretical limitations of increasing negative asphericity. *Invest Ophthalmol Vis Sci.* 2002;43:941-948.)

Effect on Stability of Refractive Outcome

It has been shown that epithelial hyperplasia seems to have an important role in the regression of refractive effect after PRK[86-91] and LASIK.[92,93] Spadea and associates[74] used a 50 MHz ultrasonic pachymeter or an ultrasound biomicroscope to measure central epithelium thickness and found that after LASIK the epithelium showed a tendency toward hyperplasia starting from the first day, becoming statistically significantly thicker in the first week, and continuing to increase up to the third month postoperatively before becoming stable.

Gatinel and associates[94] generated a mathematic model of aspheric myopic corneal laser surgery to investigate the influence of the initial corneal apical radius of curvature, initial asphericity, intended dioptric correction, diameter of treatment, and intended change in corneal asphericity on the maximal depth of ablation.[94] Figure 25-6 illustrates that in addition to its effects on the apical power, an increase in central corneal thickness during wound healing could induce a modification in the corneal asphericity. The extent of epithelial and stromal thickening during wound healing after PRK are greater than those after LASIK.[86,87,90,95] The in vivo clinical observations that epithelial hyperplasia is more common in eyes treated with small ablation zone diameters or with high magnitudes of treatment are consistent with findings predicted by this model.[90]

Stromal remodeling may also play an important role in determining predictability and stability of refractive outcomes. It has been histopathologically documented that after uncomplicated keratomileusis, there is minimal production of new extracellular matrix in the posterior stromal corneal flap interface.[96-99] However, there are numerous evidences that implicate the corneal keratocyte and the process of keratocyte transformation to fibroblast or myofibroblast phenotype as playing a pivotal role in determining the outcome of refractive surgery.[100] In addition, using confocal microscopy, Moller-Pedersen and associates[95] reported that the stromal keratocyte-mediated regrowth of the photoablated stroma appears to be the main cause of myopic regression in humans treated with a 6 mm diameter PRK, whereas hyperopic shifts appear to be a direct consequence of stromal thinning.

Modulation of Corneal Wound Healing After Refractive Surgery

The development of haze following refractive surgery may vary in its occurrence from 2 days to 2 months, may peak in intensity from 1 to 6 months, and can take as long as 18 months to resolve.[101] It is widely accepted that haze is modulated by the events surrounding stromal wound healing. The factors that induce haze formation are epithelial and surface irregularities, activated keratocytes, subepithelial deposits, and keratocyte loss.

The hastening of epithelial healing in PRK and LASEK may modulate stromal responses, thereby minimizing the occurrence of haze. Work on rabbit eyes demonstrated that topical interferon–α eye drops applied QID for 5 weeks reduced haze formation after PRK,[102] the addition of topical dexamethasone to the regimen improved the haze reduction even more. Topical EGF has been demonstrated to have an effect on epithelial wound healing in the treatment of traumatic corneal ulcers.[103] Topical FGF-2 applied to rabbit eyes treated with PRK until epithelial closure also showed decreased corneal haze at 5 to 13 weeks.[104] Plasmin inhibition, resulting in the modulation of fibronectin and laminin, may also hasten epithelial healing. The clinical effects and benefits from these have yet to be firmly established.

> The hastening of epithelial healing in PRK and LASEK may modulate stromal responses, thereby minimizing the occurrence of haze.

Topical corticosteroids are postulated to interfere with DNA synthesis, decreasing collagen synthesis, and reduce cellular activity, resulting in the inhibition of activated keratocytes. Corticosteroids have been used to minimize haze development post-PRK. Although effective, its efficacy in preventing haze formation is limited and transient.[10,12,13] Diclofenac sodium decreases prostaglandin E and inflammatory cells within the corneal stroma and post-PRK. Prolonged exposure to these drugs, however, has its own drawbacks.[105]

Mitomycin C in combination with topical erythromycin and steroids decreases the fibrosis associated with healing after PRK in rabbits.[36] Treatment of patients with subepithelial scarring post-PRK using mitomycin C (0.02%) improved corneal clarity throughout a follow-up period of up to 25 months.[106] We have also reported beneficial effects of using annular filter paper discs soaked in 0.02% mitomycin-C in the prevention of corneal scarring after excimer laser keratectomy based on our experiments done on rabbit eyes.[107] Such an approach has many promising treatment implications and is worth further investigation.

> Treatment of patients with subepithelial scarring post-PRK using mitomycin C (0.02%) improved corneal clarity throughout a follow-up period of up to 25 months.

Wilson and associates postulated that if the initial steps of the keratocyte apoptosis could be inhibited or blocked, the subsequent events in the wound healing cascade would be adequately attenuated.[40] Recent studies demonstrated that a well-known caspase-inhibitor, zVAD-FMK, inhibits keratocyte apoptosis.[108] However, transmission electron microscopy also revealed that superficial keratocytes were dying by necrosis. Further investigation is required in order to search for inhibitors that block apoptosis without triggering necrosis. Gene therapy is another exciting and viable strategy to control apoptosis in the cornea.[40,109]

References

1. MacRae SM. Supernormal vision, hypervision, and customized corneal ablation. *J Cataract Refract Surg*. 2000;26(2):154-157.
2. Marshall J, Trokel SL, Rothery S, Krueger RR. Long-term healing of the central cornea after photorefractive keratectomy using an excimer laser. *Ophthalmology*. 1988;95(10):1411-1421.
3. Pallikaris IG, Papatzanaki ME, Siganos DS, Tsilimbaris MK. A corneal flap technique for laser in situ keratomileusis. Human studies. *Arch Ophthalmol*. 1991;109(12):1699-1702.
4. Buratto L, Ferrari M, Rama P. Excimer laser intrastromal keratomileusis. *Am J Ophthalmol*. 1992;113(3):291-295.
5. Pallikaris IG, Kymionis GD, Panagopolou SI, et al. Induced optical aberrations following formation of a laser in situ keratomileusis flap. *J Cataract Refract Surg*. 2002;28(10):1737.
6. Azar DT, Ang RT, Lee JB, et al. Laser subepithelial keratomileusis: electron microscopy and visual outcomes of flap photorefractive keratectomy. *Curr Opin Ophthalmol*. 2001;12(4):323-328.
7. Azar DT, Ang RT. Laser subepithelial keratomileusis: evolution of alcohol assisted flap surface ablation. *Int Ophthalmol Clin*. 2002; 42(4):89-97.
8. Camellin M, Cimberle M. LASEK technique promising after 1 year of experience. *Ocular Surgery News*. 2000;18(1):14-17.
9. Seiler T, Wollensak J. Myopic photorefractive keratectomy with the excimer laser. One-year follow-up. *Ophthalmology*. 1991;98(8):1156-1163.
10. Baldwin HC, Marshall J. Growth factors in corneal wound healing following refractive surgery: a review. *Acta Ophthalmol Scand*. 2002; 80(3):238-247.
11. Liu JC, Steinemann TL, McDonald MB, Beuerman RW, Sunderland G. Effects of corticosteroids and mitomycin c on corneal remodeling after excimer laser photorefractive keratectomy (PRK). *Invest Ophthalmol Vis Sci*. 1991;32(suppl):1248.
12. Corbett MC, O'Brart DP, Marshall J. Do topical corticosteroids have a role following excimer laser photorefractive keratectomy? *J Refract Surg*. 1995;11(5):380-387.
13. O'Brart DP, Lohmann CP, Klonos G, et al. The effects of topical corticosteroids and plasmin inhibitors on refractive outcome, haze, and visual performance after photorefractive keratectomy. A prospective, randomized, observer-masked study. *Ophthalmology*. 1994;101(9):1565-1574.
14. Malley DS, Steinert RF, Puliafito CA, Dobi ET. Immunofluorescence study of corneal wound healing after excimer laser anterior keratectomy in the monkey eye. *Arch Ophthalmol*. 1990;108(9):1316-1322.
15. Kommehl EW, Steinert R, Puliafito CA, Reidy W. Morphology of an irregular corneal surface following 193 nm ArF excimer laser large area ablation with 0.3% hydroxy propyl methylcellulose 2910 and 0.1% dextran 70, 1% carboxymethyl cellulose sodium or 0.9% saline. *Invest Ophthalmol Vis Sci*. 1990;31:245.
16. Del Pero RA, Gigstad JE, Roberts AD, et al. A refractive and histopathologic study of excimer laser keratectomy in primates. *Am J Ophthalmol*. 1990;109(4):419-429.
17. Marshall J, Trokel S, Rothery S, Schubert H. An ultrastructural study of corneal incisions induced by an excimer laser at 193 nm. *Ophthalmology*. 1985;92(6):749-758.
18. Seiler T, Frantes T, Waring GO, Hanna KD. Laser corneal surgery. In: Waring GO, ed. *Refractive Keratotomy*. St. Louis, Mo: Mosby-Year Book; 2001:669-745.
19. Talamo JH, Steinert RF, Puliafito CA. Update on laser corneal surgery. *Int Ophthalmol Clin*. 1991;31(1):13-23.
20. Taylor DM, L'Esperance FA Jr, Del Pero RA, et al. Human excimer laser lamellar keratectomy. A clinical study. *Ophthalmology*. 1989;96(5):654-664.
21. L'Esperance FA Jr, Taylor DM, Del Pero RA, et al. Human excimer laser corneal surgery: preliminary report. *Trans Am Ophthalmol Soc*. 1988;86:208-275.
22. L'Esperance FA Jr, Taylor DM, Warner JW. Human excimer laser keratectomy. Short-term histopathology. *Bull N Y Acad Med*. 1989;65(5): 557-573.
23. Hanna KD, Chastang JC, Asfar L, et al. Scanning slit delivery system. *J Cataract Refract Surg*. 1989;15(4):390-396.
24. Gipson IK, Spurr-Michaud S, Tisdale A, Keough M. Reassembly of the anchoring structures of the corneal epithelium during wound repair in the rabbit. *Invest Ophthalmol Vis Sci*. 1989;30(3):425-434.
25. Gipson IK. The epithelial basement membrane zone of the limbus. *Eye*. 1989;3(Pt 2):132-140.
26. Gipson IK, Spurr-Michaud SJ, Tisdale AS. Hemidesmosomes and anchoring fibril collagen appear synchronously during development and wound healing. *Dev Biol*. 1988;126(2):253-262.
27. Gipson IK, Spurr-Michaud SJ, Tisdale AS. Anchoring fibrils form a complex network in human and rabbit cornea. *Invest Ophthalmol Vis Sci*. 1987;28(2):212-220.

28. Anhalt GJ, Jampel HD, Patel HP, et al. Bullous pemphigoid autoantibodies are markers of corneal epithelial hemidesmosomes. *Invest Ophthalmol Vis Sci.* 1987;28(5):903-907.

29. Tisdale AS, Spurr-Michaud SJ, Rodrigues M, et al. Development of the anchoring structures of the epithelium in rabbit and human fetal corneas. *Invest Ophthalmol Vis Sci.* 1988;29(5):727-736.

30. Azar DT, Spurr-Michaud SJ, Tisdale AS, Moore MD, Gipson IK. Reassembly of the corneal epithelial adhesion structures following human epikeratoplasty. *Arch Ophthalmol.* 1991;109(9):1279-1284.

31. Azar DT, Gipson IK. Repair of the corneal epithelial adhesion structures following keratectomy wounds in diabetic rabbits. *Acta Ophthalmol Suppl.* 1989;192:72-79.

32. Azar DT, Spurr-Michaud SJ, Tisdale AS, Gipson IK. Decreased penetration of anchoring fibrils into the diabetic stroma. A morphometric analysis. *Arch Ophthalmol.* 1989;107(10):1520-1523.

33. Azar DT, Spurr-Michaud SJ, Tisdale AS, Gipson IK. Altered epithelial-basement membrane interactions in diabetic corneas. *Arch Ophthalmol.* 1992;110(4):537-540.

34. Matsubara M, Zieske JD, Fini ME. Mechanism of basement membrane dissolution preceding corneal ulceration. *Invest Ophthalmol Vis Sci.* 1991;32(13):3221-3237.

35. Zieske JD, Bukusoglu G, Gipson IK. Enhancement of vinculin synthesis by migrating stratified squamous epithelium. *J Cell Biol.* 1989; 109(2):571-576.

36. Talamo JH, Gollamudi S, Green WR, et al. Modulation of corneal wound healing after excimer laser keratomileusis using topical mitomycin C and steroids. *Arch Ophthalmol.* 1991;109(8):1141-1146.

37. Hanna KD, Pouliquen YM, Savoldelli M, et al. Corneal wound healing in monkeys 18 months after excimer laser photorefractive keratectomy. *Refract Corneal Surg.* 1990;6(5):340-345.

38. Foutain TR, Azar DT, De La Cruz F, Green WR, Stark WJ. Reassembly of corneal epithelial adhesion structures following human excimer laser keratectomy. *Invest Ophthalmol Vis Sci.* 1992;33(suppl):345.

39. Seiler T, Matallana M, Sendler S, Bende T. Does Bowman's layer determine the biomechanical properties of the cornea? *Refract Corneal Surg.* 1992;8(2):139-142.

40. Wilson SE, Mohan RR, Hong JW, Lee JS, Choi R. The wound healing response after laser in situ keratomileusis and photorefractive keratectomy: elusive control of biological variability and effect on custom laser vision correction. *Arch Ophthalmol.* 2001;119(6):889-896.

41. Zieske JD. Extracellular matrix and wound healing. *Curr Opin Ophthalmol.* 2001;12(4):237-241.

42. Fini ME. Keratocyte and fibroblast phenotypes in the repairing cornea. *Prog Retin Eye Res.* 1999;18(4):529-551.

43. Sivak JM, Fini ME. MMPs in the eye: emerging roles for matrix metalloproteins in ocular physiology. *Prog Retin Eye Res.* 2002;21(1): 1-14.

44. Jester JV, Barry-Lane PA, Cavanagh HD, Petroll WM. Induction of alpha-smooth muscle actin expression and myofibroblast transformation in cultured corneal keratocytes. *Cornea.* 1996;15(5):505-516.

45. Li DQ, Tseng SC. Three patterns of cytokine expression potentially involved in epithelial-fibroblast interactions of human ocular surface. *J Cell Physiol.* 1995;163(1):61-79.

46. Rocha G, Schultz GS. Corneal wound healing in laser in situ keratomileusis. *Int Ophthalmol Clin.* 1996;36(4):9-20.

47. Desmouliere A, Geinoz A, Gabbiani F, Gabbianai G. Transforming growth factor-beta 1 induces alpha-smooth muscle actin expression in granulation tissue myofibroblasts and in quiescent and growing cultured fibroblasts. *J Cell Biol.* 1993;122(1):103-111.

48. Rockey DC, Housset CN, Friedman SL. Activation-dependent contractility of rat hepatic lipocytes in culture and in vivo. *J Clin Invest.* 1993;92(4):1795-1804.

49. You L, Kruse FE. Differential effect of activin A and BMP-7 on myofibroblast differentiation and the role of the Smad signaling pathway. *Invest Ophthalmol Vis Sci.* 2002;43(1):72-81.

50. Ronnov-Jessen L, Petersen OW. Induction of alpha-smooth muscle actin by transforming growth factor-beta 1 in quiescent human breast gland fibroblasts. Implications for myofibroblast generation in breast neoplasia. *Lab Invest.* 1993;68(6):696-707.

51. Maltseva O, Folger P, Zekaria D, Petridou S, Masur SK. Fibroblast growth factor reversal of the corneal myofibroblast phenotype. *Invest Ophthalmol Vis Sci.* 2001;42(11):2490-2495.

52. Kretzschmar M, Liu F, Hata A, Doody J, Massague J. The TGF-beta family mediator Smad1 is phosphorylated directly and activated functionally by the BMP receptor kinase. *Genes Dev.* 1997;11(8):984-995.

53. Kretzschmar M, Doody J, Massague J. Opposing BMP and EGF signalling pathways converge on the TGF-beta family mediator Smad1. *Nature.* 1997; 389(6651):618-622.

54. Lawler S, Feng XH, Chen RH, et al. The type II transforming growth factor-beta receptor autophosphorylates not only on serine and threonine but also on tyrosine residues. *J Biol Chem.* 1997;272(23): 14850-14859.

55. Masur SK, Dewal HS, Dinh TT, Erenburg I, Petridou S. Myofibroblasts differentiate from fibroblasts when plated at low density. *Proc Natl Acad Sci USA.* 1996;93(9):4219-23.

56. Zimmerman CM, Padgett RW. Transforming growth factor beta signaling mediators and modulators. *Gene.* 2000;249(1-2):17-30.

57. Ye HQ, Maeda M, Yu FS, Azar DT. Differential expression of MT1-MMP (MMP-14) and collagenase III (MMP-13) genes in normal and wounded rat corneas. *Invest Ophthalmol Vis Sci.* 2000;41(10):2894-2899.

58. Ye HQ, Azar DT. Expression of gelatinases A and B, and TIMPs 1 and 2 during corneal wound healing. *Invest Ophthalmol Vis Sci.* 1998; 39(6):913-921.

59. Azar DT, Hahn TW, Jain S, Yeh YC, Stetler-Stevensen WG. Matrix metalloproteins are expressed during wound healing after excimer laser keratectomy. *Cornea.* 1996;15(1):18-24.

60. Fini ME, Girard MT, Matsubara M. Collagenolytic/gelatinolytic enzymes in corneal wound healing. *Acta Ophthalmol Suppl.* 1992;202:26-33.

61. Vincenti MP, Coon CI, Mengshol JA, et al. Cloning of the gene for interstitial collagenase-3 (matrix metalloproteinase-13) from rabbit synovial fibroblasts: differential expression with collagenase-1 (matrix metalloproteinase-1). *Biochem J.* 1998;331(Pt 1):341-6.

62. Schorpp M, Mattei MG, Herr I, et al. Structural organization and chromosomal localization of the mouse collagenase type I gene. *Biochem J.* 1995;308(Pt 1):211-217.

63. Vaalamo M, Matilla L, Johansson N, et al. Distinct populations of stromal cells express collagenase-3 (MMP-13) and collagenase-1 (MMP-1) in chronic ulcers but not in normally healing wounds. *J Invest Dermatol.* 1997;109(1):96-101.

64. Fini ME, Parks WC, Rinehart WB, et al. Role of matrix metalloproteins in failure to re-epithelialize after corneal injury. *Am J Pathol.* 1996;149(4):1287-1302.

65. Okada A, Tomasetto C, Lutz Y, et al. Expression of matrix metalloproteins during rat skin wound healing: evidence that membrane type-1 matrix metalloproteinase is a stromal activator of pro-gelatinase A. *J Cell Biol.* 1997;137(1):67-77.

66. Knauper V, Smith B, Lopez-Otin C, et al. Activation of progelatinase B (proMMP-9) by active collagenase-3 (MMP-13). *Eur J Biochem.* 1997;248(2):369-373.

67. Maeda M, Vanlandingham BD, Ye H, et al. Immunoconfocal localization of gelatinase B expressed by migrating intrastromal epithelial cells after deep annular excimer keratectomy. *Curr Eye Res.* 1998; 17(8):836-843.

68. Sato H, Seiki M. Membrane-type matrix metalloproteins (MT-MMPs) in tumor metastasis. *J Biochem (Tokyo).* 1996;119(2):209-215.

69. Smine A, Plantner JJ. Membrane type-1 matrix metalloproteinase in human ocular tissues. *Curr Eye Res.* 1997;16(9):925-929.

70. Wilson SE, Li Q, Weng J, et al. The Fas-Fas ligand system and other modulators of apoptosis in the cornea. *Invest Ophthalmol Vis Sci.* 1996;37(8):1582-1592.
71. Mohan RR, Liang Q, Kim WJ, et al. Apoptosis in the cornea: further characterization of Fas/Fas ligand system. *Exp Eye Res.* 1997; 65(4):575-589.
72. Wilson SE, He YG, Weng J, et al. Epithelial injury induces keratocyte apoptosis: hypothesized role for the interleukin-1 system in the modulation of corneal tissue organization and wound healing. *Exp Eye Res.* 1996;62(4):325-327.
73. Hutcheon AE, Guimaraes MF, Zieske JD. Kertocyte proliferation in response to epithelial debridement. *Invest Ophthalmol Vis Sci.* 1999; 40(suppl):622.
74. Spadea L, Fasciani R, Necoziione S, Balestrazzi E. Role of the corneal epithelium in refractive changes following laser in situ keratomileusis for high myopia. *J Refract Surg.* 2000;16(2):133-139.
75. Gauthier CA, Holden BA, Epstein D, et al. Role of epithelial hyperplasia in regression following photorefractive keratectomy. *Br J Ophthalmol.* 1996;80(6):545-548.
76. Gauthier CA, Holden BA, Epstein D, et al. Factors affecting epithelial hyperplasia after photorefractive keratectomy. *J Cataract Refract Surg.* 1997;23(7):1042-1050.
77. Anderson JA, Binder PS, Roch ME, Vrabec MP. Human excimer laser keratectomy. Immunohistochemical analysis of healing. *Arch Ophthalmol.* 1996;114(1):54-60.
78. Bansal AK, Veenashree MP. Laser refractive surgery: technological advance and tissue response. *Biosci Rep.* 2001;21(4):491-512.
79. Kato T, Nakayasu K, Hosoda Y, Watanabe Y, Kanai A. Corneal wound healing following laser in situ keratomileusis (LASIK): a histopathological study in rabbits. *Br J Ophthalmol.* 1999; 83(11):1302-1305.
80. Vesaluoma M, Perez-Santonja, Petroll WM, et al. Corneal stromal changes induced by myopic LASIK. *Invest Ophthalmol Vis Sci.* 2000;41(2):369-376.
81. Gabler B, Windkler von Mohrnefels C, Dreiss AK, Marshall J, Lohmann CP. Vitality of epithelial cells after alcohol exposure during laser-assisted subepithelial keratectomy flap preparation. *J Cataract Refract Surg.* 2002;28(10):1841.
82. Chen CC, Chang JH, Lee JB, Javier J, Azar DT. Human corneal epithelial cell viability and morphology after dilute alcohol exposure. *Invest Ophthalmol Vis Sci.* 2002;43(8):2593-2602.
83. Durrie DS, Lesher MP, Cavanaugh TB. Classification of variable clinical response after photorefractive keratectomy for myopia. *J Refract Surg.* 1995;11(5):341-347.
84. Hanna KD, Pouliquen Y, Waring GO 3rd, et al. Corneal stromal wound healing in rabbits after 193-nm excimer laser surface ablation. *Arch Ophthalmol.* 1989;107(6):895-901.
85. Reinstein DZ, Silverman RH, Sutton HF, Coleman DJ. Very high-frequency ultrasound corneal analysis identifies anatomic correlates of optical complications of lamellar refractive surgery: anatomic diagnosis in lamellar surgery. *Ophthalmology.* 1999;106(3):474-482.
86. Wu WC, Stark WJ, Green WR. Corneal wound healing after 193-nm excimer laser keratectomy. *Arch Ophthalmol.* 1991;109(10):1426-1432.
87. Fagerholm P, Hamberg-Nystrom H,Tengroth B. Wound healing and myopic regression following photorefractive keratectomy. *Acta Ophthalmol (Copenh).* 1994;72(2):229-234.
88. Balestrazzi E, De Molfetta V, Spadea L, et al. Histological, immunohistochemical, and ultrastructural findings in human corneas after photorefractive keratectomy. *J Refract Surg.* 1995;11(3):181-187.
89. Wilson SE, Klyce SD, McDonald MB, Liu JC, Kaufman HE. Changes in corneal topography after excimer laser photorefractive keratectomy for myopia. *Ophthalmology.* 1991;98(9):1338-1347.
90. Gauthier CA, Epstein D, Holden BA, et al. Epithelial alterations following photorefractive keratectomy for myopia. *J Refract Surg.* 1995;11(2):113-118.
91. Siganos DS, Katsanevaki VJ, Pallikaris IG. Correlation of subepithelial haze and refractive regression 1 month after photorefractive keratectomy for myopia. *J Refract Surg.* 1999;15(3):338-342.
92. Lohmann CP, Guell JL. Regression after LASIK for the treatment of myopia: the role of the corneal epithelium. *Semin Ophthalmol.* 1998; 13(2):79-82.
93. Chayet AS, Assil KK, Montes M, et al. Regression and its mechanisms after laser in situ keratomileusis in moderate and high myopia. *Ophthalmology.* 1998;105(7):1194-1199.
94. Gatinel D, Malet J, Hoang-Xuan T, Azar DT. Analysis of customized corneal ablations: theoretical limitations of increasing negative asphericity. *Invest Ophthalmol Vis Sci.* 2002;43(4):941-948.
95. Moller-Pedersen T, Cavanagh HD, Petroll WM, Jester JV. Stromal wound healing explains refractive instability and haze development after photorefractive keratectomy: a 1-year confocal microscopic study. *Ophthalmology.* 2000;107(7):1235-1245.
96. Kezirian GM, Gremillion CM. Automated lamellar keratoplasty for the correction of hyperopia. *J Cataract Refract Surg.* 1995;21(4):386-392.
97. Baumgartner SD, Binder PS, Refractive keratoplasty. Histopathology of clinical specimens. *Ophthalmology.* 1985;92(11):1606-1615.
98. Jakobiec FA, Koch P, Iwamoto T, Harrison W, Troutman R. Keratophakia and keratomileusis: comparison of pathologic features in penetrating keratoplasty specimens. *Ophthalmology.* 1981;88(12):1251-1259.
99. Jester JV, Rodrigues MM, Willasenor RA, Schanzlin DJ. Keratophakia and keratomileusis: histopathologic, ultrastructural, and experimental studies. *Ophthalmology.* 1984;91(7):793-805.
100. Jester JV, Petroll WM, Cavanagh HD. Corneal stromal wound healing in refractive surgery: the role of myofibroblasts. *Prog Retin Eye Res.* 1999;18(3):311-356.
101. Corbett MC, Prydal JI, Verma S, et al. An in vivo investigation of the structures responsible for corneal haze after photorefractive keratectomy and their effect on visual function. *Ophthalmology.* 1996;103(9):1366-1380.
102. Morlet N, Gillies MC, Crouch R, Maloof A. Effect of topical interferon-alpha 2b on corneal haze after excimer laser photorefractive keratectomy in rabbits. *Refract Corneal Surg.* 1993;9(6):443-451.
103. Scardovi C, De Felice GP, Gazzaniga A. Epidermal growth factor in the topical treatment of traumatic corneal ulcers. *Ophthalmologica.* 1993;206(3):119-124.
104. Rieck P, David T, Hartmann C, et al. Basic fibroblast growth factor modulates corneal wound healing after excimer laser keratomileusis in rabbits. *Ger J Ophthalmol.* 1994;3(2):105-111.
105. Gartry DS, Muir MG, Lohmann CP, Marshall J. The effect of topical corticosteroids on refractive outcome and corneal haze after photorefractive keratectomy. A prospective, randomized, double-blind trial. *Arch Ophthalmol.* 1992;110(7):944-952.
106. Majmudar PA, Forstot SL, Dennis RF, et al. Topical mitomycin-C for subepithelial fibrosis after refractive corneal surgery. *Ophthalmology.* 2000;107(1):89-94.
107. Azar DT, Jain S. Topical MMC for subepithelial fibrosis after refractive corneal surgery. *Ophthalmology.* 2001;108(2):239-240.
108. Kim WJ, Mohan RR, Wilson SE. Caspase inhibitor z-VAD-FMK inhibits keratocyte apoptosis, but promotes keratocyte necrosis, after corneal epithelial scrape. *Exp Eye Res.* 2000;71(3):225-232.
109. Stechschulte SU, Joussen AM, von Recum HA, et al. Rapid ocular angiogenic control via naked DNA delivery to cornea. *Invest Ophthalmol Vis Sci.* 2001;42(9):1975-1979.

Clinical Science Section

Chapter 26

Customized Ablation Using the Alcon CustomCornea Platform

George H. Pettit, MD, PhD; John A. Campin, BSc; Marguerite B. MacDonald, MD; and Ronald R. Krueger, MD, MSE

Introduction

CustomCornea is the Alcon (Fort Worth, Tex) approach to wavefront-guided laser refractive surgery. It comprises two technology components, which are shown in Figure 26-1. The LADARWave (Alcon) device uses a Shack-Hartmann wavefront sensor to detect the preoperative aberrations present in the eye.[1] The LADARVision (Alcon) system employs an active closed loop eye tracking module to compensate for eye motion and a small diameter flying spot excimer laser to deliver the customized ablation profile.[2] These two devices work together in a coordinated fashion to provide an effective customized treatment.

In this chapter, we will describe these instruments in some detail and discuss their performance in controlled clinical testing. As an overview, this technology is based on four guiding principles. These are:

1. One consistent reference axis on the eye should be used for both measurement and treatment. This point should be readily identifiable and clinically appropriate
2. The aberration data should be consistent and accurate over an area that completely encompasses the naturally dilated pupil
3. The wavefront profile should be carefully registered to the anatomy of the eye, so that the ablative treatment can be properly positioned. This registration should include cyclotorsional information
4. The algorithm that converts the aberration data into the ablation profile should be optimized for greatest effectiveness. Outside the optical zone, the annular blend zone should also be customized to taper the corneal ablation gracefully in every direction

The following pages elaborate on these four points.

Reference Axis

The first guiding principle is that a consistent reference axis should be used throughout the customized treatment process. Figure 26-2 shows simplified views of the fixation and video alignment subsystems in the LADARWave aberrometer and LADARVision system. For either instrument, as the patient stares at an internal fixation target, a video camera looks at the eye along the same optical axis. This common design greatly facilitates the definition and use of a consistent axis on the eye.

The reference axis used is the natural line of sight. The line of sight is defined as the line connecting the point of fixation and the center of the pupil.[3] The natural (undilated) rather than dilated pupil is used as the reference because dilation, particularly pharmacological dilation, can occasionally cause a significant shift in the pupil center.[4]

The reference axis used is the natural line of sight. The line of sight is defined as the line connecting the point of fixation and the center of the pupil.[3] The natural (undilated) rather than dilated pupil is used as the reference.

The LADARWave unit records the natural line of sight as a preliminary step in the wavefront examination. The instrument captures a video image of the eye as the patient looks at an internal fixation target under daytime illumination conditions. This video snapshot is presented on-screen to the device operator, and he or she aligns two software reticles over the pupil margin and limbus. From this time onward, the device software knows where the natural pupil center sits on the eye relative to the limbus. Thus, after the patient is dilated, the eye can still be centered along this axis for the actual wavefront measurement. This centration information is also passed on to the LADARVision system in the electronic transfer file, so that the ablative treatment can be centered over the natural pupil as well.

Aberration Data

The second guiding principle is that accurate aberrometry must be made over a region that encompasses the naturally dilated pupil. This requires good fixation on the part of the patient, dilation of the eye with pharmacological agents, and high fidelity wavefront measurement by the LADARWave device.

Fixation

The patient must know exactly where to look during the wavefront exam in order to provide the best possible data. While the aberrations of the eye are relatively constant over small field angles,[5] the most relevant wavefront data will be obtained when the probe beam illuminates a central foveal region. Yet most patients do not have good unaided visual acuity before surgery, and therefore have difficulty seeing a static target at infinity focus.

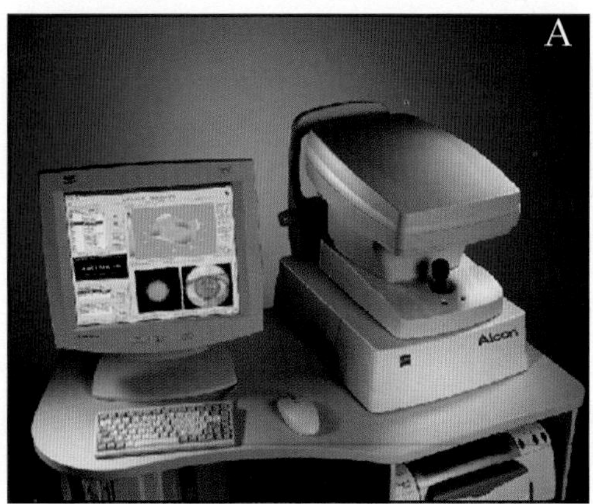

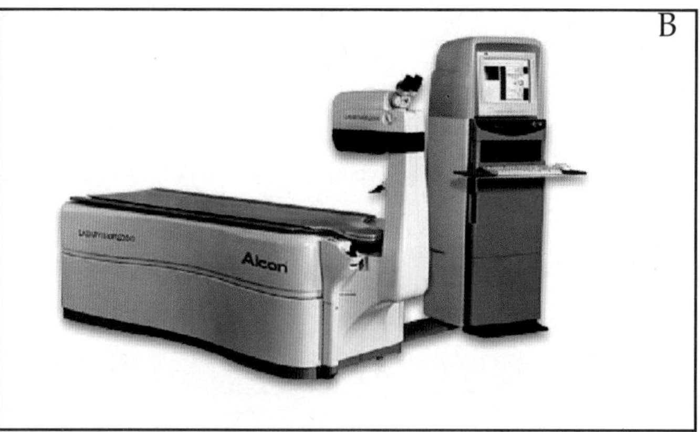

Figure 26-1. The Alcon CustomCornea technology components. (A) The LADARWave aberrometer measures the optical characteristics of the eye using the Shack-Hartmann wavefront sensing approach. (B) The LADARVision system treats the measured aberrations using an active eye-tracking system and a small flying-spot excimer laser.

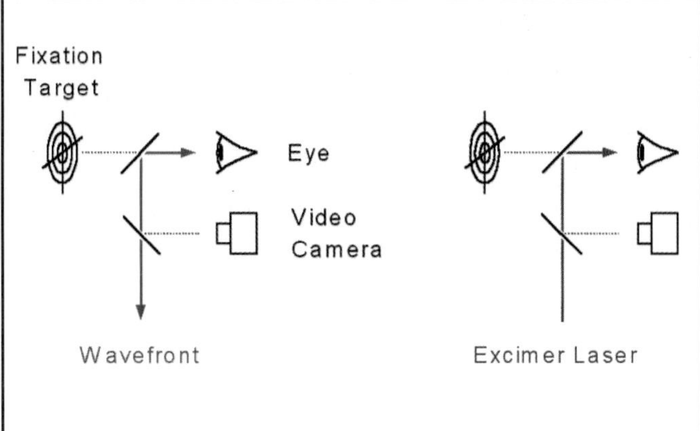

Figure 26-2. Fixation and video schemes for the LADARWave (on the left) and LADARVision systems. The commonality of these two designs allows a consistent geometric reference axis to be defined on the eye and used throughout the measurement and treatment steps.

Some people may find the target by accommodating, but this will substantially alter the wavefront profile.[6] The fixation path, therefore, must have adjustable compensating optics, so that each patient can visualize the target with the eye in a relaxed state.

The LADARWave device clarifies the target automatically for each eye by adjusting spherocylindrical lenses to correct for conventional refractive errors. The software accomplishes this task by analyzing preliminary wavefront data in real time at the beginning of the exam. The instrument can compensate for spherical errors over the range +15 diopters (D) to -15 D, and astigmatic errors up to -6 D. (Patients with somewhat larger refractive errors can still be measured, but the target clarity will not be optimal.) Once the target is clear, the software "fogs" it slightly (ie, moves it in the hyperopic direction to minimize accommodation). (The cylinder compensation is particularly important in ensuring that the correct fogging is provided to astigmatic patients.) This automatic process works well and lessens the workload on the device operator considerably. The automatic fogging routine is also used during the centration step discussed in the previous section.

The LADARWave device clarifies the target automatically for each eye by adjusting spherocylindrical lenses to correct for conventional refractive errors.

Dilation

The pupil is the limiting aperture for the wavefront measurement, meaning that we cannot obtain aberration data beyond the pupil margin. In fact, we cannot even obtain valid data over the entire pupil extent because the iris aperture partially distorts the peripheral measurements. Yet, the higher-order aberrations we are specifically trying to measure typically become more pronounced near the pupil periphery.

Pharmacologically dilating the eye expands the region of valid wavefront data to completely encompass the largest natural pupil. Alcon has conducted careful clinical testing to study effects of drug dilation on the aberration profile.[7] The only notable pharmacological effect on the wavefront is a small hyperopic shift in the defocus term. (This defocus shift is more common with hyperopic patients.) The higher-order aberrations are unaffected by the dilating agent. This consistency has been observed in every eye tested, demonstrating the validity of measuring the wavefront under drug dilation.

The higher-order aberrations are unaffected by the dilating agent.

Wavefront Measurement

The LADARWave device utilizes the Shack-Hartmann approach to measure the aberrations in the eye. This method is described in great detail elsewhere in this book. The actual Shack-Hartmann measurement data is simply a camera image showing a pattern of dots, which are the individual wavefront pieces divided up and focused by the lenslet array. The device software measures the displacement of each focused dot from its ideal location (ie, the pattern generated by a perfectly flat plane wave) and uses this information to calculate the slope of the intact wavefront at each lenslet location. The software then uses

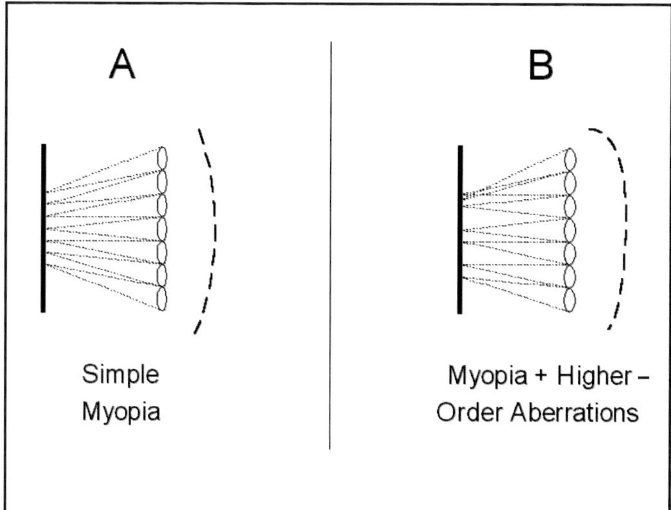

Figure 26-3. Shack-Hartmann detection of two different myopic wavefronts. The wavefronts are propagating from right to left in the picture. (A) Simple myopic wavefront with no higher-order aberrations. The spacing between individual focused wavefront elements on the charged-coupled device (CCD) is uniform, but smaller than the lenslet array spacing. (B) Complex wavefront including higher-order aberrations. The focused dot pattern here is no longer uniform. In addition, the two wavefront elements at the top have crossed over each other in traveling from the lens array to the screen. This measurement is compromised in this region.

this slope data to generate a mathematical description of the original wavefront profile.

This is simple in concept, but much care must be taken in building a clinical aberrometer that is reliable, easy to operate, and highly accurate in measuring the wide variety of visual aberrations found among refractive surgery patients.

Figure 26-3 shows the detection of two significantly myopic wavefronts by a Shack-Hartmann sensor. In a good clinical device, the software must be able to analyze large spot displacements in the charged-coupled device (CCD) camera image (as shown in both parts A and B of the figure). In addition, the optical hardware design must minimize the chance of spot crossover occurring (as shown in part B).

After much clinical testing and engineering innovation, Alcon has been able to address issues such as these and has produced an instrument that provides both high accuracy and a large dynamic range, along with high density sampling of the wavefront across the pupil. While some details are proprietary, the performance characteristics are not. The LADARWave unit utilizes a square lenslet array geometry, and samples the eye every -420 microns (µm) at the corneal plane. For a 7 millimeter (mm) diameter pupil, this results in more than 200 wavefront samples at the Shack-Hartmann sensor. This large body of data allows calculation of wavefront aberrations up to the eighth order. The device can measure wavefronts with a maximum curvature in any meridian lying between +8 D and -14 D (defined for an 8-mm pupil). The unit can also measure up to 8 D of astigmatism. The sphere and cylinder accuracy over this measurement range is 1% of the actual value or 0.05 D (whichever is larger). On top of the classical refractive error, the device can also measure large amounts of higher-order aberrations.

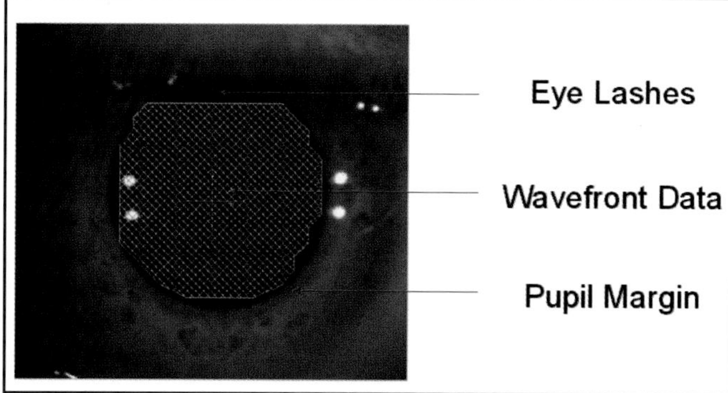

Figure 26-4. Frozen video image taken simultaneously with a wavefront measurement. The crosshatched region in the picture is the area providing wavefront data, as determined by the device software. Because the pupil is the limiting aperture for a good measurement, the crosshatched area should closely approximate that of the pupil. In this instance, the top of the pupil is partially occluded by the eyelashes.

> The LADARWave unit utilizes a square lenslet array geometry, and samples the eye every -420 µm at the corneal plane. For a 7 mm diameter pupil, this results in more than 200 wavefront samples at the Shack-Hartmann sensor.

A typical wavefront examination consists of five individual measurements. The LADARWave software compares the five wavefront profiles automatically, and the three in closest agreement are then averaged together to generate a composite final wavefront. This eliminates transient fluctuations in the aberration content due to microsaccadic eye movements or dynamic action of the lens.

The LADARWave device utilizes the synchronized video imagery to help the operator determine the validity of the wavefront measurement. Figure 26-4 shows a video image frozen at the instant a wavefront measurement was made. In this example, the patient has begun to blink just as the probe beam fires. Maintaining an intact tear film is essential to the wavefront exam,[8] so the instrument must accommodate normal blinking by the patient. Therefore, the upper lid will occasionally get in the way. By automatically projecting the wavefront data region onto the picture, the device software provides a clear indication that this measurement is not representative of the full pupil, and thus should be rejected. Intracorneal or intraocular opacities (eg, cataracts, vitreous strands) may also obscure part of the re-emitted wavefront, and such conditions will also be revealed in this synchronized video display.

Registration

The third guiding principle is that the wavefront data must be accurately registered to the anatomy of the eye, so that the ablative correction can be applied to the correct corneal location. On the wavefront measurement side, this registration is accomplished again using synchronized video imagery. Both the video and Shack-Hartmann cameras are looking at the pupil of the eye along the same optical axis. Therefore, there is a direct one-to-one correspondence between each point in the video and wavefront

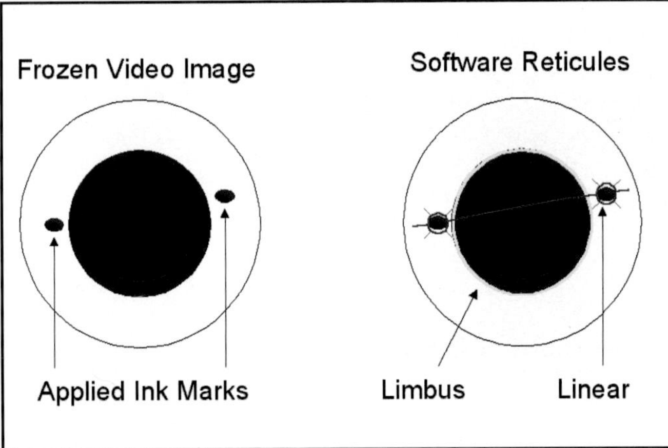

Figure 26-5. Method of registering the wavefront geometry with the anatomy of the eye. Just prior to the wavefront exam, multiple ink marks are applied to the sclera. In the frozen video image of the eye (taken simultaneously with the wavefront measurement), software reticles are aligned to these marks and the limbus. This provides the system with accurate position and cyclotorsion information.

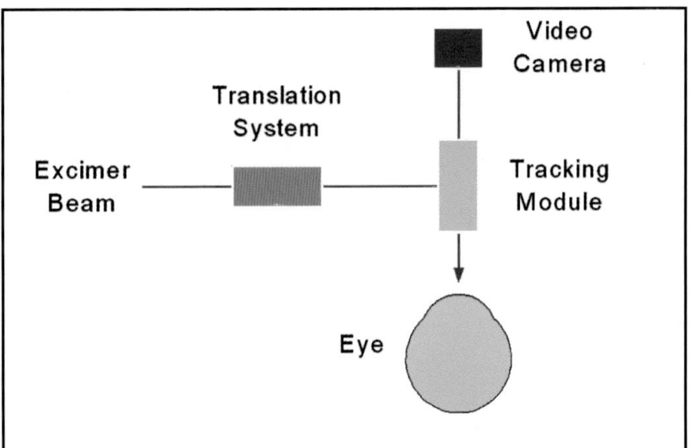

Figure 26-6. Optical strategy employed in the LADARVision system. The tracking module contains a dedicated set of mirrors, tasked solely with compensating for detected eye motion. Both the video and excimer subsystems are optically coupled into the tracking module, so that both of these interact with a space-stabilized eye. The translation system contains a second set of mirrors, whose only job is to deliver the excimer beam in a predetermined pattern of pulses based on the patient's aberration data.

camera images. At the instant that a wavefront measurement is taken, the LADARWave software freezes the video picture of the eye. The device operator aligns two reticles (limbus and linear) in the frozen video image, as shown in Figure 26-5, and this tells the software the exact position and cyclotorsional state of the eye at the instant the wavefront was captured. The process is repeated for each of the five measurements in the complete examination, and the reticle data is then used in calculating the composite wavefront profile. The reticle information is also transmitted in the electronic file over to the LADARVision system, so that the ablative treatment can be properly aligned.

The device operator aligns two reticles (limbus and linear) in the frozen video image, as shown in Figure 26-5, and this tells the software the exact position and cyclotorsional state of the eye at the instant the wavefront was captured. The reticle information is also transmitted in the electronic file over to the LADARVision system, so that the ablative treatment can be properly aligned.

On the treatment side, the registration process takes advantage of the LADARVision system's closed loop eye tracking device/system. The optical block diagram of the treatment device is shown in Figure 26-6. The video camera looking through the tracking mirrors sees the eye after any motion has been compensated for. The LADARVision graphical user interface presents this "space stabilized" video image to the system operator along with registration reticles identical to those used during measurement by the LADARWave system. The operator repositions the on screen reticles over the appropriate anatomical landmarks to ensure accurate delivery of the excimer ablation profile.

Cyclotorsion is a key but often overlooked part of the complete wavefront registration. With conventional surgery it is well known that torsional alignment of the ablation is important in correcting conventional ("second-order") astigmatism. It has been shown that a torsion error of 10 degrees results in a residual astigmatism that is approximately one-third of the initial astigmatism magnitude.[9] With higher-order treatments, the required torsional accuracy becomes even more critical, dependent on the azimuthal frequency of the wavefront aberration.

This statement merits a brief explanation. Zernike polynomials increase in complexity with increasing order. Only a small fraction of these polynomials are rotationally symmetric (ie, have no angular dependency). Examples of rotationally symmetric Zernike shapes include defocus and spherical aberration. Non-rotationally symmetric terms, such as coma or tetrafoil, have an undulating height around their perimeter. The azimuthal frequency is directly related to the number of these up/down undulations. If we attempt to treat one of the rotationally symmetric aberrations, the presence of a torsion error will have no effect because the shape stays the same upon rotation. In contrast, a torsional error will have a substantial effect on the treatment of non-rotationally symmetric aberrations, as is shown in Figure 26-7.

Cyclotorsion takes on additional significance if we consider that the aberration exam is performed with the patient sitting upright. He or she must then lie down for surgery, and the apparent rotational state of the eye may change significantly. Unless this rotation is accounted for, it will degrade the wavefront-based correction. Thus, we have to register the wavefront very accurately in position and angle relative to the anatomy of the eye. With the LADARWave/LADARVision system technology, we can do just that.

Conversion

The fourth guiding principle behind CustomCornea concerns the algorithm that converts the aberration data into the ablation profile. This algorithm should be optimized to provide best optical performance over the optical zone and graceful tapering of the ablation in the surrounding blend zone.

The treatment algorithm resides on the LADARVision system. As it is proprietary, we cannot provide a detailed explanation here. A "first-order" approximation is shown in Figure 26-8. The optical path difference approach shown here represents a good

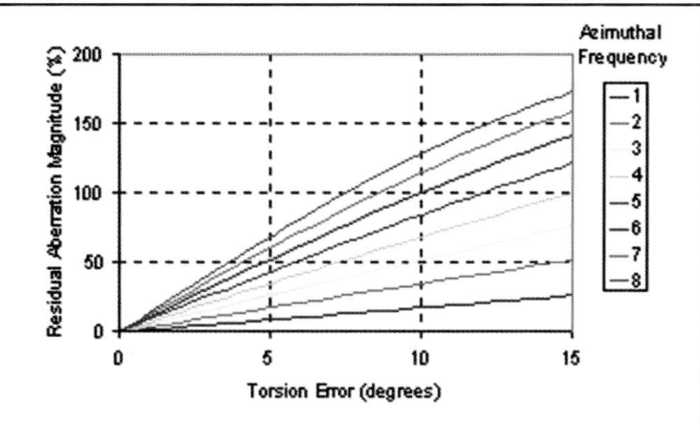

Figure 26-7. Effect of torsional error on the correction of nonrotationally symmetric aberrations. The horizontal axis indicates the rotational error in delivering an ablation profile to the eye. The vertical axis indicates the percentage of a particular aberration that will be left after the surgery. The different colored plots indicate the relationship for aberrations with different azimuthal frequencies, according to the legend at the right of the plot. Note that the vertical axis goes beyond 100%, indicating that some aberrations may actually be increased by a poorly registered customized ablation.

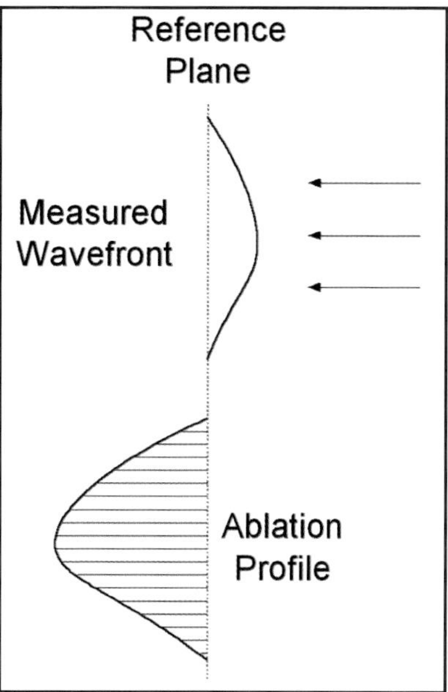

Figure 26-8. "First-order" approach in determining the appropriate ablation profile from the wavefront shape. The upper part of the figure shows a generally myopic wavefront (traveling to the left) compared to the idealized (flat) reference plane. The difference between the real wavefront and ideal plane is calculated at each point in the examination plane. This optical path difference (OPD) profile is then multiplied by -1 and then divided by the refractive index difference between cornea and air. Because light travels slower in corneal tissue than in air, ablating the most cornea centrally will "speed up" the central wavefront with respect to the edges. This produces a flatter aberration profile.

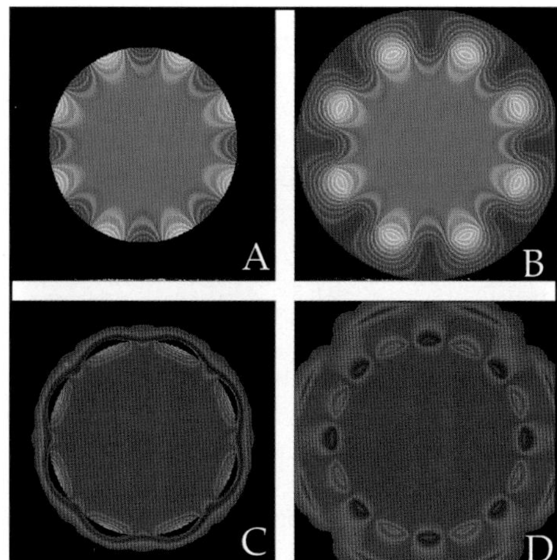

Figure 26-9. Effect of a customized blend zone on the treatment accuracy. (A) Color map indicating the ablation profile needed to correct a particular eighth-order aberration over a 6.50 mm circular optical zone with no blend. (B) Map showing the same treatment with a 1.25 mm blend zone annulus added around the optical zone. (C) Simulated corneal treatment of the ablation profile shown in A, using a small diameter (750 mm full width at half maximum [FWHM]) excimer laser. Accurate correction is indicated by the uniform blueish color near the center of the image. Residual corneal height errors are indicated by the other colors. (D) Simulated corneal treatment of the ablation profile shown in B. Inclusion of the customized blend zone significantly improves the treatment accuracy.

starting point in determining the correction needed; however, it is not the complete method used in CustomCornea treatments. Additional factors, such as corneal curvature[10] and corneal biomechanics,[11] must be taken into account in optimizing the ablative treatment.

Additional factors such as corneal curvature[10] and corneal biomechanics[11] must be taken into account in optimizing the ablative treatment.

Figure 26-9 shows the importance of surrounding the optical zone with a customized blend annulus. Both ablation profiles are attempting to treat the Z_8^8 "flower" aberration over a 6.50-mm diameter optical zone. This aberration is relatively flat centrally, with eight undulating ripples evenly spaced around the perimeter. Without a blend zone, the resulting corneal surface (see Figure 26-9C) has finite height errors within the optical zone and significant irregularities just outside it. Adding the blend zone obviously produces a more regular corneal surface in the periphery. However, it also improves the peripheral treatment accuracy within the optical zone. Because "flying spot" excimer ablation relies on the cumulative effect of many partially overlapping pulses, shots delivered just outside the optical zone contribute to the correction just inside it. The wavefront RMS error corresponding to the ablation outcome in Figure 29-6C is 70% of the pretreatment value. In contrast, if a blend zone is included in the ablation profile, the root mean square (RMS) wavefront error afterward is only 36% of the preoperative level.

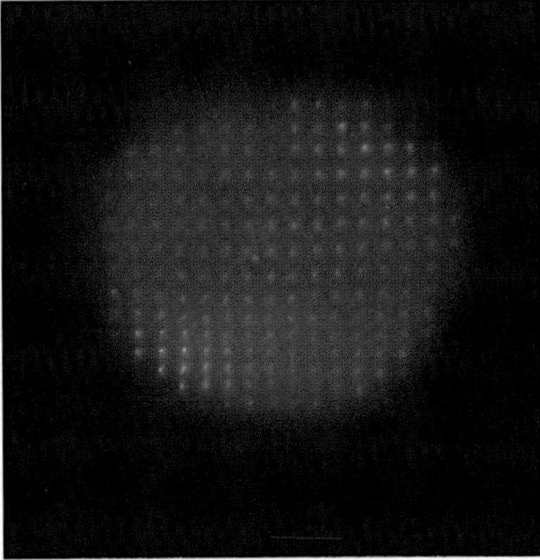

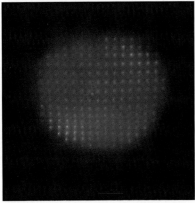

Figure 26-10. Shack-Hartmann CCD camera image from an eye with keratoconus. The focused wavefront pieces appear as white dots in the picture. The general pattern of dots is due to the square arrangement of lenses in the microlens array. Deviations in individual dot positions from a perfect square array alignment are due to aberrations in the eye. Note that the dot density is greatest in the lower central part of the pattern, due to the local myopia of the keratoconic bulge. The roughly elliptical boundary of the dot pattern is due to the pupil of the eye, which is the limiting aperture for the measurement.

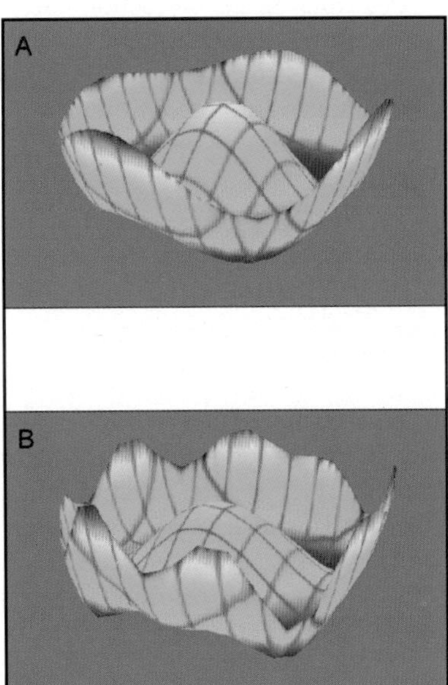

Figure 26-12. Three-dimensional (3-D) wavefront displays for an eye with prior eight-incision radial keratotomy surgery. (A) Wavefront reconstruction using up to fourth-order Zernike polynomials. (B) Wavefront reconstruction using up to eighth-order Zernike terms. The wavefront diameter in both A and B is 6.50 mm.

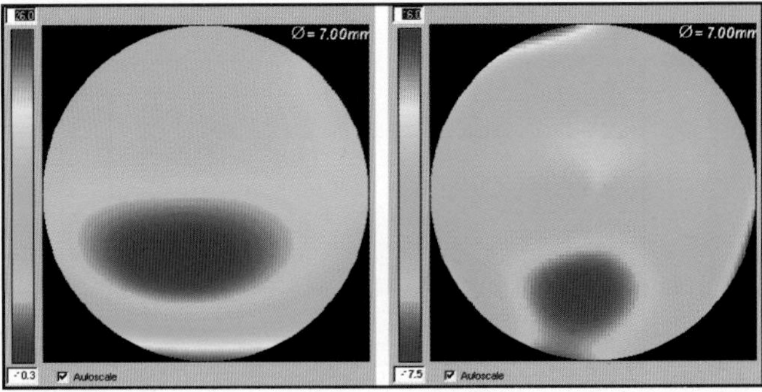

Figure 26-11. LADARWave system wavefront analysis for the keratoconus patient introduced in Figure 26-10. (A) Two dimensional pseudocolor display of the wavefront profile. The eye is below the plane of the figure. The color scale is shown on the left side of the panel, with the units being in microns. Red indicates the highest points in the profile, while blue shows the deepest depressions. (B) Instantaneous power map calculated directly from the wavefront axial curvature. Here the colors indicate instantaneous refractive power in diopters, with red indicating the most hyperopic and blue the most myopic regions. Both maps cover the same 7 mm diameter circle at the cornea and are based on an eighth-order Zernike polynomial reconstruction.

Clinical Data

All this sounds fine in theory, but how well does CustomCornea actually work on real human eyes? In this last section, we discuss clinical aberration measurements by the LADARWave unit and wavefront-guided surgeries by the LADARVision system.

Aberration Measurement

In order to illustrate the measurement capability of the LADARWave unit, we present two case examples: one patient with moderate keratoconus and another with prior eight-incision radial keratotomy surgery. We choose these eyes in particular because they have substantial amounts of very different higher-order aberrations.

In the keratoconic eye, the bulge in the inferior cornea increases the local curvature and hence the refractive power in that region. Thus, the eye is more myopic inferiorly than superiorly, producing substantial vertical coma. Coma can roughly be described as one half of the pupil being more myopic and the other half more hyperopic than the overall average. Figure 26-10 shows the LADARWave Shack-Hartmann camera image from an eye with moderate keratoconus. Note that although the dots are more closely spaced in the region of the keratoconic bulge, they remain distinct, easily resolvable by the device software. Figure 26-11 shows wavefront analysis for this eye. Note in the power map (B) that the maximum myopic power exceeds -17 D and is rapidly changing over the lower pupil. This patient example demonstrates that the instrument is able to measure marked aberrations without difficulty.

Our radial keratotomy example is an eye with a prior eight-incision surgery. Figure 26-12 shows two 3-D wavefront reconstructions for this case. Notice that both profiles have a general "sombrero" shape. This is due to spherical aberration, which is the most significant single term for this eye. However, note also that there are obvious differences between wavefront descriptions A and B. The eighth-order reconstruction (B) looks almost

Table 26-1
Mesopic Uncorrected Visual Acuity Changes for Both Myopic LASIK Treatment Populations.

UCVA	Initial Spherical Treatment Group (N = 139)	Refined Treatment Group (N = 141)
20/16 or better	58%	69%
20/20 or better	80%	91%
20/25 or better	91%	96%

like a flower. This is due to the nature of the surgical procedure. The eight relaxing incisions lie at the edge of this measurement region. Those cuts cause general but nonuniform flattening of the central cornea. The eight-incision pattern in fact produces a slight periodic ripple in the surface. If we could look at topographic data just along the circumference of this measurement circle, we would see eight local peaks and valleys. The fluctuations produce refractive undulations with an azimuthal frequency of 8, and these are described by two eighth-order Zernike terms. The LADARWave device is able to provide a fine level of detail by allowing analysis to very high Zernike order.

Customized Treatment

Dr. Marguerite MacDonald initiated Alcon's United States CustomCornea clinical trials in New Orleans in October 1999. These cases were the first wavefront-based excimer laser treatments in the United States, and the first in the world with the Alcon wavefront system. To date, more than 600 eyes have been treated in the United States and Canada as part of the trial. These patients included both myopic and hyperopic eyes, treated with either laser in-situ keratomileusis (LASIK) or photorefractive keratectomy (PRK). In the fall of 2002,the study was expanded to include therapeutic treatments (ie, wavefront-guided surgery for patients with pronounced visual symptoms due to large higher-order aberrations). At the end of October 2002, Alcon received the first Food and Drug Administration (FDA) approval for wavefront-guided refractive surgery: CustomCornea treatment of simple myopia (ie, myopia with less than 0.50 D of astigmatism).

Various Alcon trials are ongoing at the time of this writing, as we refine algorithms and treatment techniques to obtain the best possible outcomes and broaden the FDA approval. The treatment group with the most number of patients and the longest-term follow-up data is the myopic LASIK cohort. That treatment data is summarized here.

Four hundred twenty-six myopic eyes were treated in what is referred to here as the "initial treatment group." The results showed mild undercorrection of the spherical component and over-correction of the cylinder component, as discussed below. The treatment algorithm, the software routine that converts the wavefront data into the ablation profile, was adjusted accordingly, and an additional 141 myopic eyes were treated in the "refined treatment group." Preoperatively, the initial treatment group had a mean spherical refraction of -3.10 D ± 1.38 D, with a range of 0 to -7 D. Cylinder ranged from 0 to -4 D, with a mean of -0.77 ± 0.74 D. The spherical equivalent for the initial treatment group was -3.48 D ± 1.33 D, with a range of -0.50 to -7.125 D.

The initial treatment group contained a spherical subset (ie, a group with less than 0.50 D of conventional astigmatism preoperatively), which was studied separately and is also reported on here. For this spherical subset the mean preoperative spherical equivalent refraction was -3.23 D ± 1.31 D.

The refined treatment group of 141 eyes had slightly less preoperative myopia. The mean preoperative sphere was -2.65 ± 1.18 D, with a range of 0 to -5.50 D. The mean preoperative cylinder was -0.77 D ± 0.63 D, with a range of 0 to -2.50 D. The spherical equivalent for the refined treatment group was -3.03 D ± 1.18 D, with a range of -0.50 to 5.50 D.

All treatments were based on wavefront aberrations up to and including the fourth Zernike order. A composite of five wavefront measurements were taken on each eye; two "outliers" were discarded based on a statistical analysis, and the three remaining measurements were averaged to generate a composite aberration map. This composite wavefront was then used to calculate the ablation profile. All patients received a 6.50 mm diameter optical zone with a 1.25 mm wide blend zone, for a total 9 mm circular ablation region on the eye.

Table 26-1 shows the mesopic uncorrected visual acuity (UCVA) 6 months after CustomCornea LASIK surgery for the spherical subset of the initial treatment group and the entire refined treatment group. Note that while both groups had good UCVA outcomes the refined population results were significantly better, despite the fact that the latter group included substantial astigmatic corrections. For the initial spherical treatment group, 69% of all eyes were within 0.50 D of emmetropia at 6 months and 94% were within 1 D. However, the mean 6 month manifest refractive spherical equivalent (MRSE) for the initial group was -0.40 D, meaning that not all of the preoperative myopia was addressed in the treatment. The treatment algorithm was adjusted to address the mild undercorrection before the second round of surgeries. For the refined group at 6 months, the mean MRSE was -0.03 D, 94% of patients were within 0.50 D and 99% were within 1 D.

Both populations did well by other objective clinical measures. Best-corrected visual acuity (BCVA) results are shown in Table 26-2. For the initial treatment group, four times as many eyes had a gain of greater than or equal one line than had an equivalent loss. Contrast sensitivity testing was also performed before and after surgery. A clinically significant change in contrast sensitivity was defined as greater than 0.3 log units (ie, a difference preop to postop of at least two test intervals) at two or more spatial frequencies. By this criterion, in the initial group under photopic conditions, 2% of the eyes had clinically significant loss from the preoperative state and 2% had a clinically significant gain in contrast. Under mesopic conditions, 5% of the

Table 26-2
Mesopic Best-Corrected Visual Acuity Changes for Both Myopic LASIK Treatment Populations

BCVA	Initial Spherical Treatment Group (N = 139)		Refined Treatment Group (N = 141)	
	Preoperative	Six Months	Preoperative	Six Months
20/12.5 or better	18%	32%	21%	42%
20/16 or better	86%	92%	77%	93%
20/20 or better	99%	100%	99%	99%

Table 26-3
Changes in Higher-Order Aberrations for Different Myopic LASIK Treatment Populations

Wavefront Parameter	Conventional LASIK (N = 138)	Initial Treatment Group (N = 426)	Refined Treatment Group (N = 141)
Total Higher Order	+60%	+24%	+19%
Coma	+53%	+23%	+24%
Spherical Aberration	+136%	+11%	+1%

initial treatment group eyes lost contrast sensitivity and 15% gained. Contrast sensitivity testing in the refined treatment group indicated that 2% lost but 5% gained contrast under photopic conditions, and 8% lost but 18% gained under mesopic conditions. Thus, in general, photopic contrast sensitivity was virtually unchanged, but mesopic performance generally improved after treatment.

Table 26-3 summarizes the changes in higher-order aberrations for these treatment groups. For comparison the chart also includes data for a group of patients who received conventional LASIK surgery. This conventional group comprised 138 eyes with preoperative refractive errors and wavefront aberrations similar to the wavefront-guided treatment populations. The conventional LASIK procedures were performed using the same optical and blend zone dimensions as the customized surgeries. While the two custom treatment populations had similar outcomes by these measures, the aberration differences between wavefront guided and conventional surgery were statistically significant ($p < 0.05$) for all three parameters shown. Conventional outcomes exhibited a marked aberration increase, while custom results were only slightly larger than preoperative levels. Optical analysis suggests this significant difference in postoperative higher-order aberrations between wavefront-guided and traditional LASIK corresponds to an equivalent value of about 0.20 D of defocus error.

The results shown in Table 26-3 are average values for the different groups of eyes. On an individual patient basis, the higher-order wavefront error actually decreased in 38% of the wavefront guided treatments vs only 19% of the conventionally treated eyes. Spherical aberration was reduced in 46% of the custom surgeries vs in only 12% of the conventional group. This data further supports the optical benefit of the customized approach.

On an individual patient basis, the higher-order wavefront error actually decreased in 38% of the wavefront-guided treatments vs only 19% of the conventionally treated eyes.

Psychometric testing was performed in order to assess the CustomCornea outcomes subjectively. Patients rated changes in various symptoms after surgery versus before treatment using a five-interval scale ("significantly better," "better," "same," "worse," and "significantly worse"). Results indicated that the vast majority of patients felt that they were the same or significantly better with regard to glare, halos, night driving difficulty, blurring of vision, and fluctuation of vision. With the initial treatment group, 3.4% of patients felt that they were significantly worse in regard to blurring of vision, which was correlated to undercorrection of the myopic treatment. None of the patients in the refined group rated blurring of vision as significantly worse. Notably, only 1.4% of patients in the refined group rated night driving difficulty as significantly worse.

Summary

The ability of CustomCornea to measure the wavefront accurately and treat the appropriate location on the eye has led to impressive clinical results. The data shows excellent visual acuity, as well as more gain and less loss of mesopic contrast sensitivity. The higher-order aberrations for customized eyes are increased in magnitude, but remain modest and are significantly less than those seen with conventional eyes. As compared to conventional surgery, a much larger percentage of customized eyes show a reduction in higher-order aberrations.

Acknowledgments

The authors would like to thank the CustomCornea clinical investigators for their many contributions to the development of this technology. In addition to Dr. MacDonald, this group includes Dr. Steve Brint in Metairie, Louisiana; Dr. Dan Durrie in Overland Park, Kansas; Dr. Omar Hakim in Waterloo, Ontario; and Dr. Brock Magruder in Orlando, Florida.

References

1. Liang J, Grimm B, Goelz S, Bille JF. Objective measurement of wave aberrations of the human eye with the use of a Hartmann-Shack wave-front sensor. *J Opt Soc Am A*. 1994;11:1949-1957.
2. Campin JA, Housand BJ, Liedel KK, Pettit GH. Technology requirements for customized refractive laser surgery. *Invest Ophthalmol Vis Sci*. 1999;40:S891.
3. Atchison DA, Smith G. *Optics of the Human Eye*. Oxford, United Kingdom: Butterworth Heinemann; 2000:31.
4. Yang Y, Thompson K, Burns SA. Pupil location under mesopic, photopic, and pharmacologically dilated conditions. *Invest Ophthalmol Vis Sci*. 2002;43:2508-2512.
5. Roorda A. Adaptive optics ophthalmoscopy. *J Refract Surg*. 2000; 16:S602-S607.
6. Gray GP, Campin JA, Pettit GH, Liedel KK. Use of wavefront technology for measuring accommodation and corresponding changes in higher order aberrations. *Invest Ophthalmol Vis Sci*. 2001;42:S26.
7. Liedel KK, Campin JA, Pettit GH, Gray GP. Effect of cycloplegic agents on wavefront aberrations. ARVO 2002 Annual Meeting.
8. Tutt R, Bradley A, Begley C, Thibos LN. Optical and visual impact of tear break-up in human eyes. *Invest Ophthalmol Vis Sci*. 2000; 41:4117-4123.
9. Alpins NA. Vector analysis of astigmatism changes by flattening, steepening, and torque. *J Cataract Refract Surg*. 1997;23:1503-1514.
10. Mrochen M, Seiler T. Influence of corneal curvature on calculation of ablation patterns used in photorefractive laser surgery. *J Refract Surg*. 2001;17:S584-S587.
11. Dupps WJ, Roberts C. Effect of acute biomechanical changes on corneal curvature after photokeratectomy. *J Refract Surg*. 2001;17: 658-669.

Chapter 27
Customized Ablation Using the VISX WaveScan System and the VISX S4 ActiveTrak Excimer Laser

Junzhong Liang, PhD and Douglas D. Koch, MD

Introduction

Wavefront sensing technology, combined with advances in refractive lasers, promises to add a new dimension to the practice of refractive surgery. Wavefront-guided refractive surgery creates treatments tailored to the individual eye based on the total wavefront error, rather than on the conventional manifest refraction. Surgeons are no longer limited to traditional spherocylindrical corrections, but have the means to assess and treat higher-order ocular aberrations as well.[1-4]

Creating wavefront-guided customized ablations requires integrating the diagnostic wavefront device and the surgical laser into a cohesive system. This chapter describes each element of the VISX (Santa Clara, Calif) platform for refractive surgery, from measurement on the WaveScan device, to testing the treatment plan with the PreVue lens (VISX), through surgery on the STAR laser system. It concludes with surgical outcome data from VISX clinical studies and a discussion of the implications of these study results.

VISX Custom Ablation System

The VISX custom ablation process begins with measurement of the eye's wavefront aberration on the WaveScan Wavefront System. The proprietary software housed in the device computes a customized corrective treatment, which is transferred to the VISX laser system for surgery. The VISX STAR S4 ActiveTrak Excimer Laser System recreates the treatment, first on PreVue lenses so that the patient can see with the new vision prior to the procedure, and finally, on the patient's eyes.

WaveScan Wavefront Sensor

The WaveScan System employs a Shack-Hartmann wavefront sensor to measure the refractive error and aberrations of the eye.[5,6] A light source from the WaveScan is focused on the retina, and the light reflected from the retina forms a wavefront at the pupil. One hundred eighty lenslets focus the wavefront into the aberrated spot pattern within a 6.0 millimeter (mm) pupil area. The WaveScan System measures the wavefront and generates two aberration maps. One map shows total wavefront errors of the eye, including conventional spherical and cylindrical refractive errors, and the other map isolates the higher-order aberrations. From the total wavefront error map, the WaveScan proprietary Variable Spot Scanning (VSS) software calculates the best treatment table for a customized ablation.

The VISX WaveScan System can measure spherical refractive errors between -8 diopter (D) and +6 D; cylindrical refractive errors up to 5 D; and higher-order aberrations up to sixth- order Zernike terms. Figure 27-1 shows the high correlation between the subjective manifest refractive spherical equivalent (SE) and the SE predicted by the WaveScan System for 96 eyes of 57 patients. (Forty-three of the eyes had not had previous surgery. Fifty-three eyes had had previous refractive surgeries.[7]) The difference between the two techniques (manifest refraction - WaveScan refraction) was -0.16 ± 0.49 D for sphere, -0.24 ± 0.36 D for cylinder, and -0.28 ± 0.41 D for SE.

Measurements of higher-order Zernike aberrations by the WaveScan System were validated by testing an artificial eye with known optical aberrations. The artificial eye consists of a biconvex lens with an artificial retina. By changing the lens position, the magnitude of coma (a third-order Zernike aberration), spherical aberration (a fourth-order Zernike aberration), and astigmatism could be controlled in the artificial eye. Figure 27-2 shows coma, spherical aberration, and astigmatism of an artificial eye measured with the WaveScan Wavefront System and those obtained from a simulation using ZEMAX optical design software (ZEMAX Development Corp, San Diego, Calif). Agreement between the measurement and the simulation is excellent.

Generation of Treatment Tables

After obtaining the wavefront maps for the refractive correction, the VISX algorithm computes the best configuration of pulses for an optimum fit. The algorithm begins the computation with a coarse fit, selecting larger pulses to ensure that the maximum amount of tissue is removed in the minimum amount of time. Next, the algorithm refines the fit by adding smaller pulses. In this way, the program finds the best corrective shape while keeping the treatment time to a minimum.

The VISX algorithm begins the computation with a coarse fit, selecting larger pulses to ensure that the maximum amount of tissue is removed in the minimum amount of time. Next, the algorithm refines the fit by adding smaller pulses.

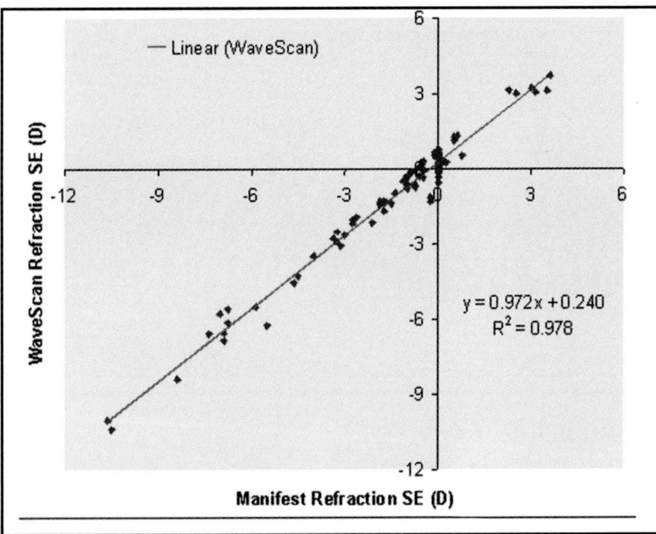

Figure 27-1. Correlation of manifest refractive spherical equivalent (MRSE) and refractive SE determined by the WaveScan wavefront system. Sixty-four percent of eyes had WaveScan SE within +0.50 D of MRSE, and 97% had WaveScan SE within +1 D of MRSE.

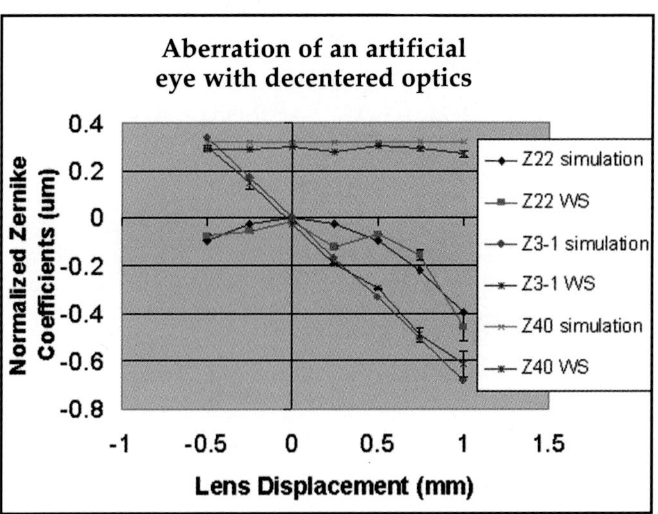

Figure 27-2. Calibration of a WaveScan system for the measurement of higher-order Zernike aberrations in an artificial eye. Coma (Z^3_{-1}), spherical aberration (Z^4_0) and astigmatism (Z^2_2) of a model eye measured with the WaveScan wavefront sensor vs those obtained from a simulation using ZEMAX optical design software. Error bar for the measurement with WaveScan was plus and minus one standard deviation.

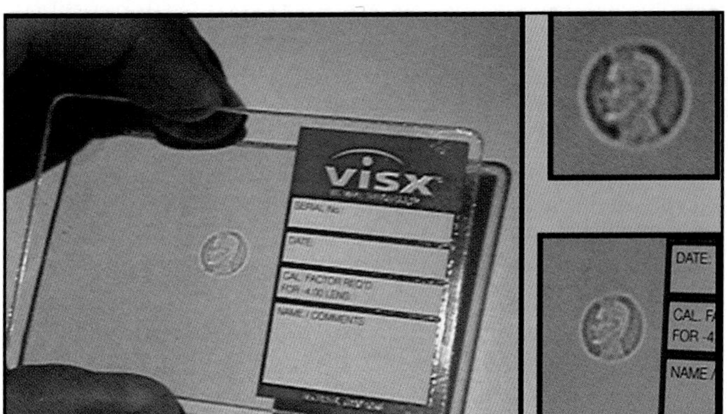

Figure 27-3. The 3-D profile of Abraham Lincoln from a penny recreated by the laser using VSS.

The software creates two treatment tables—one for calibration plastic and one for corneal tissue. The treatment data are transferred by diskette to the STAR S4 ActiveTrak Excimer Laser system, eliminating the possibility of transposition occurring during data entry.

Variable Spot Scanning on the Laser System

The customized treatment is completely dependent upon having a laser system capable of delivering the ultraviolet (UV) light pulses accurately according to the treatment table. The WaveScan VSS software creates the shape for the laser to ablate directly from the wavefront measurement while taking into account optical effect, laser tissue interaction, structural effect, and other software features that improve outcome. The STAR laser system then uses its own software to recreate the treatment by scanning a series of variably sized pulses over the corneal surface.

The ablation diameter is not limited by the size of the beam. Pulses range from a diameter of 0.65 to 6.50 mm, but, depending on the type of treatment, they can be applied over an area as large as 9.50 mm in diameter. VSS gives the laser the flexibility to duplicate virtually any shape—while using no more pulses than necessary.[8,9] Figure 27-3 shows the three-dimensional profile of Abraham Lincoln, which was recreated from the image on the penny using VSS.

Treatment Preview

The current VISX system allows the patient to test the treatment through ablated plastic lenses before surgery. Before performing the laser treatment on corneal tissue, the physician can create a PreVue lens on plastic. When aligned in a frame and fitted on the patient, this lens can be used to validate the treatment plan. To create the PreVue lens, a technician aligns the plastic on the calibration platform and fires the laser. The lens is then put into a frame and fitted on the patient. Doctors report that being able to look through the PreVue lens can give the patient a psychological boost and allay residual fears about the procedure. Plans call for replacing PreVue lenses with a system of integrated adaptive optics in the WaveScan System.[10]

The PreVue lens concept arose during the development of the VISX custom ablation system. A validation testing system was devised to verify that the WaveScan System could accurately assess higher-order aberrations and that the excimer laser system could accurately ablate the surfaces needed to correct the aberrations. The STAR S4 laser system was programmed to ablate single and dual Zernike terms, and flat plastic was ablated with these terms. Following ablation, the plastic phase plates were measured on the WaveScan device and with a Phase Shift Technology MicroXAM Interferometric Surface Profiler (ISP) (ADE Corp, Westwood, Mass). Figure 27-4 shows the wavefront maps of three typical phase plates. Excellent agreement among all three devices proves the following:

1. The STAR S4 laser accurately ablates higher-order terms as programmed
2. The WaveScan device accurately measures higher-order terms as proved by the agreement with ISP
3. The WaveScan device accurately measures higher-order aberrations not normally seen in conventional optics

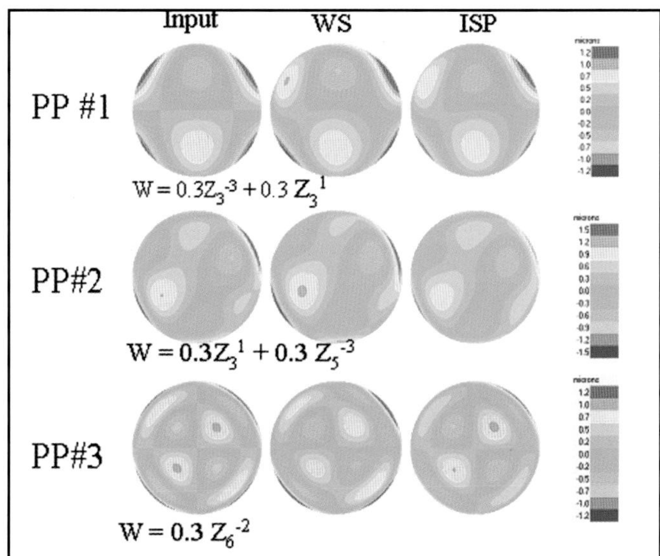

Figure 27-4. Wavefront maps of phase plates (special PreVue lenses) with individual Zernike terms. Phase plates were generated on plastic flats with a VISX STAR S4 laser and measured with a WaveScan system and an Interferometric Surface Profiler (ISP). Left: input to the laser with individual and combined Zernike aberrations up to the sixth order. Center: wavefront map measured with a WaveScan system. Right: wavefront maps obtained by measuring ablation depth profile with a Phase Shift Technology MicroXAM ISP.

Eye Tracking and Registration

In addition to being flexible enough to create a complex shape, the laser system must be capable of placing and keeping that shape exactly registered to the diagnosed treatment area. Precise registration involves compensating for the tiny eye movements that take place during surgery, as well as any cyclotorsional eye movement that occurs between the transition from a seated position at the measuring device to a supine position under the laser. Proper registration of a customized ablation is crucial for obtaining the best possible results.

Tracking Eye Movement During Surgery

The ActiveTrak Eye Tracking System tracks eye movement in three dimensions.[11,12] In addition to tracking horizontal (x) and vertical (y) movements of the eye, it tracks up and down motion (z) as well. An active, three-dimensional eye tracker is instrumental in the performance of wavefront-guided ablations because the importance of eye motion is magnified when the procedure is wavefront guided. Wavefront-guided ablations must be registered accurately on the cornea to achieve the intended refractive results. Therefore, eliminating the effects of eye motion is critical to achieving the best results.

In addition to tracking horizontal (x) and vertical (y) movements of the eye, it tracks up and down motion (z) as well.

The ActiveTrak System allows the laser beam to follow eye movements that occur during surgery by locking onto the natural pupil while the patient fixates on a flashing light-emitting diode (LED). The tracker monitors eye movements 60 times a second, or six times for every pulse of the laser, while the laser system's beam-deflection module steers the laser beam to keep up with the pupil's movements. The software program continually retrieves the pupil position from the eye tracker, adjusting the position of the laser beam to follow the eye's movements.

If the pupil briefly strays more than 1.50 mm beyond the starting point, the tracker remains active, but stops the laser from firing until the pupil moves back into range. The reason for stopping the laser from firing has to do with the angle of the beam in relationship to the eye as it rotates. If the beam follows the rotation of the eye beyond a certain point, the spot begins to elongate, which decreases its effectiveness. VISX has determined the acceptable cutoff distance to be 1.50 mm. In this case, the doctor merely waits until the laser begins to fire again. The ActiveTrak System can detect the eye movements and stop the laser much faster than the surgeon can.

There is no need for pharmaceutical dilation because illumination is off the visual axis and the pupil remains dark. The cameras determine eye position by measuring motion along the x- and y-axes as well as up and down (z- axis) motion. As with any tracker that follows the pupil, it is important that the patient maintain excellent fixation to avoid ablation errors due to parallax. Maintaining fixation on the VISX system is easier for patients because the pupil is not dilated for the procedure.

Overcoming Cyclotorsional Motion: Iris-Based Solution

Human eyes often undergo torsional movements about their axes during normal activities. The amount of rotation may be influenced by what they are viewing, the motion of the subject, and head and body orientation. When the wavefront measurement is taken, the patient is sitting up. For surgery, the patient is seated in a chair and then lowered to a supine position. Cyclotorsion has been shown to occur with these kinds of movements. If cyclotorsion is not compensated for, the resulting rotational errors could have a significant negative impact on results.[13]

At this writing, doctors must document points of reference with manual techniques such as inking the limbus just before surgery or sketching the iris area or local blood vessel formations. These methods are time consuming and lacking in accuracy. Fortunately, development of a reliable method of image matching is progressing well.

VISX has recently developed and applied for a patent for a noninvasive, automated alignment method that effectively eliminates the registration problems presented by cyclotorsional movement between wavefront measurement and surgical procedure.[14] This method captures the images of the eye with cameras on both the measurement and the treatment devices. Immediately before treatment, the features of the iris from both images are matched, and the laser adjusts to compensate for cyclotorsional position.

Similar technology to cyclotorsional registration is currently under development for tracking cyclotorsional movements during surgery. The pupil characteristics under the laser are continually matched during surgery by the tracking system.

Table 27-1
Multicenter Cohort Study

Gender	Mean Age	Preoperative Refractive Error
56 M, 45 F	34.9 ± 7.5 years	Sphere: -3.5 ± 1.4 D (-0.8 – -6.5) Cylinder: +0.5 ± 0.5 D (0.0 – +2.8) MRSE: -3.2 ± 1.3 D (-0.8 – -6.0)

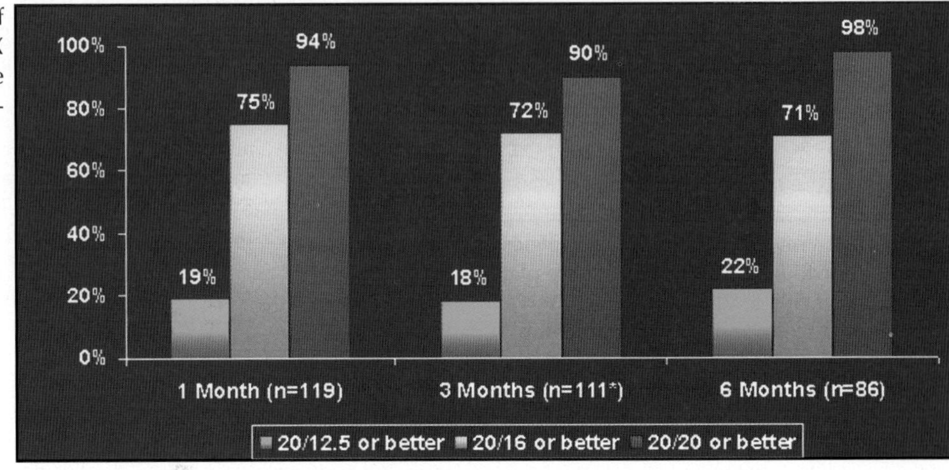

Figure 27-5. Uncorrected visual acuity of patients after refractive surgery with VISX wavefront-driven treatment. Data are from 176 eyes of 101 patients in a multicenter wavefront-driven LASIK trial.

Clinical Results With Wavefront-Guided Laser In-Situ Keratomileusis

What exactly do wavefront-guided ablations mean for the field of refractive surgery? The term *super vision* has been used extensively to describe the hoped-for results, but, in view of the results of early studies, what should be considered realistic expectations?

Human vision is limited by diffraction, retinal cone spacing, and aberrations. Briefly, there is nothing we can do about diffraction or retinal cone spacing limits. Cone spacing holds improvement to 20/8 at the maximum. However, research indicates that by surgically reducing higher-order aberrations that could not be measured previously, we can consistently obtain levels of vision correction exceeding those previously achieved by correcting spherocylindrical errors.

The results of the multicenter study related on the following pages were predictive of the outcomes physicians are now seeing in clinical practice.

Six centers participated in the study of 176 eyes of 101 patients.[1] All of the centers used the VISX custom ablation system consisting of the WaveScan Wavefront System and the VISX STAR S4 ActiveTrak Excimer Laser System using the WavePrint of each subject. Treatments were bilateral laser in-situ keratomileusis (LASIK) with 6 mm optical zones blended to 8 mm. There were no nomogram adjustments, and the target was emmetropia. Follow-up data were collected at 1, 3, and 6 months. Table 27-1 describes the study.

Refractive Outcomes

Overall, study results were very encouraging. Figure 27-5 shows UCVA at 1-, 3-, and 6- months. At the 6-month postoperative vision test, 47% of the eyes had uncorrected visual acuity (UCVA) better than their pre-op best-spectacle corrected visual acuity (BSCVA); 98% of eyes were at 20/20 or better; 71% of eyes were at 20/16 or better; and 22% of eyes were at 20/12.5 or better. No eye lost more than three letters of BSCVA, and no eye had a postoperative BSCVA lower than 20/20.

MRSE was -0.20 D at 6 months. Ninety-nine percent of eyes achieved refractive stability between the 1-, 3-, and 6-month visits. At six months, 94% of eyes treated were within ±0.50 D of their intended correction, and 100% were within 1.00 D (Figure 27-6).

Higher-Order Aberrations

One significant trend in the study was the improvement in higher-order aberrations. In the past, LASIK has been known to induce higher-order aberrations.[15,16] In this study, at 6 months 33% of eyes experienced a reduction in higher-order aberrations for a 6 mm pupil; 32% of eyes experienced increased higher-order aberrations by less than 0.10 microns (μm) root mean square (RMS) wavefront error for a 6 mm pupil; and 35% of eyes experienced increased higher-order aberrations greater than 0.10 μm RMS for a 6 mm pupil. Preoperative higher-order RMS wavefront error was 0.28 ± 0.12 mm while 6-month postoperative RMS wavefront error was 0.33 ± 0.10 mm for a 6 mm pupil. More than 70% of eyes (n = 64) either improved or changed by less than 0.10 mm in coma, trefoil, and spherical aberration terms. Results are shown in Figure 27-7.

Case Study

Figure 27-8 shows the wavefront maps of one eye before and after the wavefront-guided treatment. The best-corrected visual acuity of this patient before treatment was 20/20. After surgery,

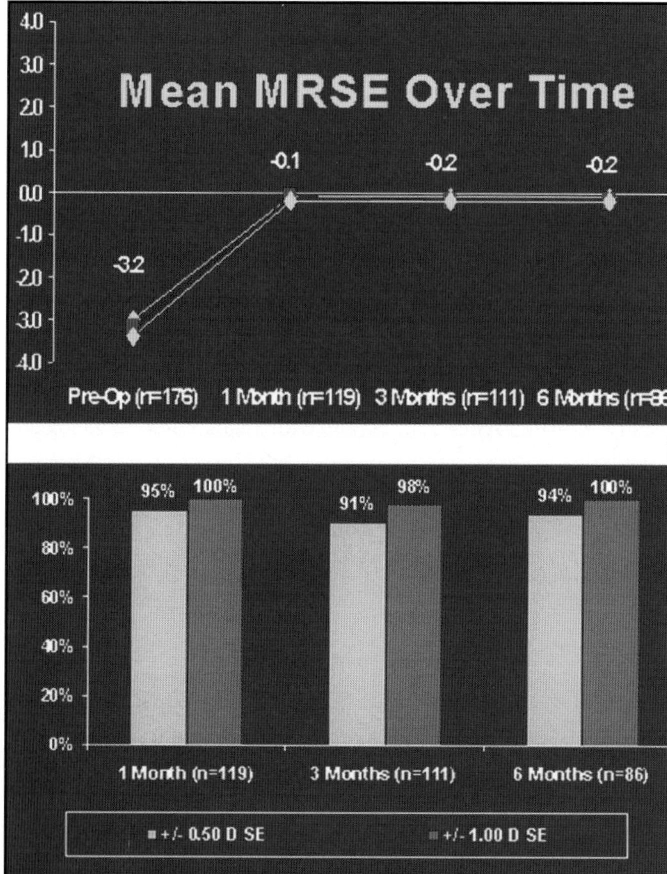

Figure 27-6. Lower-order refractive outcomes with VISX wavefront-guided LASIK. Top: Mean MRSE over time. Bottom: Percentage of eyes within ±0.5 D ± 1 D of desired SE. Data are from 176 eyes of 101 patients in a multicenter wavefront driven LASIK trial.

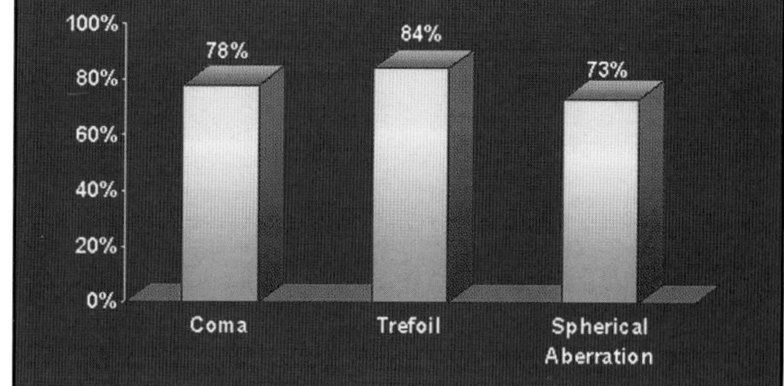

Figure 27-7. Percentage of eyes with improvement or a change of < 0.10 μm (n=64) at 6 months.

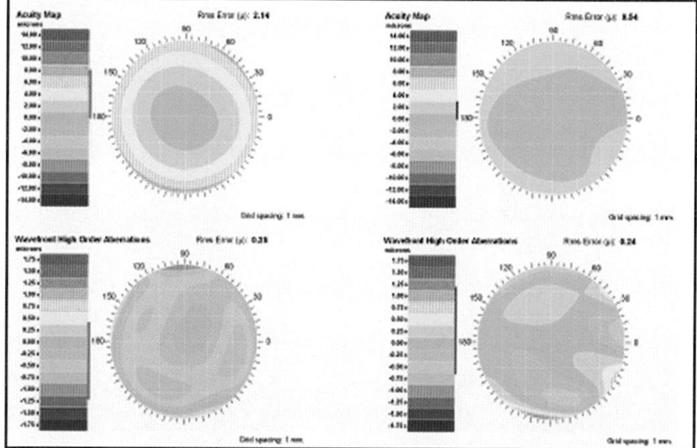

Figure 27-8. Wavefront maps of one eye measured preoperatively (left) and postoperatively (right). Top: Total wavefront error of the eye. Bottom: Higher-order aberrations of the eye. Reduction of spherical aberration was from 0.16 mm preoperatively to 0.02 mm postoperatively and trefoil from 0.11 mm preoperatively to 0.02 mm postoperatively. Total RMS of higher-order aberration was about the same (preoperative: 0.25 mm, postoperative: 0.24 mm). The surgery induced some local irregular aberration, which can be seen at the edge of the wavefront map.

this patient's UCVA was 20/16 at the 1-, 3-, and 6-month exams. With a 6 mm pupil size, spherical aberration was reduced from 0.16 μm to 0.02 μm and trefoil was reduced from 0.11 mm to 0.02 mm. Total RMS of higher-order aberrations was about the same because the surgery induced some local irregular aberration that can be seen at the edge of wavefront map.

> In this study, at 6 months 33% of eyes experienced a reduction in higher-order aberrations for a 6 mm pupil; 32% of eyes experienced increased higher-order aberrations by less than 0.10 μm RMS wavefront error for a 6 mm pupil; and 35% of eyes experienced increased higher-order aberrations greater than 0.10 μm RMS for a 6 mm pupil.

Subjective Questionnaire Results

Patients were given subjective questionnaires preoperatively and postoperatively regarding their relative satisfaction with their vision under different lighting conditions. At 6 months postoperatively, 96% of the respondents said they were "very satisfied" under bright conditions, 2% were "unsure," and 2% were "somewhat dissatisfied."

Patients experienced quite a lot of night vision improvement over their preoperative perceptions. Under night vision conditions, 87% said they were "very satisfied" or "satisfied" postoperatively as contrasted with 69% who indicated this preoperatively. The somewhat dissatisfied group decreased from 21% to 6%, and those who were "very dissatisfied" with their night vision prior to surgery dropped from 1% to 0%. Ten percent stated that they were unsure about their satisfaction with their night vision prior to surgery. This group decreased slightly to 8% at 6 months. Details are shown in Figure 27-9.

Patients' satisfaction with night vision under glare conditions also improved. The "very satisfied" group increased from 62% to 73%. The preoperative "very dissatisfied" group dropped from 4% to 0%. The "somewhat dissatisfieds" decreased from 21% to 6%. The "not sure" group increased from 13% to 21%. Results are shown in Figure 27-10.

Halo incidence overall also decreased postoperatively. Patients who never or rarely experienced halos preoperatively increased from 76% to 88% postoperatively. The percentage of those who sometimes saw halos decreased by more than half —

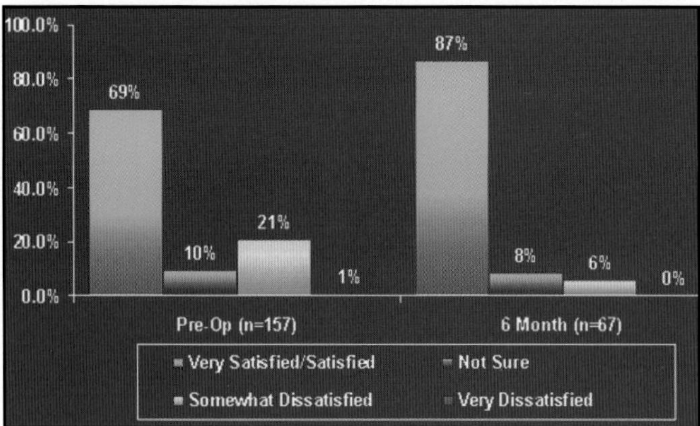

Figure 27-9. Patient satisfaction with night vision.

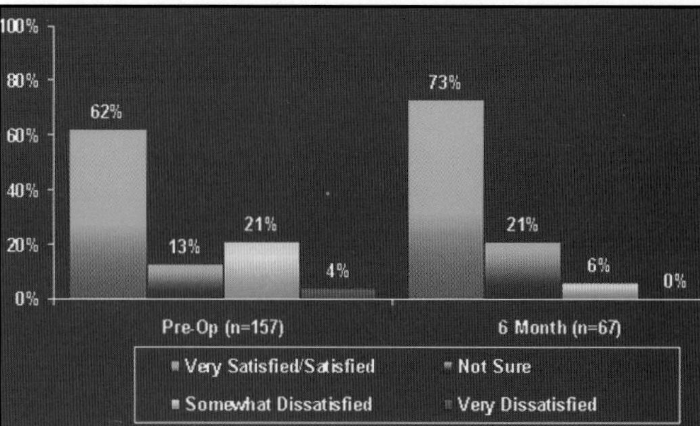

Figure 27-10. Patient satisfaction with night vision under glare conditions.

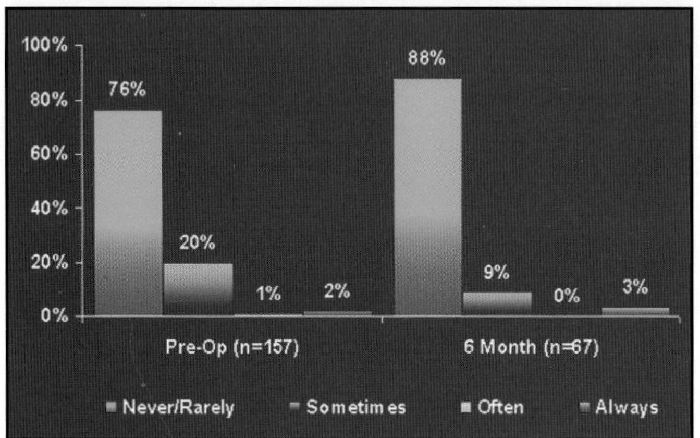

Figure 27-11. Report of halo by patients preoperatively and 6 months postoperatively.

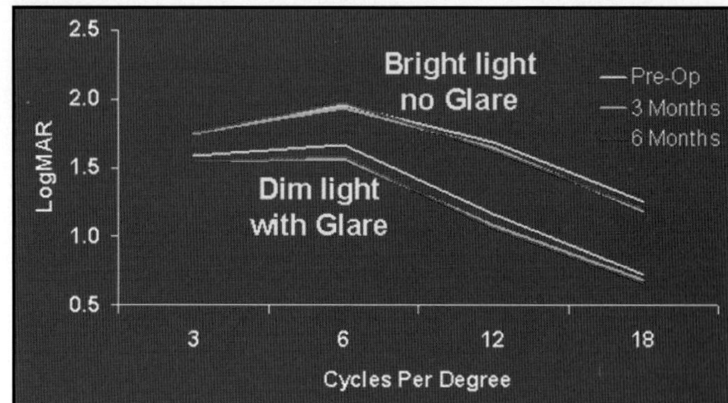

Figure 27-12. Contrast sensitivity preoperatively, and at 3 and 6 months postoperatively.

from 20% preoperatively to 9% postoperatively. The segment that often saw halos decreased from 1% to 0%. The segment that reported always seeing halos increased from 2% to 3%. Details are shown in Figure 27-11.

Contrast Sensitivity

Patients' contrast sensitivity was tested in dim light with glare and in bright light with no glare. At 6 months, 81% had the same or better contrast sensitivity in dim light with glare, and 96% had the same or better level under bright conditions. Results are shown in Figure 27-12.

Complications

Three adverse events were reported, but they all resolved satisfactorily. One eye experienced an epithelial defect. At the 6-month visit, this patient's UCVA was 20/12.5, and there was no loss in BSCVA. In another patient, one eye developed diffuse lamellar keratitis (DLK). At the 1-week visit, this patient's UCVA was 20/16 and the event resolved with no loss in BSCVA. The third adverse event was an incomplete LASIK flap in one eye. The flap was repositioned and no laser treatment was applied. The patient's manifest refraction did not change from baseline.

Longer-Term Low Myopia Results

One of the centers taking part in the multicenter studies, the Kraff Eye Institute in Chicago, had gathered 12-month data at the time of this writing.[17] Of the 19 subjects, 24% had attained 20/12.5 or better UCVA, and 64% had attained 20/16 or better UCVA. All patients had achieved 20/20 or better UCVA. The number of patients with BSCVA of 20/12.5 preoperatively increased fourfold with the surgery.

Conclusion

In the study cited above, at six months, 98% of eyes had achieved UCVA of 20/20 or better; 94% of eyes had come within 0.50 D of emmetropia, and no eyes had lost more than three letters of BSCVA at 6 months. Although there is still much to resolve regarding the nature and role of higher-order aberrations in vision, in our opinion, these results indicate that the promise of wavefront-guided ablations will be fulfilled and that a new standard for refractive surgery is in the process of being established.

Acknowledgments

The authors are thankful to Drs. S. Coleman, W. Culbertson, M. Hamill, N. Jabbur, C. Kraff, M. Kraff, R. Maloney, T. O'Brien, S. Pflugfelder, B. Seibel, W. Stark, and S. Yoo for providing the clinical data from the VISX-sponsored multicenter trials for the wavefront-guided LASIK; and to Drs. D. Chernyak, C. Harner, K. Yee, and E. Gross, R. Hofer, J. Persoff and many other employees at VISX and at 20/10 Perfect Vision who are instrumental in developing various technologies for the VISX platform. The authors are also thankful to Ms. C.E. Hunt and Dr. L. Wang for their assistance in preparing this manuscript.

VISX, WaveScan Wavefront System, VISX STAR S4 ActiveTrak Excimer Laser System, WavePrint, and PreVue Lens are registered trademarks of VISX Incorporated, Santa Clara, California.

References

1. O'Brien T. Six-month results of the multi-center wavefront LASIK trial. ASCRS 2002. Philadelphia, Pennsylvania.
2. Seiler T, Mrochen M, Kaemmerer M. Operative correction of ocular aberrations to improve visual acuity. *J Refract Surg.* 2000;16:S619-S622.
3. MacRae S, Williams DR. Wavefront guided ablation. *Am J Ophthalmol.* 2001;132:915-919.
4. Krueger R. Technology requirements for customized corneal ablation. In: MacRae S, Krueger R, Applegate R, eds. *Customized Corneal Ablation: The Quest for Super Vision.* Thorofare, NJ: SLACK Incorporated; 2001:133-147.
5. Liang J, Grimm B, Goelz S, Bille JF. Objective measurement of the wave aberrations of the human eye using a Hartmann-Shack wavefront sensor. *J Opt Soc Am A.* 1994; A11:1949-1957.
6. Liang J, Williams DR, Miller D. Supernormal vision and high resolution imaging through adaptive optics. *J Opt Soc A.* 1997; A14:2884-2892.
7. Wang L, Wang N, Koch D. Evaluation of refractive error measurements of the WaveScan Wavefront system and Tracey Wavefront aberrometer. *J Cataract Refract Surg.* 2003;29:970-979.
8. Gross E, Yee K. Method for Generating Scanning Spot Locations for Laser Eye Surgery. US patent application (PCT# :WO 01/67978).
9. Watson J, Shimmick J, Cutrer B, et al. Method for wavefront driven custom ablations. In: Bille J, Harner C, Loesel F, eds. *New Frontiers in Vision and Aberration Free Refractive Surgery.* New York, NY: Springer Verlag; 2003:85-101.
10. Bille JF. Preoperative simulation of outcomes using adaptive optics. *J Refract Surg.* 2000;16:S608-S610.
11. Shimmick J, Yee K, Cutrer B. The VISX STAR S4 ActiveTrak eye tracker. In Bille J, Harner C, Loesel F, eds. *New Frontiers in Vision and Aberration Free Refractive Surgery.* New York, NY: Springer Verlag; 2003:71-83.
12. Yee K, Munnerlyn C. Two-camera off-axis eye tracker for laser eye surgery. US patent #6322216, 2001.
13. Guirao A, Williams D, Cox I. Effect of rotation and translation on the expected benefit of an ideal method to correct the eye's higher-order aberrations. *J Opt Soc Am A.* 2001;A18:1003-1015.
14. Harner C. Cyclotorsional tracking technology. Paper presented at: ASCRS; June 5, 2002;Philadelphia, Pa.
15. Seiler T, Kaemmer M, Mierdel P, Krinke HE. Ocular optical aberrations after photorefractive keratectomy for myopia and myopic astigmatism. *Arch Ophthalmol.* 2000;118:17-27.
16. Applegate RA, Howland HC, Klyce SD. Corneal aberrations and refractive surgery. In: MacRae S, Krueger R, Applegate R, eds. *Customized Corneal Ablation: The Quest for Super Vision.* Thorofare, NJ: SLACK Incorporated; 2001:239-246.
17. Kraff C. Results of wavefront-guided LASIK studies using the VISX WaveScan system and STAR S4 ActiveTrak Excimer Laser system to create custom ablations. *J Cataract Refract Surg.* In press.

Chapter 28

Customized Ablation Using the Bausch & Lomb Zyoptix System

Scott M. MacRae, MD; Steven Slade, MD; Daniel S. Durrie, MD; and Ian Cox, PhD

The treatment of the eye with wavefront-driven customized ablation represents a fundamental shift in eye care practitioners' approach to the correction of refractive errors. Wavefront-driven correction attempts to correct higher-order aberrations in addition to the conventional treatment of sphere and cylinder. These higher-order aberrations are minimal in some patients but may be considerable in others. Preliminary studies have been encouraging, suggesting that the correction of higher-order aberration is possible but certain higher aberrations, such as spherical aberration, are more difficult to treat.[1-5]

This chapter will present our experience using wavefront-guided customized ablation in a large cohort of eyes involved in an United States Food and Drug Administration (FDA) clinical trial.

Methods

Three hundred forty eyes were treated using wavefront driven customized ablation as part of a prospective FDA investigational device exemption multicentric clinical trial. All patients were given and agreed to an informed consent that met the requirements of each local institutional review board and the Declaration of Helsinki. The study was Internal Review Board (IRB) monitored at each of three investigational sites: the University of Rochester, Rochester, New York; The Laser Center, Houston, Tex; and Hunkeler Eye Center, Kansas City, Mo. The treatments were up to -7 diopters (D) of myopia with up to -3.50 D of astigmatism.

Inclusion Criteria

Manifest refraction and mesopic pupil diameter measurements were performed on each eye. Measurements taken with the Orbscan II Cornea Mapping System (Bausch & Lomb Diagnostics, Salt Lake City, Utah) yielded corneal thickness and curvature readings, which were used to rule out keratoconus suspects. The Orbscan corneal thickness measurement was also used to screen for corneas that were too thin relative to the predicted thickness of the ablation.

The subjects were required to be in good health with no major systemic diseases that might affect outcome, such as collagen vascular disease or diabetes. We required them to have a visual acuity correctable to 20/40 or better in both eyes. The patients needed to have a stable refractive error for at least 12 months and be 21 years or older.

Exclusion Criteria

Patients were excluded if their baseline corneal thickness and planned operative parameters for the laser in-situ keratomileusis (LASIK) procedure would result in less than 250 microns (μm) of remaining posterior corneal thickness below the flap, postoperatively. Eyes were excluded if the 2.5% neosynephrine dilated (noncycloplegic) Zywave refraction (Predicted Phoropter Value) and the cycloplegic (1% tropicainamide) refraction exhibited a difference of 0.75 D or greater in sphere power, or a difference of greater than 0.50 D in cylinder power, or a difference in cylinder axis of more than 15 degrees when compared to the manifest or cycloplegic (1% tropicamide) refraction.

Patients were excluded if they had active chronic eye or eyelid disease or any corneal abnormality (including recurrent corneal erosion, basement membrane disease, or keratoconus). Eyes with previous surgery were excluded.

Examination Methods

The preoperative examinations included manifest, 2.5% neosynephrine "dilated manifest," and a cycloplegic (1% Cyclogel) refractions. We collected standardized distance visual acuity by using a Vector Vision backlit ETDRS chart with incident illumination of 74 to 125 foot candles adjusted for either 13 feet (4 meters) or 8 feet.

Corneal topography and pachymetry were also determined using the Orbscan. Contrast sensitivity was done with the Vision Sciences Research Corporation (San Ramon, California) CST-1500 FACT test system. Contrast sensitivity was measured at five spatial frequencies: 1.5, 3, 6, 12, and 18 cycles/degree in both photopic and mesopic testing conditions according to the manufacturer's recommendations at the preoperative, 1 week, 1 month, 3 month, and 6 month postoperative exams.

Rigid contact lens and soft lens wearers were required to discontinue their contact lenses prior to the preoperative evaluation for a minimum of 3 weeks and 1 week, respectively.

Wavefront Sensing

Five Shack-Hartmann wavefront sensings using the Zywave aberrometer (Figure 28-1) (Bausch & Lomb, Rochester, NY) were performed after the eyes were dilated with 2.5% neosynephrine until the pupil diameter was a minimal of 6.00 millimeter (mm) diameter. The Zywave system measures up to and including the fifth Zernike order. The Zywave system measures sphere from

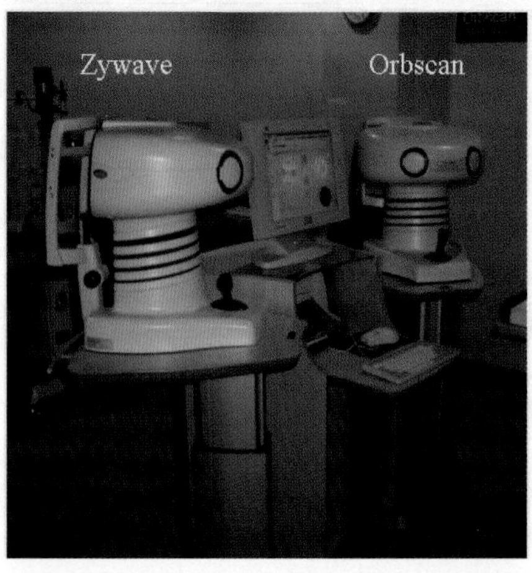

Figure 28-1. Bausch & Lomb Dual Work Station which combines the Zywave Shack-Hartmann Wavefront Sensor with the Orbscan Corneal Topographer. The Dual Workstation Zylink Software generates a customized excimer treatment profile that is driven by the Zywave Wavefront Sensor.

+6 to -12 D and cylinder from 0 to 5 D with pupil diameters ranging from 2.5 to 8.5 mm. The system uses a 785 nanometers (nm) infrared laser pulse that reaches a minimum beam diameter of 15 μm in focus on the retina with u 100 millisecond (ms) exposure period. A minimum of five Zywave measurements were taken. The wavefront sensing that had the closest correspondence to the manifest and cycloplegic refraction was selected for the laser treatment. The Orbscan and the Zywave readings were entered in the Zylink Software (Bausch & Lomb, Rochester, New York) and the ablation pattern was calculated (see Figure 28-1). The Zylink software uses the corneal pachymetry obtained from the Orbscan, the wavefront error data determined by the Zywave, and the surgeon's preferred ablation optical zone to construct the ablation pattern. No adjustments were made to the Zywave wavefront values for treatment. (Eyes were not treated with a monovision undercorrection and no correction factors were added.) A postoperative 2.5% neosynephrine-dilated Zywave measurement was performed at 1 week, 1 month, 3 months, and 6 months.

The Bausch & Lomb Dual Workstation combines the Orbscan corneal topographer with the Zywave wavefront sensor into one system, called Zylink, which creates the computer shot pattern for Zyoptix.

In the data analysis of higher-order aberration, we examined the percentage of eyes that had less than 0.10 μm of increase in root mean square (RMS) wavefront error from their preoperative value because we have noted that an increase of 0.10 μm or less of higher-order RMS wavefront error is not clinically significant.

Surgical Procedure

All eyes were marked with a methylene blue pen at the 3:00 and 6:00 limbal positions at the slit lamp. That position was confirmed when the patient first lay down on the operating table, and again prior to ablation, using an ocular reticule on the operating microscope. A superior hinged LASIK flap was then created using the Hansatome microkeratome (Bausch & Lomb, Rochester, New York).

The ablation was performed with the Bausch & Lomb Technolas 217Z excimer laser, which uses a 1 mm and a 2 mm spot size. A 120 hertz active eye tracker was used with a passive automatic shut-off system if the eye moved more than 0.5 mm. The system allows the surgeon to monitor the eye tracker while performing the procedure to ensure centration. The majority of the treatment is done with a 2 mm spot and the transition zone and higher- order aberration are treated with a 1 mm spot.

Patients were seen at 1 day, 1 week, and 1 month, 3 months, and 6 months postoperatively. They were asked to fill out a questionnaire quantifying their subjective symptoms and their response to the surgery at the 6-month visit.

Statistical Analysis

Comparisons of preoperative values to postoperative values were done using the McNemar test. Chi-squared tests were performed to compare the proportion of patients who reported improvement to the proportion who reported worsening for each symptom parameter. (Patients reporting "no change" were excluded from the analysis.)

Results

Demographics/Accountability

The mean age of the participants was 34.4 ± 8.29 years and there were 46.1% males and 53.9% females. The accountability was 100% with all 340 eyes being evaluated at the 6-month postoperative interval.

Preoperative Measurements

The mean preoperative mesopic pupil diameter was 5.60 mm ± 1.07 mm. The population was reflective of a representative myopic population where 54.3% of eyes had a preoperative best-corrected visual acuity (BCVA) of 20/16 or better and 98.2% of eyes were 20/20 or better, which is similar to our previous study on the Bausch & Lomb Technolas 217 using conventional treatment. This indicates that our preselection techniques did not bias our study population toward eyes that saw 20/16 or better.

Efficacy

The mean preoperative myopic sphere was -3.32 ± 1.54 (Table 28-1.) The mean postoperative sphere was +0.29 ± 0.55 at 6 months postoperatively. Refractive stability was obtained at 1 to 3 months with the mean postoperative spherical values ranging between +0.33 ± 0.63 at 1 day postoperatively and +0.29 ± 0.55 D at 6 months postoperatively (see Table 28-1).

Of the 340 eyes, 91.5% of eyes had 20/20 or better uncorrected visual acuity (UCVA), while 70.3% had 20/16 and 30.9% had 20/12.5 or better UCVA 6 months after surgery. Most (99.4%) eyes had 20/40 or better vision without correction 6 months after surgery. When 117 eyes treated for sphere only were analyzed, 94% of eyes were 20/20 or better.

Table 28-1
Refractive Status of Eyes Preoperatively and Postoperatively With Regard to Manifest Refraction Sphere and Cylinder

MANIFEST SPHERE (D)	N	MEAN	MINIMUM	MAXIMUM	STANDARD DEVIATION
Zyoptix preoperative sphere	340	-3.32	-7.00	-0.50	1.54
Zyoptix 3M sphere	340	0.30	-1.25	2.00	0.53
Zyoptix 6M sphere	340	0.30	-1.50	2.75	0.55
Zyoptix preoperative cylinder	340	-0.67	-3.25	0.00	0.62
Zyoptix 3M cylinder	340	-0.29	-1.75	0.00	0.32
Zyoptix 6M cylinder	340	-0.26	-1.50	0.00	0.32

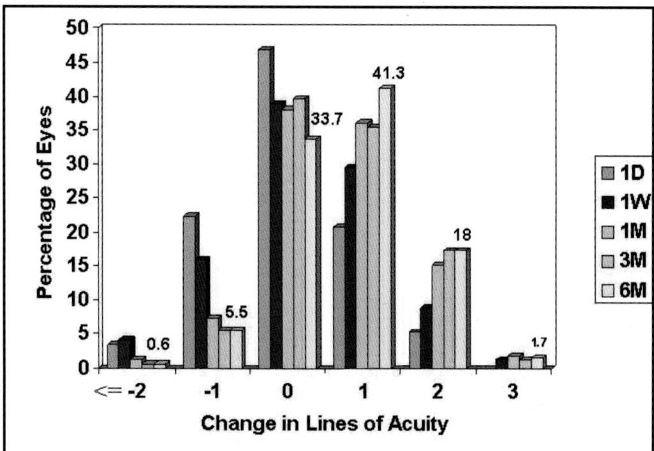

Figure 28-2. Comparison of BCVA preoperatively, 1 day, 1 week, 1 month, 3 months, and 6 months postoperatively. At 6 months, 60% of eyes gained one or more lines of vision while 0.6% of eyes lost two lines of vision. No eyes lost more than two lines of vision.

Of the 340 eyes, 91.5% of eyes had 20/20 or better UCVA, while 70.3 had 20/16 and 30.9% had 20/12.5 or better uncorrected vision 6 months after surgery.

Predictability

Of the 340 eyes, 258 (75.9%) were within ±0.50 D of plano while 319 (93.8%) of eyes were within ±1 D of plano.

Astigmatism

Preoperatively, the mean astigmatism was -0.68 ± 0.59 D, while the postoperative mean astigmatism was -0.29 ± 0.32 D at 6 months postoperatively (see Table 28-1). The mean intended refractive cylinder (IRC) was 0.68 D, while the surgically induced astigmatism (SIRC) was 0.75 D. The SIRC/IRC ratio is 1.10 ± 0.74 D, indicating a slight overcorrection of the astigmatic component.

Safety

At 6 months after surgery, 78.3% of eyes had UCVA that was either as good as or better than the BCVA measured preoperatively. Sixty percent of eyes gained one or more lines of BCVA and 19.7% of eyes gained two lines or more lines of BCVA (Figure 28-2). Ninety-nine percent of eyes had 20/20 or better BCVA at 6 months postoperatively. There were no eyes that lost more than two lines of BCVA at 6 months postoperatively. Two eyes lost two lines of BCVA vision 6 months after surgery. One eye had a preoperative BCVA of 20/12.5, which decreased two lines to 20/20 at 6 months postoperatively. The second eye had a preoperative BCVA of 20/16 that was reduced to 20/25 at the 6-month interval.

At 6 months after surgery, 73% percent of eyes had UCVA that was either as good as or better than the BCVA measured. Sixty percent (60%) of eyes gained one or more lines of vision of BCVA and 19.7% gained two lines of BCVA.

Wavefront Analysis

Preoperative

The preoperative wavefront testing demonstrated a variation in the amount of preoperative higher-order aberration with a normal distribution about the mean of 0.414 µm ± 0.162 µm of RMS wavefront error (Figure 28-3). There was no correlation between the amount of preoperative sphere or cylinder and the amount of higher-order aberrations, nor was there any correlation between the amount of sphere or cylinder and the amount of the individual Zernike modes tested (Figure 28-4). The preoperative higher-order aberration was predominantly third-order aberration (coma and trefoil) (Figure 28-5). There was very little fifth-order aberration noted preoperatively or postoperatively on average.

Postoperative

Postoperatively, there was a decrease or insignificant increase in 69% (Figure 28-6), 36% and 96% of eyes with third-, fourth-

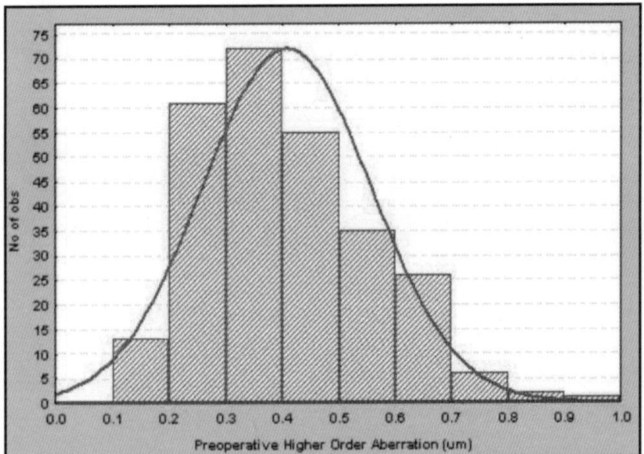

Figure 28-3. The preoperative distribution of the higher-order wavefront aberration. Note that higher-order aberration is being presented as root mean square (RMS). This is the square root of the sum of the individual Zernike terms squared. This makes the values always positive and allows comparison of the magnitude of wavefront aberration from eye to eye. A higher-order RMS value of zero indicates a perfect optical system. The typical amount of preoperative higher-order aberration measured using the Bausch & Lomb Zywave is about 0.40 µm for a 6 mm pupil.

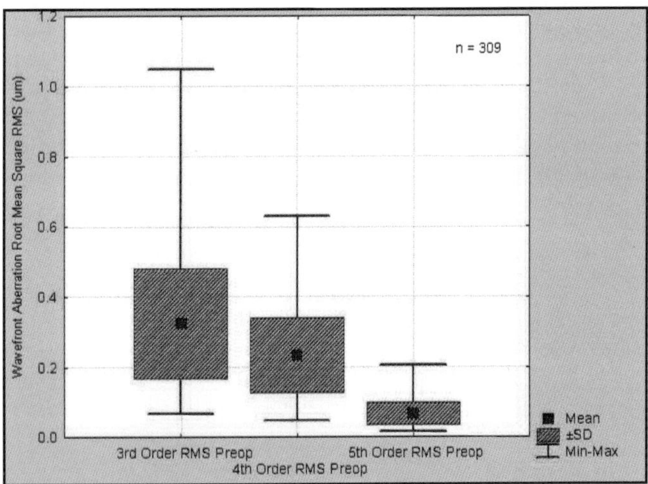

Figure 28-5. Profile of preoperative higher-order aberrations: third, fourth, and fifth expressed in RMS of wavefront error. Note that third-order aberrations dominate. Coma and trefoil are third-order aberrations. Fourth-order (including spherical aberration) and fifth-order aberrations are not as predominant preoperatively.

and fifth-order aberrations when compared to higher-order aberrations preoperatively with a 6.00 mm aperture. When total higher-order aberrations were analyzed, 49% (Figure 28-7) (6 mm aperture or pupil diameter) and 70% (5 mm aperture) of eyes either showed a decrease or insignificant increase (<0.10 µm root mean square [RMS]) increase in higher-order aberration when compared to preoperatively. Twenty-eight percent of eyes showed a reduction in total higher-order aberrations at 6 months postoperatively, when compared to preoperatively, with a 6 mm aperture or pupil diameter.

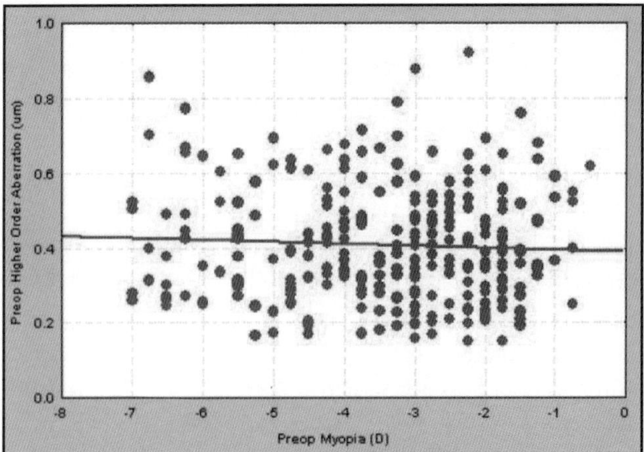

Figure 28-4. The relationship between degree of myopia and higher-order RMS. Note that there is no correlation between myopia and higher-order aberration. Some have speculated that higher degrees of myopia will have more higher-order aberration, but this was not noted in the current study.

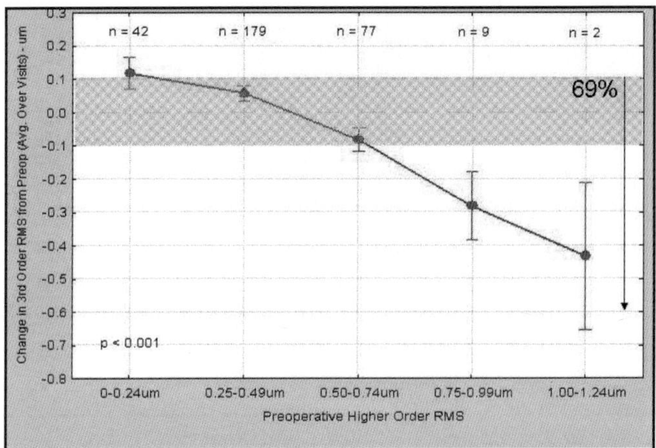

Figure 28-6. Third-order aberrations in RMS values (including trefoil and coma) 6 months postoperatively compared to preoperatively. Note that if the eye has 0.3 or more µm of higher-order RMS error, on average, preoperatively, it is likely to have a reduction in third-order aberration. The gray portion of the graph represents the limits of detection of change in the higher-order aberrations for the typical patient (ie, a typical patient would not notice a decrease or increase of higher-order aberrations by approximately 0.1 µm of higher-order RMS). In the 340 eye cohort, 69% of eyes either had a decrease or insignificant increase (<0.1% increase RMS) in third-order aberration when compared to preoperative mean values.

> Postoperatively, there was a decrease or insignificant increase in total higher-order aberration in 49% of eyes with a 6 mm pupil and 70% of eyes with a 5 mm pupil. Third-order aberrations improved the most, with 69% of eyes either having an improvement or insignificant increase in third-order aberrations.

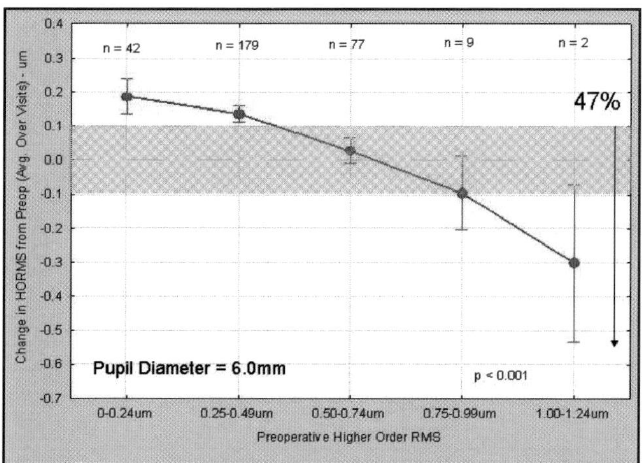

Figure 28-7. Total higher-order aberrations at 6 months postoperatively in RMS values compared to preoperatively. Eyes with 0.5 µm or more RMS error preoperatively were statistically more likely to have either a reduction or insignificant increase in higher-order aberration compared to eyes with less than 0.5 µm of RMS preoperatively. Nearly half (49%) of eyes studied had a decrease or insignificant increase (<0.1 µm RMS) in total higher-order aberration when compared to mean preoperative values.

Postoperatively, there was a mean increase in higher-order aberration in eyes with 0.50 µm or less of RMS wavefront error preoperatively (see Figure 28-7). For eyes that had more than 0.50 µm RMS wavefront error preoperatively, there was a mean decrease in RMS of higher-order aberration.

Contrast Sensitivity

The mean contrast sensitivity measures improved from preoperative to 6 month postoperative values by one patch or 0.15 log units for all spatial frequencies tested (1.5, 3, 6, 12, and 18 cycles/degree), which includes low, mid, and high spatial frequencies (Table 28-2). The one patch postsurgery improvement is a 29% average increase in contrast for the entire population noted at all spatial frequencies under low (mesopic) and high (photopic) illuminations. This was noted to be more striking when larger ablation optical zones were used (6.5 and 7.0 mm compared to 6.0 mm).

Under photopic (daylight) conditions, 25% of eyes were >0.30 log units (two patches) improved compared to preoperatively, while 71% were unchanged and 4.1% were >0.30 log units worse. Under mesopic (nighttime) conditions, 22.1% of eyes were improved >0.30 log units, while 75.9% of eyes were unchanged from preoperative and 2.1% were worse than preoperative.

Mean contrast sensitivity improved 0.15 log units when compared to preoperative values for all spatial frequencies tested (1.5, 3, 6, 12, and 18 cycles/degree).

Table 28-2

Percentage of Patients With Clinically Significant Change in Contrast Sensitivity at 6M Postoperative*

Eyes >0.3 Log Units	Photopic Daylight	Mesopic Nighttime
Better than preoperative	25.0%	22.1%
Same as preoperative	71.0%	75.9%
Worse than preoperative	4.1%	2.1%

*Contrast sensitivity data demonstrating two patch units (>0.3 log units) change comparing the preoperative evaluations with the evaluation at 6 months postoperatively. A change of 0.15 log units (one patch unit) represented a 29% contrast improvement in the postoperative eye cohort overall for both photopic and mesopic conditions.

Complications

The following complications occurred at the time of surgery: the microkeratome stopped halfway through the cut (case excluded from the study), one eye had a thin flap associated with an epithelial defect (case excluded from the study), one eye had a small (<2 mm) flap hinge tear that healed uneventfully, and one treatment had a laser energy problem that was treated as planned after a laser gas refill. The most common complication postoperatively was debris in the interface. This was noted in 7.9% (27/340) of eyes one day after surgery but only 2.0% (7/340) of eyes had interface debris noted at the 6 month visit. We found that 5.8% (19/340) of eyes had stage 2 or less interface keratitis. Two eyes were taken back to the operating room and the interface washed out for lamellar keratitis. These eyes recovered without sequelae. One eye was noted to have a corneal recurrent erosion at 6 months.

Optical Zone Efficacy

We found a strong relationship between improved outcomes and the use of larger ablation optical zones. The was a statistically significant better outcome in UCVA, photopic and mesopic contrast sensitivity, reduction in higher-order aberrations, and improvement in subjective symptoms when larger ablation optical zones (specifically 6.5 to 7 mm) were used when compared to smaller optical zones (6 mm). The use of a larger ablation optical zone tended to minimize an increase in higher-order aberration. We recommend the use of a larger optical zone if feasible while balancing this with other considerations like corneal thickness and pupil size.

Subjective Surveys

Nine of 18 subjective symptoms surveyed before and after the surgery were significantly improved overall after surgery, including bright light vision, dim light vision, and difficulties with night driving (Table 28-3 [shown in yellow]). Seven of the 18

Patients noted an significant improvement in eight of the 18 subjective categories surveyed including an improvement in dim light vision and in difficulties with night diving

Table 28-3. Subjective patient symptoms demonstrating symptoms that had no statistically significant change in grey. Patient categories that had a significant improvement are noted in yellow. Patient categories that were significantly worse postoperatively are shown in white. Only two categories were worse, dryness and fluctuation in vision. Nine of the 18 categories surveyed were improved compared to preoperatively. The unchanged group is not shown for simplicity sake but can be derived by subtracting from 100% the sum of the worse and better categories. For instance, light sensitivity was better than preoperative in 36.8% of eyes and worse in 7.6% for a total of 44.4% that were better or worse, while 55.6% were unchanged.

	Better Than Preop	Worse Than Preop	p-value
Light Sensitivity	36.8% (125)	7.6% (26)	<0.001
Headaches	25.3% (86)	5.3% (18)	<0.001
Pain	6.2% (21)	2.1% (7)	0.008
Redness	23.2% (79)	10.9% (37)	<0.001
Excessive Tearing	12.1% (41)	3.8% (13)	<0.001
Burning	14.4% (49)	7.9% (27)	0.012
Bright Light Vision	23.9% (81)	10.6% (36)	<0.001
Dim Light Vision	25.4% (86)	17.4% (59)	0.025
Difficulties with Night Driving	40.3% (137)	10.3% (35)	<0.001
Normal Light Vision	9.4% (32)	11.2% (38)	0.473
Grittiness	8.5% (29)	6.2% (21)	0.258
Glare	20.9% (71)	15.3% (52)	0.087
Halos	13.5% (46)	14.4% (49)	0.758
Blurry Vision	22.4% (76)	18.5% (63)	0.270
Double Vision	1.5% (5)	3.2% (11)	0.134
Ghost Images	4.4% (15)	4.4% (15)	1.000
Dryness	19.7% (79)	31.2% (106)	0.003
Fluctuation in Vision	7.5% (25)	24.2% (81)	<0.001

Post op Better — No Difference — Preop Better

subjective symptoms at the 6 month interval were not significantly different when compared to preoperatively (see Table 28-3 [shown in grey]). There were two categories that were worse: fluctuation in vision and dryness. The dryness change was primarily caused by shift from 62.1% of eyes reported as an absence of dryness preoperatively to 48.5% at 6 months. The percentage of mild dryness increased 15.6% from 30.0% preoperatively to 45.6% at 6 months. Interestingly, there was no increase in moderate or marked dryness when comparing the preoperative to 6 months postoperative evaluation. Thus, most of the increase in dryness symptoms occurred when eyes moved from the absent category preoperatively to the mild category at 6 months.

Most (98.6%) patients noted moderate to extreme improvement in vision and of these, 84.7% noted extreme improvement. Most (98.8%, 336/340) patients were either very satisfied (90.9%, 309/340) or moderately satisfied (7.9%, 27/340). A few (1.2%, 4/340) patients were neutral in satisfaction and no patients (0/340) were dissatisfied with their results in the study. Most (98.2%, 334/340) would choose the surgery again when asked 6 months after the surgery, 1.2% (4/340) were unsure, and 0.6% (2/340) would choose not to have the surgery.

Discussion

Our study noted a similar pattern of higher-order aberration compared to other studies that evaluated normal populations.[6-8] We did not find a tendency for increasing higher-order aberrations with increasing myopia (see Figure 28-4). The current large population FDA study demonstrates the efficacy and safety of treatment guided by a Shack-Hartmann wavefront sensor, that treats lower- and higher-order aberrations.[9] This result is better than the 87.3% 20/20 or better UCVA noted in eyes treated with conventional sphere and cylinder (using the Bausch & Lomb Technolas) in a previous FDA study.[9] The current results indicate that 91.5% of eyes achieved 20/20 or better, while 70.3% of eyes achieved 20/16 or better uncorrected vision. Preoperatively, only 54.3% of eyes had a best corrected vision of 20/20 or better, indicating that this population was similar to that encountered in the similar populations previously tested.[9]

We also noted excellent safety results with 60% of eyes gaining one or more lines of vision and 78.3% of eyes obtaining UCVA that was either as good as their BCVA preoperatively. The worst visual loss was one eye, which went from 20/16 to 20/25 BCVA at the 6 month postoperative visit.

The postoperative wavefront analysis indicated that there was a decrease or insignificant increase in higher-order aberrations in 47% of eyes treated when analyzing with a 6 mm aperture (or pupil size). Third-order aberrations (trefoil and coma) were more prominent preoperatively and these aberrations seemed to be those most profoundly reduced with Zyoptix treatment. Fourth-order aberrations are not as large preoperatively, and a smaller percentage of eyes (36%) had either a decrease or insignificant increase. This is because there is minimal fourth-order aberrations preoperatively, particularly spherical aberration. We have found in a previous study of the microkeratome flap biomechanics that the flap causes a minimal increase in spherical aberration, when 17 eyes were followed after a flap cut.[10] When the flap was lifted, after 2 months of observation, and a conventional Bausch & Lomb Planoscan ablation was performed, there was a 40% increase in spherical aberration, indicating that spherical aberration is primarily caused by the laser ablation (Figure 28-8). The current software does not attempt to compensate for the laser-induced spherical aberration. Future studies will incorporate software modification that alters the ablation to further compensate for the laser induced spherical aberration component.

Our current study also noted an improvement in contrast sensitivity. We were also encouraged by the one patch improvement in contrast sensitivity results for low, mid and high spatial frequencies including 1.5, 3, 6, 12, and 18 cycles/degree. An improvement in contrast of more than one patch (0.15 log units) is clinically significant and is associated with images being clearer or sharper. We noted a two patch improvement in up to 25% of eyes, photopic conditions being slightly better than mesopic.

We also noted that patients reported a 98% moderate or very satisfied rate when surveyed after the surgery. When surveyed regarding subjective symptom categories, 9 of 18 patient symptom categories were improved significantly after the treatment including improvement in dim light vision and difficulties with

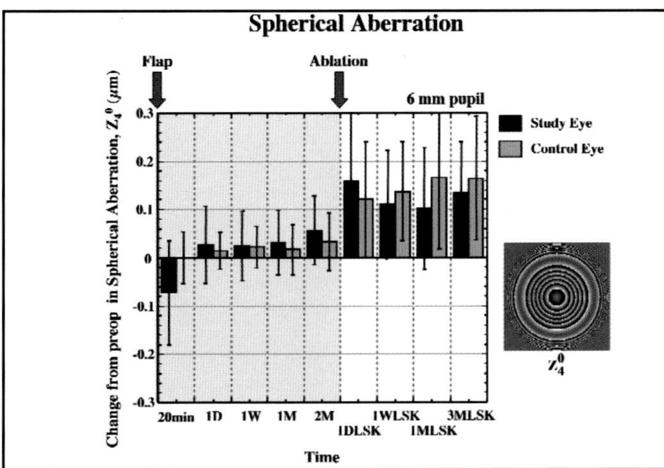

Figure 28-8. Spherical aberration changes after creating a microkeratome flap (180 µm Hansatome) and following the eye for 2 months and then lifting the flap and ablating the cornea with a conventional ablation. The contralateral eye served as an untouched control for two months and then underwent a conventional LASIK. Note that spherical aberrations changes minimally after the flap only but increases 40% to 67% after the ablation in both eyes.[10] (Reprinted with permission from Porter J, MacRae S, Yoon G, Roberts C, Cox IG, Williams DR. Separate effects of the microkeratome incision and laser ablation on the eye's wave aberration. *Am J Ophthalmol.* 2003;136(2):334, with permission from Elsevier.)

night vision at 6 months postoperatively. Only two symptom categories were worse: dryness and fluctuation in vision at 6 months. Both of these symptom categories are frequently reported as increased after post-LASIK studies and are not unique to this particular study.[9,11] We suspect that this symptom is primarily caused by the microkeratome incision and not the type of ablation. The dryness symptom category change was driven by a 13.6% shift from an absence of dryness symptoms preoperatively to mild dryness at the 6-month interval. Interestingly, there was no increase and even a slight nonsignificant decrease in the moderate and marked dryness categories. The marked dryness (worst category) decreased from 1.5% (5/340) preoperatively, to 0.0% at the 6 month postoperative interval. This suggests that the dryness that developed after LASIK was mild in most patients in this study and not severely debilitating.

Summary

The Bausch & Lomb Technolas 217Z Zyoptix results are encouraging. Patient with greater levels of higher-order aberration preoperatively are more likely to benefit from higher-order aberration correction. We noted a high level of patient satisfaction and these results suggest that wavefront driven ablation is a viable option for the correction of myopic refractive error.

References

1. Mrochen M, Kaemmerer M, Seiler T. Clinical results of wavefront-guided laser in situ keratomileusis 3 months after surgery. *J Cataract Refract Surg.* 2001;27(2):201-207.
2. Seiler T, Mrochen M, Kaemmerer M. Operative correction of ocular aberrations to improve visual acuity. *J Refract Surg.* 2000;16(5):S619-S622.
3. Nuijts R, Nabar V, Hament W, Eggink F. Wavefront-guided versus standard laser in situ keratomileusis to correct low to moderate myopia. *J Cataract Refract Surg.* 2002;28(11):1907-1913.
4. Nagy Z, Palagyi-Deak I, E EK, Kovacs A. Wavefront-guided photorefractive keratectomy for myopia and myopic astigmatism. *J Refract Surg.* 2002;18(5):S615-S619.
5. Vongthongsri A, Phusitphoykai N, Naripthapan P. Comparison of wavefront-guided customized ablation vs. conventional ablation in laser in situ keratomileusis. *J Refract Surg.* 2002;18(3):S332-S335.
6. Porter J, Guirao A, Cox I, Williams D. Monochromatic aberrations of the human eye in a large population. *J Opt Soc Am A.* 2001;18(8): 1793-1803.
7. Castejon-Mochon J, Lopez-Gil N, Benito A, Artal P. Ocular wavefront aberration statistics in a normal young population. *Vision Res.* 2002;42(2002):1611-1617.
8. Bradley A, Hong X, Thibos L, et al. The statistics of monochromatic aberrations from 200 healthy young eyes [ARVO Abstract 862]. *Invest Ophthalmol Vis Sci.* 2001;42(4):S161.
9. FDA/CDRH. FDA-Approved lasers for LASIK. CDRC, 2002. http://www.fda.gov/cdrh/PDF/P970043S010.html.
10. Porter J, MacRae S, Yoon G, Roberts C, Cox IG, Williams DR. Separating the effects of the microkeratome incision and laser ablation on the eye's wave aberration. *Am J Ophthalmol.* 2003;136(2):327-337.
11. FDA/CDRH. PMA Summary information on Alcon Laboratories, Inc. LADARVision 4000 excimer laser system, P970043/S010. FDA, CDRH, 2002. Accessed October 27, 2003 from: http://www.fda.gov/cdrh/PDF/P970043S010.html.

Chapter 29
Customized Corneal Ablation Using the Carl Zeiss Meditec Platform: CRS-Master, WASCA, TOSCA, MEL70, and MEL80 Excimer Lasers

Dan Z. Reinstein, MD, MA (Cantab), FRCSC; Daniel R. Neal, PhD; Hartmut Vogelsang, PhD; Eckhard Schroeder, PhD; Zoltan Z. Nagy, MD, PhD; Michael Bergt, PhD; James Copland, MS; and Daniel Topa

INTRODUCTION

Historical Perspective

The eye can be thought of as a sophisticated optical instrument that automatically adapts to its environment. It has automatic systems for adjusting the light level (pupil/iris) and focus (accommodative lens). The eye can also have a range of common optical errors that limit its performance. The dominant errors in most eyes are myopia (near-sightedness), hyperopia (far-sightedness), and astigmatism (asymmetrical focal power). These errors have been, for centuries, corrected by adding a lens in front of the cornea (glasses or contact lenses). Modern laser refractive surgery has been driven by efforts to modify the structure of the cornea itself. Traditionally, the amount of these errors in the eye has been measured by a trial-and-error process. A trial corrective lens is placed in front of the eye and patient feedback gives information about whether the vision is better or worse. The phoropter, trial lens kit, and, to some extent, the autorefractor are the primary instruments used to gather this refractive error information. The subjective refraction (or manifest refraction) method is the primary means for determining the proper patient corrective lens prescription, and has, for the last 15 years or so, formed the basis for calculating ablation profiles to be applied to the cornea. The errors in the eye's optical system, however, are not always limited to focus and astigmatic errors. For example, it is possible for the focal power to change at different locations across the pupil. These effects cannot be described purely in terms of focus or astigmatism since they relate to changes in the focus and astigmatism as a function of position. Thus they are called "higher-order" aberrations, while focus and astigmatic error are defined as "lower-order" aberrations. Examples of higher-order aberrations are changes in the focal power as a function of pupil diameter (predominantly spherical aberration), increased power in the upper half of the pupil, decreased power in the lower half (vertical coma), or increased/decreased power left to right (horizontal coma). These effects can be small and have relatively little effect, or they can dominate visual quality, causing starburst, glare, image ghosting, or even monocular diplopia. Until recently, it was only possible to measure the higher-order aberrations of the eye in controlled laboratory conditions, in vivo. Thanks to the advent of modern aberrometers, it is now not only possible to measure these higher-order aberrations routinely in a doctor's office, but to enable physicians to base corneal refractive surgery on this information.

Definition of Wavefront

The wavefront of the light that is transmitted through an optical system is an imaginary surface that remains normal to the direction of propagation at all cross sectional points within the optical pathway. For a perfect eye focused at infinity, the wavefront of the light collected by the optics of the eye would be part of an aspheric surface, which would converge on the back of the eye to create a (diffraction-limited) spot on the retina. Because of the reciprocal behavior of light (ie, it traverses the same path in either direction), it is possible to measure this wavefront from light that is scattered or reflected from the retina (after it has been projected onto it). This is the primary measurement principle of the Carl Zeiss Meditec Wavefront Supported Customized Ablation (WASCA) device, produced jointly with WaveFront Sciences (Albuquerque, NM), who market the same device as the Complete Ophthalmic Analysis System (COAS) in the United States. In operation, the WASCA emits a small beam of light, projecting this onto the retina. The light scatters from the retinal surface (fovea), it is collected by the lens and cornea, and is then "projected" out of the eye. A perfect, emmetropic eye would completely collimate this light. The resulting wavefront would be a perfect flat plane wavefront, perpendicular to the direction of propagation. Any deviations from a perfect plane wave are the result of optical errors in the optical system (ie, the eye), and as a result are called the *wavefront error of the system.*

Custom Ablation: Definition

We define custom ablation as an ablation profile designed to specifically meet optical correction requirements for a specific individual eye. The recent introduction of diagnostic aberrometry into refractive surgical practice has put higher-order optics into the standard vocabulary of refractive surgeons. This has also raised new issues concerning the design of ablation profiles. For example, aberrometry has now made it possible for us to study what aberrations are being induced by current treatment profiles.[1] As such, in our view, wavefront-guided ablation comprises an important component but not the total sum of custom ablation. In addition, we must also consider a number of independent variables contributing to a scheme designed to give us control over the modification of corneal shape. These will include

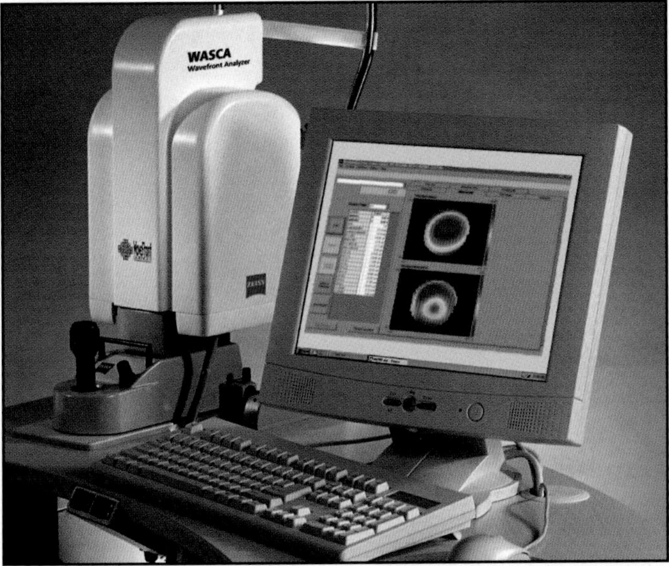

Figure 29-1. WASCA aberrometer unit showing narrow head design that enables fellow eye to "see past" the device to minimize instrument myopia and enable fellow eye targets to study dynamic accommodation.

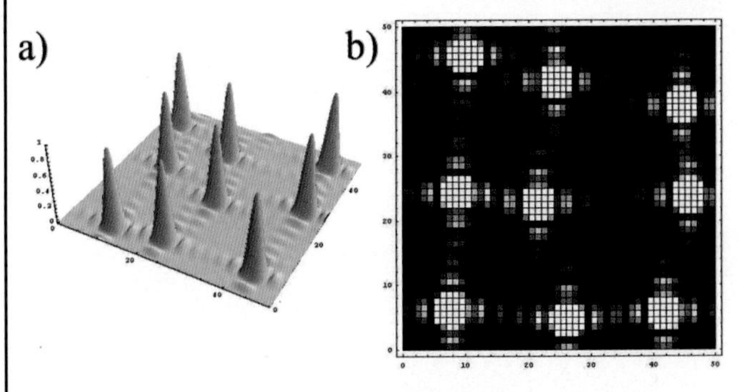

Figure 29-2. Small portion of the image from a lenslet array. (A) shows the irradiance distribution incident on the CCD detector, and (B) is the resulting CCD image pixel-by-pixel. The location of these spots is the key information that is used to determine the wavefront.

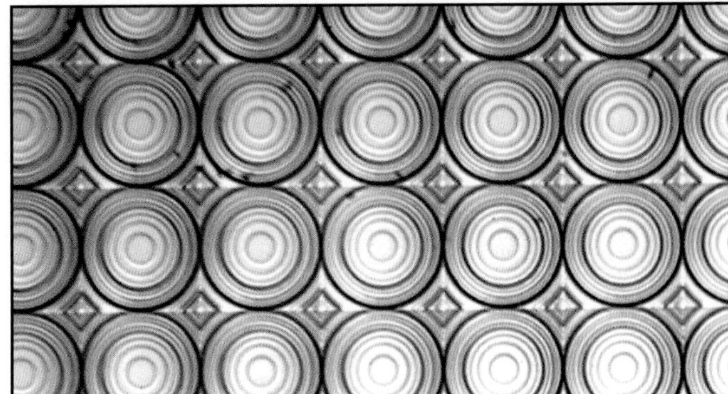

Figure 29-3. Scanning electron micrograph of a portion of the WASCA lenslet array. Each lenslet is in fact square and comprises a depression of approximately 1.6 micron (μm) with a diameter of 144 μm. Note the 100% fill (ie, no gap) between lenslets.

knowing the factors affecting the accuracy of laser energy delivery to the cornea and ablation biophysics, as well as epithelial and biomechanical responses within the cornea. This chapter will describe the current and near-future components of the Carl Zeiss Meditec system, designed to achieve true custom ablation within the cornea.

Aberrometry: WASCA

The WASCA aberrometer is based on the Shack-Hartmann wavefront sensing principle (Figure 29-1). The basis of this technology has been described elsewhere in this textbook (Chapter 14) and is based on a large body of research. Briefly, a lenslet array collects incident light emerging from the eye. Each lenslet then creates a focal projection onto a charged-coupled device (CCD) camera array. The position of the spots on the CCD array relative to a reference location (as would be produced by a flat wavefront) is used to determine the actual wavefront slope of the incident light onto a particular lenslet. The combination of this array of slopes in a topographic manner leads to the calculation and digital reconstruction of the incident wavefront. This wavefront can then be either displayed directly from the raw data (as a result of the very high resolution of the WASCA) by zonal reconstruction or broken down into a collection a shapes of varying amplitude (eg, the Zernike expansion series). We will now delineate some of the specific design features of the WASCA that provide increased accuracy and reproducibility of wavefront measurement in practice.

Lenslet Array Resolution and Spot Quality

Simply stated, lenslet resolution directly impacts the accuracy of wavefront detection, the dynamic range within a wavefront to be detected, and the reproducibility of detection. Thus, resolution will certainly affect the concordance between the measured and actual wavefront, but it will also significantly influence whether a wavefront measurement can even be obtained from a particular aberrated eye.

The lenslet array incorporated within the WASCA is based on the core patented technology of WaveFront Sciences, Inc and is comprised of the most compact lenslet array (highest resolution) available worldwide. It is constructed using methods similar to those for creating modern integrated circuits. That is, they are designed using a computer-generated mask, which is transferred to the surface of a fused-silica substrate using photolithography and reactive-ion etching. This results in an extremely accurate lenslet array with known and extremely accurate characteristics. Figure 29-2 shows some examples of the focusing data for a small portion of the incident light. Figure 29-3 shows a small portion of the actual lenslet array. The full array consists of lenslets arranged in a rectangular array 44 x 33 (1452 lenslets). The shape of each lenslet surface is spherical, but each lenslet is a 144 microns (μm) square section of this surface. In this way, there is 100% fill of the focusing array, so that no light can "leak" through between lenslets. This reduces stray light that could cause interference or background effects that reduce spot localization accuracy. The full array measures 6.5 x 4.8 millimeters (mm). The WASCA lenslet array enables approximately 800 lenslets to collect light from a 7 mm entrance pupil, with an effective lateral resolution of 210 μm. Comparison of the number of lenslets collecting from a 7 mm entrance pupil and the effective lateral resolution created by several commercial ocular aberrometers is shown in Table 29-1.

Table 29-1

Table Comparing Commercially Available Aberrometers With Respect to the Number of Lenslets (or Equivalent) Collecting Light Within a 7-mm Entrance Pupil and the Effective Resolution Enabled by Each Array

System Name (Manufacturer)	Type	Spots in 7 mm Pupil	Effective Resolution (μm)
WASCA/COAS (Carl Zeiss Meditec)	Shack-Hartman	800	210
WaveScan (VISX)	Shack-Hartman	240	350
LADARWave CustomCornea (Autonomous)	Shack-Hartman	188 to 195	400
Wavefront Analyser (WaveLight)	Tscherning	ca. 100	500
Zywave (Bausch & Lomb)	Shack-Hartman	70 to 75	700
WASCA/COAS HD Array (WaveFront Sciences, Inc)	Shack-Hartman	3300	100

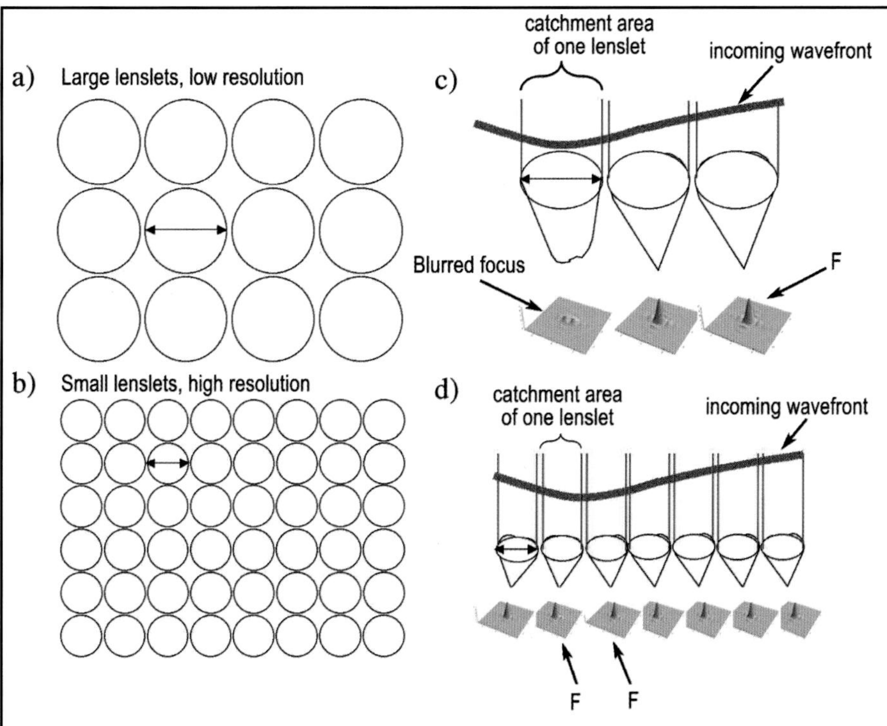

Figure 29-4. (A) and (B) The smaller the diameter of the lenslet, the more that can be contained in an array and hence the greater the number of lenslets collecting light from the entrance pupil. (C) Shows a portion of wavefront containing a nonlinear slope entering the catchment of the left-most lenslet, but effectively a linear slope entering the middle and right-most lenslets. The sample of the wavefront in the case of the left-most lenslet has a nonlinear structure; therefore, the lenslet will scatter light over a large region, causing a diffuse and irregular focal spot. In the case of the middle and right-most lenslets, light will be properly focused (F), producing a sharp peak. (D) Increasing the number of lenslets or decreasing the diameter of the lenslets allows more frequent sampling. Now each lenslet is picking up effectively linear slopes from the same wavefront as in (C); Because of the smaller sampling area the non-planar portion of the incoming wavefront is now divided into quasi-planar segments to produce well-focused projections (F), onto the CCD array.

The WASCA lenslet array enables approximately 800 lenslets to collect light from a 7 mm entrance pupil, with an effective lateral resolution of 210 μm.

The other most common method of creating lenslet arrays is by production of molded monolithic lenslet modules. These are made by an embossing process in plastic. Some of the weaknesses of this method are that the lenslet shape is less predictable, and it cannot produce a 100% fill, thus potentially enabling stray light to "leak" between lenslets.

To understand why lenslet size affects resolution and how this in turn affects the accuracy of wavefront detection, we present the illustration shown in Figure 29-4. Essentially, the smaller the lenslets, the more of them can be fit into the catchment area of the pupillary zone, and hence the higher the resolution. Smaller lenslets have smaller diameters and therefore collect a smaller sample of the incoming wavefront. The smaller the sampled area from the incoming wavefront, the less "averaging" of the wavefront slope within one lenslet occurs, and thus the more focused the spot projected onto the CCD detector. The more focused the spot on the CCD detector, the more likely that (A) it can be detected with good positional accuracy and (B) it is a true representation of the slope of the incoming wavefront into that lenslet.

Figure 29-5 demonstrates the CCD capture output obtained from a mild keratoconic eye, using either a 400 or 200 μm resolution lenslet array. This example clearly demonstrates how lenslet size/resolution affects the quality of data acquired and hence the reliability of the wavefront calculated.

Smaller lenslets have smaller diameters and therefore collect a smaller sample of the incoming wavefront. The smaller the sampled area from the incoming wavefront, the less "averaging" of the wavefront slope within one lenslet occurs, and thus the more focused the spot projected onto the CCD detector. The more focused the spot on the CCD detector, the more likely that (A) it can be detected with good positional accuracy and (B) it is a true representation of the slope of the incoming wavefront into that lenslet.

Spot Quality and Wavefront Detection Accuracy

If the position of these focal spots cannot be accurately determined, the entire accuracy of the device will suffer. The focal spot is sampled by a fixed number of pixels on the CCD camera, digitized, and stored (see Figure 29-2). The digital image is then broken up into a number of areas of interest (AOIs), encompassing one focal spot in each AOI. These AOIs are then processed to determine the position of the spot using an algorithm. The thresholded centroid algorithm used has been shown to have the accuracy of a fraction of a pixel when the spot covers several pixels.[2-4]

In order for the centroid to be accurately determined, the light incident on the detector must form a distinct grid of spots. To this end, as demonstrated above, the lenslet must sample a portion of the light that has low-enough aberrations (essentially a wavefront of constant slope) to form an ideal detectable focal spot. If, however, the incident light on a particular lenslet has a complex wavefront, the focal spot peak intensity is reduced, and the spot will be significantly blurred and spread out (see Figure 29-4). In this case, the centroid algorithm may not be accurate, or it may not be able to determine a spot position at all. An algorithm that is optimized to accurately measure the location of a distinct spot will perform poorly on blurry spots. Conversely, an algorithm that is optimized for detecting centroids in blurry spots will not be optimal for measuring distinct spots. The best overall system, then, will be one that optically makes each spot distinct. The way this is achieved is to use as many lenslets as possible over a given wavefront so that the wavefront is as close to being planar as possible over each lenslet.

Spot Crossing

In Shack-Hartmann sensing, the range of motion of the focal spot on the detector is correlated to the dynamic range. Thus, if the focal length of the lenslets is large compared to the diameter of the lenslet, focal spots can actually cross over when the presenting wavefront possesses a large change in the gradient from one lenslet to the next. The WASCA has been specifically designed with a very fine-pitch lenslet array and an extremely short focal length to match, in order to provide a very large dynamic range (6 diopters [D]). A patented system forces a lenslet focused spot to "drop out" before it can cross over to the detector field of the adjacent lenslet. Hence, spot crossing is, in fact, impossible with the WASCA aberrometer.

These features (ie, the large dynamic range and spot crossing elimination) explain why the WASCA is robust in its ability to provide a detectable, reproducible wavefront measurement even in highly aberrated eyes.

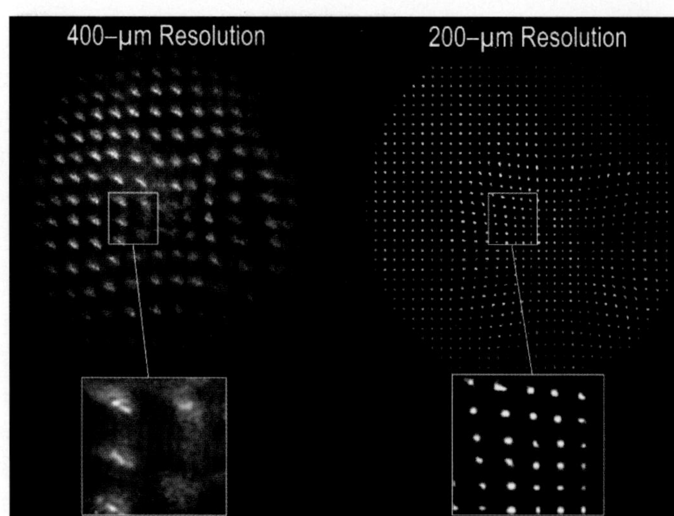

Figure 29-5. Shack-Hartman lenslet array CCD images from an eye with mild keratoconus using either a 400- or a 200-μm resolution array. The same central area of each image is sampled and zoomed x3 to demonstrate the difference in spot quality afforded by increased resolution. In this example, the lower resolution array can produce spot projections that would lead to inaccurate cen-

A patented system forces a lenslet focused spot to "drop out" before it can cross over to the detector field of the adjacent lenslet. Hence, spot crossing is, in fact, impossible with the WASCA aberrometer.

Zonal Reconstruction

The wavefront analysis process consists of three main steps: detecting the centroids of each focal spot, comparing the positions to a reference to produce a slope map, and finally, reconstructing the wavefront.

The reconstruction of the wavefront may be displayed as a point-by-point integration of the two-dimensional (2-D) raw slope map—a zonal reconstruction (Figure 29-6). Or, it may be reconstructed according to a defined mathematical fit to the Zernike polynomial series—a modal reconstruction. If the zonal resolution is low, the zonal reconstruction method will yield highly pixelated data. If, however, the zonal resolution is high (as with the WASCA), this raw pixel density is sufficient to provide graphic 2-D representation of the wavefront without resorting to artificial smoothing of the raw data. The advantage of viewing a zonal reconstruction representation is in the lack of smoothing produced by the "binning" of raw data into a defined polynomial series (particularly if only lower analyzing—only up to the sixth or eighth Zernike order). Modal reconstruction has certain advantages in that each polynomial possesses specific optical connotations and as such can provide quantization of clinical data. However, zonal reconstruction has the advantage of producing much higher spatial frequency and therefore less smoothing (Figure 29-7). Thus, zonal reconstruction may provide a better starting point for calculating customized ablation profiles in highly aberrated eyes.

Seidel Method for Predicting Manifest Refraction

It is understood that higher-order aberrations can be partially compensated for in the visual system by the use of sphere and cylinder lenses. That is why some eyes become more myopic at night when the pupil becomes larger—increasing pupil size

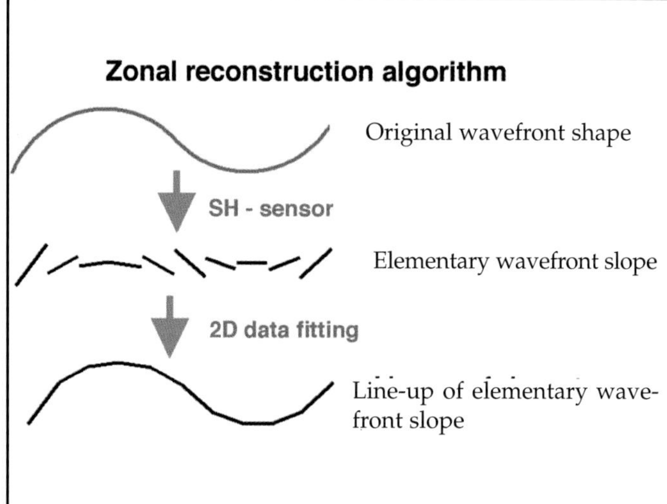

Figure 29-6. Drawing showing a wavefront being converted by the Shack-Hartman sensor into a 2-D grid of individual wavefront slopes (done as a function of spot displacement on the CCD image). These elementary wavefront slopes can be "lined-up" to produce a reconstruction of the original wavefront. If the resolution is high (ie, consisting of a large number of elementary wavefront samples) the reconstruction is smooth and of good fidelity.

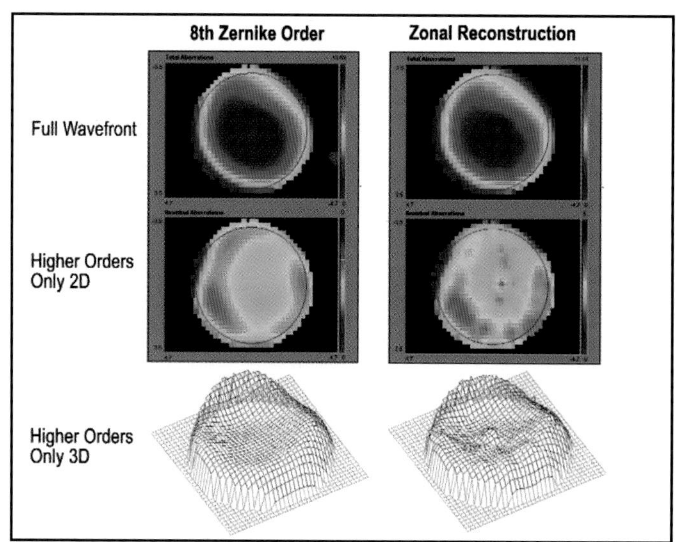

Figure 29-7. Full wavefront and higher-order 2-D and three-dimensional (3-D) displays for a single wavefront measurement acquired from an eye with a visually significant "central island" post-PRK. The plots in the left column are based on a Zernike expansion representation of the wavefront including up to the eighth order, while those on the right column are based on direct zonal reconstruction from the raw slope data. Detection of the optical irregularity produced by the central island is smoothed out by description of the wavefront data with Zernike polynomials, while zonal reconstruction with high spatial resolution (equivalent to a Zernike reconstruction to the 24th order) enables detection of the optical irregularity. (Courtesy of Gunter Grabner, MD, Salzburg, Austria.)

increases the amount of spherical aberration in the eye—which in turn can be partially compensated for by increasing the power of a spherical lens placed in front of the eye. The influence of similar, higher order astigmatic terms, such as Z(4,2) and Z(4,-2) will have an effect on the total cylindrical power that a patient will call for in manifest refraction. In brief, the Seidel method provides a basis for calculating the manifest equivalent spherocylindrical refraction based upon combining the lower order Zernike terms for sphere and cylinder (ie, sphere: Z(2,0), and cylinder: Z(2,-1) and Z(2,-1)) with the relative influence of higher order (3rd and above) polynomials. The use of the Seidel method effectively makes the WASCA into an accurate "autorefractor" (see clinical data below).

Specific Design Features That Improve Performance

In order to optimize the quality of the light focused on the retina, the WASCA is designed to maintain full wavefront sensor resolution and accuracy at all magnitudes of hyperopia and myopia (+6 D to -15 D) through a patented precorrection of the "injected" light into the eye.

The multiple display options provided are summarized in Table 29-2.

The WASCA is negligibly affected by vibration as it acquires a complete data set within 13 milliseconds (ms).

The eye's optical system is not static and is constantly shifting or focusing. Using the rapid acquisition time and proprietary high-speed analytical systems, the WASCA is capable of obtaining multiple full wavefront measurements per second. Software enables the user to acquire wavefronts at 15 hertz (Hz) over a period of up to 30 seconds. The WASCA is designed to be able to acquire a total of 450 independent wavefront measurements within a period of 30 seconds. These may be viewed as a continuous movie clip, providing an appreciation for the stability and reproducibility of the ocular wavefront. This provides a dynamic analysis of the wavefront and enables determination of the true average prescription, which may not necessarily be just the average of a few measurements. Algorithms will be shortly released that enable automatic multiple wavefront acquisition, instantaneous statistical analysis, and the delivery of the "best" wavefront, for the purposes of planning customized ablation (personal communication, Daniel R. Neal, PhD).

This rapid sequence acquisition also enables dynamic aberrometry to be performed. Vogelsang, Panagopoulou, and Pallikaris have studied the dynamic changes in higher-order aberrations occurring during the accommodation process. Dynamic study of aberrations will become increasingly important, particularly as the use of aberrometry may aid in understanding optical performance for specific tasks (eg, optimizing distance vision at night versus optimizing near and midrange vision indoors). It may be that complex superposition of particular aberrational states of the eye may allow us to induce asymptomatic multifocality (eg, for the treatment of presbyopia). Realistic classification of such intermediate states can only be characterized by true real dynamic studies since averaging between static measurements is unlikely to provide adequate answers. Figure 29-8 shows an example of how dynamic higher-order aberrations can be even in the resting state of the eye.

Using the rapid acquisition time and proprietary high-speed analytical systems, the WASCA is capable of obtaining multiple full wavefront measurements per second. Software enables the user to acquire wavefronts at 15 Hz over a period of up to 30 seconds.

Table 29-2
Summary of the Display Options Available From the WASCA Aberrometer

DISPLAY OPTIONS

- Wavefront map
  - Zernike decomposition
  - Zonal elevation
- Power map
  - Either modal or zonal maps provide direct reading in diopters
- Displays for data interpretation
  - Point-spread-function
  - Visual acuity
  - Modulation transfer function
  - Gradient vectors
- Dynamic analysis features built in
  - Movie modes for raw and saved data
  - Temporal plots for trend analysis
- Open data format for export
  - Direct output of Zernike coefficients
  - ASCII files and numerous data formats

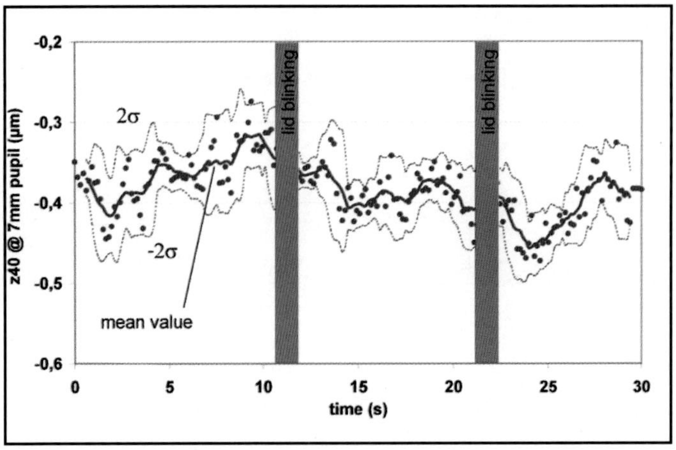

Figure 29-8. Time based (x-axis) measurement of Z(4,0) variation in a nonaccommodating eye. Wavefront measurements were acquired at a rate of 7 Hz for a period of 30 seconds with a patient looking at a distance target with the fellow-eye. All instantaneous values of Z(4,0) are shown (blue dots), surrounding a running average (solid blue line) and the 95% confidence limits of variation (two standard deviations) (dashed blue line). It can be appreciated how a single instantaneous measurement of Z(4,0) does not necessarily provide a reliable measure of the overall mean value and may be significantly different from the optimal value to be used for planning customized ablation.

Accuracy and Reproducibility

Lower-Orders and WASCA as an Autorefractor

Salmon et al formally studied the accuracy and reproducibility of the COAS (WASCA) in young myopic patients with respect to predicting sphere and cylinder obtained by autorefractor and manifest refraction.[5] For lower-order aberrations, in Seidel mode, WASCA was compared to manifest refraction, dry and cycloplegic. The reproducibility of multiple measurements of the same eye under cycloplegia was tested by 30 repeated measurements, including head repositioning. A single case example of reproducibility is shown in Figure 29-8. Including blinks, the standard deviation of the sphere term was <0.05 D, with the cylinder <0.09 D. A summary of the study results is shown in Table 29-3. The repeatability coefficient for cycloplegic data acquisition was 0.15 D.[6] These studies show that WASCA is at least as accurate as subjective refraction (the standard of comparison), but more reproducible.

Higher-Orders and WASCA Reproducibility for Higher-Order Measurements In Vivo

The higher-order terms, as measured by the Zernike polynomials, showed similar reproducibility to the lower-order measurements. Figure 29-9 shows the standard deviation (in µm) of each Zernike coefficient for higher-order aberrations measured for a single case. The repeatability of in vivo measurement was better than 0.05 µm.

SURGEON CONTROLLED CUSTOM ABLATION: THE CARL ZEISS MEDITEC CRS-MASTER

Overview

Surgeon Control

To date, for the most part, laser manufacturers have designed ablation profiles by starting with a theoretical, spherocylindrical-based ablation profile (cf. Barraquer[7] and Munnerlyn[8]), which was adjusted through experimental iteration ("nomogram adjustment") to achieve the desired effect on ocular defocus. For the past decade of excimer laser corneal refractive surgery, the surgeon's control of the ablation profile has been relatively limited. Most manufacturers have allowed surgeon control only of the intended diameter of the fully corrected optical zone and/or the size of the "transition" zone. The function of the CRS-Master (Carl Zeiss Meditec, Dublin, Calif) is to offer further variables to be considered and controlled by the surgeon—including wavefront, topography, and tissue safety limits.

Using this software application, the surgeon integrates patient clinical examination data with corneal surface data (Topography Supported Customized Ablation [TOSCA]) and wavefront (WASCA) data, providing surgeon control over the ablation profile for each individual eye.

Table 29-3
Accuracy and Reproducibility of "Autorefraction" by WASCA/COAS Compared to Both Dry and Cyloplegic Manifest Refraction

	MEAN ERROR/D	STANDARD DEVIATION/D
Dry Manifest	-0.14 -0.20 x 011	0.32
Cycloplegic	-0.06 -0.18 x 001	0.26

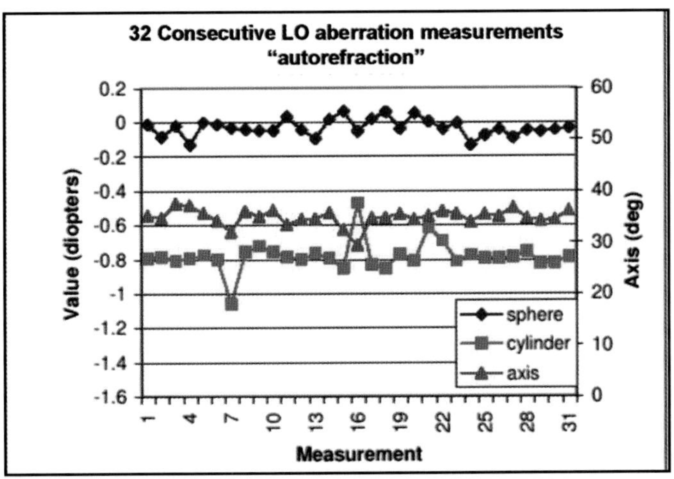

Figure 29-9. Thirty-two consecutive "autorefraction" measurements made by WASCA showing sphere (blue), cylinder (pink), and axis (red) for each consecutive independent measurement after head repositioning. Major deviations coincide with blinks. The standard deviations for these measurements are sphere: 0.049 D, cylinder: 0.089 D, and axis: 1.57 degrees.

The CRS-Master release (non-US) was envisaged during 2003. Below follows an overview of the current beta-version features, many of which will be available in the first release. Graduated clinical studies documenting efficacy and safety will be used to determine the release sequence of particular features.

Safety

Barraquer taught in his 1980 textbook on keratomileusis that to prevent progressive keratectasia following keratomileusis, the corneal cap should not be thicker than 300 µm.[9] In the average 550 µm cornea, this would leave a residual stromal thickness (RST) of 250 µm. If the human cornea had an average thickness of 900 µm, any patient would be able to safely have their refractive error, wavefront, and asphericity optimized within these safety limits. In reality, the human cornea has a mean thickness of 515 µm with 95% of it lying between 440 and 590 µm when measured with very high frequency (VHF) digital ultrasound.[10] Therefore, based on the individual optical errors and corneal thickness constraints of each particular patient, certain compromises will need to be made on the degree of prolateness, or the flattening of the wavefront. Compromises in surgery require clinical judgment. Clinical judgment is the function of surgeons. Therefore, the CRS-Master was developed to integrate a sophisticated, theoretical optical application with clinical judgment, effectively allowing surgeons into the loop of ablation profile design. Given specific desired outcome variables (eg, optimization for night vision or tissue-saving algorithms [TSA]), preset buttons enable the surgeon to instantly review suggested profiles. The CRS-Master custom mode enables the surgeon to individualize the amount of asphericity and wavefront data incorporated into the desired ablation profile, and to design the optimum distinct ablation profile for a specific eye. Ablation profile design is assisted by 3-D maps that allow the surgeon to visualize each step of the optimization process.

> Editor's note:
> Since the elimination of spherical aberration in an ablation profile results in deeper ablation than in a conventional profile, the CRS-Master software enables the surgeon to alter the amount of asphericity corrected in accordance with the residual corneal thickness as a tissue saving measure.
> R. Krueger, MD, MSE

Data Integration

Wavefront Data

The CRS-Master wavefront component is based on the WASCA system.

Corneal Surface Shape Data

The extended range of the original Meditec TOSCA functions will be included in the CRS-Master, incorporating all the commercially available (except in the United States) algorithms already implemented for the MEL70, for the correction of decentrations,[11,12] and small optical zone enlargement.

Moreover, the corneal surface data will be used to compute, according to beam angular-dependence, the laser energy adjustment required to deliver a constant fluence to the corneal surface (see below). This will ensure that the delivery of excimer laser pulses is optimized for achieving accurate shape changes on the stromal surface.

Patient Clinical Data

Pupil size, corneal thickness, and subjective refraction form clinical input components. By integrating clinical constraints into the ablation profile design, the surgeon is able to make informed decisions regarding the patient's particular anatomy and visual requirements. In addition, the CRS-Master allows individualized microkeratome precision data to be entered (mean and standard deviation), and provides the surgeon with a statistical analysis predicting the probability of crossing the 250 µm barrier under the flap for a particular ablation profile set-up.

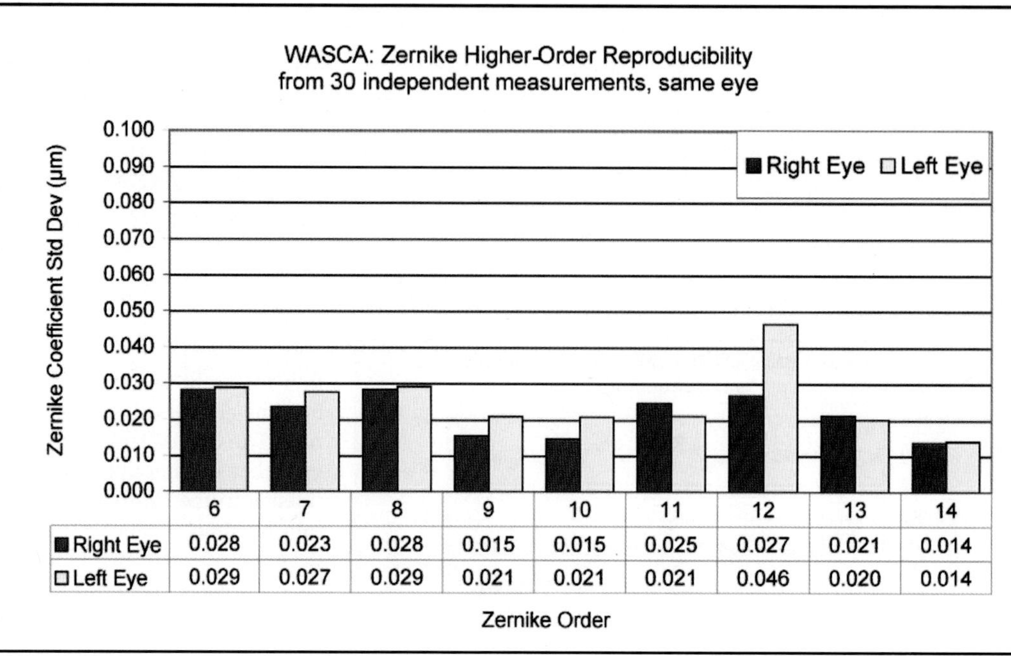

	6	7	8	9	10	11	12	13	14
Right Eye	0.028	0.023	0.028	0.015	0.015	0.025	0.027	0.021	0.014
Left Eye	0.029	0.027	0.029	0.021	0.021	0.021	0.046	0.020	0.014

Figure 29-10. Zernike polynomial coefficient reproducibility (standard deviation) for a sequence of 30 measurements of right and left eyes after head repositioning. The x axis shows the Zernike ordinal number. Reproducibility is shown in microns.

Background Principles

Achieving the "perfect" ablation: Customized ablation of the cornea can be divided into two main issues:

1. Optimization of ablation profiles: Are we getting the ablation profile that we think we are getting?
2. Customization of ablation profiles: What kind of ablation profile is required by this particular eye?

Optimization of Ablation Profiles

Laser Fluence Control

Projection correction: Standard, theoretically determined, nomogram adjusted profiles employed to date in corneal refractive surgery have been shown to induce far more higher-order aberration than theoretically predicted. Mrochen et al. have reported and calculated the influence of the effective illumination area and possible reflection losses that occur during laser-tissue interaction.[13] When a laser spot is projected onto the curved corneal front surface, moving a scanning-spot from the center of the cornea toward the limbus results in increased effective illumination area and hence less fluence. Reflective losses should also be accounted for to optimize energy delivery to the surface. These effects in turn lead to a decrease in the intended ablation depth per laser pulse (Figure 29-10). These phenomena, if not accounted for, result in effectively smaller fully corrected ablation zones and optical distortion of the intended spherocylindrical profile, leading to increases in higher-order aberrations, particularly fourth-order (spherical) aberration. Optimization of the ablation profile will be necessary to ensure that lasers are indeed removing the tissue volume intended. For this to happen, laser delivery systems will have to be able to take into account the actual shape of the cornea when calculating an ablation profile. The CRS-Master uses the integrated TOSCA module to calculate the fluence correction factor required at each location on the cornea and ensure the accuracy of transferring the desired ablation energy to the cornea.

Optimization of the ablation profile will be necessary to ensure that lasers are indeed removing the tissue volume intended. For this to happen, laser delivery systems will have to be able to take into account the actual shape of the cornea when calculating an ablation profile.

Reflection correction: The stromal surface denuded of epithelium or exposed under a flap is appreciably shiny. That is because it is reflecting light. Therefore, not surprisingly, not all of the excimer laser energy delivered to the cornea is consumed in photoablation; a small, but not negligible, proportion (in the region of 2.5%) is reflected from the surface of the cornea. The angle of the incident laser beam onto the curved corneal surface will be a factor in determining the magnitude of these losses. The reflectivity of the surface also changes over time, particularly during ablation, as a function of evaporation and fluid shock waves within the tissue. The CRS-Master is designed to consider these effects and compensate for them in optimizing the delivery of spots to achieve the desired stromal curvature change.

Control for Tissue Responses

Fourth-order spherical aberration and third-order coma are the major higher-order aberrations induced by corneal refractive surgery.[14,15]

Epithelial changes: Using VHF digital ultrasound arc scanning (Artemis, Ultralink LLC, St. Petersburg, Fla)[16-18] in conjunction with Orbscan II (Bausch & Lomb, Salt Lake City, Utah), Reinstein and colleagues have begun to characterize epithelial and biomechanical responses occurring as a result of laser in-situ keratomileusis (LASIK).[19,20]

For epithelium, they have recently described a nonlinear (and paradoxical) power shift in the cornea due to epithelial profile changes; the epithelium is responsible for a myopic power shift as a result of lower myopic ablations but, paradoxically, a hyperopic shift in higher myopic ablations. Knowledge of this epithelial behavior and the magnitude of these changes is helpful in understanding features of ablation profile adjustments that were hitherto only accounted for by empirical (nomogram or iterative)

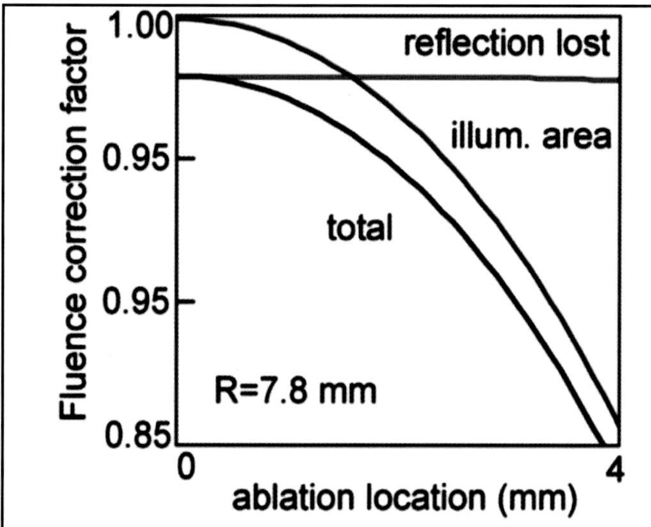

Figure 29-11. Graph showing how projected laser spot fluence drops off as a function of distance from the center (blue line) for a spherical surface of radius 7.8 mm; at 4.0 mm from the center there is a 15% loss of fluence. Reflection losses are shown (red line) and amount to approximately a 2.5% loss of energy.

adjustments. The effect and design of transition zones is also important to the understanding of epithelial profile responses after profiled photoablation.

Control for biomechanical changes: Biomechanical changes are responsible for thickening of the cornea peripheral to the ablation zone and flap (Figure 29-11).[16] Roberts has proposed a model for this effect[21] and concludes that biomechanical considerations will have to be taken into account for accurate wavefront-guided correction of the cornea.[22] This increase in thickness occurs peripherally, but, due to crosslinking of corneal lamellae, also has an effect centripetally within the cornea. The result is a centrifugal progressive reduction of intended tissue removal, and hence a radially progressive effective loss of intended flattening. This leads to an increase in spherical aberration and an effective reduction in the fully corrected optical zone as described by many.[23,24]

Prolate Optimization Function

Spherical aberrations followed by coma are the major higher-order aberrations that present in normal eyes.[25] However, they are present, for the most part, with an order of magnitude considerably less in amplitude than the aberrations induced by current ablation profiles. Therefore, in order to reach the point of being able to offer an improvement on the natural aberrational structure of a virgin cornea, we will first have to minimize the induction of aberrations when treating the defocus (spherocylindrical) component.

Power vs shape: Barraquer's method of keratomileusis was based primarily on the central corneal shape, while wavefront methods consist of measuring and altering power within the entrance pupil. The induction of aberrations by sub-optimal shape change are related within the understanding of ideal corneal asphericity; in Barraquer's keratomileusis, myopic refractive error was treated by modifying the radius of curvature of the outer surface of the cornea. From a theoretical standpoint, removing a spherically-based ablation profile should not significantly increase spherical aberration. However, in keratomileusis, Barraquer did notice and consider that these higher-order aberrations were being induced and published on aspheric (parabolic) keratomileusis.[26] In 1993, Patel and Marshall[27] reported on a model to predict the ideal postoperative shape of the cornea for minimizing spherical aberration. They mathematically predicted that the postoperative corneal contour should conform to a flattening ellipse with a shape factor (p) = 0.65 to 0.85, corresponding to an asphericity factor (Q) of -0.35 to -0.15 or an average Q of -0.25. Flattening ellipses are prolate surfaces, and hence the CRS-Master offers a tool, namely the *prolate optimization function* (POF), to optimize the postoperative asphericity of the cornea, and hence reduce the induction of higher-order aberrations.

Compensation for induced spherical aberration: Spherical aberration is induced for the most part as a result of biomechanical shifts (discussed above), effectively producing a radially progressive degradation of the intended ablation profile. This degradation induces an asphericity change that can be counteracted by increasing the ablation depth as a function of radius. This was achieved by the use of aspheric profiles as suggested and compared to standard Munnerlyn profiles by Seiler.[28]

The POF is therefore a tool that is designed to produce a variably aspheric ablation profile so as to optimize the postoperative asphericity and hence minimize postoperative spherical aberration. Because increasing the asphericity of an ablation profile—while maintaining the central radius of curvature constant—requires a deeper ablation centrally, the CRS-Master will provide the option for switching this off and returning to a standard Munnerlyn profile. We are currently testing a version that will provide the surgeon with a slider that allows control over the degree of prolate optimization for a particular cornea. If the slider is set to 100%, this signifies that the ablation profile asphericity is maximally optimized. A setting of 0% would denote that the postoperative asphericity factor would be the result of a simple conventional spherocylindrical ablation. In conjunction with tissue constraints and individual patient visual requirements, the surgeon will be able to vary the percentage of POF included in the ablation profile to provide a particular eye with it's individualized "best option" ablation profile asphericity.

Compensation for the effect of the flap: Surgically induced coma will be mainly a function of ablation centration and flap induced changes (due to the incomplete nature of the keratectomy to hinge the flap). This raises the question as to whether flap-induced aberrations could be characterized and used in ablation profiles. Reinstein and Goes[29] studied two different microkeratomes (Hansatome [Bausch & Lomb, Rochester, NY] and the M2 [Moria, Doylestown, Pa]) in a prospective, randomized, controlled evaluation. The Hansatome and M2 were found to induce significantly different aberrations. Although the mean response for flap-induced aberrations could be characterized for each microkeratome, the variances (standard deviation [SD]) from eye to eye of these changes were very large. Thus, the predictions that could be based on these data would be ineffective for customizing the treatment of a particular normal eye with initially relatively low amplitudes of higher-order aberrations.[29] Perhaps the newer generation of femtosecond-based keratomes will enable more predictable flap architecture and, hence, more predictable mechanical changes within the cornea, enabling flap induced aberrations to be more predictable and thus accounted for in ablation profile design.

Customization of Ablation Profiles

Practical Considerations

Compared with PRK of the early and mid-90's, LASIK has become the patient's procedure of choice, providing clear advantages in terms of patient comfort and rapid visual recovery. Improvements with respect to pain management and the prevention (or treatment) of post-PRK haze have led to a resurgence in the popularity of surface ablation. It appears, however, that in expert hands, the safety of the two procedures is comparable.[30] The induction of higher-order aberrations by the creation of the flap itself in LASIK has been reported now by many.[31] It remains to be seen if surface ablation carries advantages with respect to customized ablation. However, the difference in simplicity for enhancement surgery may still keep the bias toward LASIK, given that the correction of higher-order aberrations even by surface ablation may often require more than one treatment.

Treating Inherent Higher-Order Aberrations

Once there has been a reduction (ideally, elimination) of the higher-order aberrations induced by surgery, it is reasonable to consider the correction of innate naturally occurring higher-order aberrations of the eye, which, as discussed, tend to be of relatively low amplitude.

The WASCA system, as discussed previously, is specifically designed to enable the acquisition of wavefront data from highly aberrated eyes. It is therefore reasonable to include ablation profile characteristics based on higher-order aberrations with high amplitude, such as are encountered in corneas that have undergone refractive surgery previously.

The MEL80 Excimer Laser

The MEL80 excimer laser was designed specifically from the ground up to meet the requirements of higher-order customized ablation. The MEL80 operates with a distinct Gaussian beam profile by means of a passive stabilization system (patented), with a 0.8 mm effective ablation spot size at a shot frequency of 250 Hz and a proprietary nonrandom shot-distribution pattern based on thermography studies to minimize cumulative surface heating. The MEL80 possesses a patented Gaussian beam profile stabilization system that ensures a constant beam profile that does not require user calibration. The shot frequency affords a considerably foreshortened ablation time; a -5 D, 6 mm zone spherical ablation takes only 15 seconds. Myopic treatments may be performed up to a 7 mm fully corrected ablation zone. The corneal ablation range extends to the 10 mm zone, to ensure optimization of hyperopic and other blend zones. The infrared active video tracking system with automatic thresholding and pupil center detection samples at 250 Hz, and the physical delay time for the total system is 2.0 to 3.0 ms. It has a small footprint (3.30 m^2 including bed) and was designed to withstand being wheeled repeatedly over a 2 centimeter (cm) bump without the need for servicing or mirror realignment. Many aspects of the laser delivery system have been optimized to ensure that energy is delivered as efficiently from the laser head to the cornea; features include a very short and very direct beam path length, vacuum (not inert gas) pathway, and the patented cone for controlled atmosphere (CCA), which produces a virtual environmental cone for the path between the laser aperture and the corne, ensuring consistent air-flow and tissue debris removal.

Validation of the MEL80 for Use in the Correction of Higher-Order Aberrations

To validate the use of the MEL80 for the correction of higher order aberrations, Carl Zeiss Meditec performed laboratory closed loop experiments. The MEL80 was used to create transparent polymer phase plates with a defined profile that would represent a specific Zernike coefficient of determined amplitude on the polymer surface. The resulting ablated phase plate surface shape was verified independently using a profilometer and was then used to aberrate a collimated planar wavefront beam and generate a wavefront distortion to be detected by WASCA. The WASCA and profilometry measurements were used as measures of accuracy (concordance) in the ability to produce a given wavefront aberration on a phase plate. The WASCA measurement was then imported into the CRS-Master workstation to generate an ablation profile designed to reverse the specific aberration induced.

> The MEL80 possesses a patented Gaussian beam profile stabilization system that ensures a constant beam profile that does not require user calibration.

Figure 29-12 depicts a profilometer-based topography measurement and horizontal wavefront section measured after a collimated beam has passed through a phase plate ablated to produce a Z(3,-1) Zernike shape. The concordance between the measured horizontal section and the intended Zernike polynomial can be seen to be very high.

> Editor's note:
> Validation of the efficacy of the MEL80 in correcting higher-order aberrations was performed in reverse by using the laser to create a known aberration in a phase plate, and then verifying the aberrated shape with both a profilometer and the WASCA unit.
> R. Krueger, MD, MSE

Using the CRS-Master

Table 29-4 summarizes the parameters that are entered into the CRS-Master for ablation profile planning.

The surgeon imports the wavefront and topography data before being taken to the CRS-Master main control panel (Figure 29-13). Here the surgeon enters the manifest refractive error, as well as the target refraction. The treatment refraction is automatically calculated. The procedure is selected (LASIK vs surface ablation) and flap characteristics, with residual stromal thickness safety limits (generally set at 250 μm), are entered via a sub-menu window. Corneal thickness (central minimum) and scotopic pupil size are entered, while the near-scotopic pupil size obtained from the WASCA analysis (performed in the dark) is displayed for comparison.

A wavefront control panel (Figure 29-14) enables the surgeon to either deselect WASCA input or add the higher-order aberrations into the profile. There is also a submenu window that allows the surgeon to select only specific aberrations to be incorporated (eg, only spherical aberration, while excluding coma).

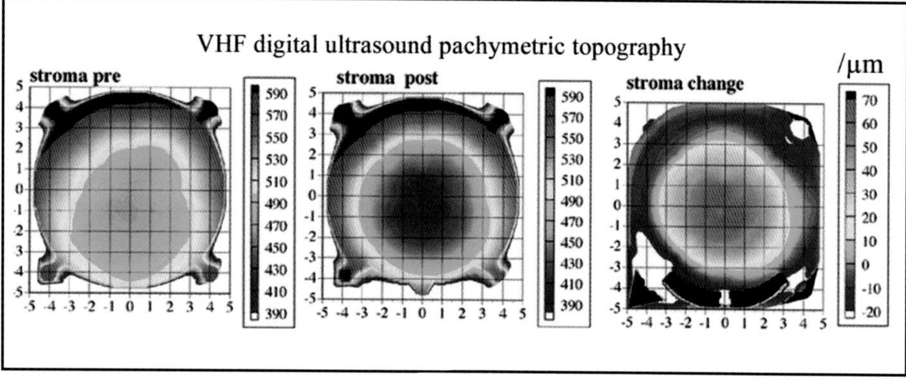

Figure 29-12. VHF digital ultrasound-based thickness profiles of the stromal component of the cornea before (2) and 6 months after (5) LASIK for correction of -5 D. Difference map (before-minus-after) demonstrates thinning in the center of approximately 70 µm consistent with the refractive ablation within a 6.5 mm zone. Peripheral to the ablation zone (within the 8 mm zone of the cornea) the stroma thickened after surgery by approximately 20 to 25 µm. (Reprinted with permission from Reinstein DZ, Silverman RH, Raevsky T, Simoni GJ, Lloyd HO, Najafi DJ, Rondeau MJ, Coleman DJ. A new arc-scanning very high-frequency ultrasound system for 3-D pachymetric mapping of corneal epithelium, lamellar flap and residual stromal layer in laser in situ keratomileusis. *J Refract Surg.* 2000;16:414-430.)

Table 29-4

Parameters Entered Into the CRS-Master for Ablation Profile Planning

The CRS-Master enables the following data to be imported, integrated, and therefore controlled by the surgeon for ablation profile design:

- Manifest refraction
- Scotopic pupil size
- Corneal thickness (central minimum)
- Flap characteristics
- Mean and standard deviation of flap thickness
- Flap diameter and location of hinge
- Corneal surface shape data (TOSCA)
- Wavefront (WASCA)
- Preoperative keratometry and asphericity (calculated by the CRS-Master from the topography)

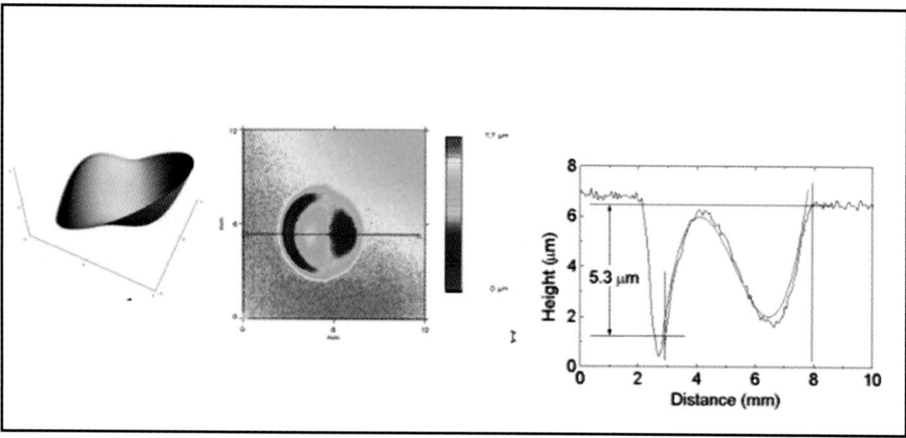

Figure 29-13. Laboratory validation of WASCA and the MEL80 excimer laser as components of a wavefront guided ablation system: 3-D plot of a planned Z(3,-1) Zernike polynomial to be ablated into PMMA (left), 3-D profilometry of the surface of the PMMA plate after ablation (middle) and a horizontal section (red line) showing the actual profile achieved (right). The attempted shape (red curve) is seen to be very close to the achieved shape (blue curve).

The surgeon now has the option of clicking on ablation profile presets to examine the profiles suggested by the CRS-Master. The standard wavefront profile preset produces an ablation profile that has a fully corrected optical zone of equal diameter to the scotopic pupil size, with a prolate optimization function setting of 100%, and inclusion of the higher-order aberrations to be corrected. Presets for "night vision" increase the fully corrected optical zone beyond the wavefront analysis pupil, while the TSA sets the fully corrected optical zone below the analysis pupil size while maintaining 100% prolate optimization function. These presets are tested by the surgeon's examination of a cross sectional corneal profile map that demonstrates the ablation profile

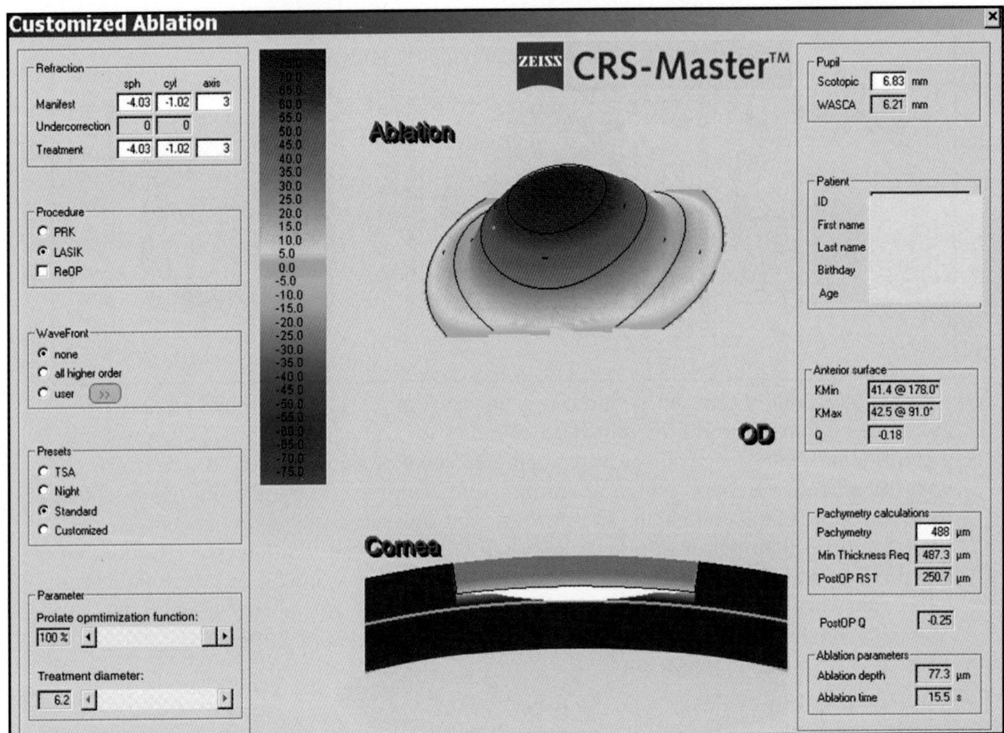

Figure 29-14. Panel for surgeon controlled custom ablation with a prototype version of the CRS-Master. This window is attained after importing WASCA and TOSCA data. The left-hand column (going from top to bottom) contains fields for entering the manifest refraction, target refraction, type of procedure, wavefront selection, or deselection (with a submenu for user defined wavefront components). Standard or preset suggested ablation profiles including TSA, night vision can be chosen, or customized surgeon control can be selected to control the POF and treatment zone diameter. The central area of the display contains a (user defined) selection of displays including 3-D representation of the ablation profile, wavefront, topography, and others, as well as a 2-D cross sectional representation of the cornea, flap, and ablation profile chosen to depict predicted total ablation depth within the cornea. Shading within this 2-D cross section represents the increased depth that may be produced by the standard deviation of the keratome being used (data that is entered by the user in a separate pop-up panel). The right-hand column (going from top to bottom) shows the WASCA derived pupil size, user entered scotopic pupil size, patient identification data, preoperative keratometry, and asphericity (Q) (from TOSCA). The pachymetry window allows user entry of the thinnest central thickness, and calculated fields showing the minimum thickness required for treatment as well as the predicted residual stromal thickness. The predicted postoperative asphericity (Q) is estimated and displayed. These fields update instantly as ablation profiles are modified by the user (eg, modification of POF, selected wavefront components, or treatment diameter).

with respect to the corneal thickness profile, flap profile, and ablation depth, and is therefore visually able to determine which preset would be safely applicable.

For the more advanced user, the surgeon selects the "customized" preset button. The fully corrected optical zone diameter and (eventually) the prolate optimization function sliders become active. The surgeon can modify these by studying the cross sectional corneal profile map to titrate the parameters and their proportion that would keep the ablation depth within safety limits. As the sliders are moved, a separate readout provides the predicted RST value in real time.

A further safety feature provides the ability to determine the 95% confidence limit for the minimum RST that can result, not based simply on the mean thickness of the keratome, but the mean and standard deviation of the microkeratome. We know that the RST limit of 250 µm is set to avoid breaching a much lower RST that would, in fact, produce a destabilized and ectatic cornea. This function, therefore, allows the surgeon to determine the actual probability that the RST will end up at or below the 180 µm, as suggested by Reinstein et al.[32]

Clinical Outcomes of Custom Ablation Using the Carl Zeiss Meditec

Wavefront Supported Custom Ablation vs Conventional Ablation

Photorefractive Keratectomy

Professor Dieter Dausch (University of Hanover, Germany) performed a prospective, consecutive, nonrandomized study to compare WASCA (30 eyes) with conventional (47 eyes) myopic PRK using the MEL70 G-scan excimer laser (1.80 mm true Gaussian flying spot, active tracker).[33] Spherical equivalent mean (±SD) myopia treated was approximately -4 (±2) D with a range extending to -8 D in both groups. Outcomes at 1 year were compared. Accuracy analysis revealed that improvements in uncorrected visual acuity (UCVA) continued between the 6 month visit and the 12 month visit. In the WASCA treated group, percentage eyes that were within ±0.5 D of intended was 87% at 6 months, reaching 97% at 12 months. In efficacy testing, 100% of WASCA treated eyes compared with 89% of conventionally treated eyes were 20/20 or better at 1 year. Similarly, 83% of WASCA treated eyes compared with 68% of conventionally treated eyes were 20/16 or better. In safety comparison, no eyes lost two lines or more in best spectacle corrected visual acuity in either group, but 6% of eyes in the conventional vs 0% of eyes in the WASCA group lost one line; again, a loss of two or more lines was observed in 53% of the WASCA group vs 6% of the conventional PRK group.

In a noncomparative study, Nagy et al reported on wavefront supported PRK for myopia and myopic astigmatism in 150 eyes.[34] The mean (±SD) preoperative spherical equivalent was -4.02 (±1.04) D (range: -1.50 D to -6.50 D spherical correction and 0.00 to -2.50 D cylindrical correction). At 6 months, 78.4% of eyes were within ±0.25 D of intended correction, and 98.6% within ±0.50 D, (100% within ±1 D). Efficacy showed UCVA of 20/20 or better in 80.7%, with 100% seeing 20/30 or better. No eyes lost lines of best-corrected visual acuity, and 20% gained one line, with 7% gaining two lines. The RMS for higher-order aberrations changed from preoperative value of 0.32 to 0.42 at 6 months.

These favorable wavefront-guided comparisons appear to also hold for hyperopic PRK (H-PRK). Nagy et al[34] reported on the comparison of WASCA (40 eyes) and conventional (40 eyes) H-PRK in a prospective, consecutive, nonrandomized study using the MEL70 G-scan excimer laser (all treatments performed by a single surgeon).[34] Spherical equivalent mean (SD) myopia treated was approximately +3 (±0.8) D in each group. The follow-up was 6 months. While the mean post-operative refraction was similar between the two groups (implying no difference in nomogram discalibration between groups), accuracy analysis showed that the percentage of eyes within ±0.50 D of intended was 82.5% and 67.5% for WASCA and conventional groups, respectively. Efficacy analysis revealed 15% of WASCA treated eyes compared with none of conventionally treated eyes were 20/15 or better. While there were similar numbers of cases losing 1 and 2 lines of best-corrected visual acuity, a gain of one line was observed in 20% of the WASCA group vs only 5% of the conventional H-PRK group.

Laser In-Situ Keratomileusis

Reinstein and coworkers compared the efficacy and safety of MEL70 G-scan LASIK with and without WASCA incorporated into the standard myopic treatment profile of consecutive patients presenting to a laser clinic in London, United Kingdom. Two consecutive series of eyes were treated by conventional ablation profile (44 eyes), followed by WASCA wavefront supported custom ablation (36 eyes). All surgery was performed by one surgeon, and all postoperative examinations were performed by a masked observer. Average follow-up was 3.2 months for all eyes. Each group had comparable starting mean (±SD) and range of spherical equivalent refraction (approximately -4 (±1.60) D, range -1.25 to -7.75 D). Efficacy was found to be similar between groups: for conventional vs WASCA treated groups, UCVA was 20/20 or better in 84% vs 83% respectively, 20/25 or better in 92% vs 91% respectively, and 20/30 or better in 100% in both groups. Six percent (2/36) of eyes in the WASCA group gained two lines of vision vs none in the conventional group, although this difference did not attain statistical significance (Fisher's exact p = 0.23). However, there were significant differences noted in safety. While no eye in the wavefront treated group lost one line of best corrected visual acuity, 13.6% (6/44) of the conventional group lost one line (Fisher's exact p = 0.03). (No eyes lost two lines or more in either group.)

Therefore, it appears that for PRK, improved efficacy as well as safety can be demonstrated by the addition of the eye's wavefront to the standard ablation profile. On the other hand, LASIK did not appear to benefit from the inclusion of WASCA data (MEL70 study). Improved PRK over LASIK results in wavefront-guided treatments could well be due to the shallower overall keratectomy in PRK (no flap), thus producing a lesser induction of higher-order aberrations due to biomechanics. In LASIK, flap-induced aberrations may overshadow the low amplitude, naturally occurring, higher-order aberrations. Perhaps preselection of those LASIK candidates with initially high amplitudes of higher-order aberrations could lead to being able to demonstrate a benefit to using the wavefront component in primary LASIK. We believe that by use of the *prolate optimization function* incorporated into the CRS-Master, a counterbalancing of the relatively high amplitude higher-order spherical aberrations induced by the flap can be achieved, allowing the naturally occurring higher-order aberrations to become less embedded.

Therefore, it appears that for PRK, improved efficacy as well as safety can be demonstrated by the addition of the eye's wavefront to the standard ablation profile. On the other hand, LASIK did not appear to benefit from the inclusion of WASCA data (MEL70 study).

Prolate Optimization Function: MEL80 Application

Preliminary investigation on the effect of prolate optimization independent of wavefront customization on the efficacy and safety of myopic LASIK data was investigated and reported by Reinstein and Srivannaboon.[35] In a prospective evaluation of LASIK for myopic astigmatism in 60 consecutive eyes, spherical equivalent mean (±SD) myopia treated was -4.51 (±1.88) D with a range extending to -9.38 D. Patients were fully evaluated at 1 week, 2 months, and 5 months by an independent observer. Accuracy analysis at 6 months showed a mean postoperative spherical equivalent of -0.05 D, with 90% of eyes within 0.25 D and 100% within 0.50 D of intended. The predictability (described by the standard deviation of the mean spherical equivalent) at 5 months was 0.18 D. Efficacy analysis reflected this level of accuracy and predictability, with 94% of eyes seeing 20/20 or better and 97% seeing 20/25 or better (100% seeing 20/32 or better). Orbscan II using software version 3.00 E, was used to derive front surface asphericity (Q factor) from the best fit central 4 mm zone before and after surgery. The mean Q-factor changed from a preoperative mean value of +0.030 to a postoperative mean value of +0.015 with a RMS change of +0.075 from before to after surgery. This is in contrast to results of a similar myopic cohort of 53 eyes treated with a conventional myopic ablation profile where the Q value changed from -0.009 to +0.089 with an RMS change of +0.531 from before to after surgery. Prolate optimization function it appears served to decrease the increase in Q, or decrease in prolateness of the cornea. This in turn would be expected to reduce the induction of higher order (mainly spherical) aberrations.

These MEL80 outcomes are significantly better than those achieved by LASIK performed with the MEL70, and it is believed that much of the improvement comes from a better understanding of corneal tissue responses to flap creation and photoablation. Such an optimized nonwavefront-guided system, we believe, forms a substantial platform for the overlay of the high quality wavefront data provided by the WASCA aberrometer. Studies to integrate all components are underway and results will be reported.

These MEL80 outcomes are significantly better than those achieved by LASIK performed with the MEL70, and it is believed that much of the improvement comes from a better understanding of corneal tissue responses to flap creation and photoablation.

Conclusion

The Carl Zeiss Meditec platform for custom ablation incorporates a suite of technology for WASCA, TOSCA, sophisticated excimer laser delivery (MEL80), and surgeon-controlled individualization of treatment protocol (CRS-Master). Together, these components promise to deliver increasingly higher accuracy and control over corneal sculpting—a dream come true for the father of keratomileusis, the late Jose Ignacio Barraquer.

References

1. Oshika T, Klyce SD, Applegate RA, Howland HC, El Danasoury MA. Comparison of corneal wavefront aberrations after photorefractive keratectomy and laser in situ keratomileusis. *Am J Ophthalmol.* 1999;127(1):1-7.
2. Neal DR, Armstrong DJ, Turner WT. Wavefront sensors for control and process monitoring in optics manufacture. *SPIE.* 1997.
3. Neal DR, Alford WJ, Gruetzner JK. Amplitude and phase beam characterization using a two-dimensional wavefront sensor. *SPIE.* 1996;72-82.
4. Pallikaris IG, Panagopoulou SI, Vogelsang H. Dynamic aberrometry and accommodation. Paper presented at: IX Congress of the European Society of Cataract and Refractive Surgery; September 2001; Amsterdam, Netherlands.
5. Salmon TO, West RW, Gasser W, Kenmore T. Accuracy, repeatability and instrument myopia with the COAS Shack-Hartman aberrometer. 3rd International Congress of Wavefront Sensing and Aberration-Free Refractive Correction; February 15, 2002; Interlaken, Switzerland.
6. Salmon TO, West RW, Gasser W, Kenmore T. Measurement of refractive errors in young myopes using the COAS Shack-Hartmann aberrometer. *Optom Vis Sci.* 2003.
7. Barraquer JI. Keratomileusis. *Int Surg.* 1967;48(2):103-117.
8. Munnerlyn CR, Koons SJ, Marshall J. Photorefractive keratectomy: a technique for laser refractive surgery. *J Cataract Refract Surg.* 1988; 14(1):46-52.
9. Barraquer JI. *Queratomileusis y queratofakia.* Bogota: Instituto Barraquer de America; 1980.
10. Reinstein DZ, Silverman RH, Rondeau MJ, Coleman DJ. Epithelial and corneal thickness measurements by high-frequency ultrasound digital signal processing. *Ophthalmology.* 1994;101(1):140-146.
11. Wygledowska-Promienska D, Zawojska I, Gierek-Ciaciura S, Sarzynski A. Correction of irregular astigmatism using excimer laser MEL 70 G-Scan with the TOSCA program—introductory report. *Klin Oczna.* 2000; 102(6):443-447.
12. Carl Zeiss Meditec AG. Data on file.
13. Mrochen M, Seiler T. Influence of corneal curvature on calculation of ablation patterns used in photorefractive laser surgery. *J Refract Surg.* 2001;17(5):S584-S587.
14. Oliver KM, O'Brart DP, Stephenson CG, et al. Anterior corneal optical aberrations induced by photorefractive keratectomy for hyperopia. *J Refract Surg.* 2001;17(4):406-413.
15. Oliver KM, Hemenger RP, Corbett MC, et al. Corneal optical aberrations induced by photorefractive keratectomy. *J Refract Surg.* 1997;13(3):246-254.
16. Reinstein DZ, Silverman RH, Raevsky T, et al. A new arc-scanning very high-frequency ultrasound system for 3D pachymetric mapping of corneal epithelium, lamellar flap and residual stromal layer in laser in situ keratomileusis. *J Refract Surg.* 2000;16:414-430.
17. Reinstein DZ, Silverman RH, Sutton HF, Coleman DJ. Very high-frequency ultrasound corneal analysis identifies anatomic correlates of optical complications of lamellar refractive surgery: anatomic diagnosis in lamellar surgery. *Ophthalmology.* 1999;106(3):474-482.
18. Reinstein DZ, Silverman RH, Coleman DJ. High-frequency ultrasound measurement of the thickness of the corneal epithelium. *Refract Corneal Surg.* 1993;9(5):385-387.
19. Reinstein DZ, Srivannaboon S, Silverman RH, Coleman DJ. The accuracy of routine LASIK: isolation of biomechanical and epithelial factors. *Invest Ophthalmol Vis Sci.* 2000;2000:S318.
20. Reinstein DZ, Srivannaboon S, Silverman RH, Coleman DJ. Limits of wavefront customized ablation: biomechanical and epithelial factors. *Invest Ophthalmol Vis Sci.* 2002;43:E-Abstract 3942.
21. Roberts C. The cornea is not a piece of plastic. *J Refract Surg.* 2000; 16(4):407-413.
22. Roberts C. Biomechanics of the cornea and wavefront-guided laser refractive surgery. *J Refract Surg.* 2002;18(5):S589-S592.
23. Hersh PS, Shah SI, Holladay JT. Corneal asphericity following excimer laser photorefractive keratectomy. Summit PRK Topography study group. *Ophthalmic Surg Lasers.* 1996;27(5 Suppl): S421-S428.
24. Holladay JT, Janes JA. Topographic changes in corneal asphericity and effective optical zone after laser in-situ keratomileusis. *J Cataract Refract Surg.* 2002;28(6):942-947.
25. Liang J, Williams DR. Aberrations and retinal image quality of the normal human eye. *J Opt Soc Am A.* 1997;14(11):2873-2883.
26. Barraquer JI. *Cirugia Refractiva de la Cornea.* Bogota: Instituto Barraquer de America; 1989.
27. Patel S, Marshall J, Fitzke FWd. Model for predicting the optical performance of the eye in refractive surgery. *Refract Corneal Surg.* 1993; 9(5):366-375.
28. Seiler T, Genth U, Holschbach A, Derse M. Aspheric photorefractive keratectomy with excimer laser. *Refract Corneal Surg.* 1993;9(3):166-172.

29. Reinstein DZ, Goes F. Prospective, controlled comparison of Hansatome vs. M2 aberrations: can we control for flap induced aberrations in primary wavefront guided LASIK? Paper presented at: XX Congress of the European Society of Cataract and Refractive Surgery; 2002; Nice, France.
30. El-Agha MS, Johnston EW, Bowman RW, Cavanagh HD, McCulley JP. Excimer laser treatment of spherical hyperopia: PRK or LASIK? *Trans Am Ophthalmol Soc.* 2000;98:59-66.
31. Pallikaris IG, Kymionis GD, Panagopoulou SI, et al. Induced optical aberrations following formation of a laser in situ keratomileusis flap. *J Cataract Refract Surg.* 2002;28(10):1737-1741.
32. Reinstein DZ, Srivannaboon S, Sutton HFS, Silverman RH, Shaikh A, Coleman DJ. Risk of ectasia in LASIK: revised safety criteria. *Invest Ophthalmol Vis Sci.* 1999;40(Suppl):S403.
33. Reinstein DZ, Dausch D, Schroder E. Custom Ablation with the Asclepion Meditec WASCA and MEL70 G-scan Excimer Laser. Paper presented at: 3rd International Congress of Wavefront Sensing and Aberration-Free Refractive Correction; February 15, 2002; Interlaken, Switzerland.
34. Nagy Z, Palágyi-Deak I, Kovács A, Kelemen E. First results with wavefront-guided photorefractive keratectomy for hyperopia. *J Refract Surg.* 2002;18(5):S620-S623.
35. Reinstein DZ, Srivannaboon S. Aberrometry and Custom Ablation Principles: Surgeon controlled custom ablation; The Carl Zeiss-Meditec CRS-Master. Paper presented at: American Academy of Ophthalmology Annual Meeting: Sub Speciality Day in Refractive Surgery; October 19, 2003; Orlando, Fla.

Chapter 30

The Allegretto Wave: A Different Approach to Wavefront-Guided Ablation

Matthias Maus, MD; Arthur Cummings, MBChB, MMed, FCS(SA) FRCSEd; and Stefan Tuess, Dip Eng

Introduction

The quality of vision a patient experiences is the ultimate gauge for the success of a refractive surgical treatment. It is believed that bright, crisp, saturated, high-contrast images actually enhance the satisfaction derived from proper refractive adjustment.[1] This area of refractive surgery continues to undergo constant development and refinement. Diagnostic procedures for the evaluation of visual quality and of the eye itself change constantly, as does surgical methodology. It is, therefore, paramount that tools such as the excimer laser be as flexible as possible in order to evolve with those changes. This was an important prerequisite for the development of the Allegretto Wave Analyzer (WaveLight Laser Technologies AG, Erlanger, Germany), with software-controlled flying-spot technology that drives a modular design that adapts easily to changes in the ablation pattern. A rapid repetition rate, high-frequency eyetracker, and a small spot size with a Gaussian beam profile are the preconditions for enabling ablation profiles to correct more than just standard spectacle prescriptions.

Wavefront-optimized and wavefront-guided treatments became possible within a very short time frame. From the day the company was founded, WaveLight Laser Technologies AG relied heavily upon the input of Theo Seiler, MD, PhD, thus incorporating clinical, as well as engineering, considerations throughout the entire product development process. This task was not an easy one. The development phase was characterized not only by adherence to strict external quality controls, but also by a commitment to flexibility and to continual reassessment in the pursuit of technology that would translate well into clinical practice. Despite being conceptually sound and "passing the muster" in the laboratory, many ideas were discarded in the early stages of development if it seemed they might not meet the high standards set for practical application. This approach helped to avert some of the "teething problems" still seen with some of the new lasers in the market today.

Technology: Measurement, Mapping, and Treatment Design

The Allegretto Wave Analyzer technology is based on the Tscherning principle of wavefront measurements. One hundred sixty-eight rays of visible light are emitted by a 660 nanometer (nm) laser diode, projecting onto the retina a grid pattern with a diameter of only 1 millimeter (mm).[2] A highly sensitive charged-coupled device (CCD) camera captures the retinal image of the grid pattern and that image is then compared to the ideal, non-aberrated image. The extent to which each spot deviates from its ideal position is calculated and that calculation is used to determine the wavefront shape (Figure 30-1).

The Allegretto Wave Analyzer ensures proper alignment of the measurement to the pupil center with an integrated eye-tracking system that tracks the pupil in x,y and the eye in a z direction during the measurement. It allows measurements in a 100 micron (µm) x,y range from the center of the pupil and in a 200 µm z range from the eye itself. It is only when the eye has been centered within this range that the data can be used for treatment.

During the measurement process, the patient's pupil should be dilated to at least 7 mm in order to obtain an optimally accurate map of all aberrations, including those in the corneal periphery. Once the eye is centered, a measurement can be taken manually or with the automatic mode. Far- and near-point accommodation can be considered by moving the accommodation target before taking the measurement. For custom laser in-situ keratomileusis (LASIK) treatments, the far-point has to be measured. To study the change of aberrations during accommodation, the patient can be measured within any part of the accommodation process. During the measurement, patients are able to see their own aberrations according to the deformation of the ideal grid pattern, which is displayed in the visible range (660 nm) (Figure 30-2).

Once the measurement has been taken, the retinal image is displayed and analyzed, and the wavefront map is determined. The Allegretto Wave Analyzer calculates Zernike coefficients up to the sixth order. The wavefront map can be displayed in several different ways: wavefront map, higher-orders map, tangential-power map, and sagittal power map. A display is possible in two- and three-dimensional maps. Also available is a chart comparison of the individual Zernike coefficients, displaying the root mean square (RMS) values for the individual orders, the total wavefront (RMS_G), and the higher orders (RMS_H).

As many as four different maps for an individual patient can be compared simultaneously in an overview window. This enables comparison of the wavefront, as well as the Zernike coefficients, for each map in order to determine reproducibility of the measurements. After review and selection of up to four meas-

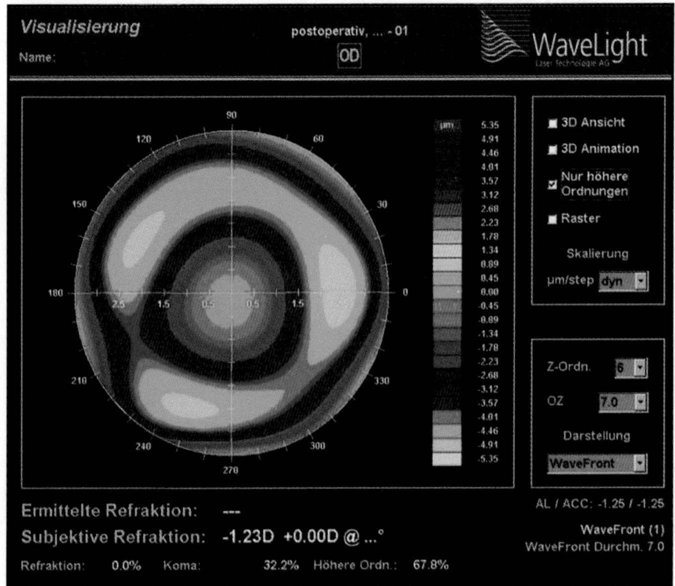

Figure 30-1. Display of colored wavefront map—higher orders only.

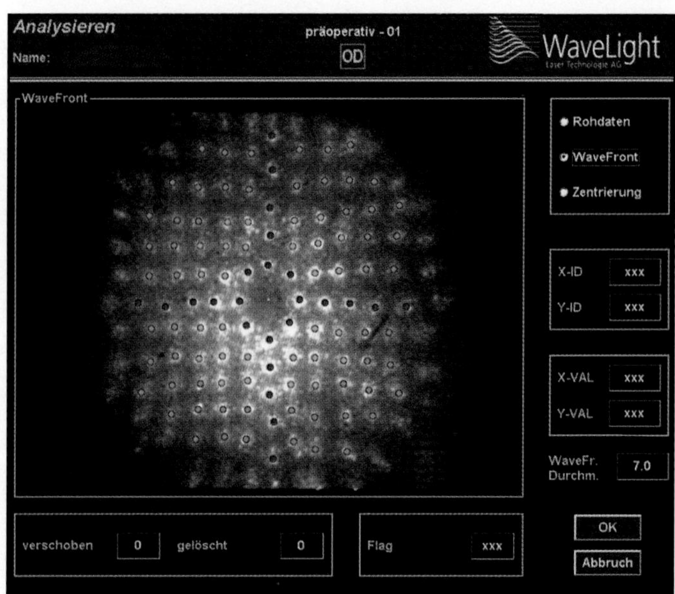

Figure 30-2. Retinal image display of a Tscherning grid pattern.

urements per patient, the data are exported onto a floppy disk that is inserted into the Allegretto Wave Excimer Laser System for a custom ablation treatment. The surgeon can devise a treatment from a single map or from an average data combination of up to four maps.

The Wavefront-Adjusted Ablation Profile

Since Watkin's introduction of the first corneal models, it has been known that the native corneal surface flattens toward the periphery.[3] When central and peripheral corneal radii are compared, measurements (in mm) toward the limbus increase and diopters of refractive power decrease. It can, therefore, be anticipated that the natural corneal contour would offset the spherical aberrations that are created with an open pupil.[4]

A two-dimensional surface plane of a meridial cut made through the corneal axis would resemble a prolate ellipsoid in shape. If the cornea were to become steeper toward the periphery, an oblate ellipsoid would be created. The issue becomes more complicated when the cornea is viewed three-dimensionally, especially since the extent to which the cornea flattens toward the individual semimeridians (nasal, temporal, superior, and inferior) can vary and, in many cases, some degree of astigmatism is present. The normal corneal contour is, therefore, a nonrotation symmetrical, toric, prolate ellipsoid, which has been described by Wilms simply as natural torus (toroid).[5,6]

Implications for Laser In-Situ Keratomileusis Surgery

Even the most modern and sophisticated laser systems are only able to emit light vertically toward the corneal center. The cornea, however, changes in both shape and radius toward the periphery. Light rays that strike an optical surface at a nonperpendicular angle are partially reflected and have less impact than rays that strike at a perpendicular angle. The degree of reflection increases with the degree of inclination of the surface, and energy density decreases as the light rays are spread over a larger surface area.[7] Naturally, this increasing reflection effect toward the corneal periphery has an impact on the ablation profile of the laser; if this is not taken into account in the design of the ablation profile, a larger amount of tissue will be removed in the center than in the periphery. Under these conditions, a spherical ablation profile will flatten the central cornea to a greater extent than the periphery, creating an oblate ellipsoid with increasing refractive power toward the corneal edges.

Light rays that enter the cornea through an open pupil toward the periphery will be refracted more strongly and will create a spherical aberration that impacts the wavefront. In the past, this was a common occurrence, causing the well-known mesopic and scotopic vision problems frequently seen with classic LASIK treatments. These effects are taken into account in the Allegretto Wave system's standard wavefront-optimized ablation profile; compensation for the energy loss in the periphery of the cornea is accomplished with a specific shot pattern based on a patent-protected algorithm.[5] As a result, the surgeon is able to achieve the desired ablation depth without creating problematic spherical aberrations.

Named for Zernike, spherical aberration is also called Zernike 12 (Z^1_2 or Z^0_4) of the fourth order and is likely the best-known of the higher-order aberration errors in geometric optics. All higher-order optical errors change the wavefront of passing light in an optical system. When these errors are corrected, the wavefront is automatically corrected as well; therefore, the ablation profile used for the correction is known as a *wavefront-optimized ablation profile*.[8]

Going one step further, WaveLight has introduced the Q-value assisted treatment mode, in which it is possible to preselect the postoperative corneal asphericity over the ablation area by choosing an appropriate Q-value.

Patient Selection

At present, complete wavefront-guided ablations with the Allegretto Wave are limited to a spherical equivalent of no greater than -7 diopters (D). At higher diopter levels, the passing point of the light rays through the natural lens deviates too greatly from the original entrance point into the optical system of the eye, thus creating additional higher-order aberrations. This is due to the change in refraction on the cornea, the first refractive plane in the eye.

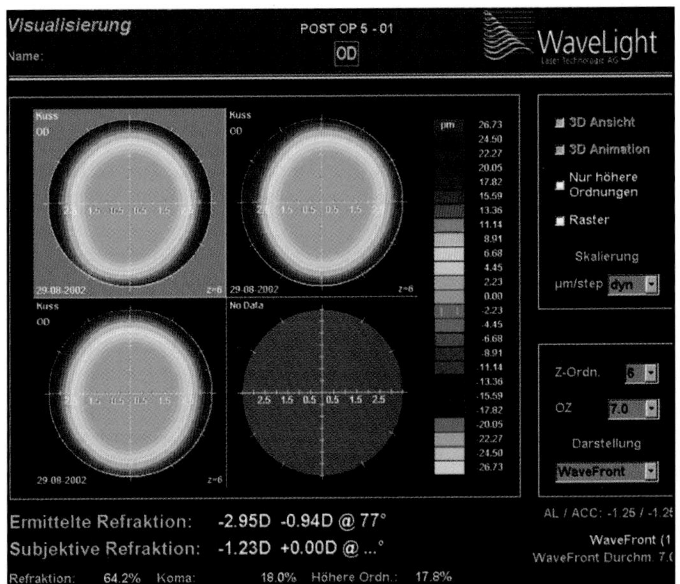

Figure 30-3. Comparison screen of multiple measurements.

As discussed previously, a successful measurement is based primarily on a centered, sharp, and wide-spread image of the dot pattern on the retina. The quality depends significantly on the transparency of the media. The dot pattern must travel undisturbed through the optical pathway from the tear film to the retina. If light is dispersed or absorbed by irregularities or opacities, the quality of the image cannot be assured. As the first optical plane of the eye, the tear film also has a strong impact on the quality of the measurement. Lack of tear film or poor quality can be improved by applying artificial tears; this in turn improves the overall result of the measurement. For standardization purposes, we routinely apply hyaluronic acid repeatedly before a measurement is undertaken.

The transparency of the media can deteriorate with age, but a specific age at which aberration measurement is no longer possible cannot be determined. Therefore, in our clinic, we measure every patient, regardless of age, as long as the patient's refraction qualifies for a wavefront-guided treatment.

Patients with limited or poor contrast sensitivity benefit most from a wavefront-guided treatment. Contrast sensitivity and glare should be evaluated along with all other preoperative measurements. If these evaluations should be repeated during the postoperative examinations, they can be used for quality control.

Most importantly, aberration measurements must be reproducible; otherwise, it will be uncertain if the measurement actually reflects true aberrations. Under no circumstances should a treatment be based on a single measurement. In fact, it is the first author's recommendation that at least four similar, validated measurements be obtained per eye. At times, the surgeon may find it advantageous to take even more qualifying measurements to enable selection of the best and most similar results for the actual treatment.

Measurement: The Diagnostic Process

As stated above, the surgeon should strive to obtain four similar, high-quality measurements of each eye, which can then be validated and averaged. While several criteria are important in this regard, some of these are not quantitatively measurable.

The essential steps involved in a measurement evaluation are as follows:

1. Evaluation of quality and point distribution of the retinal image
2. Evaluation of the colored wavefront map
3. Evaluation of the wavefront-calculated refraction and comparison of this objective refraction to the subjective refraction (at a 7 mm pupil and a 4 mm pupil)
4. Evaluation of the RMS_H value
5. Evaluation of Zernike polynomials in terms of size, distribution, and structure up to Z27 (the Zernike value structure should be within the same tolerance at all four measurements)
6. Comparison of at least four measurements, per the steps outlined above (Figure 30-3)

When evaluating individual measurements, the measured refraction and the distribution and value of the individual Zernike values are most important. Currently, there are no standardizations of fixed values that can be used for orientation. For small cylinders rather than larger cylinders, higher tolerances in the axis can be accepted. With increasing Zernike values, the importance and the size of the actual measured value decrease, as does the impact of the polynomial on the optical quality. It appears that the most important values to be considered for the diagnostic evaluation are coma (Z7 and Z8) and spherical aberrations (Z12). Our experience has shown that good, validated measurements allow even higher tolerances to the subjective refraction for sphere and cylinder. Although these deviations were originally defined as exclusion criteria and the values were adjusted toward the subjective refraction, we currently accept the measurements without further adjustments. In these cases, wavefront measurements have been shown superior to subjective measurements. The Allegretto Wave Analyzer provides the operator and diagnostic staff with extremely detailed insight into the process of image acquisition and processing. Measurements can easily be validated as optical disturbances in the optical pathway and will not result in false measurement values.

Initiating Treatment: The Therapeutic Process

Once the data have been exported to the computer that controls the laser, the operator has the opportunity to reconfirm all parameters. Again, it is possible to view the individual maps and Zernike polynomial charts for each measurement. If desired, the operator can make final adjustments to the treatment. Then when executed, the laser in-situ keratomileusis (LASIK) treatment itself is entirely wavefront-guided, meaning that the ablation algorithm does not correct higher-order aberrations in a separate pass but rather treats the entire wavefront error at once. The shot pattern is controlled in order to treat a complete optical zone from the beginning. Importantly, from a safety standpoint, an interruption in treatment results only in spherocylindrical undercorrection.

Clinical Results

It had been hoped (industry-wide) that wavefront-guided LASIK would allow surgeons to provide super vision (ie, uncorrected visual acuity of 20/12) for most or all of their patients. The approach employed by WaveLight, however, was different from the very beginning. They set out to design a laser that would provide improved quality of vision in all lighting conditions or at all of the pupil sizes encountered during the day and night.

Since improved quality of vision was already being achieved in wavefront-optimized LASIK with the Allegretto Wave, wavefront-guided LASIK would need to further improve mesopic and scotopic visual results, while also maintaining the excellent refractive and visual acuity results established with classic (ie, wavefront-optimized) LASIK.

The Allegretto Wave was engineered to optimize the optical beam path in order to produce a natural, prolate ablation pattern by increasing the number of pulses delivered to the corneal periphery. The resulting corneal contour has yielded excellent contrast sensitivity and visual performance in low-light conditions, even with the classic treatment. The challenge involved in attempting to surpass these outcomes with wavefront-guided treatment was both enormous and daunting.

> It had been hoped (industry-wide) that wavefront-guided LASIK would allow surgeons to provide super vision (ie, uncorrected visual acuity of 20/12) for most or all of their patients. The approach employed by WaveLight, however, was different from the very beginning. They set out to design a laser that would provide improved quality of vision in all lighting conditions or at all of the pupil sizes encountered during the day and night.
>
> Since improved quality of vision was already being achieved in wavefront-optimized LASIK with the Allegretto Wave, wavefront-guided LASIK would need to further improve mesopic and scotopic visual results, while also maintaining the excellent refractive and visual acuity results established with classic (ie, wavefront-optimized) LASIK.

Wavefront-Guided vs Wavefront-Optimized LASIK

Author 2 began using wavefront-guided LASIK in September 2001 and, as of November 2002, has performed more than 170 such procedures. Wavefront-optimized LASIK (referred to as classic LASIK with the Allegretto Wave) and wavefront-guided procedures performed during the same period and with the same preoperative criteria (ie, myopia <-6 D, astigmatism <-3.75 D), were compared with respect to outcomes at day 1, 6 weeks, 3 months, and 6 months post-treatment. This discussion will be limited to the visual and refractive results from 150 eyes treated with wavefront-guided LASIK and 240 eyes treated with classic LASIK. The same surgeon performed all of the procedures, and all treatments were carried out using the Hansatome microkeratome (Bausch & Lomb, Rochester, NY) (8.5 and 9.5 mm rings) and a 6.5 mm optical zone. The preoperative data from the two groups were very similar. In the wavefront-guided group, the average preoperative spherical refraction was -3.34 and the average cylindrical refraction was -0.75. In the classic LASIK group, the average preoperative spherical refraction was –3.37 and the average cylindrical refraction was -0.82. Day 1 refractive results showed an average spherical refraction of 0.23 in the wavefront-guided group and zero in the classic group. The average cylindrical refraction in the wavefront-guided group was -0.33 compared to -0.36 in the other group. Anecdotally, the glare factor was already noticeably smaller in the wavefront-guided group by day 1. Patients in the wavefront group consistently reported a reduced area of glare around a Snellen chart projected on a wall.

At the 6-week visit, the average spherical equivalent in the wavefront-guided group was +0.19 and it was -0.14 in the classic group. The cylinder in the wavefront-guided group was -0.26, almost identical to the classic group with -0.28. Uncorrected visual acuity (UCVA) was 1.07 in the wavefront-guided group versus 0.97 in the classic group.

At 3 months, the results were on average still better in the wavefront-guided group. The spherical equivalent in the wavefront-guided group was +0.105 and -0.085 in the classic group. Cylinder was identical at -0.31 in both groups. The UCVA was 1.05 in the wavefront-guided group versus 0.99 in the classic group.

At the 6-month interval, the average spherical equivalent was still slightly hyperopic in the wavefront-guided group (+0.165) and slightly myopic in the classic group (-0.11). The UCVA was very similar, with 1.02 in the wavefront-guided group and 1.03 in the classic group. This was the first interval at which the results in the classic group were marginally better than in the wavefront-guided group. It is also important to note that there were smaller numbers of patients in these groups at the 6-month interval. The 20 eyes in the wavefront-guided group were the very first 20 eyes ever treated by author 2 with wavefront-guided LASIK and they were being compared with eyes in the classic group, where the overall surgeon experience is infinitely more.

At 6 weeks and 6 months, 67.4% and 82% of eyes, respectively, were within the -0.25 D to 0.25 D range, demonstrating a high degree of accuracy in the wavefront-guided group. The results were even more accurate in the classic group, with 76.3% and 80%, respectively, being within ±0.25 D of plano. The greater degree of accuracy seen in the classic LASIK group is to be expected, since this procedure has been in use much longer than wavefront-guided LASIK. Simple nomogram adjustments will improve wavefront accuracy further (Figure 30-4).

Overall, at 6 months postoperation, only 2.4% of the classic LASIK group had lost more than one line of best-corrected visual acuity (BCVA), 5.9% had lost one line, 57% were unchanged, 35.9% had gained at least one line, and 7.1% had gained two or more lines. In the corresponding wavefront-guided group, none of the patients had lost more than one line of BCVA, 1% had lost one line, 50% were unchanged, 49% had gained at least one line, and 11% had gained two or more lines (Figure 30-5).

Closer analysis of the refractive results shows that eyes with less than -4 D benefit more from wavefront-guided LASIK as they retain the superior results over classic LASIK at every interval up to and including the 6-month mark. In the range of -4.25 D to -6 D, wavefront-guided LASIK achieves better visual results at an early stage, but between the intervals at 3 and 6 months, classic LASIK starts to outperform wavefront-guided LASIK. This may be due to corneal modeling

> Closer analysis of the refractive results shows that eyes with less than -4 D benefit more from wavefront-guided LASIK as they retain the superior results over classic LASIK at every interval up to and including the 6-month mark.

Conclusions and Outlook

The priorities of the engineers who design technology and the surgeons who rely upon that technology can sometimes be at odds. Quality of clinical results is paramount to the practitioner, while the engineer must consider a host of other factors. WaveLight has succeeded in bringing about a symbiosis of these priorities in the design of its Allegretto Wave system, as evi-

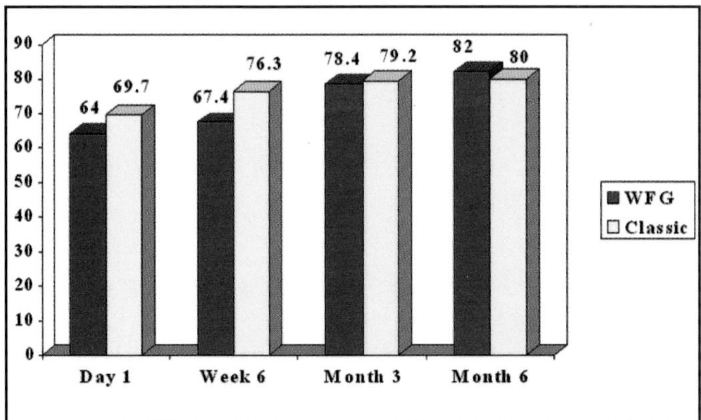

Figure 30-4. Results: Accuracy (±0.25 D) wavefront-guided vs classic LASIK.

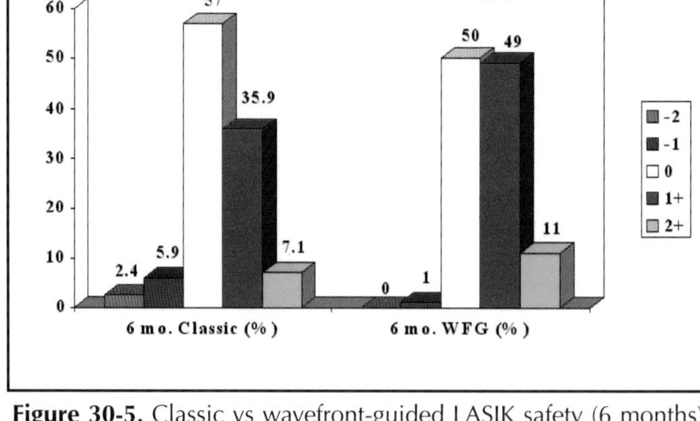

Figure 30-5. Classic vs wavefront-guided LASIK safety (6 months) (n = 170 + 100).

denced by Professor Seiler's use of the laser to conduct the world's first wavefront-guided LASIK treatment in 1999.[7]

The purpose of wavefront-guided LASIK is to improve the quality of vision, especially in mesopic and scotopic conditions. The challenge was to achieve this goal without compromising the excellent results that were being achieved with classic LASIK using the Allegretto Wave. In the authors' hands, wavefront-guided LASIK has clearly outperformed classic LASIK, both in terms of visual acuity and accuracy of refractive results.

What does the future hold? It is our belief that this technology will increasingly be used for patients with specific problems, including complaints of glare, large scotopic and mesopic pupils, and refractive errors of <6 D of myopia, especially <-4 D. We further believe that, as the technology evolves, it may find a primary role in enhancement procedures.

We can anticipate that there will be fine-tuning of existing nomograms, smaller spot sizes, faster lasers, reduction of cut impact (possibly with laser cutting), and an expansion of wavefront-guided LASIK treatments to values higher than -7.00 D spherical equivalent, accomplished by dividing aberrations into those created by the cornea and those created by the lens. Topography could play a greater role than before. Aside from central K-values, meridial eccentricities could gain a stronger impact on the algorithms.

Quality improvement and risk minimization will be critical in determining the future of refractive surgery. Wavefront-guided LASIK is a step in this direction. Measurements of vision and contrast sensitivity, as well as the subjective quality of visual perception (especially night vision), illustrate this impressively. We remain, however, far from fully understanding higher-order aberrations and their impact on the diverse visual qualities. We have yet to determine if aberration-free optics are an ideal precondition for the physics and physiology of vision, or if there are, in fact, useful aberrations that support visual comfort and physiologic perception. The goal remains to ensure the best possible results in visual quality with significantly improved predictability and minimized effort and risk.

References

1. Pinker S. *How The Mind Works*. New York, NY: WW Norton; 1997:535.
2. Mierdel P, Krinke HE, Wiegard W, Kaemmerer M, Seiler T. Messplatz zur bestimmung der monochromatischen aberration des menschlichen avgeo. *Ophthalmologe*. 1997;96:441-445.
3. Watkins JR. Corneal topography and contact lens relationship. *JAOA*. 1966;37(3):224-228.
4. Mrochen M, Seiler, T. Influence of corneal curvature on calculation of ablation patterns used in photorefractive laser surgery. *J Refract Surg*. 2001;17:584-587.
5. Wilms KH. Ein einfaches verfahren zur erfassung der corneaform mit dem klassischen pphthalmometer. *Die Kontaktlinse*. 1973;7(1): 24-30.
6. Wilms KH. Praxisnahe verfahren der corneatopometrie. *Die Kontaktlinse*. 1977;11(4):20-24.
7. Mrochen M, Kaemmerer M, Seiler T. Wavefront-guided laser in situ keratomileusis: early results in three eyes. *J Refract Surg*. 2000; 16:116-121.
8. Tscherning M. Die monochromatischen aberrationen des menschlichen auges. *Z Psychol Physiol Sinne*. 1894;6:456-471.

Chapter 31

Clinical Results With the Nidek NAVEX Platform

Arturo Chayet, MD and Harkaran S. Bains

Optical Path Difference

Device Description

The optical path difference (OPD)-Scan (Nidek, Gamagori, Japan) is a combination aberrometer and topographer that uses the principles of spatial dynamic skiascopy to measure the aberrations of the eye and placido disk topography to measure the corneal shape. The measuring principle (Figure 31-1) is a projecting system that consists of an infrared light-emitting diode housed within a chopper wheel with slit apertures.

The receiving system consists of a photodetector array that converts the time differences of stimulation in dioptric power maps. The dioptric power maps or refractive maps are displayed as OPD maps from which traditional Zernike-based maps can be derived.

The receiving system consists of a photodetector array that converts the time differences of stimulation in dioptric power maps. The dioptric power maps or refractive maps are displayed as OPD maps from which traditional Zernike-based maps can be derived. Using the traditional maps as an analogy, the OPD map is a total wavefront aberration map expressed in diopters (D) of refractive power rather than microns (μm) of light or elevation. A detailed description of this device and its advantages over traditional aberrometers is available in Chapter 19.

Nidek Advanced Vision Excimer Laser System—Scope of Treatments

The Nidek Advanced Vision Excimer Laser System (NAVEX) (Gamagori, Japan) consists of the following units:

1. The OPD-Scan aberrometer and topographer
2. The Final Fit interface software
3. The EC-5000 CX excimer laser employing both scanning slit and spot ablation capabilities to deliver the treatment onto the cornea (Figure 31-2)

The Final Fit software uses both topography and aberrometry to develop the ablation algorithms. A cyclotorsion module allows compensation for cyclotorsion that may occur between the sitting to supine positions. The spot size is 1 millimeter (mm), the optical zone can be varied to 6.5 mm and the transition zone can be varied out to 10 mm. NAVEX allows the treatment of primary refractive surgery candidates in addition to the treatment of patients who have had suboptimal outcomes for previous refractive surgery. The experience of Howard Gimbel, MD with the latter group of patients was presented at the American and European Society of Refractive Surgery Meetings in 2002. These treatments included the treatment of irregular astigmatism and decentered ablations.

The Final Fit software uses both topography and aberrometry to develop the ablation algorithms. A cyclotorsion module allows compensation for cyclotorsion that may occur between the sitting-to-supine positions.

Customized Aspheric Transition Zone

Various excimer laser manufacturers have reported large increases in spherical aberration after excimer ablation. Spherical aberration has been implicated in a variety of night vision disturbances such as halos, glare, and starburst along with a generalized decreased in best-corrected visual acuity (BCVA). The quality of vision decreases with large increases in higher-order aberration.

The customized aspheric transition zone (CATZ) method was developed to specifically address this issue. This is accomplished by an increase in the transition zone, reduction in optical zone, and a seamless transition between the two treatment zones. The advantages of this unique treatment method are the increase in the effective optical zone and the maintenance of the prolate shape of the cornea postoperatively (Figure 31-3). By moving what Vinciguerra refers to as the "red-ring" on corneal topography past the pupillary excursion diameter and reducing the severity of contour change, the spherical aberration is very effectively reduced. The red ring on instantaneous (or tangential)

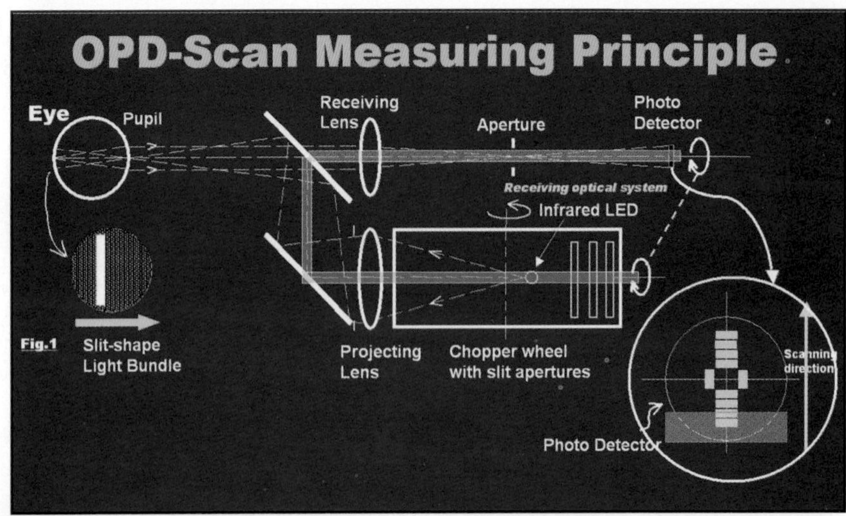

Figure 31-1. Schematic diagram of the OPD-Scan aberrometer.

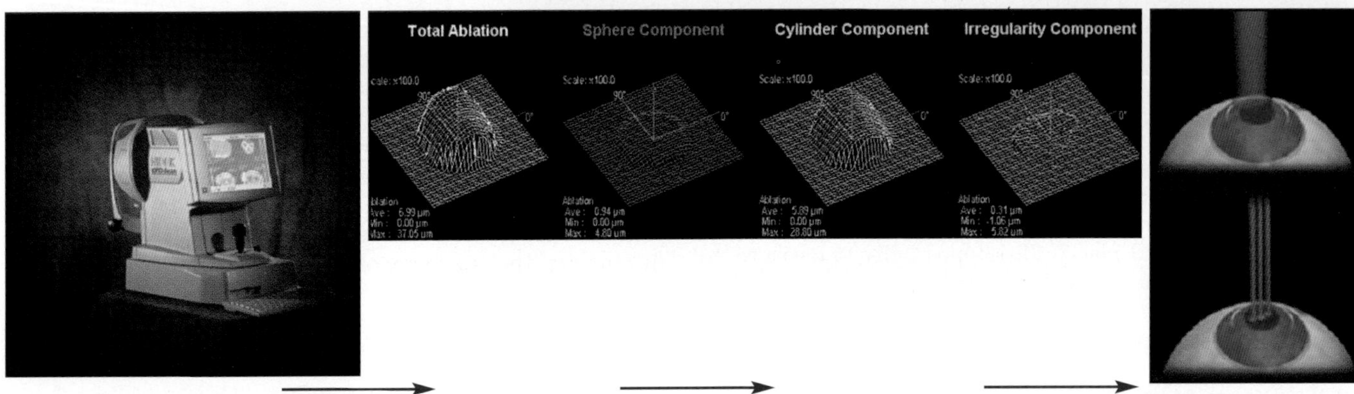

Figure 31-2. Data flow with the NAVEX.

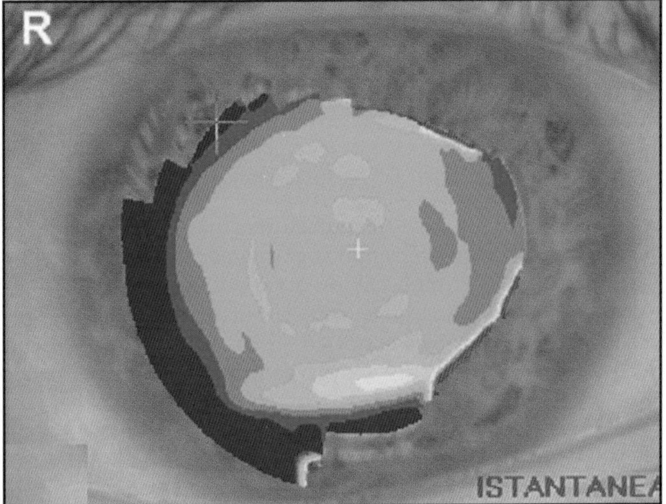

Figure 31-3. Topography post-CATZ treatment showing a large effective optical zone (no red ring). Treatment: -6 D sphere, -1.5 D cylinder, 5 mm optical zone, 10 mm transition zone. (Courtesy of Paolo Vinciguerra, MD.)

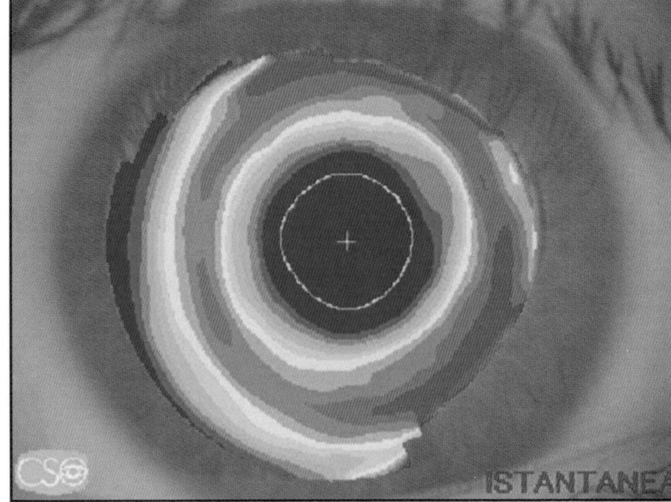

Figure 31-4. Postexcimer laser ablation topography for a -5.00 D conventional treatment showing a pronounced red ring and a small effective optical zone. (Courtesy of Paolo Vinciguerra, MD.)

topography often has a deep red ring after laser ablation (Figure 31-4). The severity of the color signifies abrupt dioptric power changes in the cornea between the optical zone, transition zone, and nascent cornea. The effective optical zone is defined within the radius of the red ring.

By introducing patented ablation algorithms in the treatment zones, the NAVEX platform reduces the abrupt dioptric power changes and consequently the spherical aberration that is induced by many conventional excimer lasers. The use of the OPD-Scan and Final Fit software allows the simulation of the postoperative aberrometry and topography maps. The cus-

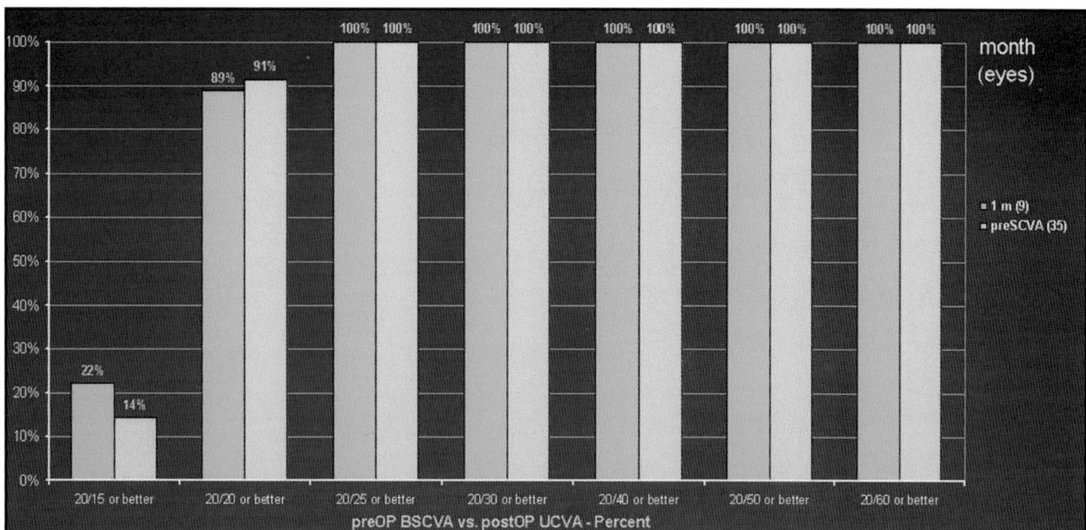

Figure 31-5. Gain in postoperative vision after CATZ treatment.

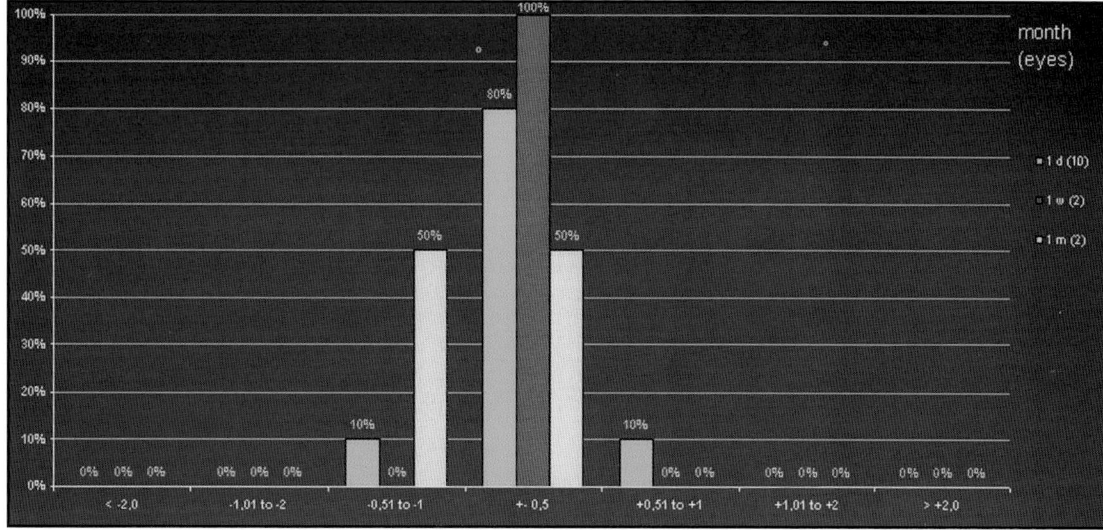

Figure 31-6. Refractive outcome. All eyes targeted for emmetropia.

tomization of the functional optical zone to a specific pupil size is also possible within the Final Fit software. The advent of this unique ablation algorithm allows refractive surgeons to taper treatments that maintain quality of vision in photopic and scotopic conditions. A more detailed explanation of CATZ is available elsewhere in this book.

> Editor's note:
> The CATZ system allows the surgeon to use an aspheric ablation that reduces the positive spherical aberration.
> S. MacRae, MD

CATZ Clinical Results

One of the authors (AC) treated 35 consecutive eyes with a preliminary version of the CATZ software. At the time of this writing, 1 month results were available. Patients with up to -5.75 D of myopia and -3.25 D of cylinder preoperatively were treated. All eyes were targeted for emmetropia. The following results are for primary treatments only.

Prior to treatment, 100% of the eyes had best spectacle-corrected visual acuity (BSCVA) of 20/40 or better, 91% of the eyes were 20/20 or better, and 14% were 20/15 or better. At 1 month postoperative 100% of the eyes had an uncorrected visual acuity (UCVA) of 20/40 or better, 89% were 20/20 or better, and 22% were 20/15 or better (Figure 31-5). As the majority of the treated patients were low and moderate myopes, magnification effects are an unlikely explanation for the gain in UCVA of 20/15 or better.

> At 1 month postoperative 100% of the eyes had UCVA of 20/40 or better, 89% were 20/20 or better, and 22% were 20/15 or better.

The accuracy of this automated platform was well within accepted criteria. For example, at the day 1 postoperative visit, 100% of the treated eyes were within +0.5 D of emmetropia; at the 1 month visit, this changed to 100% within -1 D (Figure 31-6). Thirty-three percent of the treated eyes gained at least one line of vision postoperatively and 7% lost only one line of vision (Figure 31-7). Mesopic contrast sensitivity was measured using the Vector Vision chart (Precision Vision, Inc, LaSalle, Ill) with sinusoidal gratings. At the 1 month mark, average values showed no loss of mesopic contrast sensitivity. At 6 cycles per degree, 100% of the

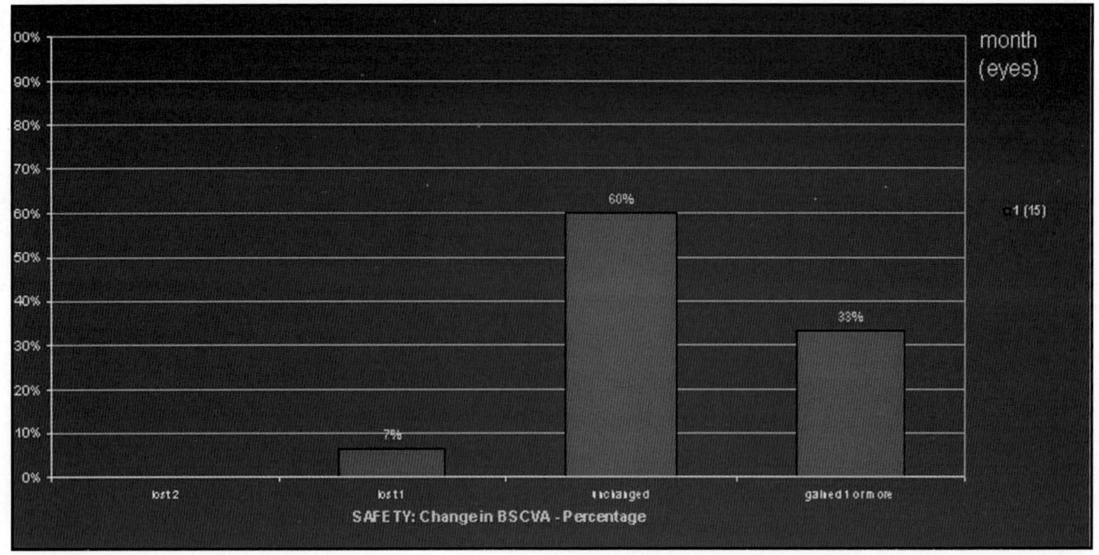

Figure 31-7. Change in BSCVA, 1 month postoperative.

patients maintained or gained lines of vision 1 month postoperatively. At 12 cycles per degree, 95% of patients either maintained or gained lines of vision. This preliminary data does demonstrate safety and efficacy of the CATZ treatment along with the added benefit of either maintaining or enhancing the quality of vision in most patients.

Section IV

Wavefront Customized Lenses

Chapter 32

Biomaterials for Wavefront Customization

Liliana Werner, MD, PhD; Nick Mamalis, MD; and David J. Apple, MD

Introduction

The development and manufacture of intraocular lenses (IOLs) for cataract surgery is evolving rapidly, and lenses that can be inserted/injected through incisions smaller than 2 millimeters (mm) will soon be marketed. However, the ability of the lens to be implanted through very small incisions is not the only feature sought by researchers, manufacturers, and surgeons. Modern cataract surgery is now in the realm of refractive surgery and patients expect almost perfect results. Thus, the most energy and funding is probably being spent on the development of new and complex IOLs that not only restore the refractive power of the eye after cataract surgery, but also provide special features, including multifocality, toric corrections, pseudoaccommodation, etc.[1] Some of these aspects may also apply to the development of new phakic IOLs, which are increasing in popularity, since they can potentially be used for the correction of different refractive errors.[2,3]

Since the development of wavefront aberrometry, it is possible to clinically measure the optical defects of the eye beyond spherical and cylindrical aberrations (lower-order aberrations). This technology can be used to quantify ocular aberrations and then design the ideal refractive correction for each patient, which may include a customized corneal ablative correction but also a customized contact lens, an IOL, or a combination of the above. It is expected that increasing understanding and availability of wavefront technology will greatly influence the manufacture of IOLs.[4]

The aim of this chapter is to present, in the first part, a brief overview of the biomaterials that can potentially be used for the manufacture of IOLs in association with wavefront technology to provide patients with a quality of vision beyond that with currently available lenses. In the second part, we describe two examples of recently developed "customized" IOLs for cataract surgery.

Biomaterials for Intraocular Lens Optics: Brief Overview

Biomaterials (polymers) currently used for the manufacture of IOL optics can be divided into two major groups, namely acrylic and silicone.[5-9] Acrylic lenses can be further divided as follows:

- Rigid (eg, manufactured from polymethyl methacrylate [PMMA]) (Figure 32-1)
- Foldable
  - Manufactured from hydrophobic acrylic materials (eg, AcrySof [Alcon Laboratories, Fort Worth, Tex] and Sensar [Advanced Medical Optics, Santa Ana, Calif]) (Figures 32-2 and 32-3)
  - Manufactured from hydrophilic acrylics also known as hydrogels (eg, Hydroview [Baush & Lomb, Rochester, NY], MemoryLens [CIBA Vision, Duluth, Ga], or Centerflex [Rayner Intraocular Lenses Ltd, Brighton-Hove, East Sussex, England]) (Figure 32-4)

Polymerization is the process by which the repeating units forming a polymer (the monomers) are linked by covalent and therefore stable bonds. Methyl methacrylate, for example, is the monomer used for the manufacture of PMMA. The latter is a rigid, linear acrylic polymer. Three-dimensional, flexible acrylic polymers can be created by a process known as *crosslinking*. When different monomers are polymerized together, the process is called *copolymerization*. Each currently available foldable acrylic lens design is manufactured from a different copolymer acrylic, with different refractive index; glass transition temperature (above this temperature the polymer exhibits flexible properties and below it remains rigid); water content; mechanical properties; etc. Hydrophobic acrylic lenses have a very low water content, lower than 1%. Most of the currently available hydrophilic acrylic lenses are manufactured from copolymer acrylics with a water content ranging from 18% to 38%. One exception is represented by a lens manufactured in Brazil (Acqua, Mediphacos, Belo Horizonte, MG, Brazil), which has a water content of 73.5%. This expandable lens is inserted in a dry state and attains its final dimensions within the capsular bag after hydration and expansion. The Collamer material (STAAR Surgical, Monrovia, Calif) can also be included in the category of hydrophilic acrylic materials. This is composed of a proprietary copolymer of a hydrophilic acrylic material and porcine collagen, with a water content of 34%.

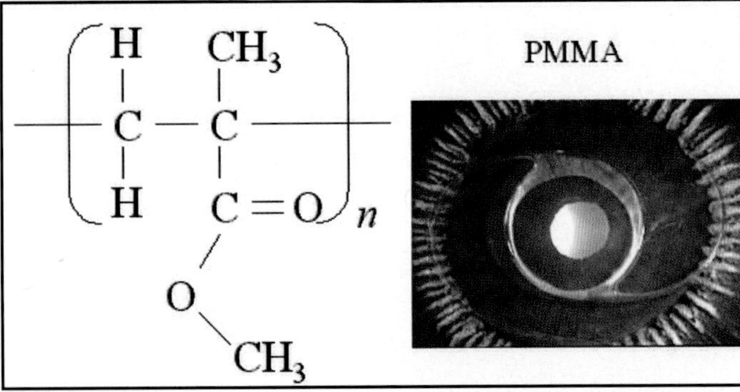

Figure 32-1. Chemical structure of polymethyl methacrylate (PMMA), and gross photograph from a human eye obtained postmortem implanted with a one-piece PMMA lens, with blue-colored PMMA haptics (posterior or Miyake-Apple view).

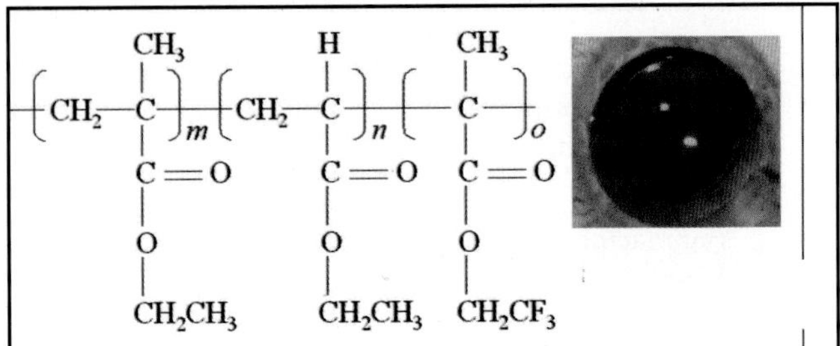

Figure 32-3. Chemical structure of the Sensar material (ethyl acrylate/ethyl methacrylate), and clinical photograph of a patient implanted with a Sensar lens. (Courtesy of Advanced Medical Optics).

Polymerization is the process by which the repeating units forming a polymer (the monomers) are linked by covalent and therefore stable bonds. Three-dimensional, flexible acrylic polymers can be created by a process known as *crosslinking*. When different monomers are polymerized together, the process is called *copolymerization*.

Silicones are known chemically as polysiloxanes based on their silicon-oxygen molecular backbone, which confers mechanical flexibility to the materials. Pendant to the silicone backbone are organic groups, which determine mechanical and optical properties. The first silicone material used in the manufacture of IOLs was polydimethyl siloxane, which has a refractive index of 1.41. Polydimethyl diphenyl siloxane is a later generation silicone IOL material that has a higher refractive index than polydimethyl siloxane (1.46) (Figure 32-5). As these polymers exhibit elastic behavior, they are also called *elastomers*. While foldable acrylics display glass transition temperatures at around room temperature, the glass transition temperature of silicones can be significantly below room temperature. Another differentiating property between foldable acrylics and silicones is the refractive index, which is higher in the first group (1.47 or greater) so acrylic lenses are thinner than silicone lenses for the same refractive power.

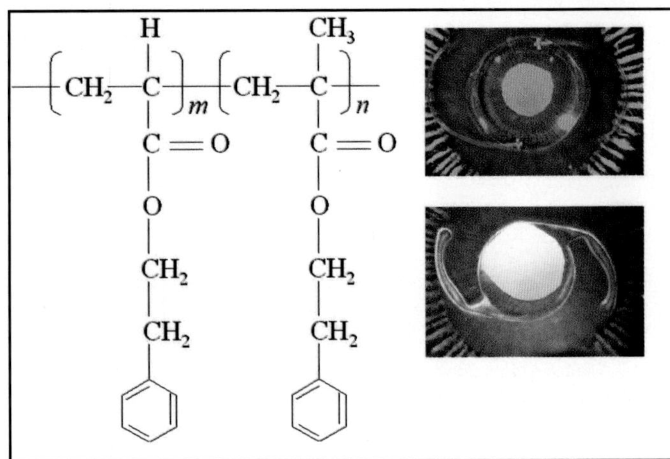

Figure 32-2. Chemical structure of the AcrySof material (phenylethyl acrylate/phenylethyl methacrylate), and gross photographs from human eyes obtained postmortem implanted with a three-piece (top), and with a one-piece (bottom) AcrySof lens.

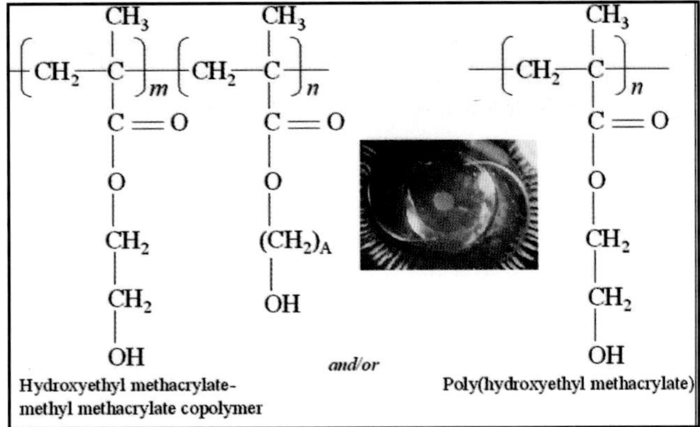

Figure 32-4. Chemical structure of a generic hydrophilic acrylic/hydrogel copolymer and gross photograph from a human eye obtained postmortem implanted with a MemoryLens. The material of the optic of this particular lens design is in fact composed of hydroxyethyl methacrylate/methyl methacrylate.

Another differentiating property between foldable acrylics and silicones is the refractive index, which is higher in the first group (1.47 or greater) so acrylic lenses are thinner than silicone lenses for the same refractive power.

Other important elements of the IOL optic component are represented by the ultraviolet-absorbing compounds (chromophores). These are incorporated to the IOL optic in order to protect the retina from ultraviolet radiation in the 300- to 400-nanometer (nm) range, a protection normally provided by the crystalline lens. Two classes of ultraviolet-absorbing chro-

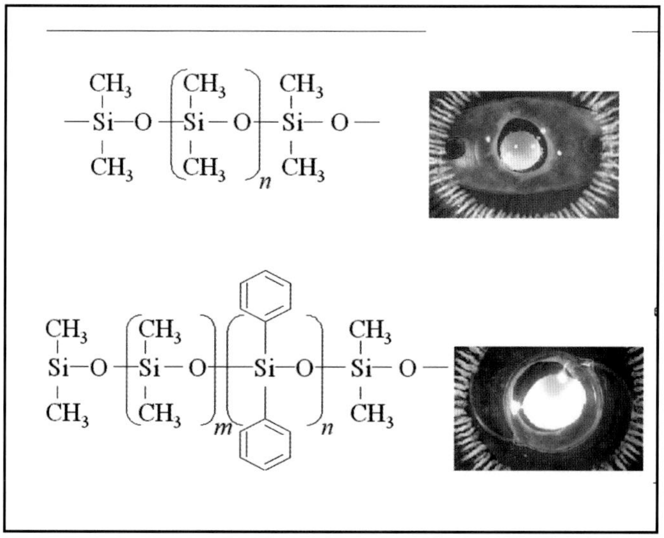

Figure 32-5. Chemical structures of two silicone elastomers used in the manufacture of IOLs, polydimethyl siloxane and polydimethyl diphenyl siloxane, and gross photographs from human eyes obtained postmortem implanted with a one-piece silicone lens with large fixation holes (STAAR Surgical, Monrovia, Calif, top), and with a 3-piece silicone optic-PMMA haptic lens (SI-40 NB, AMO; bottom).

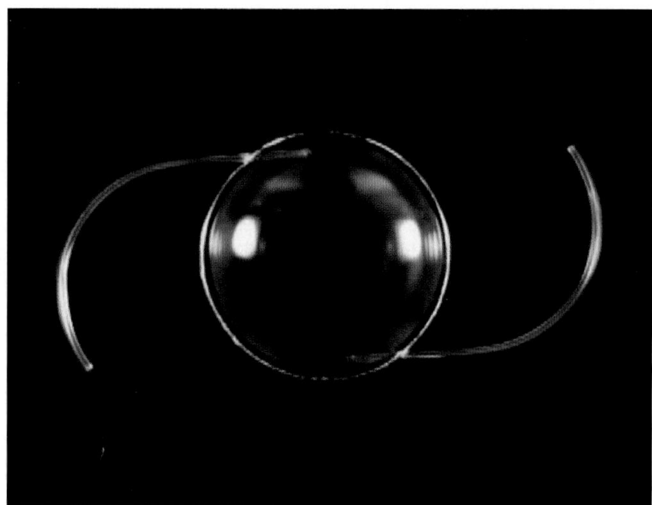

Figure 32-7. Gross photograph showing the design of the Calhoun LAL.

mophores are used in general for the manufacture of pseudophakic IOLs, namely benzotriazole and benzophenone (Figure 32-6).

"Customized" Intraocular Lenses for Cataract Surgery

Light Adjustable Lens

Calhoun Vision (Pasadena, Calif) is developing a three-piece silicone lens with photosensitive silicone subunits that move within the lens upon fine tuning with a low intensity beam of near-ultraviolet light (the Calhoun Light Adjustable Lens [LAL]).[10,11] The refractive power of the lens can be adjusted noninvasively after implantation to give the patient a definitive

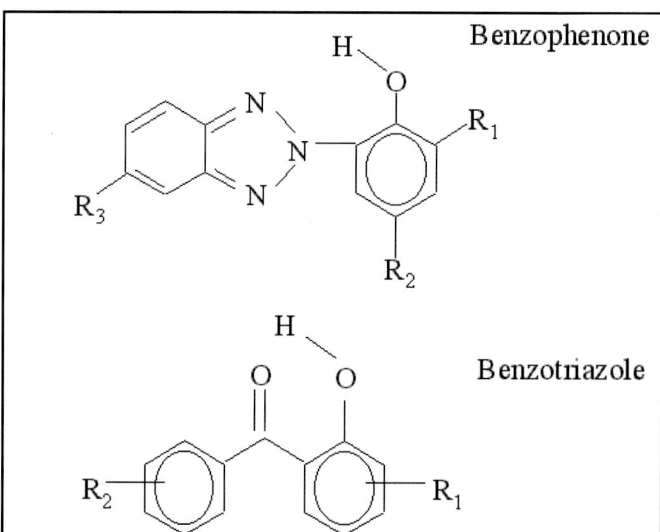

Figure 32-6. Chemical structures of two classes of ultraviolet-absorbing chromophores used in the manufacture of IOL optics.

refraction. This new technology is a potential way to correct an important postoperative complication associated with IOL implantation. Indeed, according to the American and European Societies of Cataract and Refractive Surgeons (ASCRS/ESCRS) survey on IOL explantation conducted by Nick Mamalis, MD, in the last 4 years, incorrect lens power was the most important reason for explantation of modern foldable IOLs.[12]

In the last 4 years, incorrect lens power was the most important reason for explantation of modern foldable IOLs.[12]

The Calhoun LAL is a foldable three-piece lens; the diameter of the biconvex optic is 6 mm and the overall diameter of the lens is 13 mm (Figure 32-7). The optic component is manufactured from a silicone material, polydimethyl siloxane with a refractive index of 1.43. The optic rim of this lens has square truncated edges. The haptics are manufactured from PMMA. The haptic design is a modified C, with an angulation of 10 degrees. The optic lens material has an incorporated ultraviolet absorber to protect the retina from radiation in the 300- to 400-nm range (benzotriazole).

According to Robert K. Maloney, MD, who is working with the prototype of the Calhoun LAL developed by Daniel Schwartz, MD, when the eye is healed 2 to 4 weeks after implantation, the refraction is measured and a low intensity beam of light is used to correct any residual error. The mechanism for dioptric change is akin to holography.

The application of the appropriate wavelength of light onto the central optical portion of the Calhoun LAL polymerizes the macromer in the exposed region, thereby producing a difference in the chemical potential between the irradiated and nonirradiated regions. To re-establish thermodynamic equilibrium, unreacted macromer and photoinitiator diffuses into the irradiated region. As a consequence of the diffusion process and the material properties of the host silicone matrix, the Calhoun LAL will swell, producing a concomitant decrease in the radius of curvature of the lens. This process may be repeated if further refractive change in the Calhoun LAL is desired or an irradiation of the entire lens may be applied, consuming the remaining, undif-

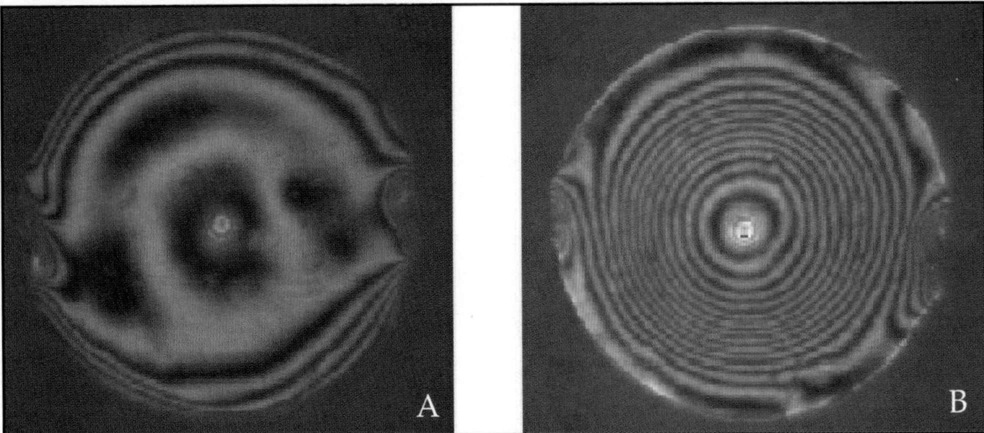

Figure 32-8. (A) Fizeau interference fringes of a Calhoun LAL immersed in water at 35°C before irradiation at best focus (double pass). The fringes present on the periphery of the Calhoun LAL are due to spherical aberration. (B) Fizeau interference fringes of the same lens 24 hours postirradiation. (Courtesy of Calhoun Vision.)

fused, unreacted macromer and photoinitiator. This action has the effect of "locking" in the refractive power of the Calhoun LAL. It should be noted that it is possible to induce a myopic change by irradiating the edges of the Calhoun LAL to effectively drive macromer and photoinitiator out of the central region of the lens, thereby increasing the radius of curvature of the lens and decreasing its power. Astigmatism is treated by using a band-shaped pattern of irradiation across the center of the lens, orienting the light beam along the astigmatic axis. After verification of the new refraction, the surgeon "locks in" the power by irradiating the entire lens optic, a procedure that does not affect the final lens power obtained. This step is very important, as some remaining photosensitive unpolymerized macromers may polymerize in ambient light. Indeed, during the interval between lens implantation and light adjustment, patients need to wear sunglasses with ultraviolet absorbers while performing outside activities. This is necessary in order to avoid unwanted, noncontrolled polymerization of the silicone macromers with unpredictable results regarding change in the IOL power. However, at least 1 hour of exposure to ambient light would be necessary for any significant polymerization to occur.

An in vitro example of the treatment process is shown in Figure 32-8. To simulate the human eye environment, a Calhoun LAL was fixtured in a water cell maintained at 35°C. The Calhoun LAL was placed one focal length away from the focus of a 4 inch (in) transmission sphere fitted to a Fizeau interferometer. Figure 32-8A displays the interference fringes of the Calhoun LAL at its best focus position prior to irradiation. The periphery of the Calhoun LAL was irradiated, causing diffusion of macromer and photoinitiator from the central portion of the lens out to the edges. Figure 32-8B displays the interference fringes 24 hours postirradiation at the original best focus position. The most striking feature is the addition of approximately 12 (in double pass) fringes of defocus (or wavefront curvature) added to the lens, which corresponds to -1.5 diopter (D) of myopic correction. After the Calhoun LAL is irradiated, it is imperative that the lens maintains a resolution efficiency that is acceptable to the patient.

The design of the device for light application is similar to a slit lamp coupled to a computer system. The preparation of the patient for the procedure involves pupil dilation and topical anesthesia. A television monitor helps to control the focus of the system, directed at the optic-haptic junctions of the lens, and a reticule target with a diameter of 6 mm is aligned with the edge of the optic component of the lens. After entering the base power of the Calhoun LAL and the correction needed, the computer selects the appropriate mask in order to deliver the light beam at the center or the periphery of the lens, as well as the intensity of the light beam and duration of the treatment. The light application for postoperative adjustment of IOL power is of short duration. For example, if a correction of -2 D for a Calhoun LAL with a base power of +20 D is necessary, a light beam with an intensity of 10.00 milliwatts per square centimeter (mw/cm^{2}) is applied for 120 seconds. The time necessary for the treatment varies slightly according to the correction necessary. For the lock-in of the IOL power, a light beam with a higher intensity is used to irradiate the whole lens, and the treatment in general lasts approximately 2 minutes.

> The light application for postoperative adjustment of IOL power is of short duration. For example, if a correction of -2 D for a Calhoun LAL with a base power of +20 D is necessary, a light beam with an intensity of 10 mw/cm^2 is applied for 120 seconds.

The biocompatibility of the lens and the reproducibility of the results after light adjustment have been evaluated in animal models. Maloney et al implanted the Calhoun LAL in rabbits after phacoemulsification.[10] The power of the lenses was then adjusted at 2 weeks postoperatively, followed by explantation. The authors reported that corrections of +2.68 ± 0.26 D, +0.98 ± 0.16 D, +0.71 ± 0.05 D, -0.64 ± 0.21 D, and -1.02 ± 0.09 D were achieved in vivo. They did not note any evidence of keratitis or chronic inflammatory reaction in the anterior chamber.

Mamalis et al also evaluated the biocompatibility of the Calhoun LAL as well as the change in power following light irradiation in a rabbit model (Figures 32-9 and 32-10).[11] In this study, the lenses underwent power adjustment using low-level light exposure, but also maximum dosage exposure was performed to assess the safety of the light exposure. The Calhoun LALs were then evaluated with optical bench testing of the power adjustment, and the rabbit eyes underwent complete histopathologic

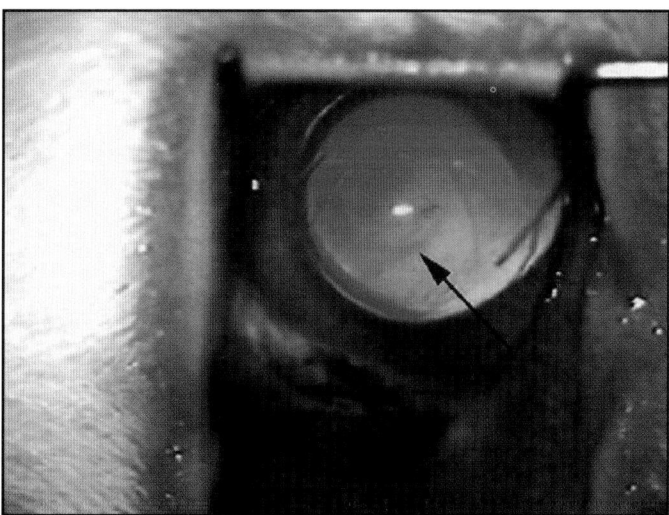

Figure 32-9. Slit lamp photograph of a rabbit eye immediately after treatment of the Calhoun LAL in its center to create a hyperopic change. The arrow shows the swelling of the irradiated area of the lens optic.

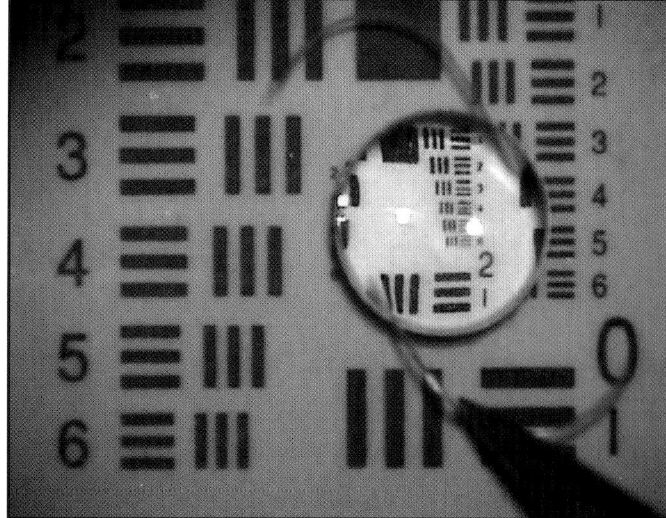

Figure 32-10. After explantation, the same lens shown in Figure 32-9 presents excellent image clarity on an Air Force test grid target.

evaluation. The authors found that hyperopic, myopic, and astigmatic adjustments of the Calhoun LALs were possible in this rabbit model. The low-level light used was well tolerated with no superficial corneal changes on slit lamp examinations and no untoward effects on the anterior and posterior segments of the globe on histopathology. According to Shiao Chang, PhD at Calhoun Vision, the neodymium:yttrium-aluminum-garnet (Nd:YAG) laser compatibility with the Calhoun LAL was evaluated. Results showed that the Calhoun LAL performs similarly to commercially available silicone lenses. The saline surrounding the Calhoun LAL during the Nd:YAG irradiation showed no leached species and no cytotoxicity.

This foldable lens will be available in different dioptric powers and can be implanted through a small incision like a standard three-piece silicone IOL. The initial clinical application will be a pseudophakic lens for use after cataract surgery, but the manufacturer believes the technology can be applied to any type of IOL, including multifocal, accommodative, injectable, or phakic lenses. Use in conjunction with wavefront scan will allow full customization of the lens. Initial human trials are expected to begin in early 2004. US clinical trials will follow only with Food and Drug Administration (FDA) approval. It is anticipated that the lens will be available commercially in Europe in late 2004 and in the United States by 2008.

Tecnis Z-9000

A recent technology invented by N.E. Sverker Norrby, PhD, at Pfizer Inc (New York, NY), named the Z-Sharp Optic Technology, is being implemented on the CeeOn Edge IOL, model 911 platform (Tecnis Z-9000 IOL).[13] The principle of this technology, which has FDA approval, is based on the fact that spherical aberrations of the human eye vary with age (Figure 32-11). The cornea has positive spherical aberration, which means peripheral rays are focused in front of the retina. This positive spherical aberration of the cornea remains throughout life. In young people, the crystalline lens corrects this defect. It exhibits many aberrations, but it is dominated by negative spherical aberration. The crystalline lens undergoes changes with age, which cause a shift of spherical aberration toward positive. The negative spherical aberration of the young lens gradually approaches zero at about age 40 and then continues to become increasingly positive as aging continues. This adds to the positive spherical aberration of the cornea, with possible increased sensitivity to glare and also reduced appreciation of contrast. Between the ages of 20 and 70 years, total aberrations of the eye increase more than 300%.[13-15]

> Editor's note:
> Although the correction of higher-order aberrations is considered in the design and/or modification of each of these two "customized" silicone-based IOLs, only the former (the Calhoun LAL) is truly "wavefront customizable." The latter (Tecnis Z-9000) is "wavefront optimized," which means it's designed to be population specific rather than patient specific. Although both can correct spherical aberration, the magnitude and sign of this term differs for each patient so that one size does not fit all.
> R. Krueger, MD, MSE

Currently available IOLs also have a positive spherical aberration. According to Sverker Norrby, when currently available IOLs are tested in laser scanning set-ups, they turn out to be almost perfect spherical lenses with positive spherical aberration, the other aberrations being close to zero. Thus, in pseudophakic patients, the spherical aberration of the eyes is increased in relation to young and old phakic eyes. Application of the Z-Sharp Optic Technology would modify the surface of IOLs to produce a negative spherical aberration that would compensate the positive aberration of the cornea.

The Tecnis lens has an aspheric surface, more specifically a modified prolate profile. It means that the lens has less refractive power at the periphery (contrary to spheric lenses, which have more refractive power at the periphery), therefore all the rays are coming to the same point, leading to a higher contrast sensitivity. The Z-Sharp Optic Technology could actually be applied to any lens biomaterial, as it is based on the modified prolate profile of the lens optic.

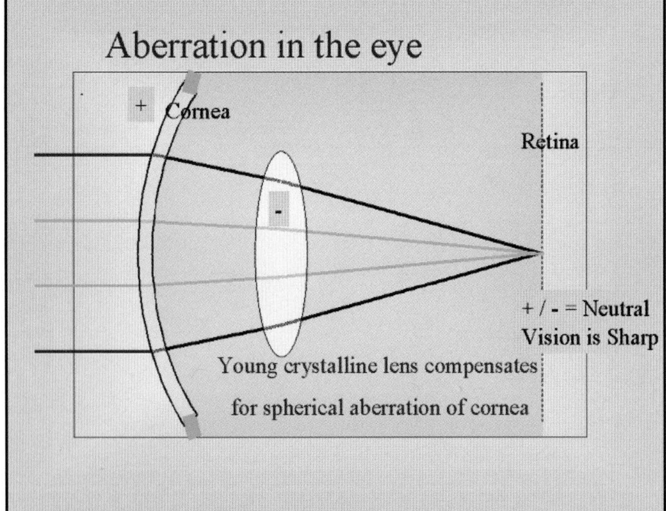

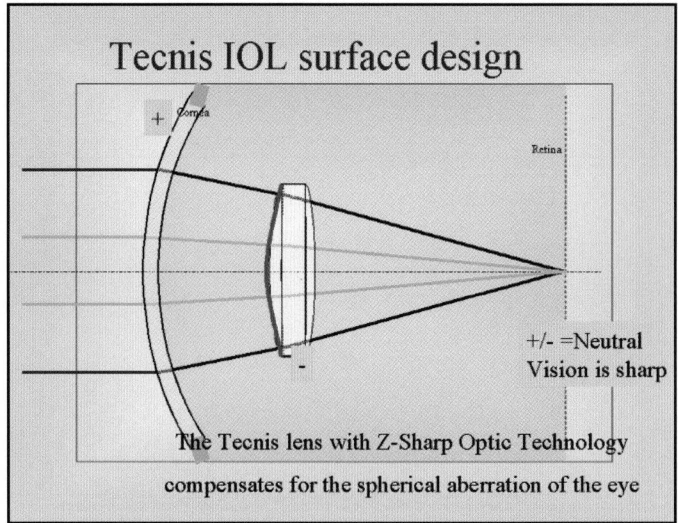

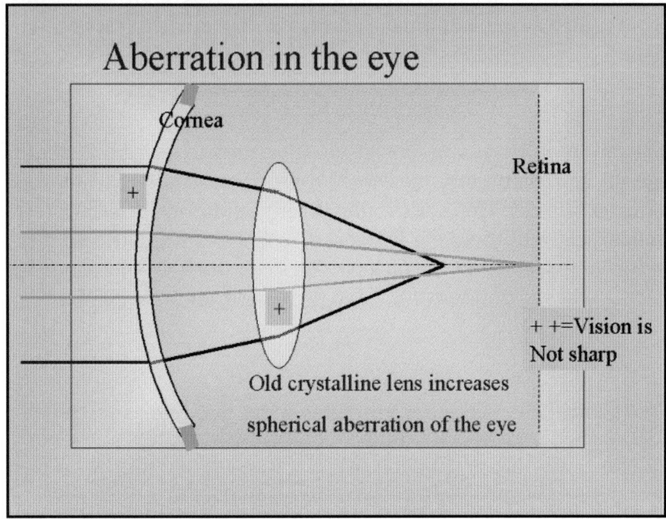

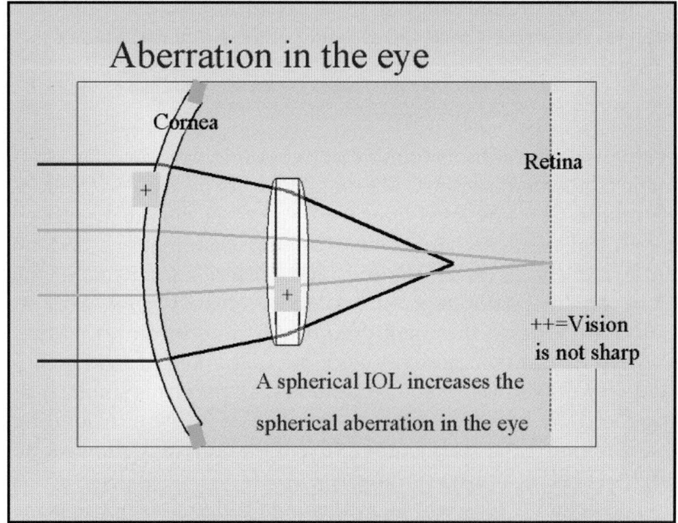

Figure 32-11. Schematic drawings illustrating the aberration observed in phakic eyes (from young and old patients) and pseudophakic eyes (implanted with the Tecnis and with other currently available lenses). (Courtesy of Pfizer.)

> The negative spherical aberration of the young lens gradually approaches zero at about age 40 and then continues to become increasingly positive as aging continues.

The Tecnis Z-9000 is a typical example of an IOL developed with the help of wavefront technology,[16] and details are provided in Chapter 34. Terwee et al measured the wavefront aberrations of the Tecnis Z-9000 and other commercially available lenses in a model eye with a Shack-Hartmann wavefront sensor.[17] The model eye also had a cornea that exhibited the spherical aberration of an average human cornea. The eye with the Tecnis IOL showed less aberrations than the eyes with other IOLs.

Initial clinical results with these lenses are encouraging, with significant improvement in contrast sensitivity under low luminance and high spatial frequencies when compared with fellow eyes implanted with conventional IOLs. In a randomized study including 40 patients, Neuhann and Mester compared the quality of vision after phacoemulsification and implantation of the CeeOn Edge model 911A in one eye and the Tecnis Z-9000 in the contralateral eye.[18] Control examinations at 1 to 2, 30 to 60, and 90 to 120 days postoperatively included contrast sensitivity, visual acuity assessment under different conditions, and wavefront analysis. The authors found that spherical aberration was markedly reduced in eyes implanted with the Tecnis Z-9000 IOL. They also found that low-contrast visual acuity and mesopic contrast sensitivity were significantly better in eyes implanted with this lens.

Corydon et al also compared the contrast sensitivity of the same lens designs in a prospective randomized study including 10 patients.[19] At 30 to 60 days postoperatively, visual acuity for near and far as well as contrast sensitivity were measured, the latter with low-contrast charts and the Contrast Sensitivity Tester model 1800 (Vision Sciences Research Co, San Ramon, Calif) for near and far. The authors found that the pupil size had an influence on the results, with patients having small pupils showing no difference between the two lenses, while patients with larger pupils had a better contrast sensitivity in the eyes implanted with the Tecnis Z-9000 IOL. Pupil size apparently plays an important role, and, taking into account the modified prolate profile of the Tecnis, no significant advantages would be expected when the pupil size is less than 3 mm.

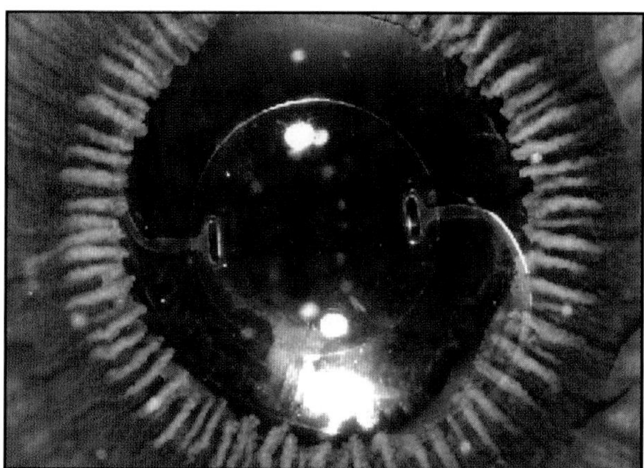

Figure 32-12. Gross photograph showing a CeeOn Edge lens experimentally implanted in a human eye obtained postmortem, prepared according to the Miyake-Apple posterior videophotographic technique.

The design of the CeeOn Edge lens appears appropriate for incorporation of the Z-Sharp Optic Technology. The CeeOn Edge IOL model 911 is a foldable three-piece lens; the diameter of the biconvex optic is 6 mm and the overall diameter of the lens is 12 mm (Figure 32-12). The CeeOn Edge is also available with an overall diameter of 13 mm, as will the Tecnis Z-9001 lens. The optic component is manufactured from a third-generation silicone material, polydimethyl diphenyl siloxane, developed and manufactured by Pfizer with a high refractive index (1.46). The optic rim has square truncated edges. The haptics are manufactured from polyvinylidene fluoride (PVDF). The haptic design is a cap C with a 90-degree exit and an angulation of 6 degrees. The lens has an incorporated ultraviolet absorber (benzotriazole) to protect the retina from radiation in the 300- to 400-nm range.

The 911 model is the first silicone IOL design with a square truncated optic edge. This has proven to provide good properties regarding posterior capsule opacification (PCO) prevention. Schauersberger et al compared the performance of the 911 and the three-piece AcrySof lens in terms of capsular bag opacification.[20] Twenty-five eyes operated on by the same surgeon were included in each lens group. After a follow up of 3 years, there was no statistically significant difference between both groups of lenses regarding PCO.

Although this lens design has square optic edges, optical phenomena are generally not associated with this lens. Indeed, these phenomena depend, among other factors, on the refractive index of the lens material. The refractive index of this lens is relatively low compared to hydrophobic acrylic lenses, which have a markedly higher refractive index. Also, opacification of the anterior capsule, which was demonstrated to be highly associated with silicone lenses, will help in the prevention of any edge-glare phenomena if the capsulorrhexis is smaller than the IOL optic diameter.

The haptic material, PVDF, was found to present good rigidity and retentive memory. Izak et al compared the shape recovery ratios of silicone lenses having different haptic materials (PMMA, polypropylene, polyimide, and PVDF) after compression (Figure 32-13).[21] Silicone-PMMA, silicone-polyimide, and silicone-PVDF lenses presented similar loop memories, which were significantly better than with silicone-polypropylene lenses

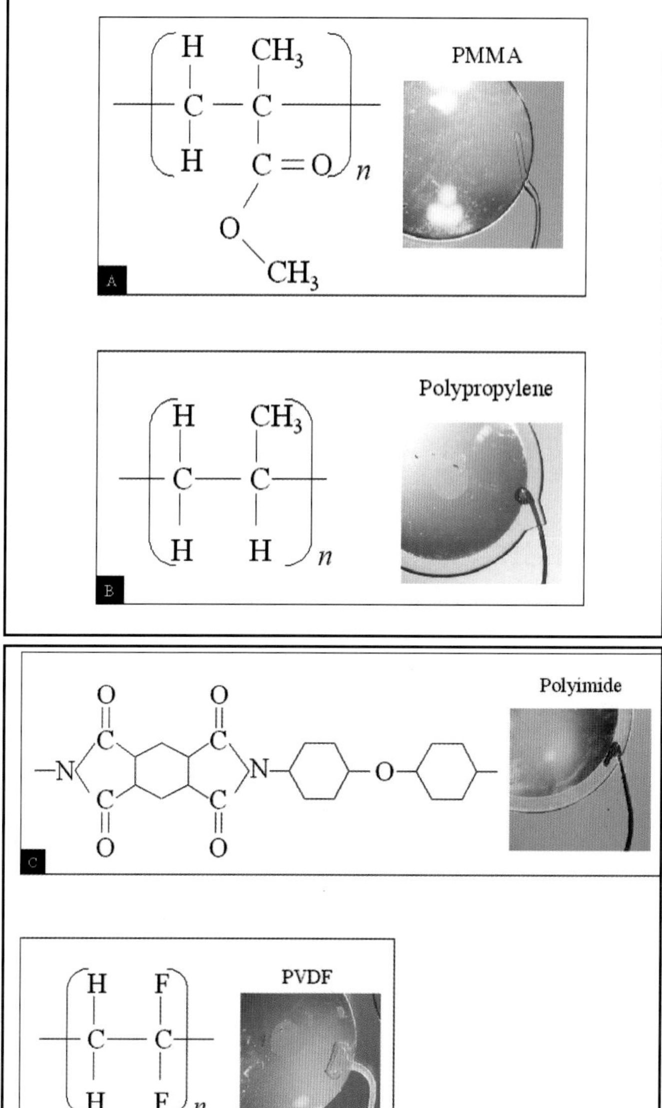

Figure 32-13. Chemical structures of the four haptic materials currently used in the manufacture of IOLs and gross photographs showing details of the optic-haptic junctions of four different three-piece silicone lenses. (A) CeeOn (912) silicone optic-PMMA haptic lens. (B) PhacoFlex II SI30 NB (Advanced Medical Optics, Santa Ana, Calif) silicone optic-Prolene haptic lens. (C) ELASTIMIDE (STAAR Surgical, Monrovia, Calif) silicone optic-Elastimide haptic lens. (D) CeeOn Edge silicone optic-PVDF haptic lens.

($P < 0.05$). The haptic cap C design is stated to maintain the shape of the capsular bag, offering more clock hours of contact between the haptics and the capsule. These characteristics help in the prevention of lens decentration and tilt in cases of capsular bag contraction. This is very important because, qualitatively, any aberration correction is sensitive to decentration and tilt. Patients will benefit from the advanced technology of Tecnis within the normal clinical limits of lens decentration inferior to 0.40 mm and lens tilt inferior to 7 degrees.

Summary

We have briefly reviewed the biomaterials currently used for the manufacture of the optic component of IOLs and presented two examples of "customized" lenses. The refractive power of the Calhoun LAL can be noninvasively adjusted in the postoperative period, correcting the major cause of postoperative explantation of modern foldable lens designs. Implementation of wavefront aberrometry on the Calhoun LAL technology will allow full customization of the lens, with correction of different ocular aberrations. The Tecnis Z-9000 lens with the Z-Sharp Optic Technology has a modified prolate profile that produces a negative spherical aberration compensating the positive aberration of the cornea. Eyes implanted with this lens presented significantly reduced spherical aberration and better contrast sensitivity in comparison to standard IOLs. We will certainly witness, in the near future, an increasing influence of wavefront aberrometry on the manufacture of different IOL designs. This will provide patients with higher quality of vision, well beyond the quality obtained with currently available lenses.

Acknowledgments

The authors would like to thank N.E. Sverker Norrby, PhD (Pfizer) and Christian Sandstedt, PhD (Calhoun Vision) for their help in the preparation of this text.

Supported in part by a grant from Research to Prevent Blindness, Inc., New York, NY, to the Department of Ophthalmology and Visual Sciences, University of Utah.

References

1. Werner L, Apple DJ, Schmidbauer JM. Ideal IOL (PMMA and foldable) for year 2002. In: Buratto L, Werner L, Zanini M, Apple DJ, eds. *Phacoemulsification: Principles and Techniques.* 2nd ed. Thorofare: NJ: SLACK Incorporated; 2002;435-451.
2. Werner L, Apple DJ, Izak A, Pandey SK, Trivedi RH, Macky TA. Phakic anterior chamber intraocular lenses. In: Werner L, Apple DJ, eds. *Complications of Aphakic and Refractive Intraocular Lenses. International Ophthalmology Clinics.* Philadelphia: Lippincott Williams & Wilkins; 2001:133-152.
3. Werner L, Apple DJ, Pandey SK, Trivedi RH, Izak A, Macky TA. Phakic posterior chamber intraocular lenses. In: Werner L, Apple DJ, eds. *Complications of Aphakic and Refractive Intraocular Lenses. International Ophthalmology Clinics.* Philadelphia: Lippincott Williams & Wilkins; 2001:153-174.
4. Applegate RA, Thibos LN, Hilmantel G. Optics aberroscopy and super vision. *J Cataract Refract Surg.* 2001;27:1093-1107.
5. Christ FR, Buchen SY, Deacon J, et al. Biomaterials used for intraocular lenses. In: Wise DL, Trantolo DJ, Altobelli DE, et al, eds. *Encyclopedic Handbook of Biomaterials and Bioengineering. Part B: applications.* Vol 2. New York: Marcel Dekker Inc; 1995:1261-1313.
6. Glazer LC, Shen TT, Azar DT, Murphy E. Intraocular lens material. In: Azar DT, ed. *Intraocular Lenses in Cataract and Refractive Surgery.* Philadelphia: WB Saunders; 2001:39-49.
7. Werner L, Legeais JM. Les matériaux pour implants intraoculaires. Partie I: les implants intraoculaires en polyméthylméthacrylate et modifications de surface. *J Fr Ophthalmol.* 1998;21:515-524.
8. Werner L, Legeais JM. Les matériaux pour implants intraoculaires. Partie II: les implants intraoculaires souples, en silicone. *J Fr Ophthalmol.* 1999;22:492-501.
9. Legeais JM, Werner L, Werner LP, Renard G. Les matériaux pour implants intraoculaires. Partie III: les implants intraoculaires acryliques souples. *J Fr Ophthalmol.* 2001;24:309-318.
10. Maloney RK, Jethmalani J, Sandstedt C, et al. Intraocular lens with light-adjustable power. Paper presented at: the ASCRS Symposium on Cataract, IOL, and Refractive Surgery; June 2002; Philadelphia, Pa.
11. Mamalis N, Chang SH, Sandstedt CA, et al. Evaluation of a light-adjustable intraocular lens. Paper presented at: the ASCRS Symposium on Cataract, IOL, and Refractive Surgery; June 2002; Philadelphia, Pa.
12. Mamalis N, Spencer TS. Complications of foldable intraocular lenses requiring explantation or secondary intervention—2000 survey update. *J Cataract Refract Surg.* 2001;7:1310-1317.
13. Norrby S. Conception of Z-sharp optic technology. Paper presented at: the ASCRS Symposium on Cataract, IOL, and Refractive Surgery; June 2002; Philadelphia, Pa.
14. Artal P, Berrio E, Guirao A, Piers P. Contribution of the cornea and internal surfaces to the change of ocular aberrations with age. *J Opt Soc Am A Opt Image Sci Vis.* 2002;19:137-143.
15. Bellucci R. Optical aberrations and intraocular lens design. In: Buratto L, Werner L, Zanini M, Apple DJ, eds. *Phacoemulsification: Principles and Techniques.* 2nd ed. Thorofare, NJ: SLACK Incorporated; 2002:454-455.
16. Holladay JT, Piers P, Koranyi G, et al. IOL design to reduce the ocular wavefront aberration in aphakic eyes. Paper presented at: the ASCRS Symposium on Cataract, IOL, and Refractive Surgery; June 2002; Philadelphia, Pa.
17. Terwee T, Barkhof J, Weeber H, Piers P. Influence of the Tecnis model Z-9000 and other IOLs on wavefront aberrations. Paper presented at: the ASCRS Symposium on Cataract, IOL, and Refractive Surgery; June 2002; Philadelphia, Pa.
18. Neuhann T, Mester U. Improvement of optical and visual quality by an intraocular lens with a correcting optical design. Paper presented at: the ASCRS Symposium on Cataract, IOL, and Refractive Surgery; June 2002; Philadelphia, Pa.
19. Corydon L, Dam-Johansen M, Winther-Nielsen A, Lundkvist T. Contrast sensitivity with the Pharmacia Tecnis Z-9000 IOL. Paper presented at: the ASCRS Symposium on Cataract, IOL, and Refractive Surgery; June 2002; Philadelphia, Pa.
20. Schauersberger J, Amon M, Kruger A, et al. Comparison of the biocompatibility of 2 foldable intraocular lenses with sharp optic edges. *J Cataract Refract Surg.* 2001;27:1579-1585.
21. Izak AM, Werner L, Apple DJ, Macky TA, Trivedi RH, Pandey SK. Loop memory of different haptic materials used in the manufacture of posterior chamber intraocular lenses. *J Cataract Refract Surg.* 2002; 28:1229-1235.

Chapter 33

Feasibility of Wavefront Customized Contact Lenses

Ian Cox, PhD and Michele Lagana, OD

The presence of higher-order aberrations in the eye has been known for several decades.[1-3] Primarily identified as spherical aberration, the significant role of nonrotationally symmetrical aberrations, such as coma, has been studied and identified more recently.[4] Current measurements using Shack-Hartmann–based wavefront sensors have opened the door to identifying the magnitude and form of higher-order wavefront aberrations in large, preoperative, physiological populations.[5]

Early descriptions of spherical aberration as the predominant monochromatic aberration of the human eye were particularly appealing to contact lens manufacturers. As early as the 1960s, contact lenses themselves were identified as having inherent spherical aberration due to their steep curvatures and relatively constant alignment with the visual axis of the eye.[6] Many manufacturers believed that it was a simple matter of using their lathing technologies to form an aspheric correcting surface on one or both sides of the contact lens to not only correct the optical aberrations of the lens itself, but also to enhance the retinal image of the eye—the first attempts at super vision.[7] Indeed, a number of manufacturers sell products today based on this concept.

Wavefront Aberrations and the General Population

Initial inspection of the average distribution of higher-order wavefront aberrations across a typical prepresbyopic population requiring refractive correction shows a distinct deviation from zero for the spherical aberration Zernike term, while all other higher-order Zernike terms have an average close to zero—a value expected of a biological optical system attempting to optimize itself across a population (Figure 33-1). This would suggest that an appropriate aspheric correcting surface would significantly reduce the wavefront aberration of the eye if it were incorporated into a contact lens. However, as Figure 33-2 shows, there is a wide range of spherical aberration values across the patient population that are not related to another variable, such as degree of ametropia. To realistically correct more than 38% of the population, spherical aberration would have to be introduced as an additional parameter in the contact lens rather than an average level of correction added into every lens. Perhaps more importantly, spherical aberration, while significant in the hierarchy of higher-order wavefront aberration of the eye, is typically not the dominant aberration in most eyes. Third-order Zernike terms, such as coma and trefoil, are the largest magnitude higher-order wavefront aberrations found in any given eye in the general population. These aberrations must be corrected by a rotationally stable contact lens and manufactured using a process capable of creating nonrotationally symmetrical surfaces. In fact, Figure 33-3 shows the Strehl ratio for a large sample of the general ophthalmic population when corrected alternatively with sphere and cylinder only; with sphere, cylinder, and spherical aberration; and with sphere, cylinder, third-order Zernike terms, and spherical aberration. Clearly, while some patients benefit from correction of spherical aberration in addition to their myopia and astigmatism, there is a substantially larger increase in retinal image quality when the third-order Zernike terms are also corrected. Therefore, a contact lens must be designed to correct both symmetrical and nonrotationally symmetrical higher-order aberrations of the eye if a true visual benefit is to be realized across a substantial proportion of the population.

> Third-order Zernike terms, such as coma and trefoil, are the largest magnitude higher-order wavefront aberrations found in a normal eye.

> There is a substantially larger increase in retinal image quality when the third-order Zernike terms are also corrected.

Rigid Gas Permeable vs Soft Contact Lenses for Customized Correction

This leads us to the question: Which type of contact lens would be ideal for neutralizing higher-order wavefront aberrations? Rigid gas permeable (RGP) lenses have been utilized for years as a method for correcting eyes with pathology or postsurgical wavefront aberration, where standard spherocylindrical spectacle lenses do not provide adequate visual acuity. However, it is the rigid nature of the lens itself, rather than innovative optics, that provides the wavefront aberration correction of these lenses. Vision of eyes with significantly distorted corneas can be improved with RGP lenses because the anterior surface of the contact lens forms the new refracting surface, with the tear film

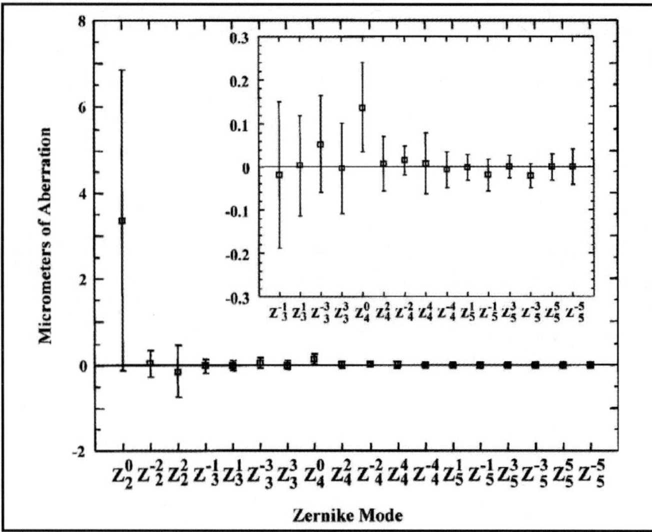

Figure 33-1. Distribution of wavefront aberrations in the patient population. Mean values of all Zernike modes in the population across a 5.7 millimeter (mm) pupil. The error bars represent plus and minus one standard deviation from the mean value. The variability of the higher-order modes is shown in the inset of the figure, which excludes all second-order modes (Z^{-2}_2, Z^0_2, and Z^2_2) and expands the ordinate. (Reprinted with permission from Porter J, Guirao A, Cox IG, Williams DR. Monochromatic aberrations of the human eye in a large population. *Journal of the Optical Society of America.* 2001;18[8]:1793-1803.)

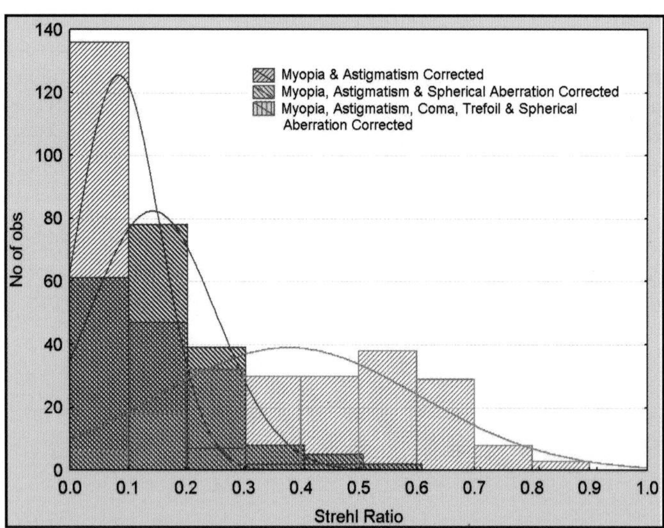

Figure 33-3. Distribution of Strehl ratios in a large physiological preoperative patient population following correction of sphere and cylinder only (blue); sphere, cylinder, and spherical aberration (red); and sphere, cylinder, coma, trefoil, and spherical aberration (green).

filling in the difference between the irregular cornea and the regular back surface of the lens. Unfortunately, the physical nature of RGP lenses—and the way they must be fit to ensure tear exchange and mobility on the eye—renders them less desirable as a method for correcting wavefront aberrations of the eye through complex optical surfaces. RGP lenses are designed to be very mobile on the eye, moving several millimeters with each blink and finding a position of rest with up to 1 millimeter (mm) difference relative to the optical axis of the eye following each blink.[8] Hence, stabilizing

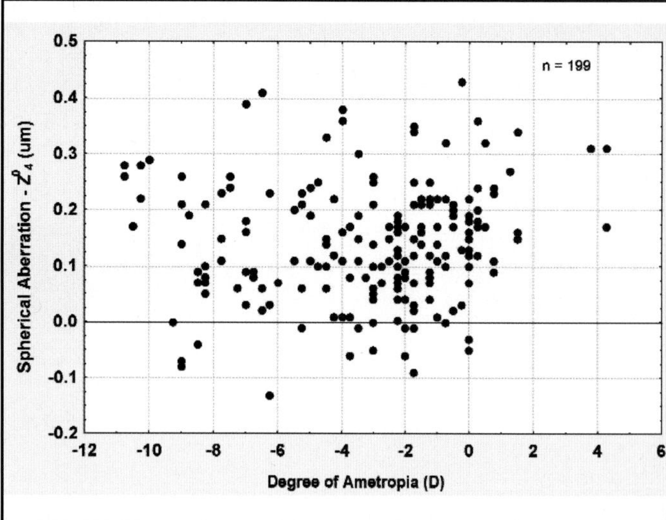

Figure 33-2. Distribution of spherical aberration (Zernike term Z^0_4) for a 5.70 mm pupil in a large physiological preoperative patient population.

an RGP lens, such that it repeatedly returns to the same horizontal and vertical location relative to the visual axis without rotating around this axis and maintaining physiologically desirable tear exchange behind the lens, is very difficult.

The physical nature of RGP lenses, and the way they must be fit to ensure tear exchange and mobility on the eye, renders them less desirable as a method for correcting wavefront aberrations of the eye through complex optical surfaces.

Soft lenses are held in position relative to the cornea by an entirely different set of forces. These lenses are always fit with a sagittal depth greater than the cornea/sclera beneath the lens. In this way, the lens is squeezed onto the cornea with the first blink and deformed to take the shape of the tissue beneath. The deformation that the lens undergoes during this process generates radial stress in the lens, and it is these forces combined with gravity that center the lens on the cornea at the position of equilibrium. When the lid blinks, the soft lens is moved away from this position of equilibrium in a vertical direction through interaction with the eyelid. As the lens is moved farther away from the center of the cornea, the radial stress within the lens increases to the point where it is greater in magnitude than the eyelid interaction. This causes the lens to reverse direction and return to its position of equilibrium on the corneal surface. Because there is only one optimal position on the corneal/scleral surface that provides the least radial stress, clinicians find that well-fitted soft lenses relocate to the same position on the cornea within 0.10 to 0.40 mm after every blink.[9] Although the lens is not centered on the visual axis of the eye, it does relocate consistently relative to that axis after every blink. Control of rotation with soft lenses has been realized for over a decade, and the current generation of sophisticated prism-ballasted designs provide rotational stability within 5 degrees between any series of blinks (Figure 33-4). It is this ability to relocate with great precision that makes soft lenses more desirable than RGP lenses for correcting higher-order wavefront aberrations.

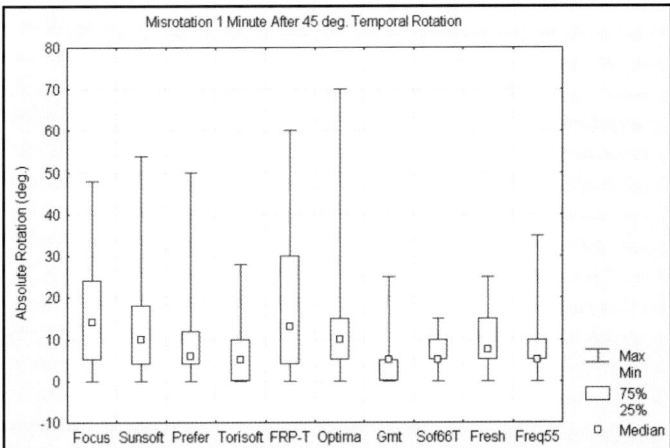

Figure 33-4. Soft toric lens rotational stability values (change from original position) based on biomicroscopic reticule measurements on 20 eyes. Lenses were misrotated 45 degrees from their position of equilibrium, and their position was remeasured 1 minute later.

> Soft lenses that fit well relocate to the same position on the cornea within 0.10 to 0.40 mm after every blink.[9]

> The current generation of sophisticated prism-ballasted designs provide rotational stability within 5 degrees between any series of blinks.

In theory, even slight changes in centration and rotation of a lens designed to correct up to fifth-order Zernike terms will significantly reduce the visual benefits experienced by that correction. Calculations to understand the tolerance:benefit ratio to decentration and rotational alignment of correcting surfaces typical of those found in the general ophthalmic population have been performed by Guirao et al.[10] They have found that Zernike terms with higher (rotational) angular orders were more sensitive to rotation of the correcting surface from the ideal position. Hence, coma is most tolerant to misrotation of the correcting surface, offering a visual benefit with misrotation up to 60 degrees; astigmatism is the next most tolerant aberration, with visual benefit with rotation up to 30 degrees; trefoil is the next most tolerant aberration, with visual benefit with rotation up to 20 degrees; and so on. Rotation from the ideal correction position that is greater than these values would provide a retinal image quality that is poorer than leaving the Zernike term uncorrected.

Decentration of the ideal correcting lens from the ideal correcting axis results in the higher-order aberrations generating a larger magnitude of lower-order aberrations. Hence, a correcting lens with coma will generate astigmatism and defocus, spherical aberration will produce coma and tilt, while defocus or astigmatism will produce only tilt (prism). In general, higher-order Zernike terms are more intolerant to decentration than lower terms. Figures 33-5A and 33-5B show the reduction in visual benefit from lenses designed to correct wavefront aberrations of a 10 eye sample population with increasing lens misrotation and decentration, respectively. Clearly the visual benefit of a lens designed to correct both lower- and higher-order wavefront aberrations is dependent on repeatable lens centration and rotation following each blink or eye movement. The values generated by Guirao's analysis suggest that a soft lens is capable of remaining within these limits.[10]

It is apparent that a contact lens designed to correct the higher-order wavefront aberrations of the eye needs to be a soft lens, prism ballasted to control rotation, with the higher order correction on the anterior surface of the lens. Because it would be extremely difficult to predict the manner in which the soft lens would distort as it is squeezed onto the cornea by the lid, the most pragmatic method would be to measure the wavefront aberrations with the contact lens in situ. Hence, a trial lens—with all the physical properties of the final custom-correcting lens but without the custom-correcting optical surface—would be placed on the eye and allowed to settle, at which time wavefront sensor measurements would be taken through the lens-eye combination. In this way, the final custom-correcting lens will compensate for any variations in the eye's higher-order wavefront aberrations introduced by the lens itself or by the tear film between the lens and the cornea.

> It is apparent that a contact lens designed to correct the higher-order wavefront aberrations of the eye needs to be a soft lens, prism ballasted to control rotation, with the higher-order correction on the anterior surface of the lens.

Alignment of the wavefront measurement is critical, and it is well known that soft lenses typically find their position of equilibrium centered on the corneal apex, which is most typically temporal and superior to the line of sight. Therefore, the line of sight as defined by the center of the pupil will be decentered relative to the geometric center of the lens. As a result, the correcting wavefront applied to the contact lens needs to compensate for the difference between these two axes. To achieve this, a marking scheme needs to be implemented on the trial lenses used for these measurements, such as that shown in Figure 33-6. These markings provide an indication of the center of the lens, as well as the rotational orientation of the lens during wavefront aberration measurements.

Customized Contact Lenses in a Disposable World

Having established the desired measurement procedure, another question that arises is how to provide a wavefront aberration correcting soft contact lens in today's paradigm of affordable frequent replacement and disposable lenses. These lenses need to be customized to an individual eye, yet the physiological needs of patients and demands of clinicians make it necessary to provide up to a year's supply of weekly to monthly replacement lenses at any one time. Figure 33-7 demonstrates one proposed model for ordering and delivery of a wavefront aberration correcting soft lens customized to an individual eye. First, the patient's eye is measured with the trial lens in place and the Zernike coefficients are uploaded to a central remote server along with other necessary data through a modem in the wavefront sensor computer. The lathing parameters necessary to cut the nonrotationally symmetrical front surface using a three-axis computer numeric controlled (CNC) lathe are calculated by the central server and downloaded into the lathe, generating the prescribed number of lenses—from a single trial lens to a 1-year supply. These lenses are then processed, packaged, sterilized,

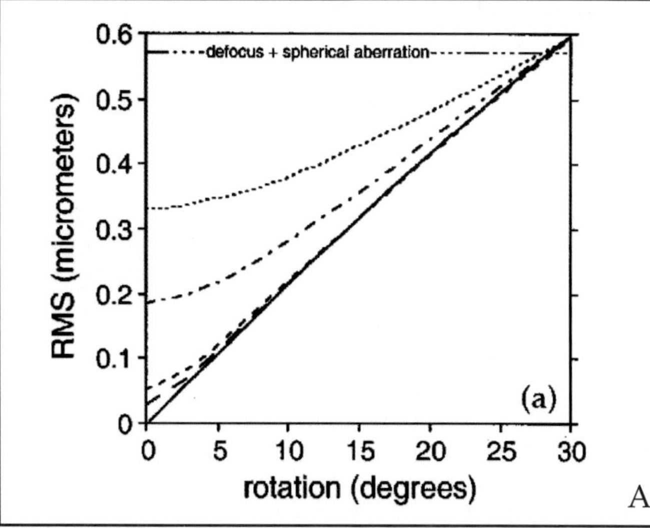

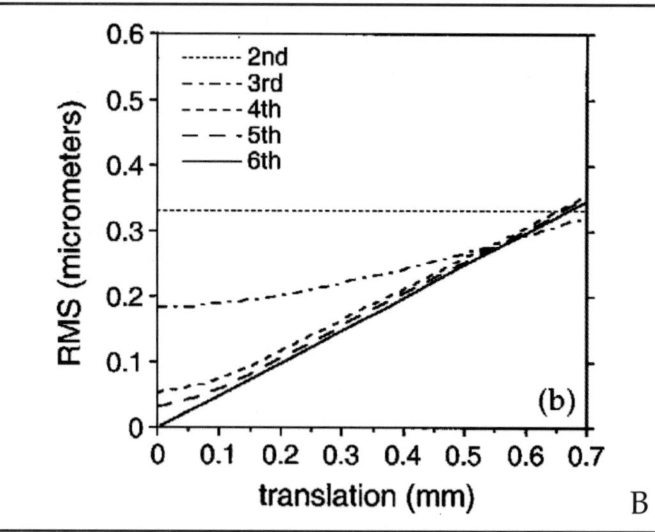

Figure 33-5. Root mean square (RMS) (mean value of a 10-eye population) of the residual wavefront aberration for a 6 mm pupil as a function of fixed rotations (A) and translations (B), when the ideal correcting surface corrects the higher-order aberrations up to second-, third-, fourth-, fifth-, and sixth-order. Results for translation are averaged across *x* and *y* axis. Also shown in Figure A, the RMS when only defocus and spherical aberration (rotationally symmetric aberrations unaffected by rotation) are corrected. (Reprinted with permission from Guirao A, Williams DR, Cox IG. Effect of rotation and translation on the expected benefit of an ideal method to correct the eye's higher order aberrations. *J Opt Soc Am.* 2001;18[5]:1003-1015.)

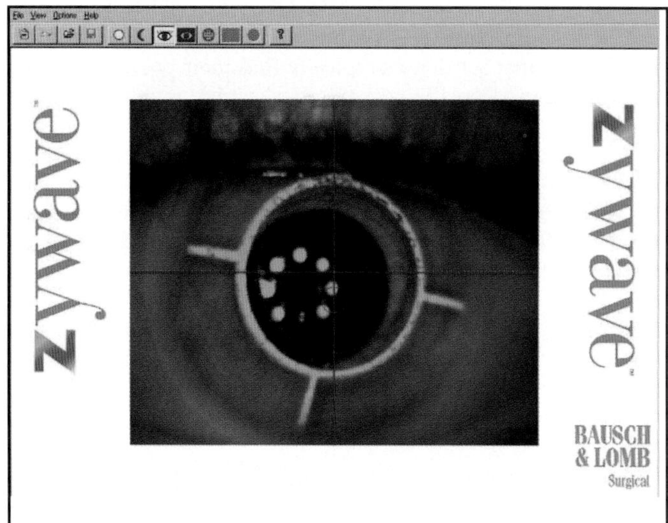

Figure 33-6. One possible marking scheme that could be used on a soft trial lens to locate the center of the lens and the rotational orientation of the lens during measurements of the wavefront aberration of the lens-eye combination.

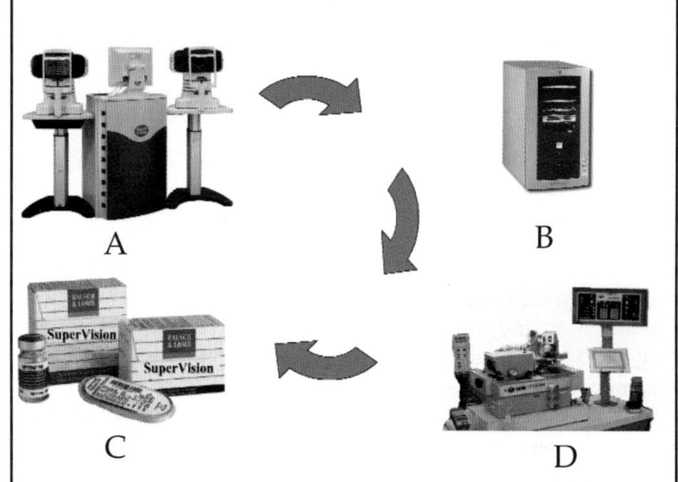

Figure 33-7. Customized contact lens order and delivery model. Wavefront aberrations are measured in the clinician's office (A), and uploaded to a remote server (B), where lathing parameters are calculated automatically and downloaded into the lathe (C). The lens is processed, packaged, sterilized, labeled, and sent back to the clinician for dispensing to the patient (D).

labeled, and returned to the prescribing clinician's office within a few days. If necessary, the process can be repeated with the new lens in situ to refine the wavefront aberration correction.

Do the currently available contact lens lathes have the capability of creating the surface profiles necessary to correct higher-order aberrations found in both the physiologic and pathologic ophthalmic population? Figure 33-8 shows a test surface created using a currently available CNC contact lens lathe for pentafoil representing a correction for fifth-order Zernike terms. This interferogram demonstrates that the CNC lathes have sufficient rotational resolution to generate the required surfaces. While this shows its capability of creating normal surfaces, there might be concern that the complex surfaces generated by pathologies, such as keratoconus, may be beyond the reach of these lathes.

Figure 33-9 shows the outcome of creating a plexiglass cylinder with a single front surface that mimics the wavefront aberration of a patient with keratoconus. Polymethylmethacrylate (PMMA) lenses with second-order Zernike correction only—and with second- through fifth-order Zernike correction—were manufactured and placed on the model eye, with the lenses centered and aligned empirically. Clearly, the majority of the higher-order wavefront aberrations were corrected by the surfaces generated by the CNC lathe manufacturing process.

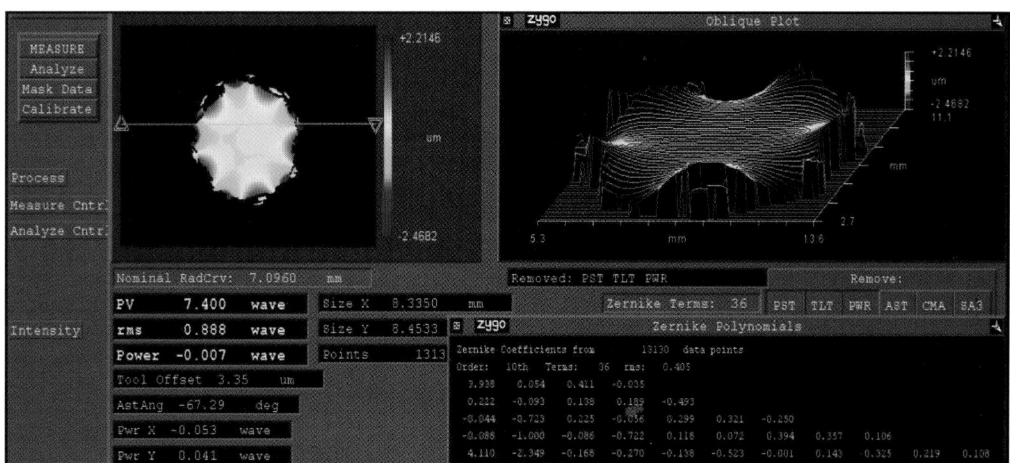

Figure 33-8. Interferogram demonstrating rotational resolution of CNC lathing technology.

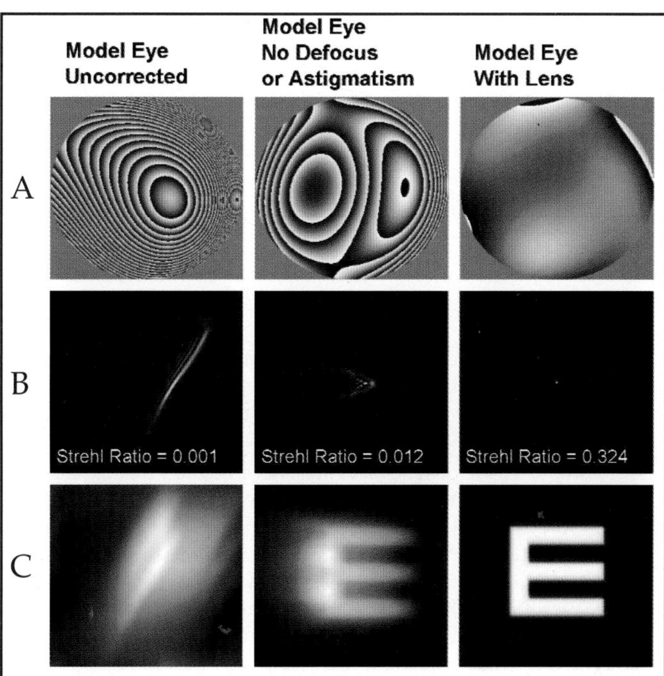

Figure 33-9. Measured wavefront aberrations (A), point spread function (PSF) (B), and image convolution (C) of a keratoconic plexiglass model eye generated by a three-axis CNC lathe. The second column represents the model eye corrected by a plexiglass contact lens generated by the same lathing technology. The third column represents the model eye corrected by a plexiglass contact lens with a front surface designed to correct up through fifth-order Zernike terms. All measurements calculated for a 5.70 mm pupil.

Experiments conducted at our research lab using this prescribing and manufacturing model have demonstrated the feasibility of a custom soft contact lens designed to correct wavefront aberrations up to and including the fifth-order Zernike terms. Measurements are made using a wavefront sensor in upstate New York, and the information is uploaded to a server in Florida where the lenses are lathed and processed. Figure 33-10 shows the results of correcting a single eye with soft, custom-correcting lenses with a variety of measured Zernike terms: second-order only (defocus and astigmatism); second-order and spherical aberration; second and third order; second-order, third-order and spherical aberration; and second- through fifth-order. Higher-order RMS, PSF, Strehl ratios, image convolutions, and high- and low-contrast logMAR visual acuities are presented. As anticipated, the results show that as the higher-order aberrations are corrected sequentially, the wavefront RMS is reduced, the Strehl ratio increases, and the low-contrast visual acuity improves up to one line with a dilated pupil. Perhaps, not surprisingly, the high-contrast visual acuity does not improve dramatically because the retinal image quality enhancement primarily affects contrast rather than resolution. These results are exciting and encouraging, although expanded studies have shown that lens alignment and rotational stability are critical to ensure the visual benefit reported in this case study.

As anticipated, the results show that as the higher-order aberrations are corrected sequentially, the wavefront RMS is reduced, the Strehl ratio increases, and the low-contrast visual acuity improves up to one line with a dilated pupil.

The concept of a customized soft contact lens designed to correct the wavefront aberration of the eye up through the fifth Zernike terms is feasible. Manufacturing technologies are available to create the complex surfaces necessary to achieve this, and a business model that provides the means of communicating the necessary individual parameters to the lab and delivering lenses within an acceptable timeframe has been demonstrated. The ability to improve wavefront aberrations, both low- and high-order Zernike terms, in a typical presurgical eye has been demonstrated, and the commensurate improvements in large pupil vision are detectable. What remains to be confirmed is the visual benefit obtained with these lenses across a wide range of physiologic and pathologic eyes, and whether this type of correction will be desirable for improved night vision to the general contact lens wearing population or confined in its appeal to that segment of the population that has significantly greater higher-order wavefront aberrations resulting from pathological or postsurgical conditions.

Definitions

CNC lathe manufacturing: A computer numeric controlled lathe that is used in the optical industry, often for manufacturing soft contact lenses.

customized soft contact lens: Soft contact lenses that correct the higher-order wavefront aberrations of an individual eye.

	Defocus	2nd Order	2nd Order & SA	2nd Ord. & Coma	2nd & 3rd Order	2nd,3rd & SA	2nd, 3rd, 4th, 5th
O/Rx Sph	1.25	0.50	0.00	0.25	0.00	-0.25	-0.25
O/Rx Cyl	-0.50	0.00	0.00	-0.50	-0.75	0.00	0.00
O/Rx Axis	155.00	0.00	0.00	60.00	96.00	0.00	0.00
Misrotation	6N	14N	4N	12N	14N	20N	18N
PPRRad	2750	2750	2750	2750	2750	2750	2750
PPRSph	0.830	0.627	0.652	0.151	0.235	0.440	0.273
PPRCyl	-0.759	-0.047	-0.456	-0.116	-0.346	-0.262	-0.117
PPRAxis	156.177	111.432	3.543	70.830	103.473	72.091	115.865
Z200	0.710	0.710	0.417	0.312	0.307	0.290	0.235
Z221	-0.437	-0.054	0.049	0.054	-0.120	0.134	-0.042
Z220	0.209	0.137	0.227	-0.218	-0.362	-0.250	-0.111
Z311	-0.347	-0.403	-0.293	-0.216	-0.255	0.006	0.063
Z310	0.140	0.134	0.414	-0.153	-0.158	0.142	0.017
Z331	0.081	0.131	0.135	0.151	0.074	0.024	-0.014
Z330	0.005	0.022	0.064	0.073	0.049	0.080	0.002
Z400	-0.163	-0.162	0.022	-0.147	-0.166	0.038	0.001
Z420	0.096	0.068	0.076	0.085	0.097	0.078	0.048
Z421	-0.003	0.011	0.003	-0.014	0.019	-0.017	0.003
Z440	-0.013	-0.026	-0.009	-0.014	-0.001	0.005	-0.020
Z441	-0.019	-0.033	-0.030	-0.007	0.006	-0.023	0.021
Z510	0.017	0.020	0.006	0.007	0.020	0.008	0.021
Z511	0.026	0.018	0.022	0.029	0.036	0.007	-0.009
Z530	-0.016	-0.012	-0.026	-0.011	-0.001	-0.018	-0.001
Z531	0.013	-0.017	-0.003	-0.024	-0.018	-0.013	0.000
Z550	0.029	-0.001	0.033	0.017	0.017	0.023	0.027
Z551	0.027	0.029	-0.003	0.037	0.047	0.044	0.010
RMS	0.96	0.87	0.718	0.527	0.62	0.45	0.279
Strehl	0.015	0.012	0.03	0.043	0.033	0.064	0.151
SphO/Rx Undilated	1.00	1.00	0.75	0.50	0.50	0.00	0.00
High Contrast	-0.28	-0.30	-0.30	-0.28	-0.20	-0.30	-0.30
Low Contrast	0.10	-0.04	0.06	0.04	0.02	-0.04	-0.06
SphO/Rx Dilated	1.25	1.00	0.50	0.50	0.50	0.00	0.00
High Contrast	-0.22	-0.28	-0.30	-0.26	-0.26	-0.28	-0.30
Low Contrast	0.18	0.02	0.14	0.08	0.12	0.04	-0.06

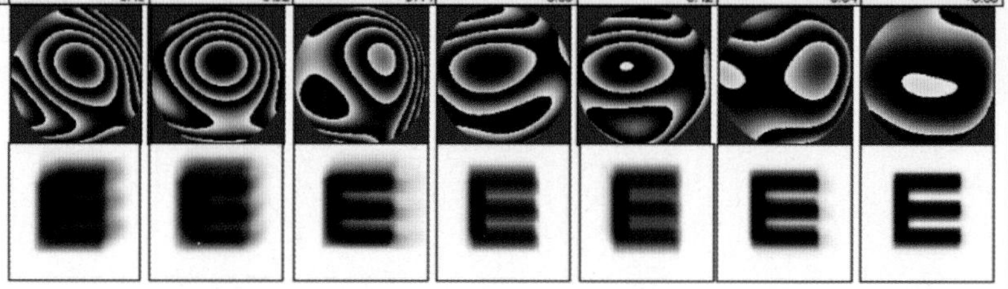

Figure 33-10. Higher-order RMS, PSFs, Strehl ratios, image convolutions, and logMAR visual acuity of an eye with a customized contact lens.

keratoconus: Noninflammatory, bilateral ectasia of the axial portion of the cornea. It is characterized by progressive thinning and steepening of the central cornea and often results in visual impairment.

nonrotationally symmetrical aberrations: Wavefront aberrations that are not symmetric around the optical axis of the optical system (eg, coma).

prism-ballasting: A design feature incorporating additional material mass into the inferior portion of a soft contact lens in order to stabilize its rotation and mislocation.

rigid gas permeable (RGP) contact lens: Rigid gas permeable contact lenses, often known as oxygen permeable lenses, are made of durable silicone or fluorosilicone-acrylate materials and provide a high level of oxygen transmissibility to the cornea.

Strehl ratio: A metric representing the quality of the PSF at the image plane of an optical system.

References

1. Ivanoff A. Letter to the editor: about the spherical aberration of the eye. *J Opt Soc Am A.* 1953;46(10):901-903.
2. Jenkins TCA. Aberrations of the eye and their effect upon vision. Part II. *British Journal of Physiological Optics.* 1963;20:161-201.
3. Koomen M, Tousey R, Scolnik R. The spherical aberration of the eye. *J Opt Soc Am A.* 1949;39(5):370-376.
4. Howland HC, Howland B. A subjective method for the measurement of the monochromatic aberrations of the eye. *J Opt Soc Am A.* 1977;67(11):1508-1518.
5. Porter J, Guirao A, Cox IG, Williams DR. Monochromatic aberrations of the human eye in a large population. *J Opt Soc Am A.* 2001;18(8):1793-1803.
6. Westheimer, G. Aberrations of contact lenses. *American Journal of Optometry and Archives of the American Academy of Optometry.* 1961;38:445-448.
7. Oxenberg LD, Carney LG. Visual performance with aspheric rigid contact lenses. *Optom Vis Sci.* 1989;66(12):818-821.
8. Knoll HA, Conway HD. Analysis of blink-induced vertical motion of contact lenses. *Am J Optom Physiol Opt.* 1987;64(2):153-155.
9. Young, G. Soft lens fitting reassessed. *Contact Lens Spectrum.* 1992;56-61.
10. Guirao A, Williams DR, Cox IG. Effect of rotation and translation on the expected benefit of an ideal method to correct the eye's higher order aberrations. *J Opt Soc Am A.* 2001;18(5), 1003-1015.

Chapter 34

Aberration-Correcting Intraocular Lenses

Patricia Piers; N.E. Sverker Norrby, PhD; and Ulrich Mester, MD

Introduction

When a patient undergoes cataract surgery, the cataractous lens is removed and replaced with an intraocular lens (IOL). During the last decade, extensive progress in the reliability and effectiveness of cataract surgery has been due not only to the introduction of new surgical techniques and new instrumentation but also to the development of next-generation IOL designs. The optical quality of isolated IOLs has received considerable attention.[1-3] However, the optical quality of the pseudophakic eye, as a whole, has only recently been examined. For example, recent studies of the contrast sensitivity of pseudophakic eyes have shown that patients implanted with spherical IOLs have contrast vision that is comparable with that of a healthy control population of the same age.[4] Similarly, Guirao et al measured the modulation transfer function (MTF) of 20 IOL patients and 20 patients with healthy control eyes of the same age and found that the MTF measured in the IOL population was similar to that measured in the normal population.[5] Similarities in outcomes are observed despite the fact that the human crystalline lens is optically inferior to an IOL. One explanation for these observations lies in the optical aberrations of the human cornea and spherical IOLs.

Recent advances in wavefront technology have enabled measurements that quantitatively describe the optical performance and aberrations of both the cornea[6,7] and the entire refractive system of the eye.[8-10] Studies have shown that the young human eye is a system in which aberrations introduced by the cornea are at least partially compensated for by the lens.[11-13] Major changes that do occur in the lens with age, such as hardening of the nucleus,[14] changes in the internal refractive index gradient,[15] and changes in lens shape,[16] produce changes in lens aberration. As a result of these structural changes in the lens, aberration compensation is gradually lost with age, leading to an increase in total ocular aberrations[10] and a corresponding loss in optical quality.[17] This reduction in ocular optical quality is at least partially responsible for a measured reduction in visual quality with age.[18]

Wavefront sensing, the technology that was used to study the aging eye, can also be applied to the on-axis optics of the pseudophakic eye. Positive spherical aberration exhibited by the cornea[6,7] occurs when rays entering the periphery of the pupil are focused in front of rays entering near the center of the pupil. Because most monofocal IOLs have one or two spherical surfaces, they also contribute positive spherical aberration,[19] and thus increase the total positive ocular spherical aberration of the average cataract patient. In a number of studies, spherical aberration data were collected in pseudophakic eyes with foldable lenses using a Shack-Hartmann wavefront sensor. Figure 34-1 shows the average and standard deviation of the Zernike coefficient Z(4,0) of the wavefront aberration (representative of fourth-order spherical aberration) measured for a 4.00 millimeter (mm) pupil in 27 eyes implanted with the AcrySof MA60BM (Alcon Laboratories, Fort Worth, Tex), 48 eyes implanted with the PhakoFlex II SI40NB (Advanced Medical Optics, Santa Ana, Calif), and 82 eyes implanted with the CeeOn Edge 911A (Pfizer, New York, NY). For these three spherical lenses of different materials and optical designs, very little difference was found in the measured pseudophakic ocular spherical aberration. The average spherical aberration present in the pseudophakic eye implanted with spherically surfaced monofocal IOLs is overwhelmingly positive.

> The average spherical aberration present in the pseudophakic eye implanted with a conventional spherically surfaced monofocal IOL is overwhelmingly positive. The Tecnis lens (Pfizer, New York, NY) uses a negative spherical aberration design to compensate for this.

Based upon these observations, a logical solution to the problem of increased positive spherical aberration in the pseudophakic eye is an IOL that compensates for the positive spherical aberration introduced by the cornea. This can be done by modifying one or both surfaces of the IOL to produce a lens that introduces negative spherical aberration to the system. To this end, Pfizer has designed the Tecnis Z-9000 lens, in which the peripheral power of the IOL is reduced by modifying the front surface, producing an IOL with negative spherical aberration. The expected result is a pseudophakic eye with very little remaining spherical aberration.

As an example of the potential benefit of aberration-correcting IOLs, the sections that follow describe the design and clinical performance of the Tecnis Z-9000.

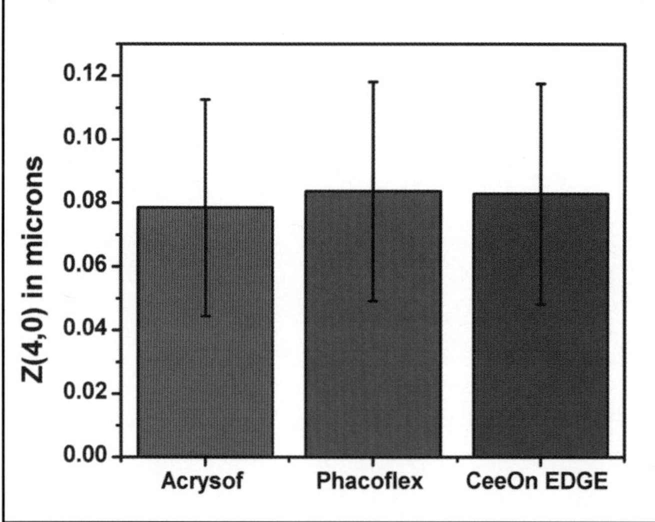

Figure 34-1. Mean root mean square (RMS) wavefront values of the Zernike coefficient Z(4,0) of the wavefront aberration for a 4 mm pupil measured in 147 pseudophakic eyes implanted with different IOL models (27 Acrysof MA60MB, 48 PhakoFlex II SI40NB, and 72 CeeOn Edge 911A). The error bars indicate plus and minus one standard deviation. This data was collected in studies conducted by Prof. Dr. U Mester, PD; Dr. HJ Hettlich; and Dr. K Gerstmeyer (Minden Eye Clinic, Germany).

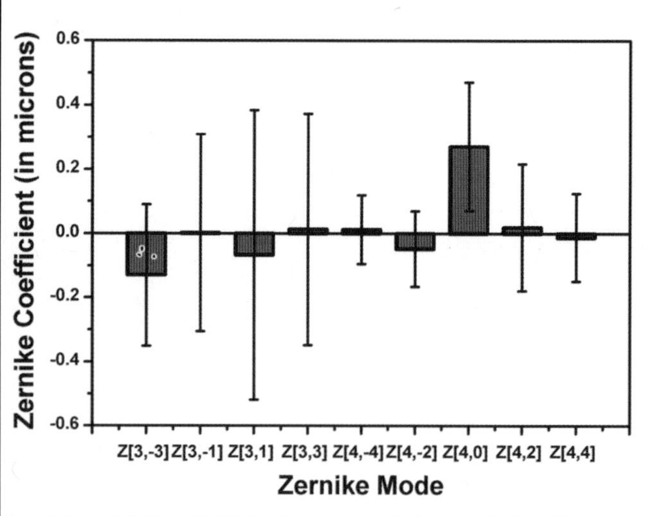

Figure 34-2. Mean RMS wavefront error values of the third- and fourth-order Zernike coefficients of the corneal wavefront aberration measured in 71 cataract patients for a 6 mm pupil. The error bars indicate plus and minus one standard deviation.

Design of a Lens for the Reduction of Pseudophakic Spherical Aberration

The Tecnis lens was designed to compensate for average corneal spherical aberration. Furthermore, because cataract surgery is predominantly performed in older eyes and uncertainty exists in the literature as to whether corneal spherical aberration changes with age (Oshika et al[6] have shown no change while Guirao et al[7] have shown that it increases slightly with age), the design of the Tecnis lens was based on the spherical aberration measured in a typical population of cataract patients.

The design population included 71 eyes of 71 subjects eligible for cataract surgery at St. Erik's Eye Hospital in Stockholm, Sweden. Their ages ranged from 35 to 94 years, with a mean age of 74. Corneal topography was recorded for all subjects using the Orbscan I (Bausch & Lomb, Rochester, NY) on the day of surgery.

The measured elevation of the anterior corneal surface and its position in the pupil were used as inputs for determining the optical properties of all corneas. A calculation of wavefront aberration of the single-surface cornea model for each subject was performed using the computational method described previously by Guirao and Artal.[20] Using a pupil centered on the subject's line-of-sight, the surface was described by fitting the elevation height data with a series of Zernike polynomials (up to and including the fourth order) after applying a Gram-Schmidt orthogonalization procedure to the height data (for a 6 mm pupil size). Knowledge of the precise shape of the anterior corneal surface allowed the wavefront aberration created by this surface to be determined using a ray trace procedure.

Like the surface shape, wavefront aberration is represented as a sum of Zernike polynomials. Figure 34-2 presents the average and standard deviation of each of the higher-order Zernike aberration terms (third and fourth order) calculated for a 6 mm diameter aperture (the ordering of the Zernike coefficients listed follows the recently standardized double-index format for Zernike coefficients for reporting the optical aberrations of eyes).[21] From this plot, it can be seen that two higher-order aberrations (trefoil Z[3,-3]) and spherical aberration (Z[4,0]) are, on average, significantly different from zero in this population. Because spherical aberration is the only rotationally symmetric higher-order aberration, it is the only aberration that can be corrected with a rotationally symmetric IOL.

A single-surface model cornea was constructed to have the same spherical aberration as the average calculated for the design population. The radius of curvature of this model cornea was the average radius determined from the Zernike fit to the elevation data, while the conic constant was adjusted until corneal spherical aberration was equal to the average for the 71 subjects. This one-surface model replaces the surfaces of the cornea and aqueous humour with one effective medium with the keratometric refractive index of 1.3375.

This new model cornea was incorporated into a pseudophakic eye model and used to design a new lens. The chosen initial starting point for lens design was an equi-biconvex lens made from high refractive index polysiloxane. This lens was placed 4.50 mm behind the anterior corneal surface (based upon measurements of IOL positioning in pseudophakic eyes).[22-24] The refractive indices used in the eye model are consistent with accepted values for the refractive indices of the ocular media at 450, 546, and 650 nanometers (nm).[25]

The anterior surface of the lens was modified in such a way that the optical path lengths of all on-axis rays within the design aperture (λ = 546) were the same. The resulting anterior surface shape can be described using the modified conicoid equation (equation 1), where R is the radius of curvature at the vertex, Q is the conic constant, and r is the radial distance from the vertex of the surface (this equation is not a simple conicoid—ad and ae are higher-order polynomial terms, and it is these terms that make the surface a modified conicoid instead of a pure conicoid). The resulting shape of the anterior surface of the Tecnis lens is a modified prolate ellipsoid (Q values between 0 and –1). Prolate surfaces are one type of aspheric surface in which the term *aspheric* is used to describe any surface that is not purely spherical (ie, having the same radius of curvature at every point on the surface).

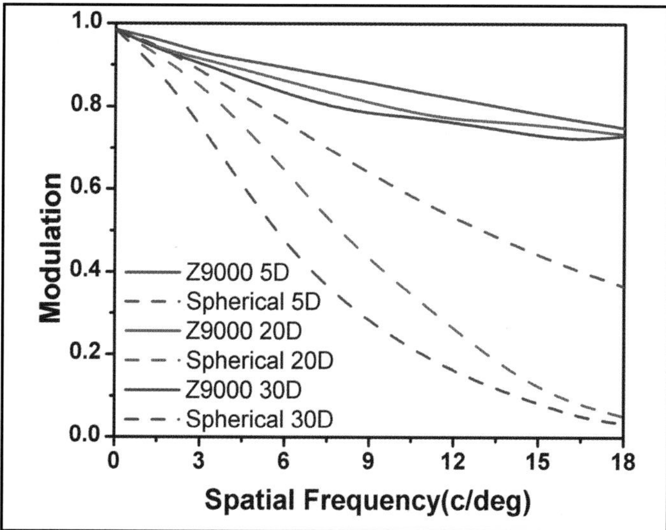

Figure 34-3. Polychromatic MTF of two pseudophakic eye models (one including an IOL with spherical surfaces and the other including the new Tecnis Z-9000 lens) calculated for 5, 20, and 30 D lenses and a 4 mm pupil.

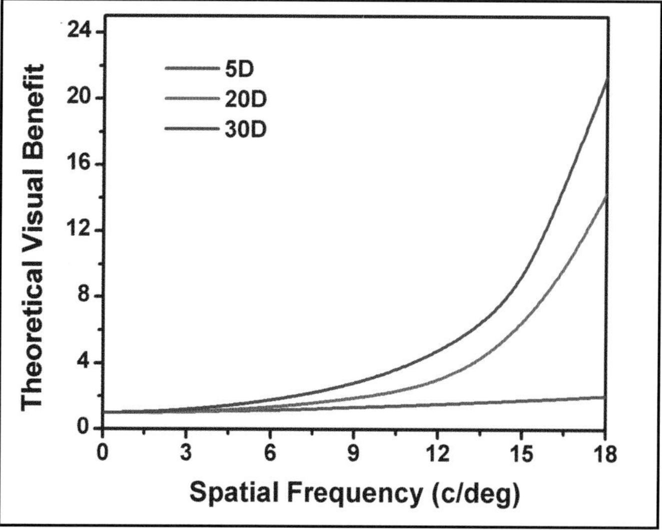

Figure 34-4. Theoretical visual benefit provided by a 5, 20, and 30 D Tecnis lens for a 4 mm pupil.

$$z = \frac{(\frac{1}{R})\, r^2}{1 + \sqrt{1 - (Q+1)(\frac{1}{R})^2 r^2}} + adr4 + aer6 \qquad (1)$$

The optical quality (MTFs) of these newly designed Tecnis lenses were calculated in the pseudophakic eye model. To provide a reference, the new modified prolate lenses were compared with an equi-biconvex lens of the same power, made from the same material but having spherical surfaces. Thus, the only difference between these two lens models is the shape of the anterior surface. The MTFs calculated for l = 450, 546, and 650 nm were weighted using the photopic spectral luminous efficiency function V(l) of the human eye to determine the polychromatic MTF. The polychromatic MTF of these two eye models, best-focused to obtain the minimum Strehl ratio for l = 546 nm, was calculated and the comparison was made for 5, 20, and 30 D lenses in Figure 34-3 (4 mm pupil).

The theoretical visual benefit (Figure 34-4) as defined by Williams et al[26] is, in this case, defined as the ratio of the polychromatic MTF calculated in the model eye with the Tecnis lens to the MTF calculated with the spherical reference lens. This value is representative of the increase in contrast present in an image on the retina for objects of different spatial frequencies (for 5, 20, and 30 D lenses). An improvement in the measured MTF translates to an improvement in image contrast. The resultant enhancement in contrast is expected to provide patients with implanted eyes with an increase in contrast sensitivity. These outcomes support the need for a clinical evaluation of a modified prolate IOL to improve the quality of vision following cataract surgery.

Clinical Results With the Tecnis Lens

In a randomized, open-label, single-center study,[27] 37 bilateral cataract patients were implanted with two different IOLs. Each patient received one Tecnis lens (modified prolate anterior surface) and one conventional IOL (spherical anterior and posterior surfaces and positive spherical aberration) both made from high refractive index silicone. These two lenses were compared intraindividually to determine if decreasing ocular spherical aberration leads to a measurable improvement in the quality of vision. All cataract surgery procedures were performed at the Department of Ophthalmology, Bundesknappschaft's Hospital, Sulzbach, Germany and every effort was made to minimize differences in the treatment in each of the patient's two eyes. To this end, all patients had both of their surgeries performed by the same doctor. The patients included in the study were cataract patients with otherwise healthy eyes. Patients with any ocular pathology (other than cataracts) or optical irregularity were excluded from the study, and the choice of which eye was to receive which lens was randomized. The surgical procedure used for implantation of both lenses has been described in detail by Mester et al.[27] Quality of vision was assessed by measuring contrast sensitivity and optical quality by wavefront aberration. The improvement in visual quality and difference in wavefront aberration were assessed using a two-sided paired t-test. A significant difference is reported for p values less than 0.01. All results reported here are from a visit conducted 3 months postoperatively.

Wavefront aberration of the whole eye was measured using a Shack-Hartmann wavefront sensor with a fully pharmacologically dilated pupil. The principles associated with this technique for measuring the ocular wavefront aberration of the eye are described in detail elsewhere.[8,28]

Wavefront aberration measurements were obtained in 30 eyes implanted with Tecnis lenses (study eyes) and 29 eyes implanted with the spherically surfaced control lens (control eyes). Figure 34-5 shows the average Zernike coefficients of the measured ocular wavefront aberration of the study eyes and of the control eyes for a 4 mm pupil. These measurements reveal that there is no statistically significant difference in any of the wavefront aberration terms except for Z(4,0), which is representative of spherical aberration. (A t-test was used to compare the sample means, $p < 0.01$.) In particular, the study eyes have, on average, no significant spherical aberration (Z[4,0] = 0.0069 ± 0.0309 mm RMS error), while the control eyes suffer from significant amounts of positive spherical aberration (Z[4,0] = 0.0813 ± 0.0258 mm RMS error).

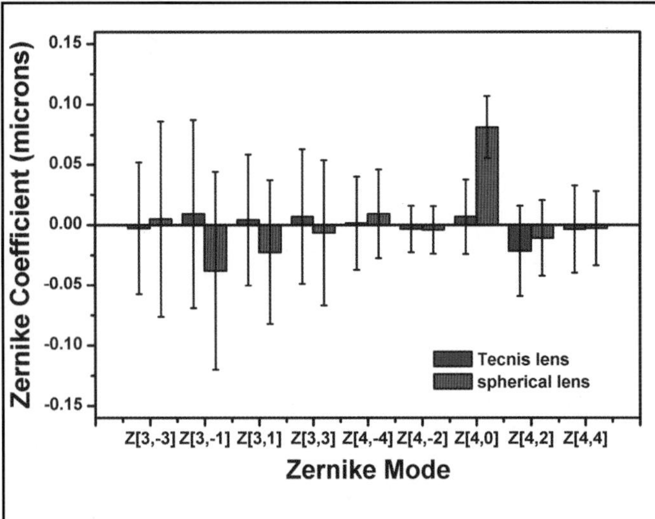

Figure 34-5. Mean RMS wavefront error values of the third- and fourth-order Zernike coefficients of the wavefront aberration measured in eyes implanted with the Tecnis lens and eyes implanted with a conventional IOL with spherical surfaces (4 mm pupil). The error bars indicate plus and minus one standard deviation.

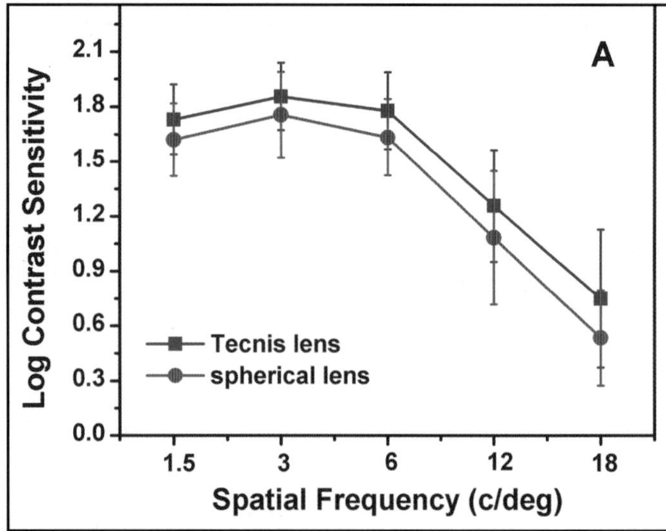

Figure 34-6A. Mean best-corrected log contrast sensitivity values measured in eyes implanted with the Tecnis lens and eyes implanted with a conventional IOL with spherical surfaces. The error bars indicate plus and minus one standard deviation. Measured under mesopic lighting conditions (6 candles/meters^2 [cd/m^2]).

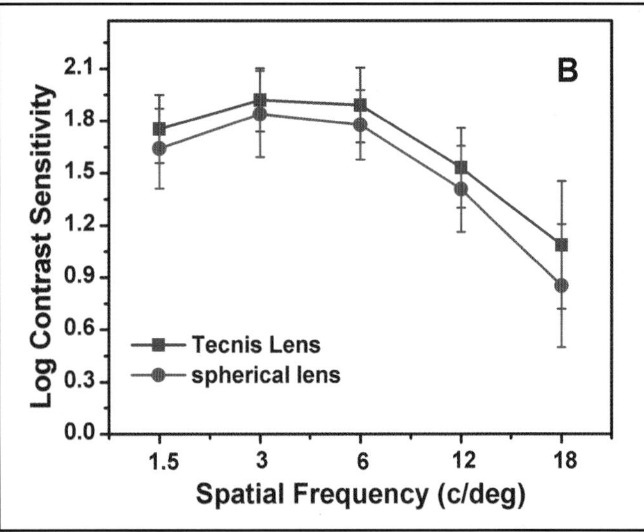

Figure 34-6B. Mean best-corrected log contrast sensitivity values measured in eyes implanted with the Tecnis lens and eyes implanted with a conventional IOL with spherical surfaces. The error bars indicate plus and minus 1 standard deviation. Measured under photopic lighting conditions (85 cd/m^2).

> The Tecnis lens on average had no significant spherical aberration, while the conventional control eye had significant residual amounts of spherical aberrations.

Best-corrected contrast sensitivity function (CSF) was measured in both eyes using the VSRC CST-1500 view-in tester with the FACT sine-wave grating (Vision Sciences Research, San Ramon, Calif) (1.5, 3, 6, 12, and 18 cycles per degree [c/deg]) contrast sensitivity chart viewed under photopic normal (85 [candles/meter^2] cd/m^2) and mesopic low light (6 cd/m^2) lighting conditions. The average photopic and mesopic log CSF values for the two groups of eyes are shown in Figures 34-6A and 34-6B. The eyes implanted with the Tecnis IOL performed significantly better for all spatial frequencies and both lighting conditions ($p < 0.01$). There was more improvement measured under mesopic conditions, due to the fact that when the pupil is wider the negative effects of aberrations are more pronounced. The measured increase in CSF indicates that the patients could detect objects of lower contrast with their Tecnis eye than with the eye implanted with the conventional control lens. For example, at 6 c/deg, the eyes implanted with the Tecnis lens had an average CSF of 67.2, while the control eyes had an average CSF of 48.3. This means that the average contrast threshold of control eyes is ~39% higher than that of the Tecnis eyes. The average measured visual benefit (Figure 34-7) is the ratio of the CSF in the study eyes to the CSF in the control eyes. A "visual benefit" of 1 means there would be no visual benefit, while a visual benefit of 2 indicates a doubling of the MTF, which means a shaper image. This factor varies from 1.1 for 3 c/deg to 1.9 for 18 c/deg for photopic conditions and from 1.2 for 3 c/deg to 2.2 for 18 c/deg for mesopic contrast sensitivity and is consistently greater than 1 (equivalent CSF).

> The Tecnis lens had a significant improvement in all spatial frequencies tested for photopic and mesopic conditions compared to the conventionally designed control lens.

Discussion

The aberration compensation provided by the Tecnis lens significantly reduces the total ocular spherical aberration in pseudophakic eyes. This reduction in ocular spherical aberration leads to an increase in the contrast of the retinal image and an increase in the CSF of patients implanted with this lens. This study reveals that wavefront aberration measurement is a valuable tool for IOL design.

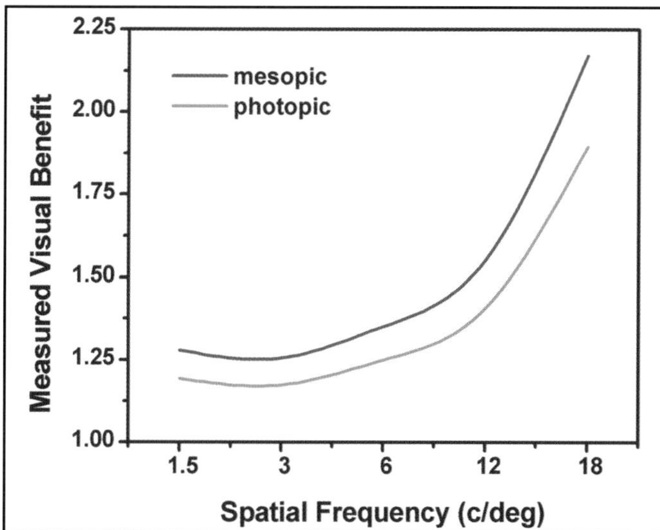

Figure 34-7. Measured visual benefit provided by the Tecnis lens for mesopic and photopic lighting conditions.

The notion of varying the surface shapes of an IOL in order to improve pseudophakic quality of vision is not new. An elegant analysis of the effects of different lens shapes on both on- and off-axis image quality of IOLs was performed by Atchison.[29,30] It was determined that the best retinal image quality is provided by a lens that is close to plano-convex, with the more curved surface facing the cornea (in this study, only plano and spherical surfaces were used). Furthermore, Lu, Smith, and Atchison have investigated the possibility of improving ocular optical quality with aspheric IOLs and it was generally agreed that a theoretical improvement is possible for well-centered implants.[31,32]

In the 1980s, ORC marketed an IOL with an aspheric anterior surface. This lens (the ORC model UV400) was designed using different principles and did not succeed in improving pseudophakic visual quality. It was premature to put such a lens on the market at a time when the surgical technique used often resulted in large amounts of tilt and decentration.[33] Manufacturing technology was also not refined enough to make the high precision surfaces that current single-point diamond turning achieves today. The only other aspheric lens on the market today that the authors are aware of is a refractive/diffractive bifocal lens sold by Acri.Tec (Berlin, Germany)—models 737D and 733D. Modifying current lens models to include aspheric surface profiles would be a natural way for other IOL producers to improve the pseudophakic visual quality provided by their lenses. Therefore, it is likely that other ophthalmic companies are developing aspheric IOLs.

As suggested above, the pseudophakic optical quality of a nonspherical lens is more sensitive to misalignments. Van der Mooren et al[34] showed, using the MTF calculated in the pseudophakic eye model (discussed in the design section of this chapter), that if the Tecnis lens is decentered less than 0.50 mm and tilted less than 9 degrees, it will exceed the optical performance of a spherical IOL. Recent studies of tilt and decentration of foldable IOLs have found average decentration values of 0.15 mm, 0.28 mm, and 0.30 mm and average tilts of 1.13 degrees, 2.83 degrees, and 2.41 degrees.[35-37] Thus, these studies confirm that modern IOL implantation is well within the decentration and tilt tolerances needed to achieve improved optical performance with the Tecnis lens.

The two lenses used in the clinical study outlined in Clinical Results With the Tecnis Lens (see p. 287) were not exactly the same—the lenses were made by different manufacturers and have different haptic designs and overall diameters. However, the major factors contributing to optical quality (ie, the refractive index of the optic material and the diameter of the optic) are very similar. In fact, the single major difference between the two lenses that contributes to intraocular optical quality is that the control lens has two spherical surfaces (resulting in a lens with positive spherical aberration) while the Tecnis lens has one spherical surface and one modified prolate surface (and thus contributes negative spherical aberration to the system). Thus, the small differences in optical quality contributed by the other differences in the two lenses are overshadowed by the larger differences contributed by the spherical aberration.

The Tecnis lens was designed to compensate for the average corneal spherical aberration of the cataract population and therefore does not provide precise compensation for each individual's corneal spherical aberration. Thus, all patients do not obtain the same benefit from the lens, and some patients may even have slightly better contrast sensitivity with a conventional spherical lens. In the clinical study described above, approximately 10% of the patients had lower mesopic contrast sensitivity in their Tecnis eye than in their control eye. In order for every patient to appreciate minimized ocular spherical aberration and thus improved contrast sensitivity, lenses customized to correct for each individual's unique corneal spherical aberration would be required. A design that compensates for all monochromatic aberrations (spherical aberration, coma, astigmatism, etc) of an individual's cornea should yield the best possible visual performance for that individual. For example, Williams et al have reported a measured average visual benefit of between 150% and 300% for a customized correction of all monochromatic aberrations in the spatial frequencies considered in our clinical study (1.5 to 18 c/deg).[26] With these possible gains, customizing IOLs to com-

In order for every patient to appreciate minimized ocular spherical aberration and thus improved contrast sensitivity, lenses customized to correct for each individual's unique corneal spherical aberration would be required. A design that compensates for all monochromatic aberrations (spherical aberration, coma, astigmatism, etc) of an individual's cornea should yield the best possible visual performance for that individual. This may be a design in future IOLs.

Editor's note:

The field of wavefront-corrected IOL is moving rapidly to minimize higher-order aberration with the first and most important step being aspheric IOLs, which are designed based on a normalized correction in spherical aberration in a normal population. It is not truly "customized" based on the individual's higher-order aberration pattern. In the future, it would be optimal to be able to adjust the IOL after insertion into the eye to compensation for subtle decentration and other higher-order aberrations measured after cataract surgery. Such wondrous systems are still under development and will take years to implement, but this first step of reducing spherical aberration in pseudophakes is an important one.

S. MacRae, MD

pensate for individual corneal monochromatic aberrations is a natural next step in improving pseudophakic visual quality.

Definitions

contrast sensitivity: The ability to detect objects with varying contrast levels. Measured with specially designed charts.

haptic: Loop attached to an IOL that is used to support the lens in the capsular bag or sulcus.

pseudophakia: The condition of having an IOL implant taking the place of a cataractous lens.

References

1. Norrby NES, Grossman LW, Geraghty EP, et al. Determining the imaging quality of intraocular lenses. *J Cataract Refract Surg*. 1998; 24:703-714.
2. Norrby NES. Standardized methods for assessing the imaging quality of intraocular lenses. *Appl Opt*. 1995;34:7327-7333.
3. Ophthalmic Implants—Intraocular lenses. Part 2: Optical properties and test methods. ISO 11979-2. ISO, Geneva, Switzerland; 1999.
4. Or H, Soylu T. The enhancement of the contrast sensitivity in cataract surgery patients with a preoperative visual acuity of 0.4-0.7 and its comparison with the normals. Paper presented at: the XXIX International Congress of Ophthalmology; April 21-25, 2002; Sydney, Australia.
5. Guirao A, Redondo M, Geraghty E, Piers PA, Norrby S, Artal P. Corneal optical aberrations and retinal image quality in patients implanted with monofocal IOLs. *Arch Ophthalmol*. 2002;120:1143.
6. Oshika, T, Klyce SD, Applegate RA, Howland HC. Changes in corneal wavefront aberrations with aging. *Invest Ophthalmol Vis Sci*. 1999;40:1351-1355.
7. Guirao A, Redondo M, Artal P. Optical aberrations of the human cornea as a function of age. *J Opt Soc Am A*. 2000;17:1697-1702.
8. Liang J, Grimm B, Goelz S, Bille JF. Objective measurement of wave aberrations of the human eye with the use of a Hartmann-Shack wave-front sensor. *J Opt Soc Am A*. 1994;11:1949-1957.
9. Porter J, Guirao A, Cox I, Williams DR. Monochromatic aberrations of the human eye in a large population. *J Opt Soc Am A*. 2001;18:1793-1803.
10. Artal P, Berrio E, Guirao A, Piers P. Contribution of the cornea and internal surfaces to the change of ocular aberration with age. *J Opt Soc Am A*. 2002;19:137-143.
11. El Hage SG, Berny F. Contribution of the crystalline lens to the spherical aberration of the eye. *J Opt Soc Am A*. 1973;63:205-211.
12. Artal P, Guirao A, Berrio E, Williams D. Compensation of corneal aberrations by the internal optics in the human eye. *Journal of Vision*. 2001;1:1-8.
13. Smith G, Cox MJ, Calver R, Garner LF. The spherical aberration of the crystalline lens of the human eye. *Vision Res*. 2001;41:235-243.
14. Glasser A, Campbell MC. Biometric, optical and physical changes in the isolated human crystalline lens with age in relation to presbyopia. *Vision Res*. 1999;39:1991-2015.
15. Smith G, Atchison DA, Pierscionek BK. Modeling the power of the aging eye. *J Opt Soc Am A*. 1992;9:2111-2117.
16. Dubbelman M, Van der Heijde GL. The shape of the aging human lens: curvature, equivalent refractive index and the lens paradox. *Vision Res*. 2001;41:1867-1877.
17. Guirao A, Gonzalez C, Redondo M, Geraghty E, Norrby S, Artal P. Average optical performance of the human eye as a function of age in a normal population. *Invest Ophthalmol Vis Sci*. 1999;40:203-213.
18. Nio YK, Jansonius NM, Fidler V, Fidler V, Geraghty E, Norrby S, Kooijman AC. Age-related changes of defocus-specific contrast sensitivity in healthy subjects. *Ophthalmic Physiol Opt*. 2000;20:323-334.
19. Barbero S, Marcos S, Llorente L, Optical changes in corneal and internal optics with cataract surgery. Abstract. *Invest Ophthalmol Vis Sci*. 2002;388.
20. Guirao A, Artal P. Corneal wave aberration from videokeratography: accuracy and limitations of the procedure. *J Opt Soc Am A*. 2000;17:955-965.
21. Thibos LN, Applegate RA, Schwiegerling JT, Webb R, VSIA Standards Taskforce Members. Standards for reporting the optical aberrations of eyes. Vision Science and its Applications, OSA *Trends in Optics and Photonics*. 2000;35:110-130.
22. Findl O, Drexler W, Menapace R, et al. Changes in intraocular lens position after neodymium:YAG capsulotomy. *J Cataract Refract Surg*. 1999;25:659-662.
23. Landau IM, Laurell CG. Ultrasound biomicroscopy examination of intraocular lens haptic position after phacoemulsification with continuous curvilinear capsulorrhexis and extracapsular cataract extraction with linear capsulotomy. *Acta Ophthalmol Scand*. 1999;77:394-396.
24. Olsen T, Corydon L, Gimbel H. Intraocular lens power calculation with an improved anterior chamber depth prediction algorithm. *J Cataract Refract Surg*. 1995;21:313-319.
25. Navarro R, Santamaria J, Bescos J. Accommodation-dependent model of the human eye with aspherics. *J Opt Soc Am A*. 1985;2:1273-1281.
26. Williams DR, Yoon GY, Guirao A, Hofer H, Porter J. How far can we extend the limits of human vision. In: MacRae SM, Kreuger RR, Applegate RA, eds. *Customized Corneal Ablation: The Quest for SuperVision*. Thorofare, NJ: SLACK Incorporated; 2001:11-32.
27. Mester U, Dillinger P, Anterist N. The impact of a modified optic design on visual function. A clinical comparative study. *J Cataract Refract Surg*. 2003;4:627.
28. Prieto PM, Vargas-Martin F, Goelz S, Artal P. Analysis of the performance of the Hartmann-Shack sensor in the human eye. *J Opt Soc Am A*. 2000;17:1388-1398.
29. Atchison DA. Optical design of intraocular lenses. I. on-axis performance. *Optom Vision Sci*. 1989;66(8):492-506.
30. Atchison DA. Optical design of intraocular lenses. II. off-axis performance. *Optom Vision Sci*. 1989;66(9):579-590.
31. Lu C, Smith G. The aspherizing of intraocular lenses. *Ophthalmic Physiol Opt*. 2000;20:323-334.
32. Atchison DA. Design of aspheric intraocular lenses. *Ophthalmic Physiol Opt*. 1991;11:137-146.
33. Auran, JD, Koester CJ, Donn A. In vivo measurement of posterior chamber intraocular lens decentration and tilt. *Arch Ophthalmol*. 1990;108:75-79.
34. Van der Mooren M, Piers P, Norrby S, Schievink H. Optical performance of the Pharmacia Tecnis Z9000 IOL designed to match the human cornea. Paper presented at: the American Society of Cataract and Refractive Surgery Annual Meeting; 2002.
35. Akkin C, Ozler SA, Mentes J. Tilt and decentration of bag-fixated lenses: a comparative study between capsulorrhexis and envelope techniques. *Doc Ophthalmol*. 1994;87:199-209.
36. Mutlu FM, Bilge AH, Altinsoy HI, Yamusak E. The role of capsulotomy and intraocular lens type on tilt and decentration of polymethylmethacrylate and foldable acrylic lenses. *Ophthalmologica*. 1998;212:359-363.
37. Hayashi K, Harada M, Hayashi H, Nakao F, Hayashi F. Decentration and tilt of polymethyl methacrylate, silicone, and acrylic soft intraocular lenses. *Ophthalmology*. 1997;104:793-798.

Chapter 35
The Calhoun Light Adjustable Lens: A Postinsertion Method for the Correction of Refractive Errors

Christian A. Sandstedt, PhD; Shiao Chang, PhD; and Daniel M. Schwartz, MD

Introduction

Cataract surgery with intraocular lens (IOL) implantation is the most commonly performed surgical procedure in patients over 60 years of age in the United States. Approximately 2.7 million cataract surgeries will be performed in the United States this year.[1] While this procedure has undergone numerous refinements over the past 25 years, certain problems remain. In particular, calculations of IOL power are sometimes imprecise because of improper preoperative measurements, postoperative astigmatism from irregular wound healing, or variability in placement of the IOL.[2-5] Of 298 emmetropic patients undergoing phacoemulsification or extracapsular cataract surgery with posterior chamber lens placement, only 45% had an emmetropic refraction postoperatively.[1] The remaining patients required spectacle correction for optimal distance vision. Ninety-four percent of patients in this group had a postoperative refractive error within 2 diopters (D) of emmetropia. In a series of patients undergoing cataract surgery with either a rigid or foldable IOL, only 35% of patients had uncorrected visual acuity of 20/25 or better. Other studies of uncorrected visual acuity after cataract surgery show that about 50% of patients require spectacles postoperatively to achieve best possible distance vision.[6]

> Of 298 emmetropic patients undergoing phacoemulsification or extracapsular cataract surgery with posterior chamber lens placement, only 45% had an emmetropic refraction postoperatively.[1]

In addition to imprecise IOL power determinations postoperatively, uncorrected visual acuity is often limited by pre-existing corneal astigmatism. Recently, STAAR Surgical (Monrovia, Calif) introduced a toric IOL that corrects pre-existing astigmatic errors. The IOL comes in only two toric powers—2 and 3.5 D—and the axis must be precisely aligned at surgery. Other than surgical repositioning, there is no way to adjust the IOL's axis, which may shift postoperatively.[7] Furthermore, individualized correction of astigmatism is limited by unavailability of multiple toric powers. An additional problem with using pre-existing astigmatic errors to gauge axis and power of a toric IOL is the unpredictable effect of the cataract wound on final refractive error. After the refractive effect of the cataract wound stabilizes, there can be a shift in both magnitude and axis of astigmatism, minimizing the corrective effect of a toric IOL. A means to postoperatively correct astigmatic refractive errors after cataract surgery would be very desirable.

Recent commercialization of multifocal IOLs in which patients can potentially be spectacle-free for both near and distance has further increased the need for precise IOL power determinations.[8-10] The Advanced Medical Optics, Inc (Santa Ana, Calif) Array multifocal IOL has concentric zones of progressive aspheric lenses, permitting simultaneous focusing at distance, near, and intermediate range. If the power calculation is correct for a multifocal IOL, the patient can be freed from using spectacles postoperatively. While some patients with multifocal lenses note glare at night and mild limitation of near visual acuity, overall patient satisfaction in early studies has been very high.[9,10] The critical feature related to patient satisfaction with the multifocal IOL is spectacle independence. In fact, a survey of patients with both monofocal and multifocal lenses indicated a willingness to pay approximately $2.00 per day to be free of spectacles after cataract surgery. Assuming a 5-year life expectancy after cataract surgery and a discount rate of 5%, this daily cost would be worth over $3000.[9] However, the ability to achieve spectacle-free vision with multifocal IOLs is limited by similar imprecision in IOL calculation noted above for monofocal IOLs.

Growing interest in phakic IOLs for refractive correction of high myopia has accentuated the need for greater precision in IOL power determination. Because of the need to ablate excessive corneal tissue to correct large refractive errors, posterior chamber, iris-fixated, or anterior chamber phakic IOLs provide better optical quality than excimer laser surgery (laser in-situ keratomileusis [LASIK] or photoreactive keratectomy [PRK]). While phakic IOLs are not associated with disabling optical aberrations, optimization of this refractive therapy remains limited by imprecision in IOL power selection.[11-13]

An additional unexpected need for improved precision in IOL power determination has recently emerged. Eyes undergoing corneal refractive procedures (approximately 1 million/year in the United States) that subsequently develop cataracts are problematic when estimating pseudophakic IOL power. Corneal topographic alterations induced by refractive surgery create imprecision in keratometric measurements.[14-16] Several series of patients who had refractive surgery (PRK, LASIK, radial keratotomy) and later required cataract surgery demonstrate surprisingly large hyperopic errors in IOL power determination.[14] As the number of myopic patients who have undergone refractive

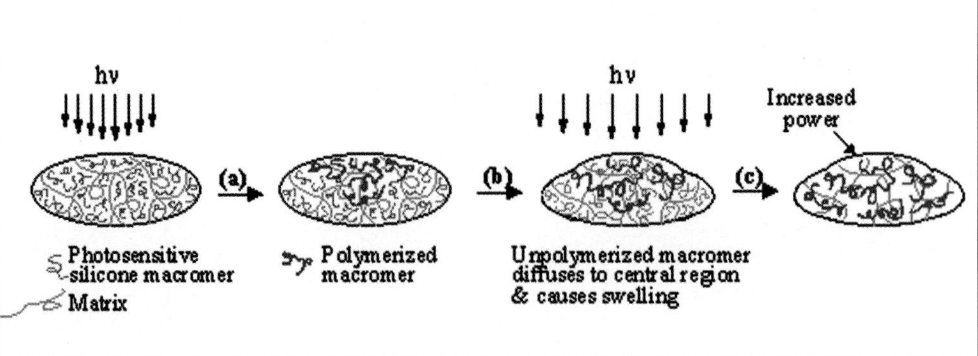

Figure 35-1. Schematic of positive power adjustment mechanism. (A) Selective irradiation of the central zone of IOL polymerizes macromer, creating a chemical potential between the irradiated and nonirradiated regions. (B) To re-establish equilibrium, excess macromer diffuses into the irradiated region, causing swelling. (C) Irradiation of the entire IOL "locks" the lens power and the shape change.

surgery increases and these patients age, difficulty in accurately predicting IOL power will become an increasingly significant clinical problem. The ability to address this problem with noninvasive postoperative IOL adjustability would be especially valuable in refractive surgery patients, many of whom are accustomed to spectacle-free vision.

As the number of myopic patients who have undergone refractive surgery increases and these patients age, difficulty in accurately predicting IOL power will become an increasingly significant clinical problem.

Therefore, despite advances in cataract and refractive surgery, imprecise IOL power determination remains an important clinical problem to address. Material and optical scientists working at Calhoun Vision, Inc (Pasadena, Calif) and the California Institute of Technology (Pasadena, Calif) have developed a light adjustable IOL that once implanted in the eye may be adjusted with safe levels of near visible radiation to effect refractive changes in the lens. This light adjustable lens (LAL) will give the cataract and refractive surgeon, for the first time, the ability to noninvasively and reproducibly correct both the lower-order (defocus and astigmatism) and some of the higher-order (spherical, coma, tetrafoil, etc) aberrations that adversely affect human vision.

Technology Description: Mechanism of Lens Power Adjustment

The Calhoun LAL contains essentially three distinct chemical entities. The first is the matrix polymer that gives the lens its basic shape, refractive index, and material properties. The second component is known as the macromer and is, by design, chemically similar to the matrix polymer. The most important difference between the two is the presence of photopolymerizable end groups on the macromer such that the application of the appropriate frequency of light will cause the macromer molecules to form chemical bonds between each other. The third major component of the Calhoun LAL is a ultraviolet (UV)-absorbing molecule that protects that retina from ambient UV irradiation.

Editor's note:

Irradiated macromer, which differs from the surrounding matrix polymer by end groups that can be chemically bound together by the light, is incorporated into the meshwork of matrix polymer, setting up a chemical concentration gradient that allows inirradiated macromer to diffuse into the irradiated area, resulting in a change in lens curvature. Wavefront customized irradiation with the appropriate frequency of light results in a wavefront customized change in lens curvature.

R. Krueger, MD, MSE

The mechanism upon which the Calhoun LAL technology is based is akin to holography and is depicted graphically in Figure 35-1. Application of light to the LAL will cause the photopolymerized macromers in the irradiated region to form an interpenetrating network within the target area of the lens. This action produces a change in the chemical potential between the irradiated and unirradiated regions of the lens. To re-establish thermodynamic equilibrium, macromers in the unirradiated portion of the lens will diffuse into the irradiated region, producing a swelling in the irradiated region that effects a change in the lens curvature. As an example, if the central portion of the lens is irradiated and the outside portion is left nonirradiated, unreacted macromer diffuses into the center portion causing an increase in the lens power and a hyperopic shift. Likewise, by irradiating the outer periphery of the lens, macromer migrates outward, causing a decrease in the lens power and a myopic correction.

By controlling the irradiation dosage (ie, beam intensity and duration), spatial intensity profile, and target area, physical changes in the radius of curvature of the lens surface are achieved, thus modifying the refractive power of an implanted Calhoun LAL to either add or subtract spherical power, adjust along toric axes, or correct higher-order aberrations. Once the appropriate power adjustment is achieved, the entire lens is irradiated to polymerize the remaining unreacted macromer to prevent any additional change in lens power. By irradiating the entire lens, macromer diffusion is prevented, thus no change in lens power results. This second irradiation procedure is referred to as *lock-in*.

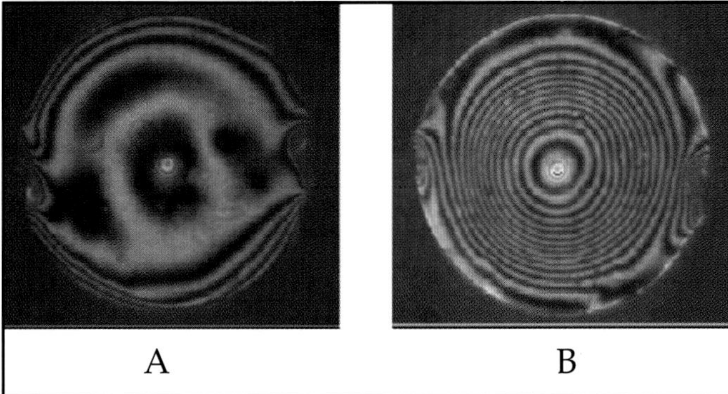

Figure 35-2. In-vitro illustration of LAL power change. (A) Fizeau interference fringes of a Calhoun LAL immersed in water at 35°C before irradiation at best focus (double pass). The fringes present on the periphery of the LAL are due to spherical aberration. (B) Fizeau interference fringes of the same lens 24 hours postirradiation.

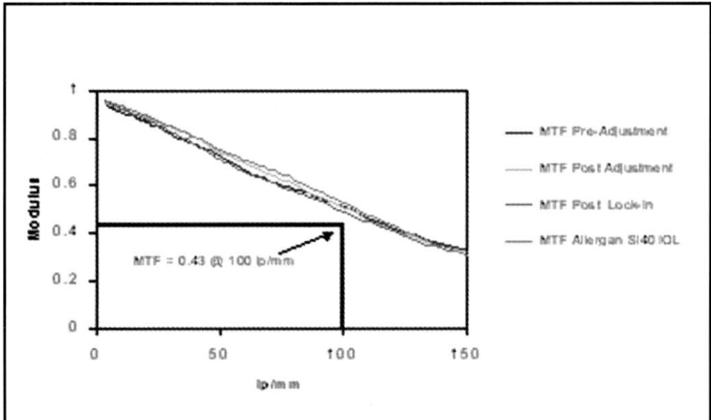

Figure 35-4. Optical quality of the irradiated lens via MTF. MTF of the Calhoun LAL measured from preirradiation through the photolocking procedure. The measurements were performed using the ISO model eye and in accordance with ISO document 11979-2. For comparison, the MTF of a PhakoFlex II SI40NB silicone IOL was measured in an identical manner and plotted on the same graph.

> Once the appropriate power adjustment is achieved, the entire lens is irradiated to polymerize the remaining unreacted macromer to prevent any additional change in lens power.

Spherical Corrections

To illustrate an in-vitro example of this process, a Calhoun LAL was fixed in a water cell maintained at 35°C. The Calhoun LAL was placed one focal length away from the focus of a 4 inch transmission sphere (f/3.3) fitted to a Fizeau interferometer (WYKO 400) (VeeCo, Tuscon, Ariz). Figure 35-2A displays the interference fringes of the Calhoun LAL at its best focus or null position prior to irradiation. The periphery of the Calhoun LAL was irradiated, causing the diffusion of macromer from the central portion of the lens out to the edges. Figure 35-2B displays the interference fringes 24 hours postirradiation at the original best focus position. The most striking feature of this figure is the addition of ~14 (in double pass) fringes of defocus (or wavefront curvature) added to the lens, which corresponds to -2 D of myopic correction.

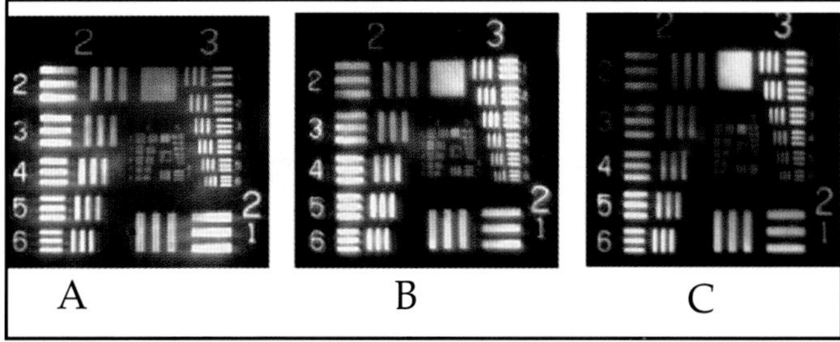

Figure 35-3. Calhoun LAL optical quality before and after power change USAF target imaged in air through (A) Calhoun LAL preirradiation and (B) the same Calhoun LAL 24 hours postirradiation after -2 D have been subtracted from the lens. (C) Commercial silicone IOL (PhakoFlex II SI40NB) (+20 D) for comparison.

After the Calhoun LAL is irradiated, it is imperative that the lens maintain a resolution efficiency that is acceptable to the patient. To monitor the resolution efficiency of the Calhoun LAL before and after irradiation, the Calhoun LAL shown in Figure 35-2 was placed on a collimation bench fitted with a standard 1951 United States Air Force (USAF) "6th root of two" resolution target. The image of the resolution target (measured in air) before irradiation is shown in Figure 35-3A. Inspection of this image shows that the Calhoun LAL, in air, can easily resolve the group 4 element 1 (G4 E1) of the target. Figure 35-3B shows the imaged target 24 hours postirradiation after inducing -2 D of change. Inspection of the images shows that the Calhoun LAL can resolve G4 E1 on the chart, indicating that resolution efficiency is not compromised after irradiation. For comparison, a standard, commercial +20 D IOL (PhakoFlex II SI40NB, Advanced Medical Optics Inc, Santa Ana, Calif) is shown in Figure 35-3C.

> The image resolution before irradiation is not compromised after irradiation.

Another metric that can be used to assess the optical performance of the Calhoun LAL is measurement of the modulation transfer function (MTF). Figure 35-4 displays the MTF of a representative Calhoun LAL through the adjustment and photolocking procedures. For comparison, the MTF of a standard +20 D PhakoFlex II SI40NB IOL is also plotted. Inspection of the data indicates that after the photolocking procedure, the Calhoun LAL still maintains an MTF above the minimum value of 0.43 at 100 line-pairs per millimeter (lp/mm) established by the International Organization for Standards (ISO) and compares quite favorably to commercially available IOLs.

Multifocality and the Calhoun Light Adjustable Lens

Accommodation, as it relates to the human visual system, refers to the ability of a person to use his or her unassisted ocular structure to view objects at both near (eg, reading) and far (eg, driving) distances. The mechanism whereby humans accommodate involves contraction and relaxation of the ciliary body, which inserts into the capsular bag surrounding the natural lens. Under the application of ciliary stress, the human lens will undergo a shape change, effectively altering the radius of curva-

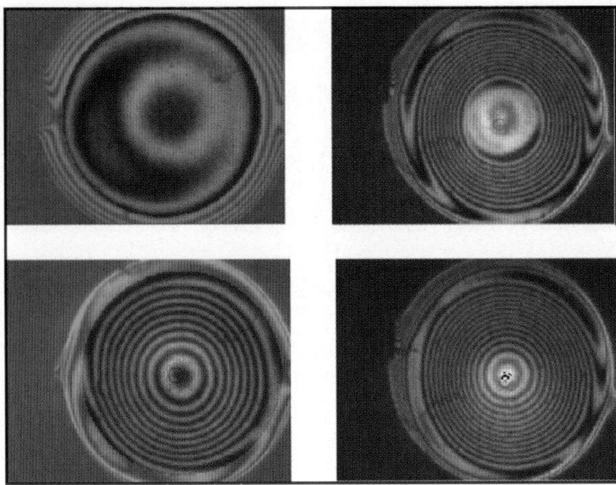

Figure 35-5. Illustration of the Calhoun LAL multifocality and multiple irradiations. The base power of the Calhoun LAL is +22.5 D. Each of these interferograms was taken at the preirradiation best focus position along the axis of the interferometer.

ture of the lens. This action produces a concomitant change in the power of the lens. However, as people grow older, the ability to accommodate is reduced dramatically. This condition is known as *presbyopia* and currently affects more than 100 million people in the United States.

To effectively treat both presbyopia and cataracts, the patient can be implanted with a multifocal IOL. The general concepts and designs of multifocal IOLs have been described in the literature. The simplest design for a multifocal IOL is commonly referred to as the "bull's-eye" configuration and consists of a small, central add zone (1.5 millimeters [mm] to 2.5 mm in diameter) that provides near vision.[17,18] The power of the central add zone is typically between 3 to 4 D greater than the base power of the IOL, which translates to an effective add of 2.5 to 3.5 D for the entire ocular system. The portion of the lens outside the central add zone is referred to as the base power and is used for distance viewing. In theory, as the pupil constricts for near viewing, only that central add zone of the lens will have light from the image passing through it. However, under bright viewing condition, the pupil will also constrict, leaving the patient 2 to 3 D myopic. This can be potentially problematic for a person who is driving in a direction with the sun shining straight at them (eg, driving west around the time of sunset). To counteract this problem, a multifocal IOL could have an annular design with the central and peripheral portion of the lens designed for distance viewing and a paracentral ring (2.1 to 3.5 mm) for near vision. This design will maintain distance viewing even if the pupil constricts.[17,18] The most widely adopted multifocal IOL currently sold in the United States is the Array lens, which consists of five concentric, aspheric annular zones. Each zone is a multifocal element and thus pupil size should play little or no role in determining final image quality.

However, as with standard IOLs, the power and focal zones of multifocal lenses must be estimated prior to implantation. Errors in estimating the needed power, as well as shifting of the lens postoperatively due to wound healing, often result in less than optimal vision. The latter effect is particularly problematic for the case of the bull's-eye lens if a transverse (ie, perpendicular to the visual axis) shift of the IOL occurred during healing. This would effectively move the add part off the visual axis of the eye, resulting in the loss of desired multifocality. The Array and paracentral IOL designs can partly overcome the dislocation problem during wound healing, although any IOL movement longitudinally (the direction along the visual axis), pre-existing astigmatism, or astigmatism induced by the surgical procedure cannot be compensated for using these multifocal IOL designs. This results in the patient having to choose between additional surgery to replace or reposition the lens or to use additional corrective lenses.

Therefore, a need exists for an IOL that can be adjusted postoperatively after implantation and wound healing to form a multifocal IOL. This type of lens can be designed in vivo to correct an initial emmetropic state and then the multifocality may be added during a second treatment. Such a lens would remove any guesswork involved in presurgical power selection, overcome the wound healing response inherent in IOL implantation, allow the size of the add or subtract zone(s) to be customized to correspond to the patient's magnitude and characteristics of dilation under different illumination conditions, and allow the corrected zones to be placed along the patient's visual axis.

This type of multifocal IOL can be designed in vivo to correct an initial emmetropic state and then the multifocality may be added during a second treatment. Such a lens would allow the size of the add or subtract zone(s) to be customized to correspond to the patient's magnitude and characteristics of dilation under different illumination conditions, and allow the corrected zones to be placed along the patient's visual axis.

An example of this capability for the Calhoun LAL is depicted in Figure 35-5. Figure 35-5A displays the interference fringes of a +22.5 D LAL at its preirradiation best focus position along the optical axis of the interferometer. Now let us assume that a cataract surgeon implanted this lens in a patient, but due to wound healing and inaccurate biometric preoperative measurements the postoperative refraction indicates that in order to bring the patient to emmetropia 2 D of power would have to be removed from the Calhoun LAL. Furthermore, let us assume that the physician initially would like the patient to be left slightly myopic post-treatment, a common practice among cataract surgeons. Figure 35-5B shows the Calhoun LAL postirradiation at the same position along the optical axis of the interferometer as in Figure 35-5A. The most striking feature of this interferogram is the appearance of 10 fringes (five waves in double pass) of spherical power change, which corresponds to a removal -1.5 D from the Calhoun LAL. Before final photolocking, the physician can then instruct the patient to try this correction and determine if he or she is satisfied or if he or she would require further adjustment. For this scenario, we shall assume that the patient would like to be brought to full emmetropia. The surgeon can retreat the Calhoun LAL to remove another -0.5 D of power from the lens. The ability of the Calhoun LAL to be treated multiple times is illustrated in Figure 35-5C, which shows the interference fringes of the Calhoun LAL after a second adjustment and the appearance of an additional four fringes (two waves) of power change corresponding to subtraction of another -0.5 D. At this point, the physician is free to impart a degree of bifocality to the Calhoun LAL by either adding or subtracting a desired amount of power in the central portion of the Calhoun LAL with a diameter that meets the patient's dilation characteristics. This is illustrated in Figure 35-5D, which shows the appearance of a 2 mm, +2 D add zone in the central portion of the Calhoun LAL as indicated by the nulled central fringe area.

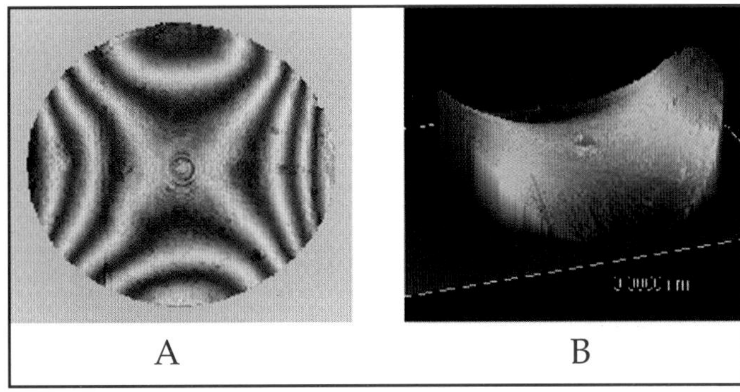

Figure 35-6. Correction of astigmatism with the Calhoun LAL. (A) Raw interference fringes of the LAL after application of astigmatic correction to the LAL. The interference fringes were recorded at the best focus position between the tangential and sagittal foci. (B) Three-dimensional (3-D) wavefront rendering of the fringes shown in A.

Astigmatic Corrections

In addition to simple defocus errors, another lower-order optical aberration that dramatically reduces vision quality is astigmatism. These toric errors are either pre-existing or induced during the cataract surgical procedure. The Calhoun LAL technology can be extended to treat these errors as well. This is accomplished by irradiating along the predetermined astigmatic meridian with a toric spatial intensity profile (Figure 35-6).

Correction of Higher-Order Aberrations With a Digital Mirror Device

As described above, the Calhoun LAL has been shown in the laboratory to be quite adequate in the correction of myopic, hyperopic, and toric errors. However, with the recent push by researchers and physicians toward more accurate determinations of the refractive state of the eye as well as the desire to measure and potentially correct higher-order ocular aberrations, it is a logical extension of the Calhoun LAL technology to address these types of corrections as well. As previously mentioned, the refractive change induced in the Calhoun LAL is dependent not only upon the intensity, wavelength, and duration of the exposure but also the spatial intensity profile of the applied light. One method that can be used to spatially profile the light across the full aperture of the Calhoun LAL is the use of apodizing filters. This approach has been used quite successfully in the correction of both spherical and toric changes in the Calhoun LAL and can be universally applied to patients to correct these lower-order aberrations. However, the main drawback to this type of approach for higher-order aberrations is that it would require a customized apodizing filter for each patient, which would not be cost or time effective. A pre-existing technology that can be applied to the LAL to address this problem is the use of a digital mirror device (DMD).

Editor's note:
The DMD allows for customization of light delivery that cannot be achieved by preset apodizing filters used in correcting lower-order aberrations. The DMD has a micromirror array that either reflects each pixel of light into or away from the projection lens, thereby customizing the light profile according a higher-order wavefront pattern.
R. Krueger, MD, MSE

A picture of a digital light delivery breadboard system is shown in Figure 35-7. At the heart of this instrument is the DMD, which is a pixilated, micromechanical spatial light modulator formed monolithically on a silicon substrate. Typical DMD chips have dimensions of 0.594 x 0.501 inches and the micromirrors are 13 to 17 microns (µm) on an edge and are covered with a reflective aluminum coating. The micromirrors are arranged in an xy array, and the chips contain row drivers, column drivers, and timing circuitry. The addressing circuitry under each mirror pixel is a memory cell that drives two electrodes under the mirror with complimentary voltages. Depending on the state of the memory cell (a "1" or "0"), each mirror is electrostatically attracted by a combination of the bias and address voltages to one of the other address electrodes. Physically, the mirror can rotate ±10 degrees. A "1" in the memory causes the mirror to rotate +10 degrees, while a "0" in the memory causes the mirror to rotate -10 degrees. A mirror rotated to +10 degrees reflects incoming light into the projection lens and onto the IOL through the eye. When the mirror is rotated -10 degrees, the reflected light misses the projection lens.

Thus, the great utility and advantage of the DMD device in its relation to the Calhoun LAL is the ability of the researcher/physician to define any spatial intensity profile that is applied to the Calhoun LAL. To assess the ability of the Calhoun LAL to correct higher-order aberrations using the DMD, the Zernike aberration known as tetrafoil and described by the equation:

$$S^4{}_4 = (4\rho^2 - 3)\rho^2\cos 2\theta$$

was programmed into the DMD and the Calhoun LAL was irradiated with this spatial intensity profile. Figure 35-8 shows the grayscale representation of the tetrafoil Zernike term that was applied to the Calhoun LAL.

Figure 35-9A depicts the raw interference fringes of the Calhoun LAL after irradiation with the tetrafoil spatial intensity profile. This figure dramatically shows that the projected spatial intensity profile was reproduced on the wavefront of the Calhoun LAL. To further illustrate this point, the 3-D wavefront calculated from the interference fringes shown in A is displayed in Figure 35-9B. This 3-D rendering shows the four-fold symmetry of the wavefront. In practice, once the Calhoun LAL has been implanted and refractive stabilization has occurred, a wavefront measurement of the eye's aberrations is made. The phase conjugate to these aberrations can then be put into the DMD device; the spatial intensity profile is created and then projected onto the Calhoun LAL to correct the aberration.

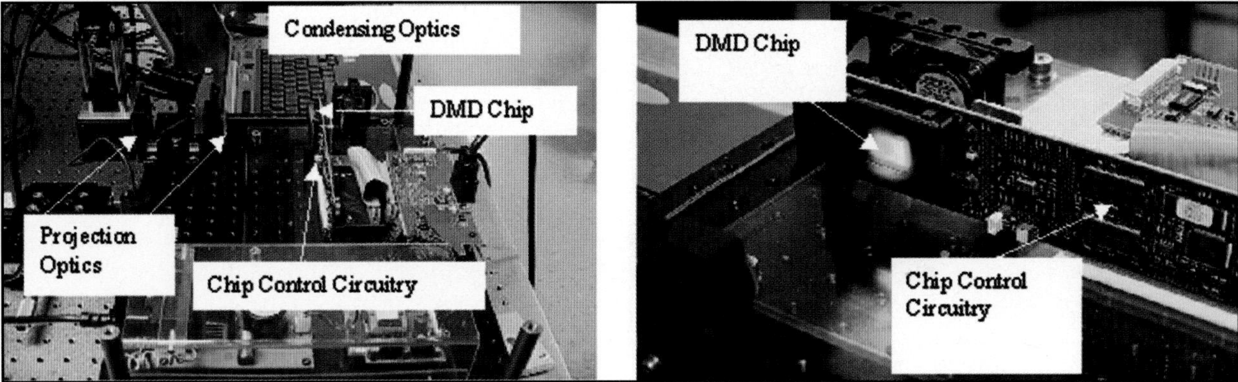

Figure 35-7. Digital light delivery breadboard system. (Courtesy of Carl Zeiss Meditec, AG.)

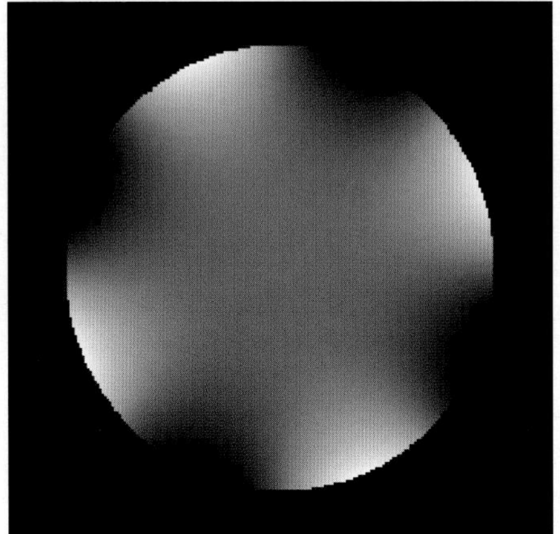

Figure 35-8. Tetrafoil greyscale spatial intensity profile programmed into the DMD.

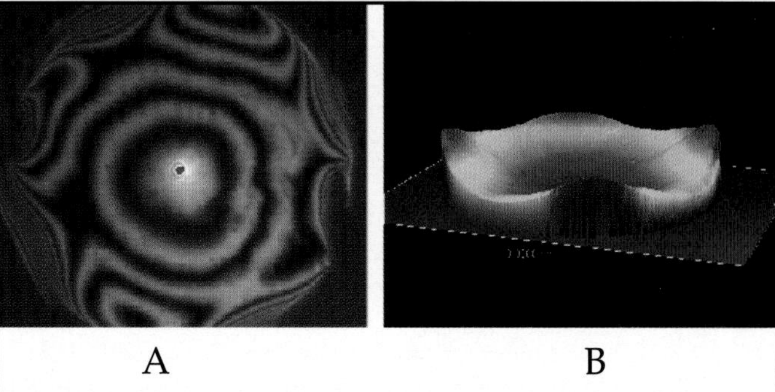

Figure 35-9. (A) Raw interference fringes of the Calhoun LAL post-irradiation with the tetrafoil spatial intensity profile. (B) 3-D wavefront rendering of the interference fringes in A.

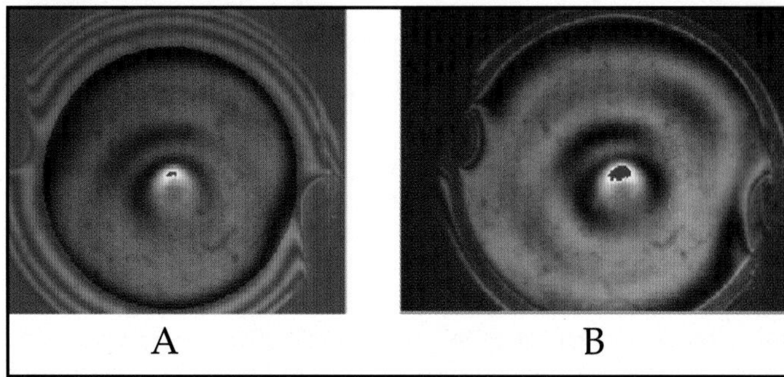

Figure 35-10. (A) Preirradiation interferogram of the Calhoun LAL with central 4 to 4.5 mm aperture of the lens at best focus. (B) Interferogram of the Calhoun LAL postirradiation at the same position along the optical axis of the interferometer.

In practice, once the Calhoun LAL has been implanted and refractive stabilization has occurred, a wavefront measurement of the eye's aberrations is made. The phase conjugate to these aberrations can then be put into the DMD device; the spatial intensity profile is created and then projected onto the LAL to correct the aberration.

A higher-order aberration that is universally common in people is the presence of spherical aberration. The wavefront of this aberration can be represented by the following Zernike polynomial:

$$C^0_4 = 6\rho^4 - 6\rho^2 - 1$$

The effect of this aberration is to cause rays of light impinging on the periphery of the lens to come to a different focus than being refracted through the central part of the optic. Applying the principles of geometric optics, one way to minimize spherical aberration is to create an aspheric lens, which in its simplest form would possess a radius of curvature difference between the central and peripheral regions. As an example of this, Figure 35-10A shows the interference fringes from a +20.50 D Calhoun LAL preirradiation. Inspection of this figure shows that the power across the central 4 to 4.5 mm of the Calhoun LAL's wavefront has been minimized. However, inspection of the interference fringes outside this region to the edge of the Calhoun LAL shows the presence of approximately four fringes (two waves) due to spherical aberration. Figure 35-10B shows the Calhoun LAL at the same position along the optical axis of the interferometer after it was irradiated on its periphery to effectively change the radius of curvature on the outside portion and reduce the amount of spherical aberration. Comparison of Figures 35-10A and 35-10B shows that the wavefront of the central 4 to 4.5 mm of the Calhoun LAL has remained unchanged due to the irradiation process; however, inspection of the periphery of the Calhoun LAL indicates the removal of two fringes (one wave) of spherical aberration. Therefore, the Calhoun LAL technology shows promise of being able to reduce the amount of spherical aberration of an implanted lens and thus the overall spherical aberration of the entire ocular system.

Conclusion

Despite advances in cataract and refractive surgery, imprecise IOL power determination and unpredictable wound healing remain important clinical problems to address. For the first time, the Calhoun LAL provides a tool for the cataract and refractive surgeon to noninvasively correct the refractive power of an IOL postimplantation. LAL formulations are useful in both pseudophakic and phakic IOLs. As additional IOLs, such as accommodative versions, become available, postoperative adjustability of IOL power will enhance value of these and other novel IOL technologies.

References

1. Leaming DV. Practice styles and preferences of ASCRS members—1999 survey. *J Cataract Refract Surg*. 2000;26(6):913-921.
2. Brandser R, Haaskjold E, Drolsum L. Accuracy of IOL calculation in cataract surgery. *Acta Ophthalmol Scan*. 1997;75(2):162-165.
3. Olsen T, Thim K, Corydon L. Accuracy of the newer generation intraocular-lens power calculation formulas in long and short eyes. *J Cataract Refract Surg*. 1991;17(2):187-193.
4. Olsen T. Sources of error in intraocular lens power calculation. *J Cataract Refract Surg*. 1992;18(2):125-129.
5. Pierro L, Modorati G, Brancato R. Clinical variability in keratometry, ultrasound biometry measurements, and emmetropic intraocular-lens power calculation. *J Cataract Refract Surg*. 1991;17(1):91-94.
6. Mendivil A. Intraocular lens implantation through 3.2 versus 4.0 mm incisions. *J Cataract Refract Surg*. 1996;22(10):1461-1464.
7. Sun XY, Vicary D, Montgomery P, Griffiths M. Toric intraocular lenses for correcting astigmatism in 130 eyes. *Ophthalmology*. 2000; 107(9):1776-81.
8. Steinert RF, Aker BL, Trentacost DJ, Smith PJ, Tarantino N. A prospective comparative study of the AMO ARRAY zonal-progressive multifocal silicone intraocular lens and a monofocal intraocular lens. *Ophthalmology*. 1999;106(7):1243-1255.
9. Javitt JC, Wang F, Trentacost DJ, Rowe M, Tarantino N. Outcomes of cataract extraction with multifocal intraocular lens implantation - functional status and quality of life. *Ophthalmology*. 1997;104(4):589-599.
10. Negishi K, BissenMiyajima H, Kato K, Kurosaka D, Nagamoto T. Evaluation of a zonal-progressive multifocal intraocular lens. *Am J Ophthalmol*. 1997;124(3):321-330.
11. Zaldivar R, Davidorf JM, Oscherow S. Posterior chamber phakic intraocular lens for myopia of -8 to -19 diopters. *J Refract Surg*. 1998;14(3):294-305.
12. Baikoff G, Arne JL, Bokobza Y, et al. Angle-fixated anterior chamber phakic intraocular lens for myopia of -7 to -19 diopters. *J Refract Surg*. 1998;14(3):282-293.
13. Rosen E, Gore C. STAAR Collamer posterior chamber phakic intraocular lens to correct myopia and hyperopia. *J Cataract Refract Surg*. 1998;24(5):596-606.
14. Seitz B, Langenbucher A. Intraocular lens power calculation in eyes after corneal refractive surgery. *J Refract Surg*. 2000;16(3);349-361
15. Seitz B, Langenbucher A. Intraocular lens calculations status after corneal refractive surgery. *Curr Opinion Ophthalmology*. 2000;11(1): 35-46.
16. Gimbel HV, Sun R, Furlong MT, van Westenbrugge JA, Kassab J. Accuracy and predictability of intraocular lens power after photorefractive keratectomy. *J Cataract Refract Surg*. 2000;26(8):1147-1151.
17. Azar DT, et al. *Intraocular Lenses in Cataract and Refractive Surgery*. Philadelphia, Pa: WB Saunders; 2001.
18. Stamper RL, Sugar A, Ripkin DJ. Intraocular lenses: basics and clinical applications. Paper presented at: the American Academy of Ophthalmology; November 15, 1993; Chicago, Ill.

Section V

Nonwavefront Customized Corrections

Basic Science Section

Chapter 36

Corneal Topography and Customized Ablation

Charles E. Campbell, BS

In a certain sense, all refractive corrections of the eye are customized because each eye has a unique refractive error and it is that unique error that must be corrected. The term *customized ablation* has come to take on a special meaning to differentiate those procedures that correct more complicated refractive errors from those more common procedures that only correct simple spherocylindrical errors. The first corneal refractive surgical procedures attempted to correct only mean spherical error. As a result, the ablation patterns exhibited a great degree of spatial symmetry and so were fairly insensitive to minor positional errors. When correction for astigmatism was added, rotational symmetry was broken and the relationship of the cylinder axis of the ablation to that of the eye became critical. However, from an optical point of view, minor positional errors in the placement of the ablation pattern on the cornea were not too important.

We find the same thing to be true in the more familiar case of spectacles lenses in which we know that the correction for astigmatism in single vision lenses remains good even as the eye turns to look through different portions of the lens, in effect simulating a decentered ablation pattern. The situation is quite different once we attempt to correct localized refractive errors and so attempt a customized ablation. If such an ablation is not precisely aligned both in position and rotational orientation, the refractive result will quite likely be worse than before the procedure, whereas if alignment is correct, vision will be improved. So when a customized ablation is to be used, it is quite important that the measurements of localized error—both magnitude and location—are precisely made. The alignment requirements will be discussed later.

It is the shape of the cornea that is altered during any type of ablative procedure and so it is only reasonable that we would wish to measure that shape prior to any surgery and use this information to attain our goal: improvement of vision through the removal of refractive error. Corneal topography is a means to measure that shape, and we shall be investigating what role corneal topography can have in obtaining this information. Before we can discuss how the information gained through corneal topography can be used to guide customized ablation procedures, it best to first establish what is measured by corneal topography, how it is presented, and what it means to the refractive state of the eye.

The Optical Role of the Cornea

The cornea is one of the principal refractive elements of the eye. It has a highly curved surface and it exists at the interface between the outside world—usually air—and the tissue of the eye itself. We may think of action of any optical refractive surface element to be primarily governed by two parameters: the curvature of the surface and the change index of refraction across that surface. The term *optical refractive surface element* is used to define an optical element where refraction occurs only at the surface, thus differentiating it from an optical element where the index of refraction changes in some continuous fashion in the bulk of the material, thereby causing refraction to occur throughout the element. This is an important consideration for the eye because the optical action of the cornea may be thought to occur solely on its surfaces whereas the refractive action crystalline lens not only comes from its surfaces but also from an index of refraction gradient throughout the bulk of the lens.

For an optical refractive surface element, the refractive power is directly proportional to the product of the change of index of refraction across the surface and the magnitude of the curvature of the surface. With these thoughts in mind, it is easy to see why the cornea is the major refractive element of the eye. It has a very highly curved surface with a radius of curvature in the vicinity of 8 millimeters (mm) and the refractive index at its anterior surface changes from 1.00 in air to 1.336 in the anterior tear film. The crystalline lens has a curvature very similar in magnitude to that of the cornea on its surfaces, but the index change is much less, changing at the surfaces from 1.336 in the aqueous humor to 1.386 at edge of the cortex of the lens. This change of 0.05 is 15% of that at the anterior tear film interface so the refractive action of the lens surface is much less than that of the cornea because it is the product of the refractive index change and the curvature that determines the refractive power of any optical element. It also suggests that any local curvature changes in lens surfaces will have proportionally less overall effect on the refractive state of the eye than changes of the same magnitude in the curvature of the cornea.

It would seem then that the curvature of the cornea and changes to that curvature are the most important parameters to consider when changing the refractive state of the eye via corneal refractive surgery. However, for the purposes of deciding how to control the action of a laser ablation system, curvature is not the most convenient parameter to use. Before explaining why this is the case, let us first consider what the corneal topographer measures at a fundamental level.

Measurements That Can Be Made by a Corneal Topographer: Curvature vs Height

If we were to talk of the topography of the surface of the earth or the topography of some three-dimensional (3-D) object, we would most likely be describing topography in terms of the height or elevation of the surface at designed locations above some fixed plane or reference surface. We would be describing the topography in terms of the 3-D coordinates of the surface. For mostly historical reasons, this is not what is generally meant when one speaks of corneal topography. Corneal measurements were first taken with instruments called *ophthalmometers* or *keratometers*. These instruments measure the curvature of small areas of the cornea by measuring the magnification of luminous targets, known as *mires*, by the highly curved corneal surface. The values thus found are curvature values, and it was in terms of curvature that ophthalmic professionals came to think of characterizing the corneal surface. It was therefore reasonable, when corneal topographers first became available, to present their topographical data in terms of curvature at various locations on the cornea. However, this created a problem in presentation because the curvature at a given location (x, y) on a surface cannot be expressed as a single value as surface elevation (z) can be. Curvature needs three values (ie, sphere, cylinder, and axis) to express it at a given location. Normal topographical maps using contour lines or colors to represent the elevation variable in terms of two position variables are inadequate to fully represent curvature. The compromise that was settled on for corneal topographical curvature maps was to pick one component of the curvature and represent it in a color-coded contour map. The component chosen was the one in the direction of the meridians of a polar coordinate system drawn on the corneal surface and centered on the corneal vertex.

> Curvature needs three values (ie, sphere, cylinder, and axis) to express it at a given location. Therefore, typical topographical maps using contour lines or colors to represent the elevation variable in terms of two position variables are inadequate to fully represent curvature.

The types of analyses customarily used in commercial corneal topographers are not the best to use when considering customized ablation. As will be seen from the discussion below, precise measurements of elevation constitute the best form of data with which to begin any analysis. Some corneal topography systems have the ability to export data of this type and only these systems, if their precision of measurement is high enough, are truly useful tools in matters dealing with customized ablation. In addition, the best methods of curvature analysis are not implemented in commercial topography systems. Consequently, to best use available corneal topography data, one needs to employ specialized analysis methods. Some of these will be mentioned next.

> Precise measurements of elevation constitute the best form of data with which to begin any corneal analysis.

Methods of Analysis Used by Corneal Topographers

How is curvature and elevation information to be obtained by the corneal topographer? Several approaches have been used, among them the keratometric analysis method, the arc step method, and calculations of curvature from analysis of elevation data. They will briefly described next.

Keratometric Analysis Method

It is possible to analyze a multiple ring corneal topographer image (Placido ring system) in the same way one analyzes a keratometer ring image. Each of the multiple rings is considered to be a keratometer ring by itself. Its size, usually expressed as the distance of a location on the ring image from the center of the total image, the corneal vertex, and representing the magnification of the ring by the corneal surface, is converted to a keratometric dioptric value using the logic used in the case of an ophthalmometer. Each chosen location on each ring, defined by the location at which a meridian intersects the ring, is then assigned a curvature value. This method only gives one curvature value at each location, and one finds upon investigation that this is not a true curvature of the surface in any mathematical sense. The keratometric analysis method does not generate corneal surface elevation information.

Arc Step Method

It turns out that there is a better method to analyze the image of a Placido ring system created by the corneal surface to assign the surface curvature than the keratometric analysis method. This method employs a form of ray tracing to follow rays backward from the charge-coupled device (CCD) detector, through the optical system of the topographer to the corneal surface. At the corneal surface, the rays are reflected and pass to their source—the luminous ring. The CCD location, found via image analysis is known as is the geometry of the optical system. This fixes the ray in space both in location and in direction of travel. At some point along its travel, initially an assumed location, the ray strikes the surface of the cornea and is reflected. Having assumed a reflection location and knowing the location of the luminous ring in space, the direction of the ray after reflection is fixed. Then, employing the laws of reflection, the direction of the surface normal (a measure of surface slope) at the point of reflection is found by dividing the angle between the incoming ray and the reflected ray. This slope information is then used to calculate values related to the local curvature of the surface at a great number of points on the corneal surface. If the method used to find these slope values is the iterative method known as the *arc step method*, the elevation of the surface is also found at each measured location along with the surface slope. The arc step method reconstructs a meridian by piecing together short circular arcs that have the characteristic that each joins to its neighbor in such a fashion that the centers of curvatures of both arcs lie on the common line that is coincident with the radii of both arcs at the point at which they join. This insures that the first derivative of the combined arc is everywhere continuous. The procedure consists of proceeding ring by ring, usually starting in the center of the cornea, in such a fashion that the new arc fulfills the joining criterion to its preceding neighbor while fulfilling the reflec-

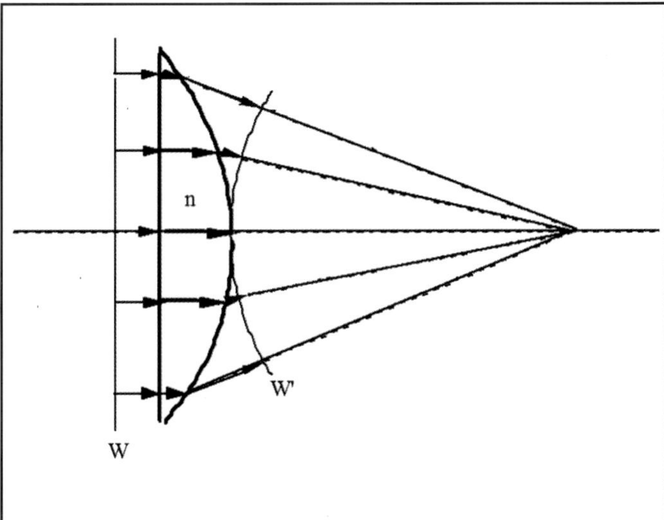

Figure 36-1. Because the OPL for edge rays is less than for central rays, they exit the lens sooner and travel some distance beyond the lens before the central rays exit. This causes the refracted wavefront to take a convex curvature, producing the focusing action of the lens.

tion criterion for the ray under analysis at the farther end. This is done with an iterative process of modifying the radius of curvature of the arc until the ray successfully strikes the end point of the arc and its directed to its proper ring to within the tolerance limits chosen for the process. In this process, the end point locations of each arc are precisely found and this provides the necessary high precision elevation information needed for use in planning and analyzing custom ablations.

Note that surface slope information is only found along the meridians and so must be termed the *meridional slope* instead of the *surface slope*. Nothing is found as to the surface slope in other directions and hence information on surface curvature is incomplete. This is because only along meridians can curvature be found when present-day corneal topographer analysis methods are employed. Such partial displays of curvature have proved extremely useful to clinicians to get an overall subjective idea of the refractive state of the cornea, but they are not particularly useful for optical analysis of the cornea via ray tracing and other analytical methods.

For full ray tracing, one needs to know the surface normal at various locations. The surface normal is a line passing through a point on the surface perpendicular to a plane tangent to the surface at that point. To know the surface normal, one needs to know not only to the surface slope along a meridian but also the slope at right angles to the meridian. So it seems that corneal topography, as currently done, is not adequate for detailed analysis of refractive error. However, if the elevation information—which is obtained in addition to slope information in certain analysis methods—is considered, the situation changes and there is a way to analyze the optical action of the cornea in great detail.

Curvature From Elevation Data

While the arc step method, as currently implemented, does not give complete curvature information on the corneal surface, it does yield very accurate surface elevation data on the surface. This information is complete in that it completely specifies the corneal shape. If the elevation is of sufficient precision, complete curvature information of the corneal surface may be found using well-known methods from differential geometry that involve finding the surface gradient at each desired location from the elevation information and then using the gradient information to find the second derivatives of the surface at each location. The surface gradients and the second derivative values are then used to find all three curvature values at each location.

Treatment of the Optical Action of a Refractive Element in Terms of its Thickness (Optical Path Length)

The optical action of a refractive element has thus far been considered to be governed by the change in index of refraction at its surfaces and by the surface curvatures. There is a very different way to treat optical action that is just as valid and useful as the more common approach. Instead of considering the refraction of light rays by a surface, one considers the change in optical path length (OPL) for different rays as they pass through an optical element and imposes the restraint that each ray as it progresses from an initial wavefront to a refracted wavefront has the same OPL. The OPL for a segment of a ray is defined as the physical distance along the ray segment multiplied by the index of refraction found in that segment:

$$\text{OPL} = \text{physical distance} \times \text{index of refraction} \quad (1)$$

The OPL for a segment of a ray is defined as the physical distance along the ray segment multiplied by the index of refraction found in that segment.

To see how this creates optical action, consider a simple positive lens. Such lenses are thicker in the middle than at the edge. This means that the OPL of a ray passing through the middle of the lens has a longer OPL than does a ray passing through the edge. Now let this positive lens have a plano front surface and a convex back surface and suppose that a plane wavefront enters the flat front surface so that all rays enter the lens at once. Because the OPL for edge rays is less than for central rays, they exit the lens sooner and travel some distance beyond the lens before the central rays exit. This causes the refracted wavefront to take a convex curvature, producing the focusing action of the lens. This is illustrated in the Figure 36-1.

This is a very simple example, but the approach is general and it allows the optical behavior to be expressed in terms of the change in thickness of a lens or other optical element as the position on the element changes. In addition, this method allows aberrations to be treated by considering them to be differences in OPL between the actual wavefront and some ideal wavefront at various positions on the wavefront. We can therefore use distance measures, in the form of elevation changes of a surface, to analyze its optical performance instead of using curvature information or surface slope information. In many ways, this is a better approach because it allows very powerful optical analysis theorems to be used to predict the quality of images without having to resort to ray tracing. Ray tracing is difficult to perform precisely in the case of the eye because of uncertainty regarding the optical characteristics of an individual crystalline lens. There is no convenient way to precisely measure the surface profile or the index of refraction gradient within this gradient index lens in the living eye. Even if precise ray tracing could be done, interpretation of ray intercepts with the fovea is not as easy as interpretation of point spread functions (PSFs) and spatial frequency spectrums, which can be directly related to contrast sensitivity and visual resolution (computed directly from wavefront error information).

For the purposes of controlling a laser ablation system, the thickness approach to characterizing a lens is the only practical one. Refractive correction is accomplished when using photorefractive keratectomy (PRK) or laser in-situ keratomileusis (LASIK) procedure by removing a tissue lens with the laser system. This tissue lens will be referred to as the *treatment lenticule*. The power of this treatment lenticule is the power of the refractive error. As the laser selectively removes tissue to remove the treatment lenticule, it needs to know how much tissue to remove at different locations. When the treatment lenticule is characterized by thickness, the information needed by the laser is immediately available. In fact, for simple refractive errors, there is no need for information on the topography of the cornea. A treatment lenticule with the correct thickness gradient to produce the desired correction is removed and the optical result is the desired one regardless of the shape of the corneal surface.

> Refractive correction is accomplished when using PRK or LASIK procedure by removing a tissue lens with the laser system. This tissue lens will be referred to as the *treatment lenticule*.

Customized Ablation

We have defined customized ablation as corneal refractive surgical procedures that correct more complicated refractive errors than simple spherocylindrical ones. We may wish to do this for a variety of reasons. An earlier procedure may have induced corneal irregularity that we wish to remove. We may wish to remove higher-order aberrations of the eye in addition to spherocylindrical error, thereby increasing the resolution of the eye. No matter what the reason for the customization, it will be necessary to measure the aberrations of the eye carefully so that they are well characterized not only in magnitude but also in location with respect to the pupil of the eye. This information must then be converted to instructions for the laser ablation system that consist of amounts of tissue to be removed at specified locations.

Wavefront Error

The most convenient form for the aberration information for the above use is in terms of wavefront error. The wavefront error is the OPL difference at each location between the desired wavefront and the actual wavefront. Because OPL is the product of the index of refraction and the physical path length, a measurement method that measures an actual surface and compares it to a desired surface in essence finds the wavefront error. In the case of the cornea, the index of refraction to use is the index of refraction of the stroma (1.376).

We now can see how information from a corneal topographer can be used if the system can measure the 3-D position of the surface. What the corneal topographer does not measure is the shape of the desired corneal surface. This must be supplied in some fashion. There are a number of reasonable approaches.

One approach uses a combination of the desired spherocylindrical correction and considerations of aberration-free surfaces. Usually, there is a spherocylindrical refractive error to be removed and the ablation profile to accomplish this can be found without any reference to the cornea surface as was noted previously. The elevation values associated with the spherocylindrical correction can then be directly subtracted from the measured corneal elevation values to give the surface that will exist after the basic correction. It is known that surfaces that minimize aberration are very smooth surfaces in the sense that their curvature changes slowly as a function of position. The cornea can exhibit fluctuations in curvature on a very local basis. If these local fluctuations can be removed, the higher-order aberrations will also be reduced. This can be done by fitting the surface found by subtracting spherocylindrical ablation pattern from the measured surface to a smooth function, such a general ellipsoid. The elevation difference between this surface and the best fit smooth surface gives the extra amount of ablation needed to remove corneal irregularities and the resulting higher-order aberrations from the eye.

> Approaches to correct the optical errors of the eye, which by design minimize corneal aberration and ignore the contributions of the crystalline lens to the total aberration of the eye, are at risk of increasing the residual higher-order aberration of the eye.

There is an even better way to assess the aberrations introduced into the optical system of the eye due to the cornea alone. This is to find a corneal surface that would introduce no aberrations at all, select this surface as a reference, and find the wavefront error induced by the cornea by subtracting the reference surface from the actual surface to create a tissue error lens. The aberrations created by this tissue error lens are the aberrations induced by the corneal surface. Such aberration-free surfaces have been known since 1637 when they were introduced by Descartes and are known as *Cartesian ovals*. These ovals take the simple form of an ellipsoid of revolution whose eccentricity is given by the ratio of the index of refraction of the incident media to the index of refraction of the media following the interface. Taking the incident index of refraction to be that of air (1.000) and the exiting index of the refraction to be that of the corneal stroma (1.376), the Cartesian oval desired has an eccentricity of 0.73 and is thus more aspheric than the mean human cornea with an eccentricity (0.55). It now remains to find the apical curvature of this ellipsoid to completely specify it. This may be done by measuring the spherical equivalent refractive error of the eye, subtracting this from the mean surface power of the central cornea and converting the remaining surface power of the cornea to a curvature value. Such a surface will insure that a central collimated pencil of light entering the eye focuses on the retina.

Corneal aberrations found in this way are particularly valuable when they are used in conjunction with aberrations found using a wavefront refractor because they give information on not only the aberrations induced by the corneal surface but also on the aberrations induced by the rest of the optical system of the eye.

When the above method is employed, there are some technical details that need to be considered. The coordinate systems of corneal topography typically use the corneal vertex as the origin. For analysis of wavefront error, it is best to use a coordinate system whose origin is the pupil center. This means that the displacement, if any, of the corneal vertex and the pupil center must be measured and the reference Cartesian oval decentered by this amount when it is subtracted from the corneal elevation data to create the tissue error lens. When this is done, tilt (prism) is invariably introduced into the tissue error lens. This tilt should be removed from the subsequent analysis, as it can have no effect on image formation. There is indeed a prismatic effect introduced by the decentration of the corneal vertex from the pupil center but it is optically removed by a simple eye turn so that the object of interest falls on the fovea.

> One eye can adjust for tilt by a simple eye turn; however, under binocular conditions, induced prism could produce a binocular imbalance.

Consideration of Alignment Precision Needed for Customized Ablations

There is no way that a hard and fast rule can be given for necessary alignment precision because of the wide variation in the size and severity of localized refractive errors found in practice. It is helpful, though, to think of the situation in this way. Suppose that there is a local corneal irregularity that degrades vision by some amount. We may think of the correction for this irregularity as the addition of second corneal irregularity that is equal but opposite to the original so that the two cancel one another. Now let us suppose that we misalign the correction so that it does not fall on the original. It then adds a refractive error similar in magnitude to the original error without causing the original to go away. In the worst case, we have essentially doubled the problem for the visual system. On the other hand, if our misalignment is only partial, then some cancellation of error will occur and the net result may be an improvement. This is a very simple approach to what in practice will be a fairly complicated optical situation, but it gives us good direction in our thinking on this matter. It must also be noted that errors of alignment can be rotational as well as translational; a concept well known from our experience in correcting astigmatism. Perhaps the most important idea, as we consider the alignment precision needed for customized ablation, is that the size of the local irregularity is not only important from the point of view of its effect on vision but also on the precision with which we must apply a correction ablation to remove its effect. A second important idea is that the magnitude of the irregularity is also important. To see this, consider the familiar case of correction for simple astigmatism and the need to correctly orient cylinder axis. The residual refractive error when axis is misaligned is proportional to the product of the axis error (the rotational positional error) and the original magnitude of the cylinder error. Much more axis error can be tolerated for a small amount of cylinder power error than can be tolerated for a large amount of cylinder power error.

To treat the requirements for alignment in an analytical manner, the following approach is suggested. Starting with 3-D information on the wavefront error function, a transformation of the coordinate system consisting of a translation and rotation of the desired amount is made, and the wavefront error function is expressed in this new system. Next, the difference between the original and the transformed wavefront error function is found, thus creating a new wavefront error function. This wavefront error function may be considered to be the aberrations induced by the misalignment. To make the approach practical, the initial wavefront error needs to be expressed as an analytical function, and this is most easily done by expressing it in terms of Zernike polynomial functions weighted by their respective coefficients. There exist fairly simple mathematical methods for performing the needed coordinate transformation on a set of Zernike polynomial functions that yield the coefficients for the transformed functions. These may then be directly subtracted from the original coefficient set to give the residual error in terms of its Zernike coefficients.

One interesting effect of applying decentered aberration corrections is that aberrations of different types and symmetries than those found in the original aberration set are generated while at the same time the original aberrations are removed. The simplest example is the well-known effect of introducing prism when a spherocylindrical correction is decentered. When one considers some of the common higher-order aberrations, one finds that decentering a coma correction generates astigmatism and defocus, decentering a trefoil correction generates astigmatism, and decentering a spherical aberration correction generates coma. In general, decentered corrections have the interesting effect of correcting the aberrations they are designed to correct while at the same time generating new aberrations of lower order than the original aberrations.

When aberration corrections are applied with a rotation or axis error, another effect occurs. Now one finds that no aberrations of lower order are introduced, but that original aberrations whose meridional index is non-zero are not completely removed so that a residual magnitude remains with the axis of that aberration (when expressed in magnitude/axis form) rotated.

> Decentered corrections remove the original error and generate lower-order aberrations of opposite meridional symmetry. Rotated corrections do not induce aberrations of different order or meridional symmetry but partially remove the original aberration and rotate its axis.

Requirements for Corneal Topographers When Used to Guide Customized Ablation

A corneal topographer must be able to measure the elevation of the corneal surface for it to be useful for planning customized ablation. Systems that only measure curvature may be useful for subjective evaluation of the corneal surface, but they are not adequate tools for planning customized ablation. For those corneal topographers that can make elevation information available, only those with sufficient precision of measurement are truly useful. To guide us on setting limits for this necessary precision, we have the characteristics of laser ablation systems and the magnitude of expected aberrations. It is best to express aberrations in terms of OPL and the appropriate unit is the wavelength of light. Therefore, errors are best expressed in microns (μm), as the midrange wavelength value for the visible spectrum is

0.55 μm. Laser ablation systems typically remove 0.25 μm of tissue per pulse. As this is stromal tissue with an index of refraction of 1.376, the OPL removed per pulse is 0.62 wave (dividing equation 1 by the wave length).

OPL = physical distance x index of refraction/wavelength

OPL = 0.25 x 1.376/0.55 = 0.62 waves

Since we are really interested in the change wavefront error caused by the ablation, what is important is the change in OPL from the case of light traveling through stromal tissue to that of light traveling through air, when the stromal tissue is removed. The change in OPL—d(OPL)—is the physical distance times the change in index of refraction. A single ablation pulse changes the OPL, in waves, by 0.17 waves:

d(OPL) = physical distance x (index of refraction in tissue - index of refraction in air)/wavelength

d(OPL) = 0.25 x (1.376 -1.000) /0.55 = 0.17 wave

There is little need to measure surface details to an accuracy greater than the minimum amount of tissue that can be removed.

To get an idea of the elevation resolution needed for custom ablation, let us first consider the variation in thickness for a tissue lens that represents a change in refractive power of 0.25 diopters (D). A change in refractive power of this magnitude can be expressed in terms of wavefront error if a pupil diameter is assumed. Using the simple approximation for sag of a sphere:

$$sag = D^2F/8 \quad (2)$$

where D is the diameter of the aperture (in mm) and F is the power (in D), the sag is expressed in microns. The wavefront error, W, from the center to the edge of the aperture given in waves is the sag divided by the wavelength of light.

$$W = sag/wavelength = D^2F/(8\ wavelengths) \quad (3)$$

If a 3 mm pupil is chosen and the wavelength is 0.55 μm, W is 0.51 waves. It should be noted in passing that this is twice the Rayleigh criterion for the amount of wavefront error that is just enough to perceptibly change image quality. This fact provides a physical reason for the observation that 0.25 D blur is just noticeable under normal visual conditions. We should also note that often the wavefront error is not expressed as the difference from the aperture center to the edge but in terms of the root mean square (RMS) wavefront error. To convert W to RMS error for simple surface forms such as spheres, ellipsoids, and toric surfaces, a good approximation is found by multiplying W by the factor 0.30:

$$RMS\ error \cong 0.3 \times W \quad (4)$$

The RMS error corresponding to the Rayleigh quarter wave criterion is 0.075 wave:

$$0.075 = 0.3 \times 0.25$$

To find out what a 0.25 D error means in terms of the variation in thickness of a corneal tissue lens, we may use the simple formula that is widely used to calculate ablation depths (equation 2 divided by n-1) :

$$d = D^2F/8(n-1) \quad (5)$$

where d is the variation in lens thickness (in μm), D is the diameter (in mm), F is the power (in D), and n is the index of refraction of the tissue. Choosing a pupil diameter of 3 mm, we find that the thickness variation from tissue lens center to edge is 0.75 μm. As this thickness is equivalent to the ablation effect of just three nominal pulses, it first shows us that customized ablation will require an ablation system to operate at the limit of its capability in any case. Interestingly, the change in measured RMS wavefront error for the higher-order aberrations found in recent LASIK studies show increases of about 0.15 wave. Removal of this error is certainly at the limit of a system that removes 0.17 waves per pulse.

It is clear that a corneal topography system needs to be able to measure surface elevation differences to better than 1 μm resolution to be useful in guiding customized ablation. This is not to say that corneal topography systems with less resolution are not useful in assessing larger corneal surface features. They are valuable in monitoring change both following corneal procedure and for other purposes. Wavefront errors beyond those of normal refractive errors are of a size that they will not be detected unless a measurement system has this resolution. Current Placido disk-based corneal topography systems using arc step reconstruction algorithms are able to resolve corneal surface elevation variations to about 0.7 μm. These systems give the best resolution available today.

> This means that highest resolution corneal topography systems available are just able to detect the presence of surface variations that will contribute to higher-order wavefront errors as 0.7 μm of tissue removal converts to 0.48 wave of wavefront change.

For those more familiar with the performance of corneal topography system expressed in axial curvature values (keratometric diopters), the following example is given to illustrate the relationship between variation in surface elevation and variation in axial curvature in a local area of the corneal surface. Let us take a circular area of the corneal 1.5 mm in diameter and let it have an axial curvature value 1 D greater that the surrounding area. Then using equation 5 and the nominal index of refraction value taken to express keratometric diopter of 1.3375, we find the variation in elevation, d, to be 0.833 μm. As we know that the better corneal topography system can detect curvature changes of this size over this area, we see that they have resolution that is in the range that is useful for customized ablation. This simple test can be used to judge the suitability of any corneal topography system as a guide for customized ablation.

Comparison of Corneal Topography to Wavefront Sensing as a Guide for Customized Ablation

When corneal topography is used as a guide for customized ablation, the desired surface is not known and some reference surface is needed to find the wavefront error so that a correcting ablation profile can be generated. Wavefront error sensing devices, such an ophthalmic Shack-Hartmann wavefront sensor, are configured to directly measure the wavefront error of the entire eye in the area of the pupil. For this area, they supply the information needed to create an ablation profile directly. In doing so, they also account for aberration induced by the lens in addition to that created by the cornea. They would therefore be superior to a corneal topographer as a guide to planning a customized ablation. However, certain characteristics of these devices must first be considered before completely accepting this view.

Wavefront sensing devices can only sample in the pupil area so it is important that the pupil be fully dilated so that areas of the pupil that are only used in low light conditions are sampled. It is also best if the accommodation is paralyzed during the measurement to remove the accommodation uncertainty in the crystalline lens. In essence, wavefront sensors are automatic refractors with a very high sample density so all the known precautions associated with obtaining good refractive information with automatic refractors applies directly to them. Corneal topographers, on the other hand, often sample over a larger area of the cornea and are unaffected by accommodation, pupil size, or other refractive effects.

Wavefront sensing devices measure the entire refractive state of the eye and cannot tell if measured aberrations are caused by the cornea or by a combination of effects of the cornea and crystalline lens. Unlike corneal topographers, they give no direct information on the state of the corneal surface.

Wavefront sensing devices sample in a different way from corneal topographers. The sample density is somewhat less, in general, and the sample pattern is different. Wavefront sensors divide the pupil in small areas, usually in a rectangular grid, and measure the average deflection of light exiting from each area. This deflection information is then processed to yield wavefront error. The most common corneal topographers sample the cornea with concentric rings and may be thought to measure the surface either only at boundaries between light and dark or averaged over the area illuminated by a ring. Because the ring images are often closer together than are the center spacing the lenslet array of the wavefront sensor and because very dense sampling is taken along a corneal topographer ring image, a higher sample density is usually obtained with a corneal topography system than can be obtained with a wavefront refractor, thereby allowing smaller irregularities to be detected. Counter balancing this view, it must also be recognized that the sample density of the polar measuring system employed by corneal topographers is nonuniform with the meridional sample density decreasing toward the periphery.

It seems that if wisely used, wavefront sensing devices serve better as guides for customized ablation than do corneal topographers. However, corneal topographers should not be neglected because they give direct information on the shape of the cornea, information that is unavailable from a wavefront sensor. They should therefore be routinely used as a "second opinion" when planning a customized ablation and to see if the desired ablation pattern was achieved. For corneal ablative procedures, subtracting postsurgical corneal elevations from presurgical elevations will reveal the nature of the obtained surgical lenticule. Comparisons of the desired lenticule to the obtained surgical lenticule contain valuable information that can be used to improve future surgeries.

Comparisons of the desired lenticule to the obtained surgical lenticule contain valuable information that can be used to improve future surgeries.

In addition, there are cases in which a wavefront sensor will not work well because wavefront sensing devices must be able to send and receive light from the retinal surface without significant interference from the ocular tissue. In cases of corneal trauma, the cornea may be compromised to the extent that it is not possible for the incoming beam of the wavefront sensing device to form a reasonably well-focused spot on the retina. When this happens, the detected spots of light may be so badly deformed that good measurements of higher-order aberrations are not possible. The corneal topographer has no such limitation. It can measure the corneal surface shape even in the presence of serious irregularity and this information is quite sufficient to plan an ablation pattern to correct this defect. Because the crystalline lens may be assumed to be a regular optical element even though its exact details are not known, its effect can safely be assumed in calculations and the major cause of the degradation of vision, the corneal irregularity, can be corrected using only corneal information. This suggests that the correlation between wavefront error measured with a wavefront sensor and wavefront error measured with a corneal topographer needs to be established so that when it is not possible to obtain wavefront error information from a wavefront sensing device, corneal topographical information can be reliably substituted.

As a first-order approximation, the crystalline lens can be assumed to be a regular optical element in calculations to assess the effects of corneal irregularities on vision.

Uses of Corneal Topography to Assist With Corneal Ablation Procedures

There are other uses of corneal topographical information in the guidance of customized ablations of the cornea. Corneal topography displays can be used to simulate an ablation graphically illustrating what can be expected with different ablation patterns. As discussed above, historical displays showing the difference in corneal shape from that expected are useful to allow the surgeon to alter procedure to get desired results.

Similarly, one can simulate the anticipated effect of a given corneal ablation procedure. A simulated ablation feature first allows an ablation pattern to be specified. This specification includes such variables as the desired ablation zone size, the refractive error to be removed, the specification of transition zones between the corrected central optical zone and the unablated peripheral cornea, and the centration of the pattern with respect to the pupil center. Alternatively, the ablation pattern may be supplied by the laser ablation system, in which case it will be referred to as the treatment pattern. In either case, the ablation pattern is removed from the corneal shape as measured by the corneal topographer by the software program to produce a new corneal shape. This new shape is then displayed using one of the display modes of the topographer. The practitioner, familiar with corneal topography map presentations and their meaning, is now in a position to judge if the proposed ablation pattern will produce the desired effect.

A second effective way to use corneal topography information to assist with laser refractive surgery procedures is to use difference maps to graphically show the difference between two corneal surfaces. The first use of such a technique was to monitor changes in the corneal shape before and after surgery and then to monitor subsequent changes over time as corneal healing progressed. A more advanced use of difference information is to consider the difference found to represent a tissue lens that creates a wavefront error and then analyze this tissue lens wavefront error as one would any wavefront, expressing the aberrations in terms of Zernike polynomials coefficients, creating point spread patterns, convolving these point spreads with images, and calculating the modulation transfer function for the difference.

In all differencing techniques, the corneal topographical information needs preprocessing before comparison can be made. This is because the ring locations will invariably be slightly different when topographic changes occur in the corneal surface, so the data locations are not at the same horizontal and vertical positions on the cornea. The best plan is to chose a common grid to be used for comparison purposed and interpolate the elevation data sets onto this grid. There are several mathematical techniques available to do this. One interesting one is to use Zernike polynomials as fitting functions. This orthogonal polynomial set is quite capable of decomposing data on a randomly spaced grid into a set of coefficients. The coefficients, once so generated, may then be used to reconstruct the surface on the chosen grid.

Such interpolation has a second desirable feature when dealing with elevation data from a corneal topographer—that of imposing surface continuity across meridians and removing noise introduced in the reconstruction process. There is always noise introduced into the data as the ring locations are found from the video images of the reflected rings. Typically, a smoothing operation is done on each ring to remove discontinuities in radial position before reconstruction is done along meridians. This has the effect of imposing some meridian-to-meridian continuity in the reconstructed surface. However, when the better reconstruction methods—such as the arc step method—are used to reconstruct the surface one meridian at a time, there is continuity in the elevation data imposed only along meridians and that only through the first derivative. No cross meridian continuity is imposed. The interpolation discussed above imposes continuity to second degree and above if a method such a using Zernike polynomial functions is used.

Another use of the differencing method is to combine it with simulated ablation. A simulated postsurgical corneal shape is created by subtracting the treatment pattern from the presurgical corneal surface. A difference tissue lens is then created by taking the difference between the simulated postsurgical corneal surface and the actual postsurgical corneal surface as measured by the corneal topographer. In this way, actual results can be compared with expected results in a visual way and the above mentioned advanced techniques may be used to analyze the differences between the achieved and planned treatment. Because actual results are often slightly different from expected results, studies of this kind can serve as a guide to alter ablation patterns to get desired results.

While differencing techniques are also valuable when dealing with aberrometer data, there is one area in which the topographical analysis is clearly superior. This is in the monitoring of changes to the corneal shape in areas outside the treatment area. It has been found that the cornea not only changes its shape in the area of the ablation but also in areas peripheral to the treatment zone. These changes can never be seen by an aberrometer, limited as it is to measurement within the pupil area; yet these changes are important in understanding the response of the cornea to treatment.

> Corneal topographers measure areas outside of the pupil, aberrometers cannot. Measurements outside the pupil are important in understanding the corneal response to surgery.

Special Uses of Curvature Information

Normally, curvature information obtained by corneal topographers and presented in the form of axial curvature or meridional curvature maps has been used clinically in a subjective way to assess the state of the corneal surface. Curvature information may be presented of other ways, as mentioned above, and these have special diagnostic advantages that are not as well known. Two types of these curvature displays will be mentioned here. They are both measures of local curvature and are true curvature measures in the sense of differential geometry as opposed to the common curvature measures, axial curvature and meridional curvature.

The first is mean local curvature. One may think of this measure as being similar to spherical equivalent power in that the mean local curvature is the mean of the maximum normal curvature and minimum local curvature at a surface location. This measure is particularly helpful in detecting power or curvature gradients on the corneal surface that may result from the type of refractive surgery performed either as an unplanned effect or as a planned treatment. Mean local power gradients are one of the indicators of a corneal surface that will in certain cases produce a variable power refractive effect (a type of presbyopic correction) or in others visual difficulties in enlarged pupil conditions.

The second special curvature display is of local Gaussian curvature. Whereas local mean curvature is the average of the maximum and minimum local curvatures, local Gaussian curvature is their product. As such, it has units of inverse area instead of units of inverse length as do other types of curvature. In effect, it measures the change in the area of a small local area of the surface from that of a plane surface that curved surface projects onto and in doing so gives a measure of how much a flat surface would have to be stretched or deformed to turn into the curved surface. This type of display can give information on corneal change following surgery if local Gaussian curvature difference maps are created. For areas of the corneal surface where ablation has not taken place but the Gaussian curvature has changed, we know that the corneal stroma has undergone stretching or compression. If precise corneal thickness measures are combined with precise anterior corneal surface measurements, posterior curvature information may be generated and so stretching and compression of the posterior stroma may be inferred from local Gaussian curvature maps.

Corneal Topography and Wavefront Refraction: Complementary Technologies

The above considerations show us that as we consider customized corneal ablation, we should consider corneal topography and wavefront refraction as complementary measurement technologies. Both should be included in any clinical practice that performs customized corneal ablation and both should be included in any program that enables laser systems for corneal reshaping to include customized ablations as an option. Whereas wavefront refraction should serve as the primary guide for planning customized ablations, corneal topography should serve as a guide for monitoring the recovery process and as a means to learn how to subtly modify the planning process so as to obtain the best final visual results. Therefore, it is important to have both preoperative and postoperative corneal topography on all patients. It is also important to analytical means to most fully use the corneal information thus obtained.

> Corneal topography and wavefront refraction are complementary measurement technologies.

Chapter 37

Combining Corneal and Ocular Wave Aberrations

Pablo Artal, PhD

Introduction

The wave aberration is a function that completely describes the image-forming properties of any optical system and, in particular, the eye. It is defined as the difference between the perfect (spherical) and the real wavefronts for every point over the eye's pupil. It is typically represented as a two-dimensional gray or color image, where each gray or color level represents the amount of wave aberration expressed either in microns or number of wavelengths. An eye without aberrations forms a perfect retinal image of a point source (Airy disk). However, an eye with aberrations produces a larger and, in general, asymmetric retinal image.

The wave aberration is a function that completely describes the image-forming properties of any optical system and, in particular, the eye.

The aberrations of the complete eye (ocular wave aberration), considered as one single imaging system, can be measured by using a large variety of wavefront sensors or aberrometers. On the other hand, the aberrations introduced only by the anterior corneal surface (corneal wave aberration) can be computed from data obtained by corneal topographers. The combined use of both corneal and ocular wave aberrations is a powerful tool to be applied in both basic and clinical studies.

Since the eye is a relatively complex optical structure, every surface contributes differently to the overall quality of the retinal image. The study of the relative contribution to the eye's aberrations of the main ocular components—the crystalline lens and the cornea—has attracted the interest of researchers for centuries. In 1801, Young[1] performed an experiment in his own eye to measure the contribution of the lens to ocular astigmatism. He neutralized the corneal contribution by immersing his eye in water. In clinical practice, it is commonly accepted that the lens compensates for moderate amounts of corneal astigmatism. Other, more recent studies continued the exploration in vivo of the sources of aberrations within the eye, although initially centered only in the spherical aberration,[2,3] or used indirect estimates of image quality.[4]

The advent of new technology (ie, wavefront sensors and corneal topographers) opened new possibilities for a more precise evaluation of the contribution of the different ocular surfaces to the overall retinal image quality. The combined use of ocular and corneal aberrations has already been used to obtain more detailed information on the relative sources of aberrations in the human eye.[5,6] If the aberrations produced by the cornea and the total aberrations are measured in the same eye, the aberrations of the internal ocular optics (ie, those produced by the posterior corneal surface and the lens) can be estimated. This approach is particularly powerful for most refractive surgery procedures where virtually any practical case would benefit from knowing the optical contribution of the ocular component that is being modified: the cornea in laser refractive surgery or the internal optics in cataract surgery.

Since the eye is a relatively complex optical structure, every surface contributes differently to the overall quality of the retinal image.

The advent of new technology (ie, wavefront sensors and corneal topographers) opened new possibilities for a more precise evaluation of the contribution of the different ocular surfaces to the overall retinal image quality.

This chapter will review how to obtain and how to combine the corneal and ocular aberrations, with special emphasis on the problems and limitations of using data obtained with different instruments. In the final part, and to demonstrate the potential of this approach, examples of ocular, corneal, and internal aberrations in different eyes will be presented.

Measuring Corneal Wave Aberrations

To determine the aberrations associated with the anterior surface of the cornea, it is necessary to determine the corneal shape with submicron precision. The need for an instrument capable of measuring with precision the corneal curvature at each point was already noted in the early 60s.[7] Many techniques have been proposed to measure the corneal shape, from interferometry to profile photography or holography. However, most instruments in

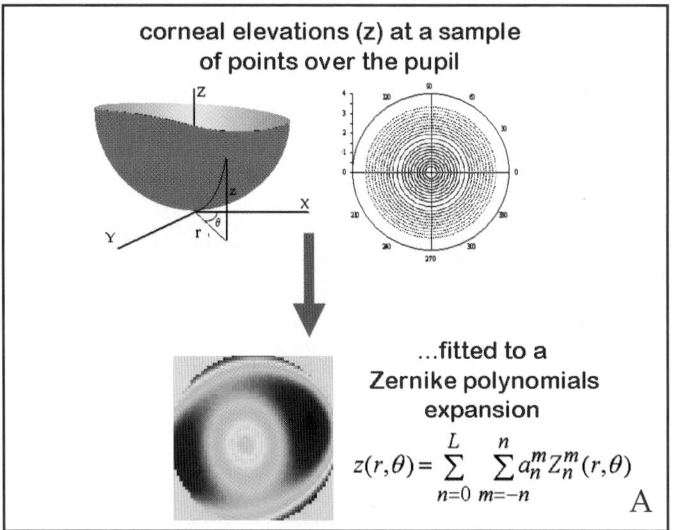

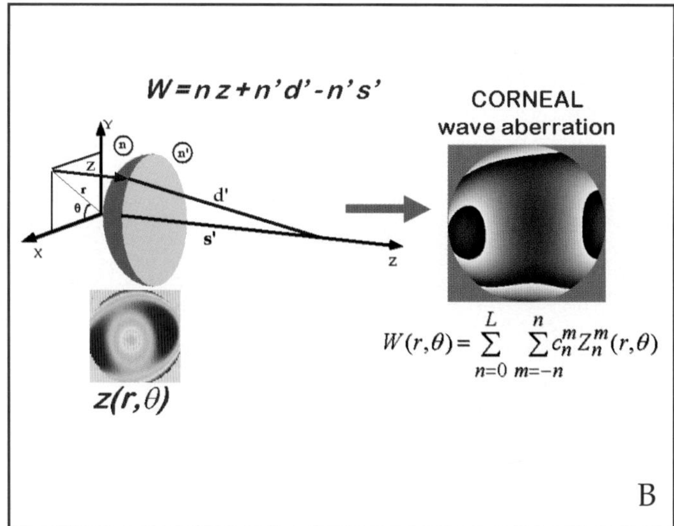

Figure 37-1. Schematic representation of the procedure used to calculate the aberrations associated with the anterior surface of the cornea. (A) Corneal elevations provided by a videokeratoscope are fitted to an expansion of Zernike polynomials. (B) A ray tracing procedure is used to calculate the corneal wave aberration as the differences in optical path between marginal and principal rays, also expressed as a Zernike polynomial expansion (see text for details).

clinical practice today (eg, videokeratoscopes) are based upon Placido's disk principle. That is, a camera images series of concentric rings reflected off the corneal first surface and the corneal first surface geometry is obtained in each meridian from the ring spacing. Since this type of apparatus is widely used in the clinic, a number of studies have evaluated their precision in estimating the corneal surface, aiming to calculate corneal aberrations.[8,9] Although it was accepted that Placido-based devices do not provide accurate topographic data in the periphery and when the surface severely differs from a sphere, a recent study[9] showed that it is possible to determine corneal aberrations from this data with enough precision for small to medium pupil diameters.

> Small to medium pupil diameters are between 4 and 6 millimeters (mm). Enough precision is defined to be between 0.05 and 0.20 microns (µm) of root mean square (RMS) error (spherical equivalent dioptric error of between 0.09 and 0.15 diopters [D]).

Even if we could measure perfectly the corneal topography, a second problem is the calculation procedure used to determinate the corneal aberrations. The direct and simplest approach is to obtain a "remainder lens" by subtracting the best conic surface fitted to the measured cornea and calculating the aberrations by multiplying by the refractive index difference.[10-12] Another option is to perform a ray tracing to the corneal surface to compute the associated aberrations.[9] Figure 37-1 show a schematic diagram of this type of procedure.

The corneal elevations, representing the distance (z_i) from each point of the corneal surface to a reference plane tangential to the vertex of the cornea, are fitted to a Zernike expansion[13] (see Figure 37-1A):

$$z\,(r,\theta)=\sum_{n=0}^{L}\;\sum_{m=-n}^{n}a^m{}_n\,Z^m{}_n\,(r,\theta) \qquad (1)$$

by using a Gram-Schmidt orthogonalization method. The wavefront aberration associated with the corneal surface (W) is obtained as the difference in optical path length between the principal ray that passes through the center of the pupil and a marginal ray (see Figure 37-1B):

$$W=nz+n'd'-n's' \qquad (2)$$

where n and n' are refractive indexes; z, d', and s' are the distances represented in Figure 37-1B. By using the Zernike representation for the corneal surface (equation 1), the corneal wave aberration is also obtained as another Zernike expansion:

$$W\,(r,\theta)=\sum_{n=0}^{L}\;\sum_{m=-n}^{n}c^m{}_nZ^m{}_n\,(r,\theta) \qquad (3)$$

where the coefficients $c^m{}_n$ are linear combinations of the coefficients $a^m{}_n$.[9]

The accuracy of this procedure to estimate the corneal wave aberration was evaluated using reference surfaces.[9] For central regions of 4 and 6 mm diameter, the RMS error between the actual and the measured aberrations were found to be around 0.05 mm and 0.2 mm, respectively, which renders the method appropriate for aberration studies.

Measuring Ocular Wave Aberrations

Many different techniques have been proposed to estimate the wave aberration of the complete eye, both subjective and objective. Although they are described more extensively elsewhere in this book, some of them are the method of "vernier" alignment,[14] the aberroscope,[15] the Foucault-knife technique,[16] calculations from double-pass retinal images,[17,18] the pyramid sensor,[19] and probably the most widely used method today, the Shack-Hartmann wavefront sensor.[20-22] This system consists of a microlenslet array, conjugated with the eye's pupil and a camera placed at its focal plane. If a plane wavefront reaches the

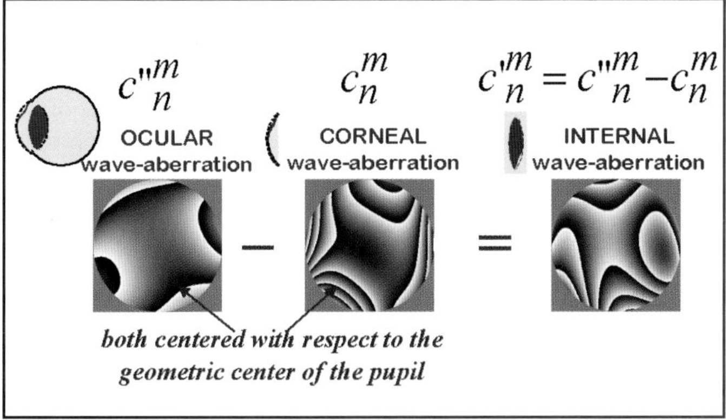

Figure 37-2. Schematic representation of the combination of corneal and ocular wave aberrations to estimate the wave aberration of the internal optics.

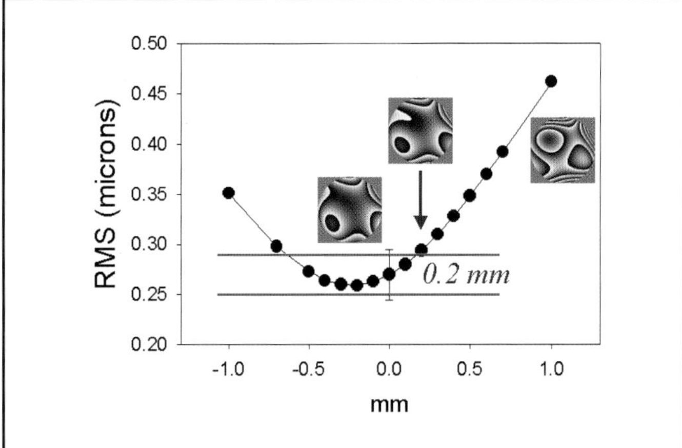

Figure 37-3B. RMS of the corneal aberrations as a function of the decentration of the pupil center in mm. The red horizontal lines indicate the average error expected in normal eyes when estimating corneal aberrations.

microlenslet array, the camera records a perfectly regular mosaic of spots. However, if a distorted (ie, aberrated) wavefront reaches the sensor, the pattern of spots is irregular. The displacement of each spot is proportional to the derivative of the wavefront over each microlens area. From the images of spots, the ocular wave aberration is computed, and in general it is also expressed as a Zernike polynomial expansion similar to that of equation 3.

Combining Ocular and Corneal Wave Aberrations

If the wave aberrations of the complete eye and the cornea are available, the relative contributions of the different ocular surfaces to the retinal image quality can be evaluated. In particular, the wavefront aberration of the internal ocular optics (ie, principally the posterior surface of the cornea plus the crystalline lens) is estimated simply by direct subtraction of the ocular and corneal aberrations. Figure 37-2 shows a schematic representation of this procedure. In a simple model, having the two series of Zernike coefficients, both for the cornea (c^n_m) and the eye (c''^n_m), the aberrations of the internal optics are obtained by direct subtraction of each pair of coefficients (c'^n_m). It is assumed that the changes in the wave aberration are small for different axial planes (ie, from the corneal vertex to the pupil plane).

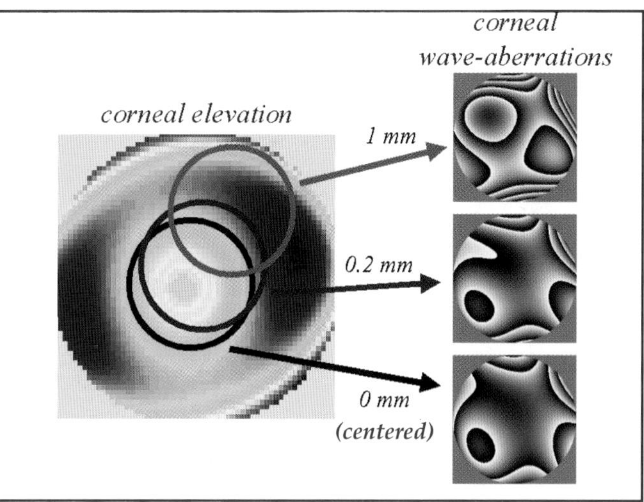

Figure 37-3A. Examples of corneal wave-aberrations calculated from the corneal elevations for different locations of the pupil center (0, 0.2, and 1 mm). The circles represent schematically the position of the pupil.

In general, when using this approach, ocular and corneal aberrations are obtained with two different instruments. Then a major problem is how to determine a correct reference centering for registration. If the corneal and ocular aberrations are obtained centered at different locations, subtraction will produce an incorrect estimate of the internal aberrations, and in consequence, an incorrect picture of the coupling of aberrations. Figures 37-3A and 37-3B show an example to clarify this point. From a given corneal elevation map (in a color representation in the figure), the corneal wave aberration was computed for different positions of the pupil center with respect to the corneal vertex. Figure 37-3A shows, as an example, three wave aberration maps, for 0, 0.2, and 1 mm, respectively, of relative decentering of the corneal vertex (where the topography is centered) to the center of the possible pupil. Figure 37-3B shows the RMS of the corneal aberrations calculated when changing the center of the pupil in a range of 2 mm along one diagonal. The two red horizontal lines indicate typical errors when estimating corneal wave aberrations from corneal topography measured with a videokeratographic instrument. These results indicate that, as anticipated, decentering can induce substantial changes in the aberrations (note the complete different map for the 1 mm decentration case in Figure 37-3A). However, in normally aberrated eyes, small misalignments (below 0.2 mm) would probably introduce errors in the calculated aberrations within the same magnitude that other errors also present in the measuring process (see Figure 37-3B). As a practical rule, an obvious choice for realignment of the ocular and corneal aberration maps is the geometrical center of the pupil. When doing this, it must be considered that the pupil center changes with dilatation.

> Typically the pupil location varies less than 0.2 mm during normal physiologic pupil dilation and constriction.

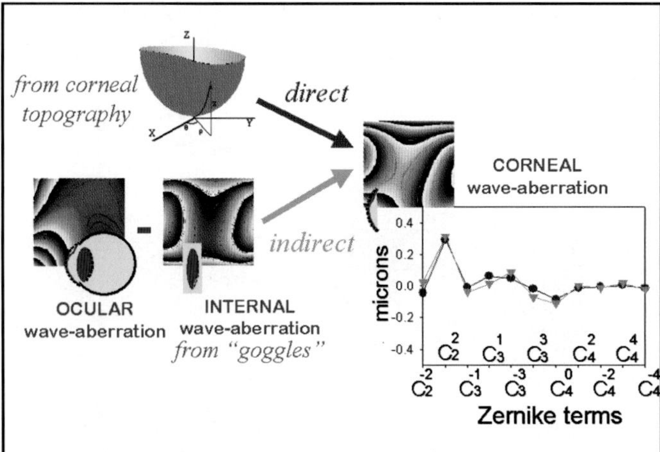

Figure 37-4. Schematic procedure to estimate the aberrations of the cornea directly and from indirect measurements (complete eye and internal optics). The box shows the Zernike coefficients of the aberrations of the cornea in one subject, obtained from the shape (circles) and by subtraction of the aberrations of the whole eye and the internal surfaces (triangles).

Although decentering in a single plane of both wave aberrations is probably the most important source of error when combining ocular and corneal aberrations, it is not the only one.[23] Most instruments measuring ocular aberrations use the line of sight as the alignment axis. However, this is not usually the case for videokeratoscopes providing the corneal elevations used to calculate the aberrations of the cornea. If this factor is not considered, the wave aberration for the cornea will be obtained for a plane forming a different angle as that of the wave aberration for the eye, introducing another potential registration problem. When this happens, it is also possible to correct computationally for the difference in axis, although this should implicate the assumption of approximate values for the angles involved in the instruments and the eyes.

Errors induced when estimating the internal aberrations by measuring the corneal aberrations in the plane tangent to the corneal apex and ocular aberrations in the plane of the entrance pupil can be minimized by referring the corneal aberrations back to the center of the entrance pupil.

An intuitive solution for these problems appearing when combining corneal and ocular aberrations is the use of one single instrument with a unique alignment axis to collect both corneal and ocular data under the same conditions. However, if the two sets of data are obtained with two apparatus, it is still possible to use different approaches to correct for the registration errors. One is to use a common pupil point, usually the geometrical center of the pupil, to calculate the aberrations of the cornea and the eye. The differences in the angle of axis may be also incorporated to the calculations. Another approach is the search of a registration position that minimizes the aberration differences between the cornea and the eye.[24] This last approach may underestimate the real contribution of the internal optics.

How Precise Are the Combination Results?

With all the potential sources of error described in the previous section, plus those related to each instrument, the important question is how precise are the data obtained from the combination of ocular and corneal aberrations? A few experiments have been performed to address this question. Artal et al,[5] in addition to measuring ocular and corneal aberrations, also directly measured the wave aberration for the internal optics, using a Shack-Hartmann wavefront sensor when the aberrations of the corneal surface were cancelled by immersing the eye in saline water using swimming goggles. This was a similar idea as that of Young[1] and more recently Millodot and Sivak,[25] but using current wavefront sensing technology. The comparison of the aberrations obtained from independent measurements is an indication of the validity of the combination approach. In particular, the aberrations of the cornea, measured both directly from its shape and by subtraction of the aberrations of the whole eye and the internal optics were compared in that study[5] and found to be similar within the experimental variability. Figure 37-4 shows this comparison schematically, together with the Zernike coefficients obtained in one eye as an example. This result provides strong proof of the consistency of this type of procedure: the combination of ocular and corneal aberrations despite the experimental and methodological difficulties that are involved.

Another interesting type of experiment performed to test the validity of the combination approach was to compare the estimates of both ocular and corneal aberrations in highly aberrated eyes where the cornea were by far the main contributor to aberrations (eg, in an eye with keratoconus).[24] In this situation, both aberrations for the eye and the cornea were quite similar, indicating again the reasonable accuracy of the combined use of corneal and aberration maps when most precautions were taken into account during data processing.

Corneal, Internal, and Ocular Aberrations in Different Eyes

By the combined use of corneal and ocular aberrations, the relative contribution to the aberrations of the cornea and the internal optics in different eyes has been evaluated in recent studies. As an example of the potential of the procedure, this section presents results for three types of eyes: normal young eyes, normal older eyes, and highly aberrated eyes due to an abnormal cornea.

Normal Young Eyes

Figure 37-5 shows an example of the wave aberrations and the associated point spread functions (PSFs) for the cornea, the internal optics, and the complete eye in a normal young eye. The magnitude of aberrations is larger in the cornea than in the complete eye. This indicates an active role of the lens for a partial reduction of the aberrations produced by the cornea. Figure 37-6 shows the Zernike terms for the aberrations of the cornea (solid symbols) and the internal optics (white symbols) for a number of young normal subjects.[5] It is remarkable that the magnitude of several aberrations is similar for the two components, but they have an opposite sign. This indicates that the internal optics may

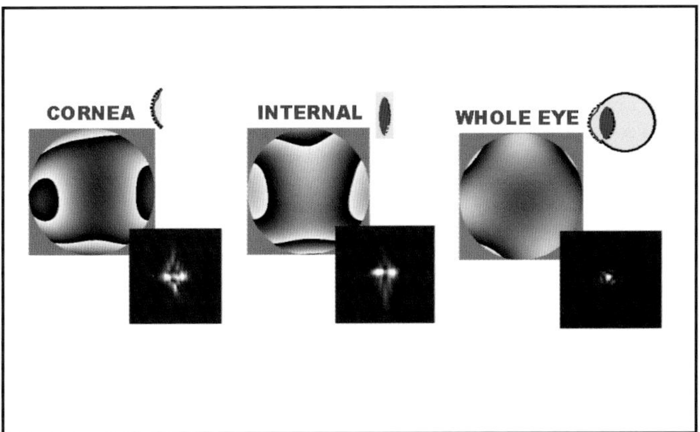

Figure 37-5. Example of wave aberrations (represented module-p) for the cornea, the internal optics and the complete eye in one normal young subject. The associated PSFs were calculated at the best image plane from the wave aberrations and subtends 20 minutes of arc of visual field. The aberrations of the internal optics compensate in part for the corneal aberrations.

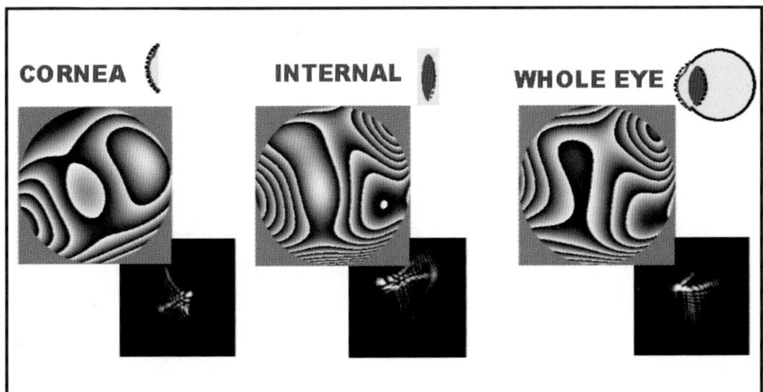

Figure 37-7. Example of wave aberrations (represented module-p) for the cornea, the internal optics, and the complete eye in one normal older subject. The associated PSFs were calculated at the best image plane from the wave aberrations and subtend 20 minutes of arc of visual field.

play a significant role to compensate for the corneal aberrations in normal young eyes. This behavior may not be present in every young eye, depending on the amount of aberrations or the refractive error.[23]

Normal Older Eyes

It is now generally accepted that the amount of monochromatic aberrations in the eye increases approximately linearly with age (also see Chapter 11). [26-28] The combined study of the aberrations of the cornea and the whole eye provides useful information on the underlying cause of the increase of ocular aberration with age.[6] While the optical aberration of the cornea increase moderately with age,[29] the aberration of the internal surfaces show variability, but with a tendency to increase in middle age and older subjects. However, neither ocular component itself isolated appears to explain the change of aberrations in the entire eye. A different coupling between corneal and internal aberrations in young and older eyes explains the optical deterioration of the eye with age. Figure 37-7 shows an example of wave

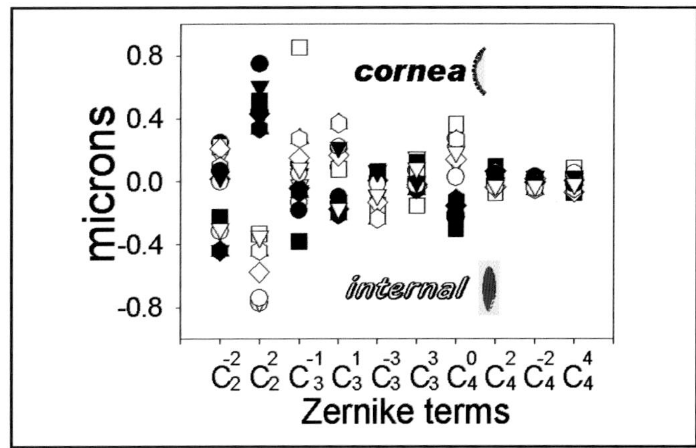

Figure 37-6. Zernike terms for the cornea (solid symbols) and the internal optics (open symbols) for number of normal young subjects.

aberrations and their associated PSFs for the cornea, the internal optics, and the complete eye in a typical older eye. In this case, contrary to the coupling of the young eye, the internal optics do not compensate the corneal optics, but instead add aberrations to those of the cornea.

Highly Aberrated Eyes

An interesting case to apply the combined measurement of aberrations is in the highly aberrated eye, in particular those with the cornea as the major contributor to the ocular aberrations. For instance, the keratoconic eye, or an eye after penetrating keratoplasty, are excellent eyes for testing the whole procedure of calculating the aberration of the internal optics from corneal and whole eye measurements. In these eyes, both wave aberrations for the cornea and the eye are similar, indicating a minor role of the internal optics to modify the high corneal aberrations.

Examples of the Clinical Impact of the Combined Use of Corneal and Ocular Aberrations

The use of the combined information of the ocular and corneal aberrations helped to explain some facts that were not well-understood previously. One example was the optical performance of eyes after implantation of intraocular lenses (IOLs). These lenses usually have good image quality when measured in an optical bench, but the final optical performance in the implanted eye was typically lower than expected.[30] One plausible reason is that the ideal substitute of the natural lens is not a lens with the best optical performance when isolated, but one designed to compensate for the aberrations of the cornea.[31] Figure 37-8 schematically shows this situation. This has important implications for ophthalmic applications. IOLs and contact lenses should be designed with an aberration profile matching that of the cornea or the lens to maximize the quality of the retinal image. In addition, procedures in refractive surgery should ablate the cornea based on the overall ocular aberrations rather than use corneal aberrations to achieve the optimum retinal image.

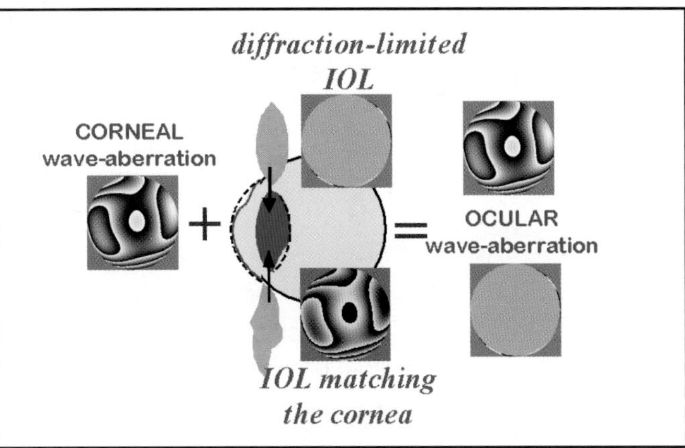

Figure 37-8. Schematic illustration of the effect of the coupling of aberrations of the cornea and the IOL (see the text for details).

Professor Artal makes two extremely important clinical points: 1) IOLs and contact lenses should be designed with an aberration profile matching that of the cornea or the lens, to maximize the quality of the retinal image; and 2) Corneal refractive surgery should ablate the cornea based on the overall ocular aberrations rather than corneal aberrations measured with corneal topography.

Acknowledgments

Parts of the research described in this chapter was supported by the Ministerio de Ciencia y Tecnología (MCyT) (Spain) and by Pharmacia-Groningen (The Netherlands). The author thanks his students, colleagues, and collaborators that participated in the different projects related to the topic of this chapter. In particular, Antonio Guirao, Antonio Benito, and Esther Berrio of University of Murcia; Patricia Piers and Sverker Norrby of Pharmacia-Groningen; and David Williams of University of Rochester played crucial roles in some of the results presented.

References

1. Young T. On the mechanism of the eye. *Phil Trans R Soc.* 1801;19:23-88.
2. El Hage SG, Berny F. Contribution of crystalline lens to the spherical aberration of the eye. *J Opt Soc Am.* 1973;63:205-211.
3. Tomlinson A, Hemenger RP, Garriott R. Method for estimating the spherical aberration of the human crystalline lens in vivo. *Invest Ophthal Vis Sci.* 1993;34:621-629.
4. Artal P, Guirao A. Contribution of the cornea and the lens to the aberrations of the human eye. *Optics Letters.* 1998;23:1713-1715.
5. Artal P, Guirao A, Berrio E, Williams DR. Compensation of corneal aberrations by the internal optics in the human eye. *Journal of Vision.* 2001;1(1):1-8.
6. Artal P, Berrio E, Guirao A, Piers P. Contribution of the cornea and internal surfaces to the change of ocular aberrations with age. *J Opt Soc Am A.* 2002;19:137-143.
7. Jenkins TCA. Aberrations of the eye and their effects on vision: part 1. *Br J Physiol Optics.* 1963;20:59-91.
8. Applegate RA, Nuñez R, Buettner J, Howland HC. How accurately can videokeratographic systems measure surface elevation? *Optom Vis Sci.* 1995;72:785-792.
9. Guirao A, Artal P. Corneal wave aberration from videokeratography: accuracy and limitations of the procedure. *J Opt Soc Am A.* 2000;17:955-965.
10. Howland HC, Buettner J, Applegate RA. *Computation of the shapes of normal corneas and their monochromatic aberrations from videokeratometric measurements.* Vision Science and Its Applications, 1994 Technical Digest Series, Vol. 2. Washington, DC: Optical Society of America; 1994:54-57.
11. Applegate RA, Howland HC, Buettner, Yee RWJ, Cottingham AJ, Sharp RP. *Corneal aberrations before and after radial keratotomy (RK) calculated from videokeratometric measurements.* Vision Science and Its Applications, 1994 Technical Digest Series, Vol. 2. Washington, DC: Optical Society of America; 1994:58-61.
12. Schwiegerling J, Greivenkamp JE. Using corneal height maps and polynomial decomposition to determine corneal aberrations. *Optom Vis Sci.* 1997;74:906-916.
13. Schwiegerling J, Greivenkamp JE, Miller JM. Representation of videokeratoscopic height data with Zernike polynomials. *J Opt Soc Am A.* 1995;12:2105-2113.
14. Smirnov MS. Measurement of the wave aberration of the human eye. *Biofizika.* 1961;6:776-795.
15. Howland HC, Howland B. A subjective method for the measurement of monochromatic aberrations of the eye. *J Opt Soc Am.* 1977;67:1508-1518.
16. Berny F, Slansky S. Wavefront determination resulting from foucault test as applied to the human eye and visual instruments. In: Dickenson JH, ed. *Optical Instruments and Techniques.* Newcastle, UK: Oriel; 1969:375-386.
17. Artal P, Santamaría J, Bescós J. Retrieval of the wave aberration of human eyes from actual point-spread function data. *J Opt Soc Am A.* 1988;5:1201-1206.
18. Iglesias I, Berrio E, Artal P. Estimates of the ocular wave aberration from pairs of double-pass retinal images. *J Opt Soc Am A.* 1998;15:2466-2476.
19. Iglesias I, Ragazzoni R, Julien Y, Artal P. Extended source pyramid wavefront sensor for the human eye. *Opt Express.* 2002;10:419-428.
20. Liang B, Grimm S, Goelz, Bille JF. Objective measurement of the wave-aberrations of the human eye with the use of a Hartmann-Shack sensor. *J Opt Soc Am A.* 1994;11:1949-1957.
21. Liang J, Williams DR. Aberrations and retinal image quality of the normal human eye. *J Opt Soc Am A.* 1997;14:2873-2883.
22. Prieto PM, Vargas-Martín F, Goelz S, Artal P. Analysis of the performance of the Hartmann-Shack sensor in the human eye. *J Opt Soc Am A.* 2000;17:1388-1398.
23. Salmon TO, Thibos LN. Videokeratoscope line of sight misalignment and its effect on measurements of corneal and internal ocular aberrations. *J Opt Soc Am A.* 2002;19:657-669.
24. Barbero S, Marcos S, Merayo-Lloves J, Moreno-Barriuso E. Validation of the estimation of corneal aberrations from videokeratography in keratoconus. *J Refrac Surg.* 2002;18:263-270.
25. Millodot M, Sivak J. Contribution of the cornea and the lens to the spherical aberration of the eye. *Vision Res.* 1979;19:685-687.
26. Artal P, Ferro M, Miranda I, Navarro R. Effects of aging in retinal image quality. *J Opt Soc Am A.* 1993;10:1656-1662.
27. Guirao A, González C, Redondo M, Geraghty E, Norrby S, Artal P. Average optical performance of the human eye as a function of age in a normal population. *Invest Ophthalmol Vis Sci.* 1999;40:197-202.
28. McLellan JS, Marcos S, Burns SA. Age-related changed in monochromatic wave-aberrations of the human eye. *Invest Ophthalmol Vis Sci.* 2001;42:1390-1395.
29. Guirao A, Redondo M, Artal P. Optical aberrations of the human cornea as a function of age. *J Opt Soc Am A.* 2000;17(10):1697-1702.
30. Artal P, Marcos S, Navarro R, Miranda I, Ferro M. Through focus image quality of eyes implanted with monofocal and multifocal intraocular lenses. *Opt Eng.* 1995;34:772-779.
31. Guirao A, Redondo M, Geraghty E, Piers P, Norrby S, Artal P. Corneal optical aberrations and retinal image quality in patients in whom monofocal intraocular lenses were implanted. *Arch Ophthalmol.* 2002;120:1143-1151.

Chapter 38

Combining Vector Planning With Wavefront Analysis to Optimize Laser In-Situ Keratomileusis Outcomes

Noel Alpins, FRACO, FRCOphth, FACS and Leisa Schmid, PhD

Introduction

Recent advances in laser technology are aimed at correcting ocular aberrations of the eye to improve visual outcomes. These new treatment paradigms, while offering advances for refractive surgery outcomes, do not take into account the possible mismatch between refractive and corneal astigmatism. Here we discuss both wavefront-guided laser in-situ keratomileusis (LASIK) surgery and the principles of vector analysis of astigmatism. The astigmatism outcomes of a series of patients treated with wavefront-guided LASIK are analyzed using the Alpins method of vector analysis.[1-3]

Principles of Wavefront Analysis

Introduction

The basic components of refraction, which are routinely measured, consist of myopia, hyperopia, and astigmatism. Traditionally, refractive surgery aims to correct errors of refraction, which are lower-order (second) aberrations. Higher-order aberrations include spherical aberration, coma, and foils. Even eyes with normal emmetropic vision can suffer from aberrations that affect vision.[4] The measurement of higher-order aberrations of the eye can be performed by wavefront analysis where the deviation of the wavefront from the ideal reference wave is measured. The quality of the visual system can also be described by determining how an object is imaged. Thus, the point spread function (PSF) or line spread function (LSF) can be used to measure the resultant blur from error in an optical system.

Shack-Hartmann Aberrometer

The aberrations of the eye can be measured using a Shack-Hartmann aberrometer to determine the wavefront. In Shack-Hartmann aberrometers, a small, focused beam of infrared light is shone into the eye (Figure 38-1A). The beam is reflected from the retina and passes through the optical system on the way out. This reflected beam is then captured by an array of lenslets and focused onto a charged-coupled device (CCD) array (Figure 38-1B). The wavefront is then measured from this reflected beam. The wavefront can be described by breaking down the map into component mathematical functions. The most commonly used system is to describe the wavefront in terms of Zernike polynomials of increasing order (Figure 38-2).

The Bausch & Lomb Zywave aberrometer (Rochester, NY) is Shack-Hartmann based. The Bausch & Lomb Zywave aberrometer is used to measure the wavefront deviation in prospective wavefront-guided (Zyoptix, Bausch & Lomb) LASIK patients both prior to and after surgery. It can also be used to determine the PSF. The Shack-Hartmann aberrometer has been used to measure the optical aberrations of the eye in patients with tear film abnormalities, corneal disease, and following LASIK.[5]

Aberrations and Visual Performance

Refractive techniques such as photorefractive keratectomy (PRK)[6] and LASIK,[7-9] while decreasing refractive errors have been shown to increase the optic aberrations of the eye. Performing LASIK surgery increases both coma-like and spherical-like aberrations, which are greater for larger myopic ablations.[9] The presence of optical aberrations after LASIK surgery may explain why some patients who have achieved 20/20 vision when measured on high contrast charts are not satisfied with their visual outcome after surgery. Since optical aberrations affect image contrast, measuring visual acuity on high contrast charts is not representative of the effect of optical aberrations on visual performance.[10]

These aberrations can result in a large PSF that reduces retinal image quality for large pupils.[5] In an optical system with aberrations, the larger the pupil, the greater the loss in image contrast.[11] Visual performance can be affected after LASIK, particularly in light conditions where a large pupil exists.[12,13]

It has been proposed that the increase in aberrations following LASIK surgery may be due to an increase in corneal asphericity, decentration of the ablation, corneal irregularities, interface corneal haze, and variability in wound healing.[9] Ocular aberrations also cause phase shifts and phase reversals that can affect image quality.[11] It was suggested in 1997 that "we need to move toward minimizing the eye's aberration at the same time we are correcting the eye's spherical and cylindrical refractive error."[14]

Wavefront-Guided Refractive Surgery

By correcting not only the spherical and cylindrical components of refraction but also the aberrations in the visual system that may affect vision performance, optimal visual outcomes beyond those currently achieved with "standard" laser ablations

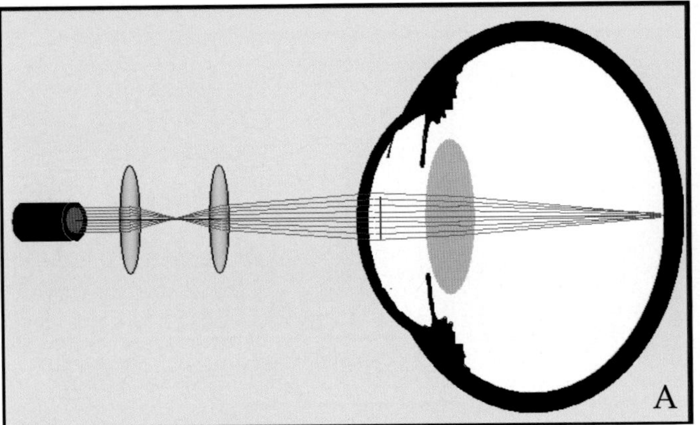

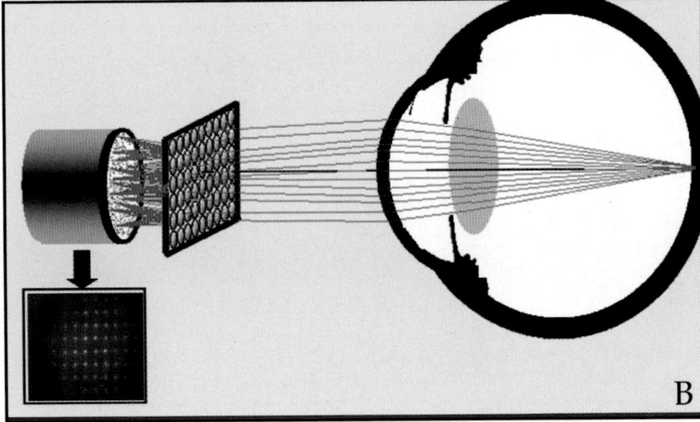

Figure 38-1. (A) A narrow beam is focused on the retina to generate a point source. (B) The outcoming rays experience the aberrations of the eye and their deviation is detected by an array of lenses. (Courtesy of Bausch & Lomb Surgical.)

may be possible. The first demonstration that the optical aberrations of the eye could be corrected was by Liang and colleagues.[15] Current laser refractive techniques have been developed to use wavefront analysis for determining LASIK customized ablations.

Recent results of patients treated with wavefront-guided LASIK are encouraging.[16-18] Mrochen and colleagues,[16] using a Tscherning wavefront sensor, reported on three eyes that had wavefront deviations reduced by an average of 27% following wavefront-guided LASIK. Consequently, uncorrected visual acuity (UCVA) of 20/12 or better was achieved. In a later series of 15 eyes by the same investigators using the Allegretto scanning spot excimer laser (WaveLight Laser Technologies AG, Erlanger, Germany), variable results were reported.[17] However, the majority of eyes gained one or more lines of best-corrected visual acuity (BCVA).

Arbelaez reported a series of patients where conventional and custom LASIK was performed using the NIDEK EC-5000 Multipoint excimer laser (Nidek, Gamagori, Japan) in which "more accuracy, better visual acuity, and more subjective satisfaction was achieved in the custom LASIK treatment group" than in the conventionally treated group.[18] Similarly, Panagopoulou and Pallikaris[19] reported that eyes that underwent Wavefront Aberration Supported Cornea Ablation (WASCA) (Asclepion-Meditec AG, Jena, Germany) demonstrated "improved outcomes" in comparison to conventionally treated eyes. Results like this have acted as a catalyst for claims of "supernormal" visual acuity and for the potential to use wavefront-guided LASIK on emmetropic eyes "aiming toward improved visual acuity only."[17]

While wavefront-guided LASIK is designed to correct higher-order aberrations, these impediments to a perfect outcome are still present after surgery. In a group of patients in which one eye was treated by conventional LASIK and the other by wavefront-guided customized ablation using the Nidek EC-5000 excimer laser system, no statistically significant difference was found in the postoperative higher-order aberrations or in the BCVA between the two groups 1 month after surgery.[20] In a study by Mrochen et al,[21] only 22.5% of eyes had a significant reduction in higher-order aberrations. On average, the optical aberrations were increased by a factor of 1.44 3 months after surgery.[21]

The limitations of refraction-based treatments only are:

1. Treatment is not regionally customized
2. There is potential for reduced contrast sensitivity, hence
3. There is potential for poor visual performance in low light conditions

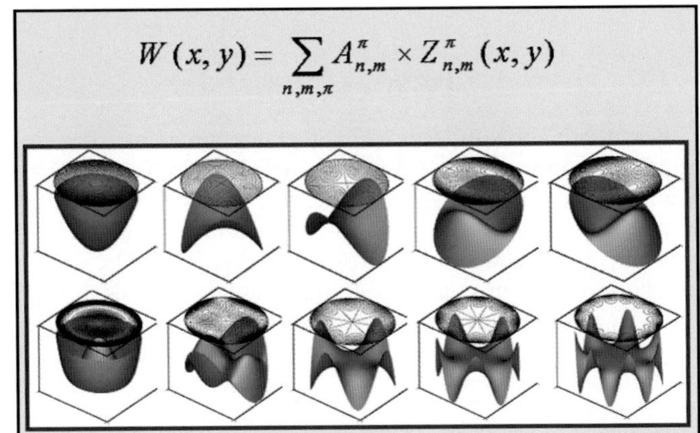

Figure 38-2. The shape of the wavefront is presented as a sum of a Zernike polynomial, each describing a certain deformation. (Courtesy of Bausch & Lomb Surgical.)

From the reported literature, it appears that wavefront-guided treatments achieve superior results to conventional treatments. The potential benefits of wavefront-guided treatments are:

1. Reduced aberrations in the optical system
2. Errors in spatial phase are corrected[11]
3. Improved contrast sensitivity and night vision
4. Better visual outcomes when compared to refraction-only based treatments

However, the potential limitations of wavefront-guided treatments are that they:

1. Do not take into account the amount of corneal astigmatism
2. Do not distinguish between corneal and lenticular aberrations
3. "Neutralize" internal aberrations of the eye onto the corneal surface
4. May increase irregularity of the cornea
5. Exclude the component of cortical perception of astigmatism, which would influence treatment with manifest refraction
6. Do not make allowances for internal aberrations that are likely to change with age

Table 38-1
Aggregate Data: Spherical Analysis of Treatment

MEASUREMENT	MANIFEST REFRACTION	ZYWAVE REFRACTION
Preoperative spherical equivalent mean ± SD (D) (spectacle plane)	-3.65 ± 1.26	-3.78 ± 1.45
Postoperative spherical equivalent mean ± SD (D) (spectacle plane)	+0.27 ± 0.43	+0.17 ± 0.57
S.IOS (corneal plane)	0.14 ± 0.23	0.14 ± 0.12
S.CI (corneal plane)	1.07 ± 1.01	1.05 ± 1.02

S.IOS = Spherical Index of Success, S.CI = Spherical Correction Index

7. Utilize ablations to correct aberrations that may be small in comparison to the changes in corneal aberrations caused by creating a corneal flap

PRINCIPLES OF VECTOR ANALYSIS OF ASTIGMATISM

Introduction

Refractive and corneal astigmatism, while usually related, seldom perfectly coincide. In many cases, they can be markedly different both in magnitude and orientation. Most current laser techniques aim for a zero refractive astigmatism outcome regardless of the amount or orientation of corneal astigmatism. Thus, the final shape of the cornea after surgery is seldom predetermined to target a spherical cornea. Surgical treatment of astigmatism determined by refractive means alone may result in an unfavorable distribution of astigmatism to the cornea.[22] Similarly, correcting astigmatism solely on corneal values could potentially lead to a gross overcorrection of manifest refraction and leave excessive refractive astigmatism remaining.

> Most current laser techniques aim for a zero refractive astigmatism outcome regardless of the amount or orientation of corneal astigmatism. Thus, the final shape of the cornea after surgery is seldom predetermined to target a spherical cornea.

By examining the relationship between surgery vectors, in particular the target-induced astigmatism vector (TIA), the surgically-induced astigmatism vector (SIA), and the difference vector (DV), outcomes of astigmatism treatment can be analyzed. In individual patients, the amount of correction achieved and the errors that occurred can be calculated. Aggregate data from a group of patients can be analyzed to determine systematic errors in laser application or surgical techniques and enable nomogram calculation for future adjustments to treatment.

ASTIGMATISM OUTCOMES IN A GROUP OF PATIENTS TREATED BY WAVEFRONT-GUIDED LASIK

The results reported here are from the first series of patients with astigmatism treated with Zyoptix (Technolas 217z, Bausch & Lomb, Rochester, NY) at The Laservision Centre in Southport, Australia by Drs. Darryl Gregor and Peter Heiner. Patients were selected for Zyoptix treatment based on a number of set criteria. They had to have myopia of between -1 diopter (D) and -7 D combined with refractive astigmatism of not more than -3 D. The mean preoperative subjective refraction was -3.65 D ± 1.26 D for the spherical component and -1.01 D ± 0.6 D for the astigmatic component of the refraction.

The goal of surgery was a plano refractive outcome. Patients had to pass the usual criteria to be suitable for laser surgery. They had to have adequate corneal pachymetry, normal topography, better than 20/30 BCVA, and no signs of ocular pathology. Orbscan corneal topography and Zywave wavefront images were taken according to the manufacturer's (Bausch & Lomb) instructions.

Bilateral Zyoptix LASIK surgery was performed in all cases, except for the very first patient to be treated. In this case, Zyoptix was performed on one eye and a standard Planoscan (nonwavefront) treatment on the other. Corneal flaps were created with a Nidek MK 2000 microkeratome with heads designed to achieve either a 130 millimeter (mm) or 160.00 mm flap thickness depending on the preoperative pachymetry. Patients were reviewed at 1 day, 1 week, and at 1 and 3 months after surgery.

This initial cohort data has been previously analyzed by Bausch & Lomb Surgical (Germany). Based on the Bausch & Lomb analysis, a nomogram adjustment was made to alter future treatments by a factor of 90% of the spherical component of the refraction (this is in agreement with the results reported here). For the purposes of this paper, the 3 month postoperative data were analyzed using the Alpins Statistical System for Ophthalmic Refractive-Surgery Techniques (ASSORT) outcomes analysis program (ASSORT Pty Ltd, Victoria, Australia). The method and terminology followed in this paper have been published previously.[3] All refractive values were converted to the corneal plane and all calculations were performed using these values. Simulated keratometry readings were taken from Orbscan computer-assisted videokeratoscopy maps and values obtained were used for the corneal astigmatism analysis.

AGGREGATE DATA ANALYSIS

Spherical Analysis

The group data were analyzed based on subjective refraction spherical equivalents (Table 38-1). On average, eyes were overcorrected by 0.27 D ± 0.43 D. The Spherical Correction Index (S.CI = 1.07) indicates an overcorrection of 7%. A Spherical Index of Success (S.IOS) of 0.14 was achieved, indicating that the spherical correction was 86% successful.

Table 38-2
Aggregate Data: Simple and Polar Value Analysis of Astigmatism

MEASUREMENT	MANIFEST REFRACTION (D)	ZYWAVE REFRACTION (D)	TOPOGRAPHY (D)	CORNEAL/ REFRACTIVE ASTIGMATISM*
Preoperative astigmatism mean ± SD	-1.01± 0.60*	-1.21 ± 0.75	1.33 ± 0.74*	1.32
Preoperative astigmatism, range	-0.25 to -3.00	-0.30 to -3.27	0.30 to 2.70	
Postoperative astigmatism, mean ± SD	-0.36 ± 0.23*	-0.43 ± 0.24	0.97 ± 0.47*	2.81
Postoperative astigmatism, range	0.00 to -0.75	-0.06 to -1.01	0.30 to 2.10	
Simple subtraction analysis mean ± SD	- 0.65 ± 0.61	- 0.78 ± 0.83	-0.36 ± 0.57	
Preoperative polar value mean ± SD	0.30 ± 1.04	0.33 ± 1.27	1.25 ± 0.86	
Postoperative polar value mean ± SD	0.25 ± 0.35	0.24 ± 0.44	0.97 ± 0.47	

Table 38-3
Aggregate Data: Surgical Vector Analysis of Astigmatic Treatment

	MANIFEST REFRACTION	ZYWAVE REFRACTION	TOPOGRAPHY
TIA, arithmetic mean ± SD	0.93 D ± 0.56	0.93 D ± 0.56	0.93 D ± 0.56
TIA, vector mean	0.22 D x 4	0.22 D x 4	0.22 D x 4
SIA, arithmetic mean ± SD	0.94 D ± 0.66	0.91 D ± 0.75	0.75 D ± 0.54
SIA, vector mean	0.11 D x 38	0.18 D x 23	0.18 D x 175
DV, arithmetic mean ± SD	0.36 D ± 0.24	0.49 D ± 0.21	0.53 D ± 0.36
DV, vector mean	0.21 D x 169	0.14 D x 157	0.08 D x 25
DV, vector mean/arithmetic mean	0.58	0.29	0.15

TIA = target-induced astigmatism, SIA = surgically-induced astigmatism, DV = difference vector

Astigmatism Analysis

Results for the group astigmatism analysis are shown in parallel for manifest refractive and Zywave measured refraction, and corneal (topographic) analysis. All patients except for one had -1.50 D or less of refractive astigmatism. The majority of patients only had a low or moderate amount of astigmatism (Table 38-2). Preoperative mean corneal astigmatism (1.33 D) exceeded mean subjective refractive astigmatism at the corneal plane (1.01 D) by a factor of 1.32. A greater reduction in refractive astigmatism (-0.65 D) than corneal astigmatism (-0.36 D) was achieved. Postoperative corneal astigmatism (0.97 D) exceeded subjective refractive astigmatism (0.36 D) by a factor of 2.81. This shows an excessive proportion of corneal, compared to refractive, astigmatism remaining. This phenomenon, which has been shown in other studies of astigmatism, is evident when employing refractive astigmatism parameters alone.[3]

Data analyzed using subjective refraction (subjective) data showed that a summated vector mean TIA value of 0.22 D x 4 (Table 38-3) was attempted. This indicates that the trend was to induce a net steepening along the horizontal meridian to result in a small net against-the-rule change. The arithmetic mean SIA by manifest refraction was 0.94 D and Zywave refraction was 0.91 D. These values were slightly lower than that aimed for (TIA = 0.93 D), suggesting a small undercorrection. An undercorrection was also evident for the corneal changes (SIA = 0.75 D). The summated vector mean values of SIA by refraction (subjective 0.11 D, wavefront 0.18 D) and topography (0.18 D) confirmed the trend for undercorrection by comparison with the TIA vector mean.

Consistent trends for treatment error are shown in both refractive and topographical measurements. The arithmetic mean magnitude of the DV by refraction (subjective 0.36 D [Figure 38-3A]; wavefront 0.49 D) was less than that by topography (0.53 D) (Figure 38-3B). When determined by subjective refraction data and topographical data, 58% and 15% of this error (0.21 D and 0.08 D, respectively) can be attributed to systematic treatment error (see Table 38-3).

Angle of error (AE) analysis for subjective refraction and topography show that both arithmetic means for the groups were close to zero (+1.57 degrees and -0.39 degrees) (slightly counterclockwise and clockwise, respectively). However, the spread of results is wide for both refractive (SD of AE = 14.45 degrees, absolute AE = 9.57 degrees) and corneal (SD of AE =

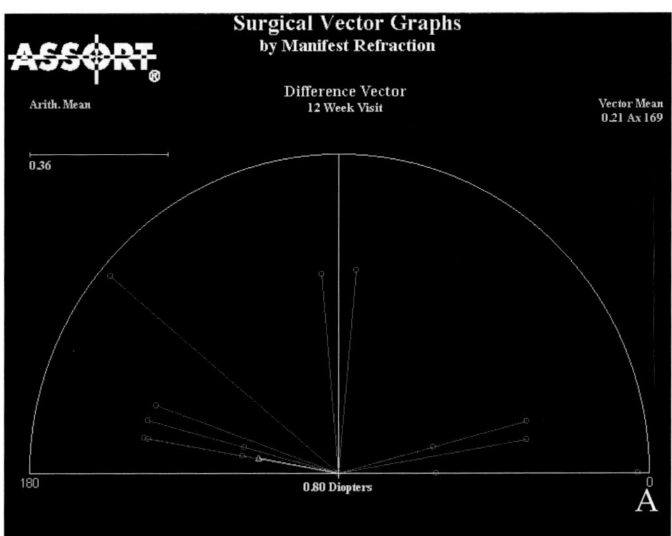

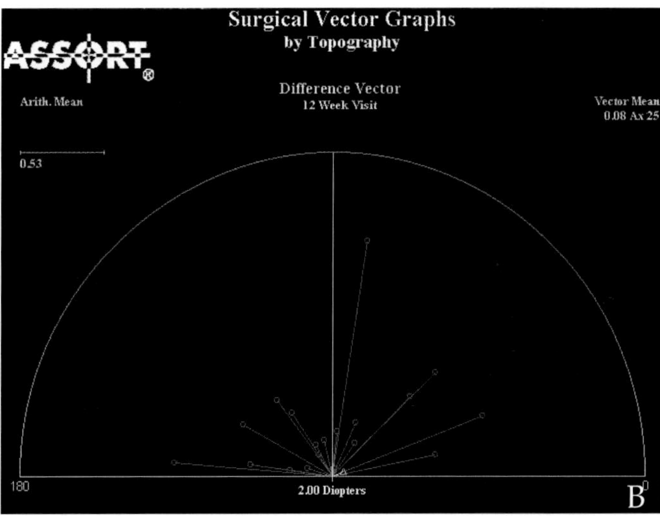

Figure 38-3. Aggregate data analyses. Surgical vector graphs for subjective refraction (A) and topography (B) are shown. Arithmetic and vectorial means are shown.

Table 38-4

Aggregate Data: Astigmatism Analysis of Vectors for Error and Treatment. A Comparison of Refractive and Topographical Values

	Manifest Refraction	*Zywave Refraction*	*Topography*
AE, arithmetic mean ± SD (degrees)	+1.57 ± 14.45	+2.07 ± 29.83	-0.39 ± 16.31
AE, absolute mean ± SD (degrees)	9.57 ± 10.93	18.81 ± 23.25	13.75 ± 8.77
ME, arithmetic mean ± SD (D)	0.01 ± 0.28	-0.02 ± 0.35	-0.18 ± 0.46
CI, geometric mean ± SD	0.96 ± 1.43	0.80 ± 1.83	0.74 ± 1.75
FI, geometric mean ± SD	0.79 ± 1.23	0.71 ± 1.28	0.62 ± 1.25
IOS, geometric mean ± SD	0.35 ± 0.12	0.61 ± 0.06	0.55 ± 0.06
CA	1.04 ± 1.43	1.26 ± 1.83	1.34 ± 1.75
ORA (D)		0.92 ± 0.47	

AE = angle of error, ME = magnitude of error, CI = correction index, FI = flattening index, IOS = index of success, CA = coefficient of adjustment, ORA = ocular residual astigmatism

16.31 degrees, absolute AE = 13.75 degrees) measures, with topographical results being more greatly spread. There was greater spread in the data when results were analyzed with wavefront-derived refractions than when analyzed with manifest refraction or corneal topography data, indicating a greater variability of wavefront measured values.

> There was greater spread in the data when results were analyzed with wavefront-derived refractions than when analyzed with manifest refraction or corneal topography data, indicating a greater variability of wavefront measured values.

The treatment (Table 38-4) was more successful when measured by subjective refractive measures (index of success [IOS] = 0.35, 65%) than by wavefront-derived refractive measures (IOS = 0.61, 39%) or objective corneal measurement (IOS = 0.55, 45%). This is supported by the correction index (CI) values of 0.96 for manifest refractive and 0.74 for topography measurements of astigmatism. It was interesting to note that wavefront-derived CI of 0.80 more closely parallels the corneal topographical value. The flattening index (FI) indicates that the treatment was less effectively applied at the treatment axis when measured by corneal (FI = 0.62) or wavefront derived refraction (FI = 0.71) than by subjective refractive (FI = 0.79) means. The values for nomogram adjustment indicate that an increase in the future magnitude of astigmatism treatment in the region of 26% (zywave) and 34% (corneal) would likely improve outcomes. However, this value should be modified down to some extent as manifest refraction showed a coefficient of adjustment (CA) of 1.04 (4%) only.

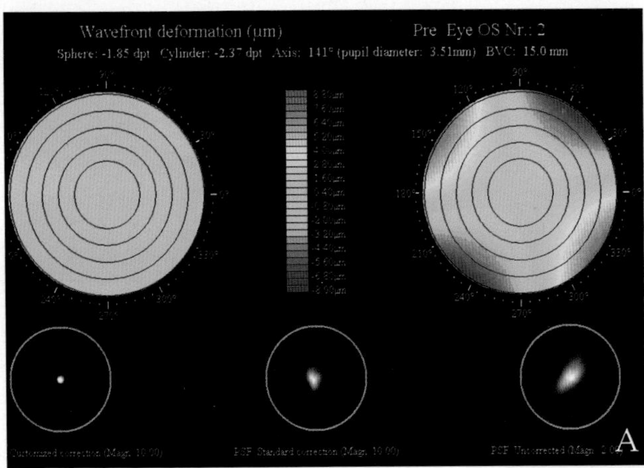

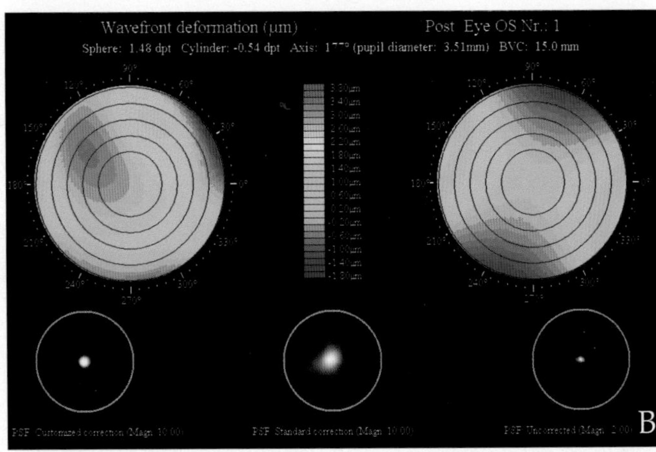

Figure 38-4. Single patient analyses. Preoperative (A) and 3-month postoperative (B) Zywave aberrometry data are shown.

Single Patient Analysis

The left eye of one patient was individually analyzed to determine changes in astigmatism. All calculations were performed on corneal plane values. The preoperative refraction was -2.00/-2.00 x 145 (UCVA = 20/200, BCVA = 20/20) and the Zywave refraction -1.85/-2.37 x 141 (Figure 38-4A). Three months after surgery, the refraction was +1.25/-0.75 x 180 (UCVA = 20/16-1, BCVA = 20/16+1) and the Zywave refraction +1.48/-0.54 x 177 (Figure 38-4B). Simulated keratometry values from the Orbscan (Figure 38-5) were 42.7/44.9 @ 67 preoperatively and 39.2/41.1 @ 90 at 3 months postoperatively.

Spherical Analysis

The preoperative spherical equivalent prior to surgery was -3 D and +0.88 D at 3 months postoperatively (Table 38-5). The S.IOS indicates that the surgery was 69% successful. The CI (1.31) shows that there has been an overcorrection in this patient of 31%.

Astigmatism Analysis

The refractive astigmatism prior to surgery was 2 D by refraction and 2.20 D by corneal values (Table 38-6). The astigmatic treatment (TIA) was 1.86 D x 145 at the corneal plane (Table 38-7). The SIA by refractive values was 1.75 D x 133 and by corneal values was 1.48 D x 124 (Figure 38-6). The DVs of 0.77 D x 0 (refractive) and 1.27 D x 171 (corneal) indicate that there was still remaining astigmatism.

Description of Astigmatism Analysis: Topography

Figure 38-6 displays corneal values for astigmatism and vectors, both on a double-angle vector diagram (DAVD). Also displayed in tables are all the astigmatism values, surgical vector values, and an analysis of errors and correction.

The DAVD is constructed by doubling all three meridian values of astigmatism and displaying these values (astigmatisms) at their respective double-angled location. The vectors are determined by joining the heads of the astigmatism displays with dashed lines.

To view the surgical vectors at their actual position, their axis value is halved and the tail of the vector is located at the origin of the polar surgical vector graph.

Both the refractive and corneal values indicate there has been an undercorrection of astigmatism. This is evidenced by CI values of 0.94 for refraction and 0.80 for corneal (Table 38-8). The AE shows that the treatment was off axis by 12 degrees clockwise for refraction and by 22 degrees clockwise when determined by corneal values. This could be due to alignment or healing factors. Thus, a significant loss of effect at the treatment meridian occurred as demonstrated by the FE (1.60 D and 1.09 D) and FI (0.86 and 0.58). The IOS shows that the treatment was 59% (0.41) successful in correcting refractive astigmatism and 31% (0.69) successful in correcting corneal astigmatism.

Torque Effect

While the FE and FI are measures of how effective the SIA has been in reducing astigmatism, the torque effect gauges the proportion of the SIA that did not reduce astigmatism. It occurs as a consequence of the effects of treatment being "off axis," and it results in the rotation of existing astigmatism and not its reduction. The torque effect is maximum when the AE reaches 45 degrees, so it is greater for corneal measurements (1.01 D) than for refractive (0.72 D) as the off-axis effect was greater (-22 degrees compared to -12 degrees).

Discussion

For the aggregate data, an average overcorrection of 7% of the spherical component of the treatment occurred (S.CI = 1.07). In comparison, the study of Alpins[3] found an undercorrection of 12% (S.CI = 0.88) for conventionally treated LASIK patients with a different laser device. This may be due to differences in individual lasers and treatment conditions. While it could indicate a trend for wavefront devices to overestimate the preoperative spherical component of refraction, this did not seem to be evident. The average spherical component was -3.65 D ± 1.26 D for the preoperative manifest refraction and -3.78 D ± 1.45 D when measured with the Zywave aberrometer.

The results reported here for a small group of patients treated with wavefront-guided LASIK compare favorably with conventional LASIK for the correction of low to moderate levels of astig-

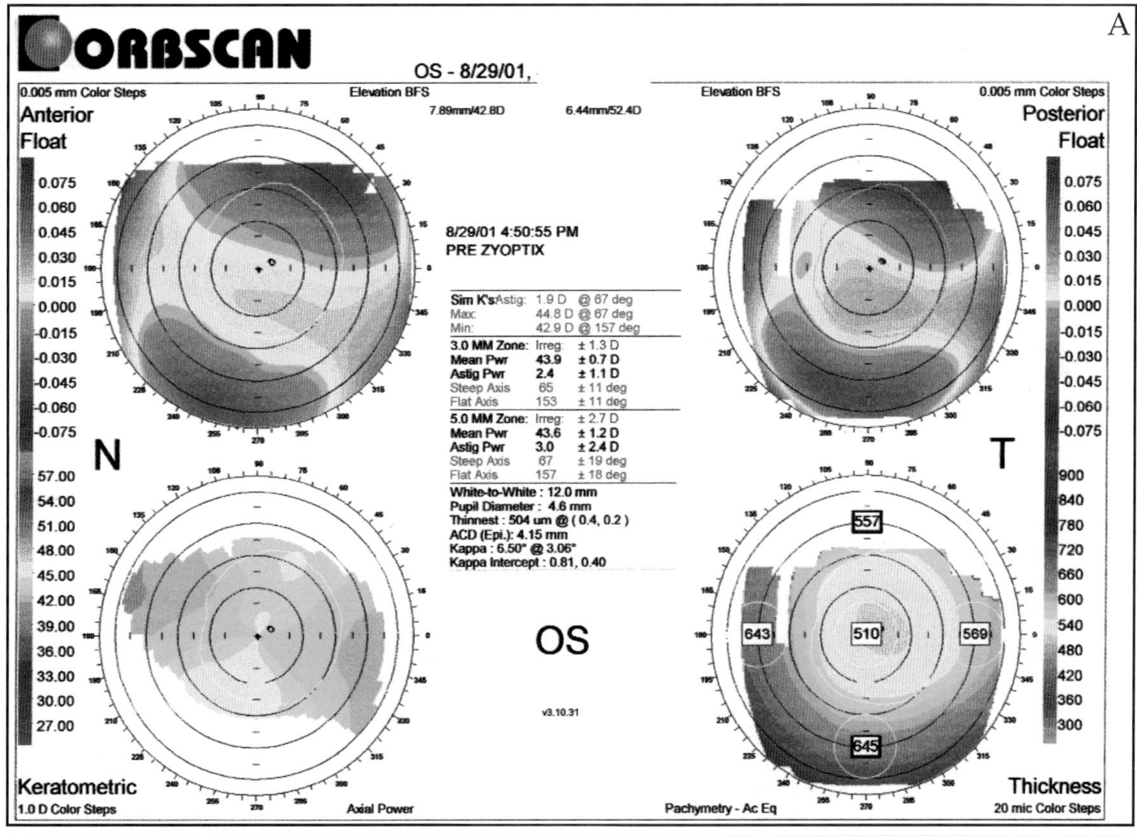

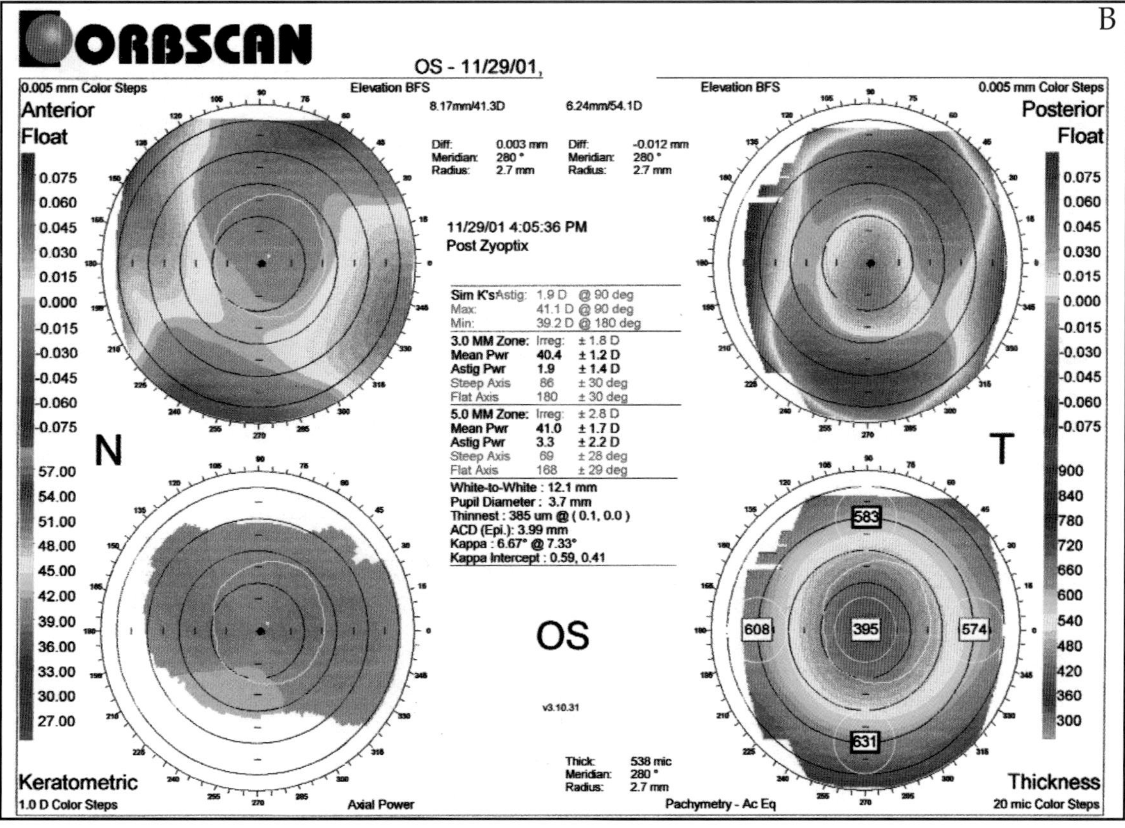

Figure 38-5. Single patient analyses. Preoperative (A) and 3-month postoperative (B) Orbscan computer-assisted videokeratoscopy maps are shown.

Table 38-5
Individual Patient Analysis: Spherical Analysis

	Refraction (Corneal plane)
Preoperative spherical equivalent (D)	-3.00 (-2.88)
Postoperative spherical equivalent (D)	0.88 (0.89)
S.IOS	0.31
S.CI	1.31

S.IOS = spherical index of success, S.CI = spherical correction index

Table 38-6
Individual Patient Analysis: Simple Astigmatism Analysis

	Refraction	Topography
Preoperative astigmatism (D)	2.00	1.90
Postoperative astigmatism (D)	0.75	1.90
Simple subtraction value	-1.25	0.00

Table 38-7
Individual Patient Analysis: Surgical Vector Analysis of Astigmatism Treatment

	Refraction	Topography
TIA (D)	1.86 x 145	1.86 x 145
SIA (D)	1.75 x 133	1.48 x 124
DV (D)	0.77 x 0	1.27 x 171

TIA = target-induced astigmatism, SIA = surgically-induced astigmatism, DV = difference vector

matism (mean astigmatism measured by manifest refraction of -1.01 D ± 0.60 D). The aggregate data show that the astigmatic treatment was more successful when determined by subjective refractive means compared to corneal measures. This trend has been reported previously for conventional LASIK treatments.[23] An analysis of 100 conventionally treated LASIK patients[3] showed a systematic undercorrection of astigmatism by 15% for refractive values and 30% for corneal values. However, when results were analyzed by wavefront-derived refraction, the success of astigmatism treatment was more similar to that determined by corneal measures. This may be due to both corneal- and wavefront-derived refraction being objective rather than subjective tests.

The aggregate data show that the astigmatic treatment was more successful when determined by subjective refractive means compared to corneal measures. This trend has been reported previously for conventional LASIK treatments.[23] When results were analyzed by wavefront-derived refraction, the success of astigmatism treatment was more similar to that determined by corneal measures. This may be due to both corneal- and wavefront-derived refraction being objective rather than subjective tests. This may also be due to intrinsic inaccuracies in this particular wavefront device.

The single patient analysis data remind us that as the amount of astigmatism increases, factors other than the treatment plan may play a role in the final surgical outcome. As astigmatism magnitude increases, a small deviation in the meridian of treatment from that planned may have a more significant effect on the amount of treatment applied at the intended axis. Where oblique astigmatism exists, it is probably more likely that the analysis will show a misalignment of axes than when compared to against- or with-the-rule astigmatism in which the principal meridia of the astigmatism lie closer to the principal poles. Healing factors may also play a role. Whether a patient is treated with conventional LASIK or wavefront-guided LASIK, these factors remain important. In this particular patient's case, the visual outcome (UCVA = 20/15-1) was still extremely good as the best sphere was close to zero and an improvement in BCVA occurred (from 20/20 to 20/15+1), masking the less than perfect astigmatic outcome revealed by vector analysis. Ultimately, the subjective evaluation of the visual outcome is the most important measure of an individual patient's success.

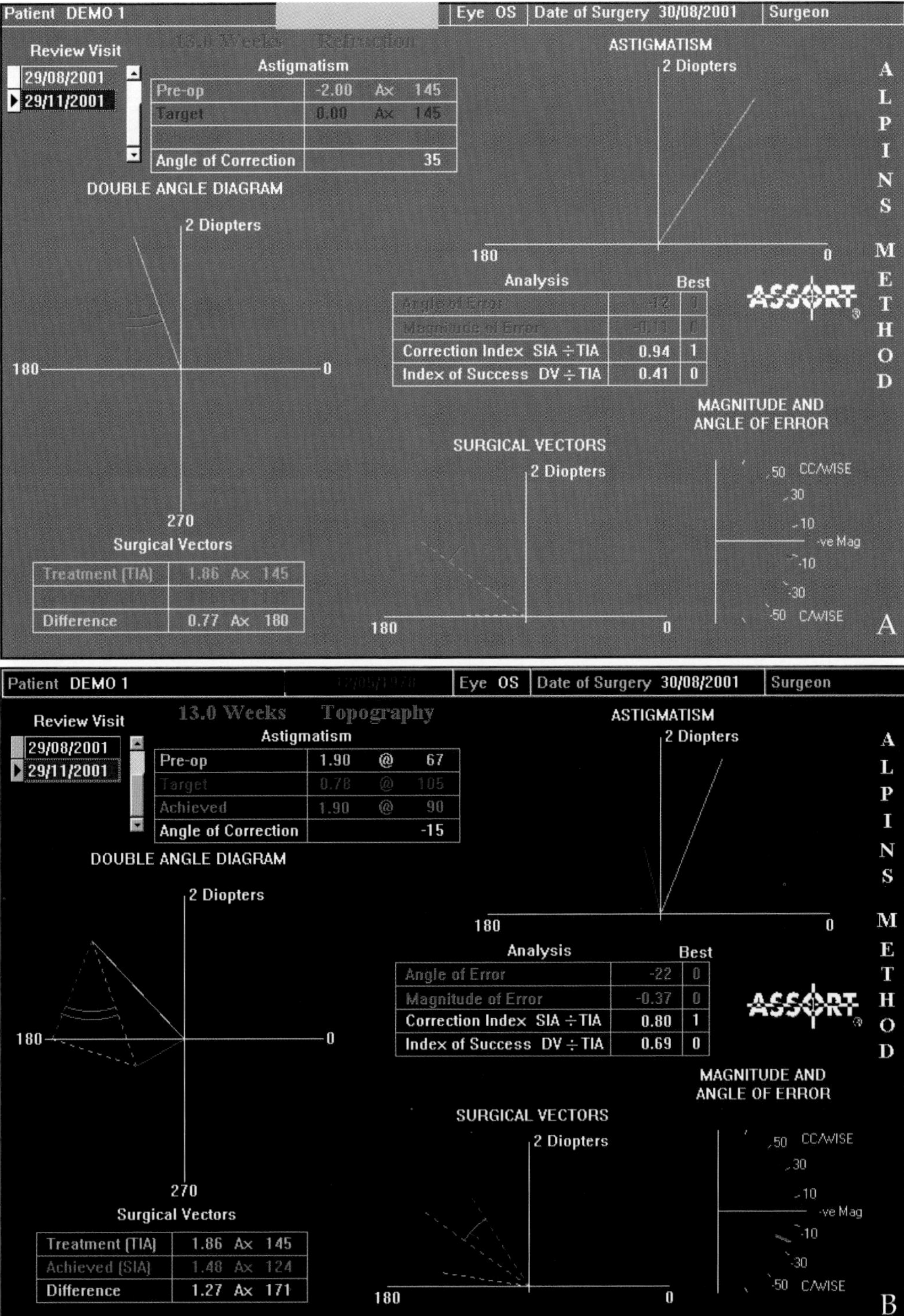

Figure 38-6. Single patient analyses. Surgical vector graphs for refraction (A) and topography (B) are shown.

Table 38-8
Individual Patient Analysis: Surgical Vector Analysis of Astigmatism Treatment. A Comparison of Refractive and Topographical Values

	REFRACTION	TOPOGRAPHY
AE	-12.00	-22.00
ME	-0.11 D	-0.37 D
IOS	0.41	0.69
CI	0.94	0.80
FE	1.60 D	1.09 D
Torque effect (CCW)	0.72 D	1.01 D
FI	0.86	0.58
CA	1.06	1.25
ORA	0.78 D x 15	0.78 D x 15

AE = angle of error, ME = magnitude of error, IOS = index of success, CI = correction index, FE = flattening effect, CCW = counter clockwise; FI = flattening index, CA = coefficient of adjustment, ORA = ocular residual astigmatism

OPTIMIZING OUTCOMES FOR TOPOGRAPHY AND WAVEFRONT

When a LASIK flap is made on the eye, changes in corneal curvature and thickness occur outside of the ablation zone.[24,25] This biomechanical response causes a FE in the treatment zone, which enhances a myopic procedure but counteracts a hyperopic ablation.[24,25]

Creating a flap on the eye changes the structure of the cornea. Applying principles of spheric corneal topography may account for the differences in relative effect of creating a flap through an elliptical or conic section. It enables differences in the relative effect of laser treatment in the presence of corneal cylinder that is either greater or less than the refractive cylinder to be incorporated into the treatment plan.

Optimizing outcomes for topography and wavefront examinations takes into account both the corneal structure and refractive function. For individual patients this means that any discrepancy between refractive and corneal astigmatism can be taken into account in the treatment plan to avoid an excess residual amount of corneal astigmatism. Changes in corneal structure induced by LASIK surgery particularly can affect the lower-order aberrations of the eye.

Guiding the TIA, the meridian of maximum ablation, closer to the principal flat corneal meridian would result in less corneal astigmatism. The process of vector planning would reduce the excess amount of corneal astigmatism remaining demonstrated in this (2.81 versus 1.32) and other studies.[3] This needs to be further investigated and then incorporated into the treatment plan if a favorable influence is identified.

The potential benefits of vector planning of preoperative corneal and refractive astigmatism values are:

1. Corneal values are included in the treatment plan
2. The treatment can be optimized and balanced between corneal and refractive parameters
3. The potential for less "off-axis" effect on principal corneal meridia and a greater reduction in corneal astigmatism
4. There is the potential to bias the treatment to a more favorable with-the-rule astigmatism outcome (which usually has the least adverse impact on distance vision) or to any other orientation preferred by the surgeon
5. Reduced corneal astigmatism is likely to provide less low-order (second) aberrations and even some high-order (third and fourth) aberrations and enhanced contrast sensitivity

CONCLUSION

Wavefront-guided laser refractive surgery holds future promise for correcting higher-order aberrations of the eye. However, we must not lose focus of the importance of correcting both the spherical and cylindrical components of refraction quantified by the lower-order (second) aberrations. Nomogram adjustment of laser treatments remains an important factor in the surgical planning process. Vector planning would potentially be a valuable adjunct to treatments that are guided by wavefront aberrometry measurements. Optimizing outcomes by incorporating both corneal and refractive values into the treatment plan are necessary challenges for the imminent future of refractive surgery.

Editor's note:
Although the content of this chapter has been primarily focused on vector analysis and planning of wavefront vs refraction vs topographic cylinder, the possibility does exist to analyze the magnitude and axis of other higher-order aberrations as well. We reserve this topic for a later time, as the complexity of vector planning and astigmatism is sufficient for now. Further practical experience is needed to bring about more widespread acceptance of this method of analysis and planning.
R. Krueger, MD, MSE

Definitions

Astigmatism Analysis

angle of error (AE): The angle described by the SIA and TIA vectors. The AE is positive if the achieved correction was counterclockwise to that intended and is negative if the achieved correction was clockwise to the intended axis.

coefficient of adjustment (CA): The coefficient required to adjust future treatments of astigmatism magnitude. It is calculated by dividing the TIA by the SIA, and is preferably 1.00.

correction index (CI): The CI is calculated by dividing the SIA by the TIA. The CI is ideally equal to 1.00. It is greater than 1.00 for an overcorrection and less than 1.00 if an undercorrection has occurred.

difference vector (DV): The induced astigmatic change needed for the initial surgery to have achieved its intended target outcome. The DV is preferably 0.

flattening effect (FE): The amount of astigmatism reduction achieved by the effective proportion of the SIA at the intended meridian.

flattening index (FI): The FI is calculated by dividing the FE by the TIA. The FI is ideally 1.00.

index of success (IOS): The IOS is calculated by dividing the DV by the TIA. The IOS is a measure of success and is preferably zero.

magnitude of error (ME): The difference between the magnitudes of the SIA and the TIA. The ME is positive for overcorrections and negative for undercorrections.

ocular residual astigmatism (ORA): The ORA represents the calculated minimum amount possible of astigmatism remaining in the system after treatment. It is the vector difference between the corneal and refractive astigmatisms.

surgically-induced astigmatism vector (SIA): The astigmatic change actually induced by the surgery.

target-induced astigmatism vector (TIA): The astigmatic change the surgery was intended to induce.

torque effect: The amount of astigmatic change induced by the SIA that has been ineffective in reducing astigmatism at the intended meridian but has caused rotation and a small increase in the existing astigmatism. Torque lies 45 degrees counter clockwise to the SIA if positive and 45 degrees clockwise to the SIA if negative.[2]

Spherical Analysis

spherical correction index (S.CI): The spherical equivalent correction achieved divided by the targeted spherical correction.

spherical difference (S.Diff): The absolute difference between the targeted spherical equivalent correction and the achieved spherical equivalent correction.

spherical index of success (S.IOS): The absolute difference between the achieved and targeted spherical equivalents divided by the targeted spherical equivalent correction.

Acknowledgments

The authors wish to thank Drs. Peter Heiner and Darryl Gregor for permission to analyze their data. Thanks also go to Mr. George Stamatelatos for performing the data analysis.

Financial Interest: Dr. Noel Alpins has a financial interest in the ASSORT vector planning and outcomes software used in the analysis of surgeries and results in this paper.

References

1. Alpins NA. A new method of analyzing vectors for changes in astigmatism. *J Cataract Refract Surg.* 1993;19:524-533.
2. Alpins NA. Vector analysis of astigmatism changes by flattening, steepening, and torque. *J Cataract Refract Surg.* 1997;23:1503-1514.
3. Alpins NA. Astigmatism analysis by the Alpins method. *J Cataract Refract Surg.* 2001;27:31-49.
4. Williams D, Yoon GY, Porter J, Guirao A, Hofer H, Cox I. Visual benefit of correcting higher-order aberrations of the eye. *J Refract Surg.* 2000;16:S554-S559.
5. Thibos LN, Hong X. Clinical applications of the Shack-Hartmann aberrometer. *Optom Vis Sci.* 1999;76:817-825.
6. Seiler T, Kaemmerer M, Mierdel P, Krinke HE. Ocular optical aberrations after photorefractive keratectomy for myopia and myopic astigmatism. *Arch Ophthalmol.* 2000;118:17-21.
7. Marcos S. Aberrations and visual performance following standard laser vision correction. *J Refract Surg.* 2001;17:S596-S601.
8. Moreno-Barriuso E, Lloves JM, Marcos S, Navarro R, Llorente L, Barbero S. Ocular aberrations before and after myopic corneal refractive surgery: LASIK-induced changes measured with laser ray tracing. *Invest Ophthalmol Vis Sci.* 2001;42:1396-1403.
9. Oshika T, Miyata K, Tokunaga T, et al. Higher-order wavefront aberrations of cornea and magnitude of refractive correction in laser in situ keratomileusis. *Ophthalmology.* 2002;109:1154-1158.
10. Marcos S, Barbero S, Llorente L, Merayo-Lloves J. Optical response to LASIK surgery for myopia from total and corneal aberration measurements. *Invest Ophthalmol Vis Sci.* 2001;42:3349-3356.
11. Applegate RA, Thibos LN, Hilmantel G. Optics of aberroscopy and supervision. *J Cataract Refract Surg.* 2001;27:1093-1107.
12. Holladay JT, Dudeja DR, Chang J. Functional vision and corneal changes after laser in situ keratomileusis determined by contrast sensitivity, glare testing, and corneal topography. *J Cataract Refract Surg.* 1999;25:663-669.
13. Applegate RA, Hilmantel G, Howland HC, Tu EY, Starck T, Zayac J. Corneal first surface optical aberrations and visual performance. *J Refract Surg.* 2000;16:507-514.
14. Applegate RA, Howland HC. Refractive surgery, optical aberrations, and visual performance. *J Refract Surg.* 1997;13:295-299.
15. Liang J, Williams DR, Miller D. Supernormal vision and high-resolution retinal imaging through adaptive optics. *J Opt Soc Am* A. 1997;14:2882-2892.
16. Mrochen M, Kaemmerer M, Seiler T. Wavefront-guided laser in situ keratomileusis: early results in three eyes. *J Refract Surg.* 2000;16:116-121.
17. Seiler T, Mrochen M, Kaemmerer M. Operative correction of ocular aberrations to improve visual acuity. *J Refract Surg.* 2000;16:S619-S622.
18. Arbelaez MC. Super vision: dream or reality. *J Refract Surg.* 2001;17:S211-S218.
19. Panagopoulou SI, Pallikaris IG. Wavefront customized ablations with the WASCA Asclepion workstation. *J Refract Surg.* 2001;17:S608-S612.
20. Vongthongsri A, Phusitphoykai N, Naripthapan P. Comparison of wavefront-guided customized ablations vs conventional ablation in laser in situ keratomileusis. *J Refract Surg.* 2002;18:S332-S335.
21. Mrochen M, Kaemmerer M, Seiler T. Clinical results of wavefront-guided laser in situ keratomileusis 3 months after surgery. *J Cataract Refract Surg.* 2001;27:201-207.
22. Alpins NA. New method of targeting vectors to treat astigmatism. *J Cataract Refract Surg.* 1997;23:65-75.

23. Alpins NA, Tabin GC. Refractive versus corneal changes after photorefractive keratectomy for astigmatism. *J Refract Surg*. 1998;14:386-396.

24. Roberts C. The cornea is not a piece of plastic. *J Refract Surg*. 2000;16:407-413.

25. Roberts C. Future challenges to aberration-free ablative procedures. *J Refract Surg*. 2000;16:S623-S629.

Clinical Science Section

Chapter 39

Custom-Contoured Ablation Pattern Method for the Treatment of Irregular Astigmatism

Gustavo E. Tamayo, MD and Mario G. Serrano, MD

Introduction

After the official release of the contoured ablation pattern (CAP method) by VISX (Santa Clara, Calif) in 1999, the technique and the method improved and evolved until its approval by the US Food and Drug Administration for use in December 2001, under a Humanitarian Device Exemption (HDE) protocol. The approval was limited to the treatment of irregular astigmatism produced by a previous refractive excimer laser surgery, and it is linked to the use of the CAP ablation planner from the Humphrey topography system (Carl Zeiss Meditec, Dublin, Calif).

The FDA exemption reflects the growing concern of a very severe problem, namely irregular astigmatism. The custom-contoured ablation pattern (C-CAP method) is the only topography-linked system with proven and safe results for the treatment of irregular astigmatism.

The method is easy to use. It allows the surgeon to manipulate the excimer laser system and set the treatment parameters, such as shape, depth, location, size, and number of ablations, based on the topographic map and the clinical judgment.

Definition of Custom-Contoured Ablation Method

C-CAP is software developed by VISX to use in conjunction with the VISX STAR S4 Excimer Laser System. It is extremely flexible and gives the surgeon a tool to produce any type of ablation, in any shape, any size, any depth, and in any location, to treat all refractive defects from regular to irregular. The software allows the user to program 20 different sequential ablations, with or without a pause between them.

The size of the beam can be varied from 0.60 millimeter (mm) (minimum) to 6.5 mm (maximum). Three different shapes can be utilized: sphere, cylinder, and ellipse. Hyperopic sphere or hyperopic cylinder can also be added as part of the treatment. Depth may go from 1 micron (μm) to 150 μm, and the beam may be directed to the center of the pupil or decentered up to 4 mm horizontally or vertically as measured from the center of the pupil, utilizing the X or Y coordinates in the laser computer (Figure 39-1).

Custom-Contoured Ablation Pattern Background

After the publication of a paper from Gibralter and Trokel in 1994[1] about the treatment of irregularities in the cornea with manual decentration of the excimer beam, we started to move the beam to treat the steepest areas of the cornea without good results. However, in 1997, the topographic difference between the steepest area and the most elevated area was noted[2] (Figure 39-2) and the beam was then deviated to ablate the areas that were elevated the most. Results improved dramatically. That was the beginning of the "manual" CAP method.[3] Several treatments were performed with promising results (Figure 39-3) until March 30, 1999 when the three first eyes were treated with the CAP method software, launched then by VISX in April 1999 during an American Society of Cataract and Refractive Surgery (ASCRS) meeting in Seattle, Wash.

In 1997, the topographic difference between the steepest area and the most elevated area was noted[2] and the beam was then deviated to ablate the areas that were elevated the most. Results improved dramatically.

Since then, thousands of eyes around the world have been treated with this method, and several investigational studies have been performed.[4] The technique was improved over the years and the advantages of beam changes such as the seven beam split, which makes the beam smaller like scanning and rotational, was then applied. The CAP method was incorporated into all the hardware and software changes. The eye tracker—one of the most prominent features of the VISX STAR S3 system—added much more precision to the decentration properties of the beam, making the CAP software more effective and safe in ablating the most elevated areas.

At the same time, elevation topography has improved and has become more precise and more exact in its calculations. It gives information about location, shape, size, and depth of the most elevated areas, allowing the surgeon to choose the best treatment for every zone. The term *topography-assisted excimer laser ablation* was created, reflecting the ability to topographically detect the irregularities and then treat them. Topography systems, such as the

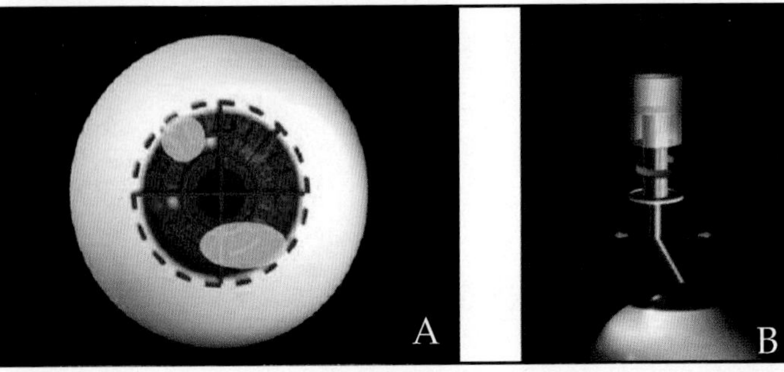

Figure 39-1. (A) C-CAP ablation on cornea demonstrating sphere and eliptical treatment. (B) Seven beam array emerges from the homogenizing and beam splitting module.

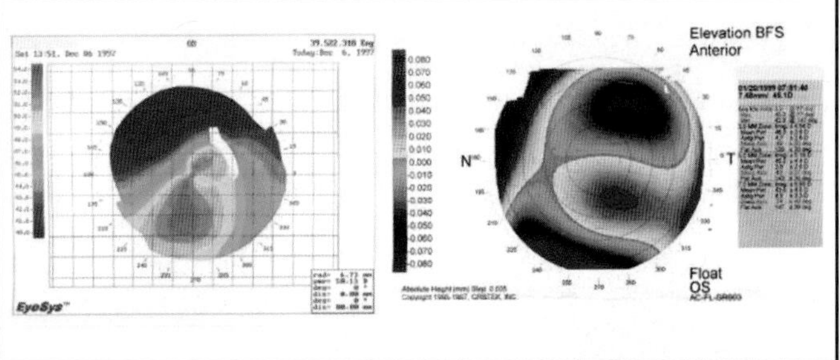

Figure 39-2. C-CAP corneal topography and elevation map.

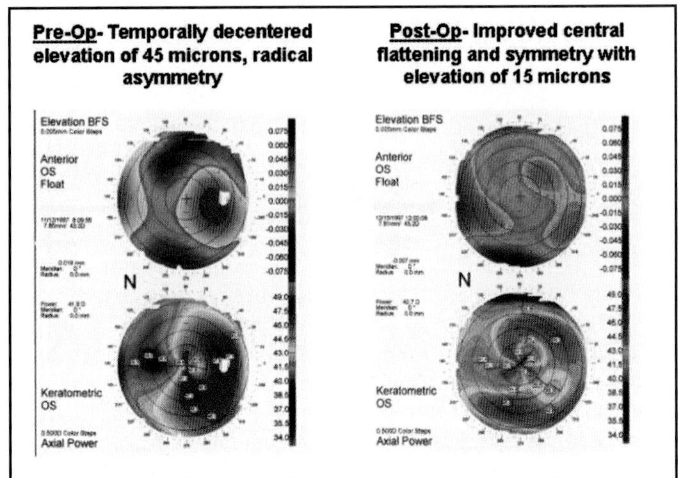

Figure 39-3. Pre- and postoperative corneal topography.

Humphrey and the Dicon, developed simulation software topographies that allow the surgeon to see the simulated topography result on the screen of the computer before the treatment is actually carried out. They have been called *CAP planners*. A section of this chapter will be dedicated to this subject (see p. 334).

Custom-Contoured Ablation Pattern Applications

For the purpose of this book, we will concentrate on the treatment of irregular astigmatism with the VISX CAP method. However, the software also has other treatment capabilities.

Regular Defects

1. Myopia
2. Myopic astigmatism
3. Hyperopia
4. Hyperopic astigmatism
5. Mixed astigmatism with or without crosscylinder technique
6. Phototherapeutic keratectomy (PTK)
7. Presbyopia (discontinued with the use of variable spot software [VSS])

Irregular Defects

These are one of the most important indications of the C-CAP method and the reason for its approval in the United States by the FDA. They are also known as *irregular astigmatism* and will be the focus of this chapter. Irregular astigmatism is a very disabling problem because of the symptoms it produces (eg, glare, halos, phantom images, multiple images). It can be produced by two main sources: nonacquired or naturally occurring, and acquired.[5]

1. Nonacquired or naturally occurring
   a. Keratoconus
   b. Pellucid marginal degeneration
   c. Congenital asymmetrical astigmatism
   d. Corneal dystrophies
2. Acquired
   a. Previous refractive treatments
      –Incisional surgery
      –Laser in-situ keratomileusis (LASIK) surgery: decentered flap complications
   b. Other types of corneal surgery
   c. Corneal trauma

Correction of Irregular Astigmatism With the Custom-Contoured Ablation Pattern Method: Topography-Assisted Excimer Laser Ablation

The treatment of irregular astigmatism with the excimer laser is based on resection of the elevated areas of the cornea that produce the irregularities. Lasers cannot add tissue to elevate the depressed zones. The method is essentially a topography-assisted ablation system; therefore, several rules must be followed in order to obtain an acceptable result.

It is extremely important to remember that the goal of the treatment is to regulate the corneal contour and not to get a complete refractive correction to allow patients to get rid of glasses.[6] Such a correction can be intended once the corneal anterior surface has been brought back to normal, provided there is enough tissue to ablate and more than 270 µm of corneal tissue remains untreated.

The C-CAP method can be used with photorefractive keratectomy (PRK) or LASIK. The election of the technique should be based on experience, thickness of the cornea, amount of tissue needed to be resected, availability for follow-up, etc.

It is extremely important to remember that the goal of the treatment is to regulate the corneal contour and not to get a complete refractive correction to allow patients to get rid of glasses.[6]

Surface Ablation: PRK or LASEK

Epithelium can be removed with the laser if the treatment fits into the central 6.50 mm optical zone. If it does not, a manual removal is selected: epithelial brush such as the Amoils brush (Innovative Excimer Solutions Inc, Toronto, Canada) or 20% or 30% alcohol. It is beyond the purpose of this chapter to explain and discuss the technique called LASEK. However, it has been used by the authors in more than 170 cases, with excellent results very similar to the PRK results.

In both surface ablation techniques, when selected, mitomycin 0.02% is applied to the exposed stroma[7] for 1 minute, as soon as the ablation is terminated, with a wet sponge. The application of this antimetabolite helps to prevent the formation of haze. It has been used very successfully by the authors in the last 1.5 years, avoiding haze in those corneas prone to scarring, post-LASIK patients treated with surface ablation, corneas with multiple incisions, etc. Mitomycin should be carefully removed from the cornea, avoiding contact with other ocular surfaces. Then the cornea should be washed thoroughly and a bandage contact lens applied and left in place for 1 week or until the epithelium is fully recovered.

For the first 2 weeks after surgery, a combination of a strong corticosteroid drop (prednisolone acetate) and an antibiotic (ofloxacin or ciprofloxacin) is used. For the next 4 weeks, the patient is switched to a mild steroid treatment such as fluorometholone and tear substitutes as needed. In the last 4 months after treatment, the patient is kept on a nonsteroidal anti-inflammatory (NSAID) drop.

The correction of the residual refractive defect, if chosen by patient and doctor, should not be attempted before 4 months after the initial treatment and the same protocol of the surface treatment must be followed.

LASIK

In the correction of irregular astigmatism, this is always the first option for treatment because patient recovery is almost immediate, there is no pain after surgery, and less postoperative care is needed. However, several considerations should be taken into account. The flap does debilitate the cornea and by no means gives strength to it. It cannot be counted in the residual non-touched stromal bed, which must be at least 270 µm. The equation (central pachymetry – flap thickness + microns of ablation) should equal 270 µm or more. The following are other considerations:

- Creating a flap in a highly irregular cornea is a challenge. The corneal curvature has been altered by the previous surgery, but the scleral curvature remains unchanged. Therefore, the ring size cannot be chosen based on the actual keratometry but on the one measured before the first surgery
- Production of irregular flaps, incomplete cuts, or buttonholes has a higher rate in these cases. The reason is the irregular protrusion of the cornea through the ring selected. When the head of the microkeratome comes to make the cut, the irregular protrusion produces an irregular flap
- Wounds from old incisional cuts can open during the flap creation, producing unexpected astigmatism that is very difficult to resolve
- When a new flap is created in a cornea with a previous flap, some complications may take place, such as cutting part of the old flap, rolling it over, etc. Those complications can cause unexpected astigmatism or undercorrection of the irregularity
- A previously treated cornea can have iatrogenic ectasia that is not recognized by the surgeon because the keratometry may no longer be a factor. Extreme care should be taken when deciding to perform LASIK in those corneas
- In corneal ectasias—iatrogenic or naturally occurring—LASIK is no longer an option; surface treatment is a must
- In some treatments, the beam must reach distant areas from the center of the pupil. Be careful to not touch the flap. To do this, it must be centered according to the proposed treatment plan

Custom-Contoured Ablation Pattern Method: The Technique

The surgical plan for a custom ablation with C-CAP is usually subjective and individual. Every cornea with irregular astigmatism has a unique and personal condition. As opposed to regular astigmatism, generalization of the treatment when irregularities are present is not possible. There is no fixed nomogram. A rationale behind every single treatment has to be applied.

The C-CAP method from VISX is a topography-assisted ablation method of treatment of irregular astigmatism. It is a link between the topography map and the VISX STAR excimer laser through the analysis and decision of the surgeon. The excimer laser beam can only remove tissue from the corneal surface; it cannot add tissue to it. Therefore, regularization of the corneal contour is based on decreasing the heights of the "bumps" of the corneal surface. Understanding a topography map is crucial in the decision-making process of these types of treatments.

First Step: Elevation Topography

Elevation topography is mandatory. Vector analysis topography, also known as curvature topography, cannot be used to decide and to make a treatment plan for irregular astigmatism. In fact, there is a strong difference between the steepest area of the cornea and the most elevated zone. They are different not only in conception and origin but also in location.[8]

The steepest area in curvature topography denotes the area where the greatest difference in dioptric power of two separate points is detected (ie, the slope of the mountain). The most elevated area is the peak of the mountain, the highest area of the cornea—in millimeters not in power—when compared to an "ideal" best fit curvature. Removing tissue from the steepest area may increase the slope of the elevation and compromise rather than improve the visual quality of that particular cornea.

There are two types of elevation topography:[9,10]

1. Placido's disk-based elevation topography systems take advantage of the reflecting properties of the cornea. They use various proprietary algorithms to produce graphic representations of corneal topography. The elevation topography from a Placido's disk unit is based on the specific program used for the adaptation of contact lenses. A mathe-

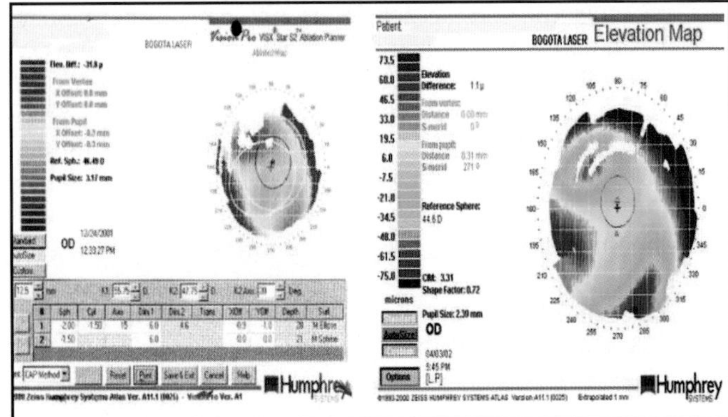

Figure 39-4. C-CAP corneal and elevation map.

matical algorithm calculates the elevation from the reflection of the concentric rings on the anterior surface of the cornea as compared to an "ideal corneal curvature," which leaves areas that are under this best fit curvature (depressed areas: cold colors) and elevated ones related to it (elevated areas: hot colors). Units with elevation topography based on Placido's disk topography are the Humphrey Atlas Unit and the Dicon-Paradigm topography unit (Paradigm Medical Industries Inc, Salt Lake City, Utah). They produce extremely accurate and reliable maps, although they are dependent on the reflecting properties of the anterior surface of the cornea, and they also depend on the quality of the tear film. Without any doubt, their great advantage is the CAP planner software present in these two systems, which is a very helpful tool in designing a treatment. The Humphrey CAP planner is the only one commercially available and approved by the FDA for its use in conjunction with the C-CAP Method and the VISX STAR S3 system

2. Slit-scan elevation topography. The only unit available with this technology is the Orbscan (Bausch & Lomb, Rochester, NY). This system produces very reliable and accurate maps, calculates the posterior surface of the cornea, and does not depend on the tear film quality. However, its great disadvantage is the lack of a computer program to help the surgeon to plan the treatment. Therefore, calculations have to be made manually

Second Step: Program of the Ablation

Ablation is based on the analysis of elevation topography. The map has to be taken very carefully and the pupil marker must be activated. There may be more than one elevated area, and it is the surgeon who decides which one should be treated first and the order of the sequential treatments. The following parameters must be determined to plan the treatment: shape, location, axis, and depth of each ablation.

Shape

The shape of the elevated area is decided by looking at the elevation map. There are three options to choose: sphere, cylinder, or ellipse.

Location

Counting from the center of the pupil on the topography, locate in X and Y coordinates (horizontal and vertical) the center of the elevated area to be ablated. Remember that in some cases the pupil center (line of sight) and corneal vertex do not match. Some topography systems show the measurements as the cursor moves along the axes. Other systems, like Orbscan, have a scale of marks that starts at 1 mm from the center in each meridian and concentric circles that measure 3, 5, 7, and 9 mm in diameter.

Axis

This must be determined any time the shape is a cylinder or an ellipse. The long axis of the irregularity is found and then translated to the center of the pupil. This is the real axis of the zone to ablate.

Depth

Elevation maps give the depth in a scale. Elevated zones are above the surface reference and are presented in hot colors (eg, red).

Third Step: The Treatment

Given the facts mentioned above, the surgeon has to decide whether the best option for the treatment of irregular astigmatism is PRK, LASEK, or LASIK. In any type of surgery, the surgeon has to remember when he or she looks through the laser microscope, he or she will find the coordinates are visually (not mathematically) rotated 180 degrees as compared to the supine position of the topography examination. When the program is made manually in the Orbscan map, this should be taken into account to make sure the treatment goes to the right location. When using the Humphrey CAP planner, this is automatically transferred to the laser.

CAP Planners

The Humphrey Atlas topography unit and the Dicon-Paradigm topography unit have developed, independently from VISX, a software program that allows the surgeon to see the topographic changes the treatment will produce in the cornea before actually doing it. The Humphrey CAP planner is the only one commercially available and approved by the FDA to be used in conjunction with the C-CAP method to treat decentered LASIK patients under the HDE protocol.

The CAP planner is extremely user-friendly software and allows the surgeon to program several ablations in the computer and see how the topography map would look if the ablation were carried out. This "simulated map" is extremely reliable when compared to the real topography postoperative maps. The possibility to know the possible topography after the planned ablations allows the surgeon to develop several plans and to change them as many times as needed until the goal of the treatment is accomplished. This is a valuable safety feature for these rather difficult and sometimes unpredictable treatments. Once the surgeon is convinced about the ablation, the treatment can be printed, the paper taken into the laser, and the data entered into the computer (Figure 39-4).

For the use of a CAP planner, several steps must be taken:

1. If the depth of the ablation is more than 30 µm, it is advisable to divide it into two or three ablations, starting from smaller to larger until the total tissue removal is obtained

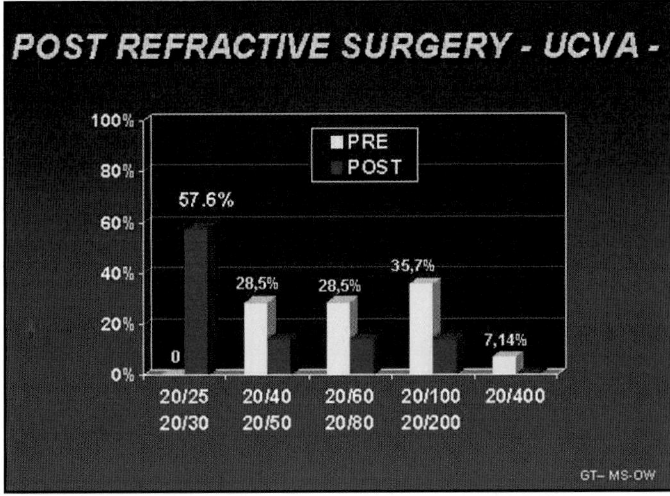

Table 39-1. Preoperative and postoperative UCVA in the postrefractive surgery group, treated with C-CAP method (36 months follow-up).

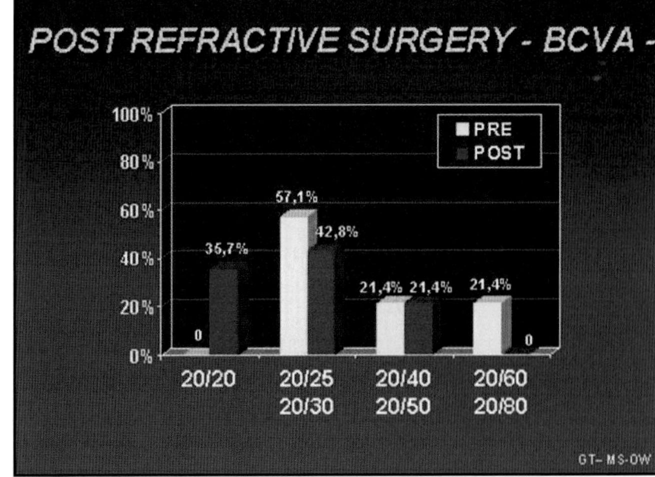

Table 39-2. Preoperative and postoperative BCVA in the postrefractive surgery group, treated with C-CAP method (36 months follow-up).

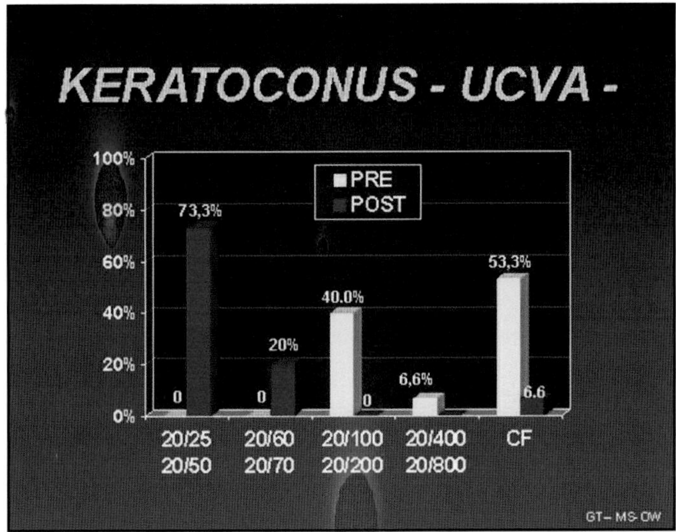

Table 39-3. Preoperative and postoperative UCVA in the keratoconus group after 31.6 months of treatment with the C-CAP method.

2. It is advisable not to have many tissue intersections among the different ablations. It is better to produce smaller ablations with less touch or less coupling between one ablation and the other
3. The least amount of tissue that is resected, the better the result. Therefore, the surgeon should try to produce a regular topographic pattern with the minimum amount of ablation
4. CAP planners can simulate the predicted corneal topography map. However, they cannot predict the final refractive result. Surgeon should be aware of "Barraquer's law," which states that any tissue resected at the periphery will produce steepening at the center of the cornea or myopic shift. Any tissue resected centrally will produce flattening at the center, or hyperopic shift

Clinical Results

Once again, the treatment of irregular astigmatism is meant to restore the regularity of the anterior surface of the cornea, not to correct a refractive defect. Of course, some steps are taken to at least decrease the refraction of the patient without compromising the main goal of regularization of corneal contour. It is the irregularity that causes the bothersome and incapacitating symptoms of those patients. They are not produced by the refractive defect.

Patients were divided subjectively into two main groups: irregular astigmatism as a result of previous surgery and "primary" irregular astigmatism/ectasias. This division depicts the large differences between these two groups not only in origin but also in results.[11,12] Ectasias are always treated by PRK and postsurgical cases are treated preferably with LASIK unless not enough tissue is found. The mean follow up is 36 months for both groups of patients. All eyes had complete preoperative and postoperative ophthalmologic evaluations. Uncorrected visual acuity (UCVA), best-corrected visual acuity (BCVA), keratometry readings, manifest refraction, and elevation topography maps were recorded.

Judging the success of this technique is very difficult, since the refraction is not what we aim to correct. In fact, it does not influence the patient's decision to have the surgery. Eighty-seven percent of patients decide to have the surgery because of the presence of symptoms and only 13% wanted to have the surgery with the goal of getting rid of their glasses. Nevertheless, when the C-CAP method is analyzed against the conventional method, marked improvement is obtained, as can be seen in Tables 39-1 and 39-2 for the postrefractive surgery group and Tables 39-3 and 39-4 for the ectasia or keratoconus group.

Postoperative topography is probably one of the best ways to measure the results of the C-CAP method. In fact, more regular topography maps are obtained after our treatment, although improvement varies among patients (Figure 39-5). Another way to judge results is the subjective answer from patients to a questionnaire regarding symptoms. Again, all patients experienced improvement to different degrees in glare, halos, burst, and mul-

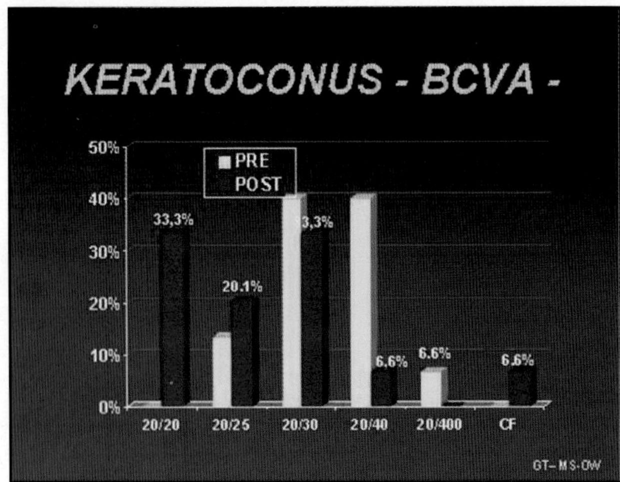

Table 39-4. Preoperative and postoperative BCVA in the keratoconus group after 31.6 months of follow-up, treated with the C-CAP method.

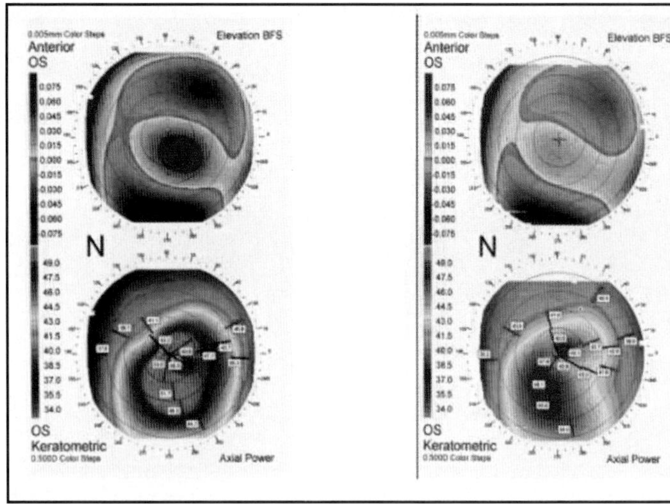

Figure 39-5. Preoperative (left) and postoperative (right) elevation and axial curvature maps.

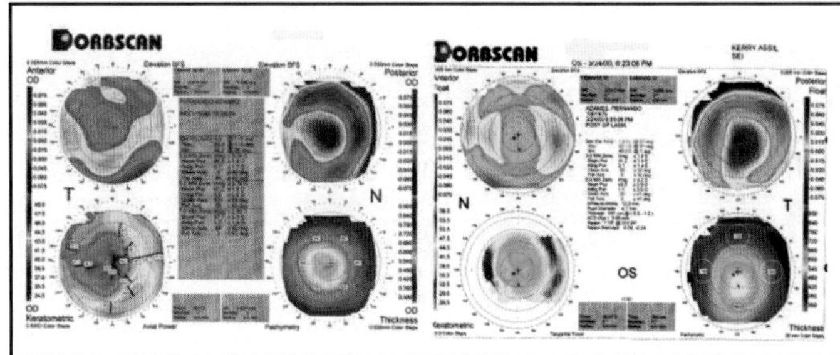

Figure 39-6. Preoperative (left) and postoperative (right) Orbscan maps using C-CAP to treat irregular astigmatism. The patient's BCVA went from 20/40 preoperatively to 20/20 postoperatively.

tiple visions. Improvement can be subtracted from these numbers: in the postsurgical group, with a follow-up of 36 months, no patient has returned to contact lens wear, 35% have returned to glasses, and 65% use no correction at all. In the ectasia group with the same 36 months of follow-up, 23% have returned satisfactorily to contact lens wear and another 45% wear glasses. The rest of the patients do not use any device for correction.

Safety

The C-CAP method has been demonstrated to be safe when lost and gained lines of BCVA are analyzed in both groups. In the postsurgical group, not one eye lost lines of BCVA. In fact, 42.5% gained one line, 18.5% gained two lines, and 7.4% gained more than two lines of BCVA.

In the ectasia group, only one eye lost one line of BCVA. This eye was treated with a BCVA of 20/400 and remained stable with a BCVA of 20/70 for 2 years. In the last 3 months, an activation of the ectatic problem was observed. This eye is ready for a corneal transplant. In terms of improvement, 52% gained one line of BCVA, 11.1% gained two lines, and 11.1% gained more than two lines.

Effectiveness

The C-CAP method is effective in the treatment of irregular astigmatism. In the postsurgical group, the mean preoperative UCVA was 20/80 while the mean postoperative UCVA was 20/40. Mean BCVA went from 20/40 preoperative to 20/25 postoperative (Figure 39-6).

In the ectasia group, mean preoperative UCVA was 20/300 and mean postoperative UCVA was 20/54. The BCVA went from 20/38 preoperatively to 20/29 postoperatively.

Stability was achieved earlier (1.2 months) in the postsurgical group than in the keratoconus group because 85% of the cases were treated with the LASIK CAP method. All patients reported subjective improvement in visual symptoms in different degrees. Satisfaction was generally rated high, although 25% of the patients reported "less improvement than expected." No patient complained of worsening of symptoms, and all of them would repeat the surgery if needed.

United States Clinical Experience

The recent approval by the FDA of the C-CAP method for the treatment of postexcimer surgery decentrations has given the US ophthalmologists this tool to correct those complicated cases. As a courtesy from Dr. Edward Manche from Stanford University School of Medicine, this is his experience with seven eyes treated with the C-CAP method and the Vision pro simulation software after a decentration from a previous LVC. The follow-up is only 3 months (see Table 39-5, a comparison of BCVA pre-LVC, pre-CAP treatment, and post-C-CAP ablation).

Not one eye lost any line of BCVA. Six out of seven eyes (86%) gained two or more lines of BCVA, and six eyes (86%) gained or maintained UCVA. Only one eye (14%) lost one line of UCVA. All patients felt a marked improvement of the debilitating symptoms from the decentration and the topography map showed the improvement in centration.

Summary

The experience from the authors, of more than 5 years treating irregular astigmatism, has been reproduced by an independent ophthalmologist. This demonstrates that this method is safe and effective in the correction of these irregular corneas.

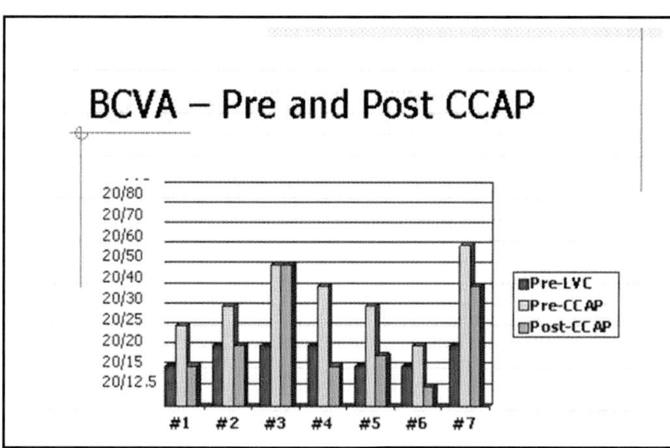

Table 39-5. US C-CAP method clinical experience. A comparison of pre LVC, pre C-CAP and post C-CAP treatment. No eye lost lines of BCVA. (Courtesy of Dr. Edward Manche.)

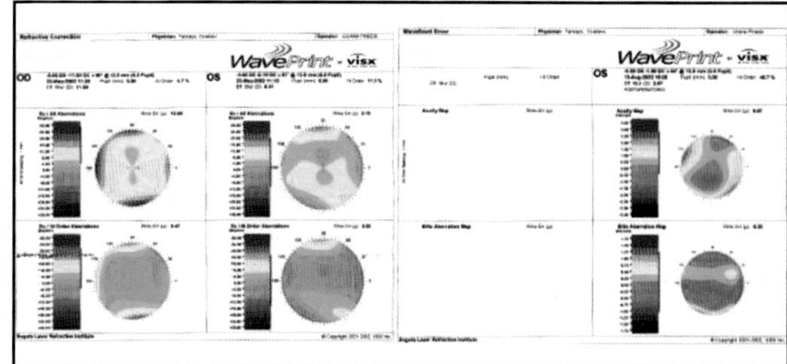

Figure 39-7. A mild case of irregular astigmatism that is being treated with customized ablation using the WaveScan (Shack-Hartmann) wavefront sensor.

The Future

Improvement in the treatment of irregular astigmatism will derive from improvement in diagnostic tools such as wavefront technology and improvement in laser systems.

Wavefront technology, because it is not an analysis of shape but instead analysis of optical properties, is the best diagnostic tool to make the "link" with the excimer laser unit.[13] Wavefront is able to make functional analysis transform the analysis into a treatment table, which when inserted into the laser dictates a change in shape to restore "normality" in optical functions. This is a real link and, of course, the future of any treatment of irregular astigmatism—provided there is enough tissue to remove from the cornea.

However, today wavefront cannot measure eyes with big irregularities and the development of a treatment table is difficult and still in its infancy. We need to learn much more about aberrations and tissue interactions before we are able to develop an algorithm for treatment with the laser. A lot of work is being carried out in this direction. VISX is working with a Shack-Hartmann device (WaveScan) (VISX, Santa Clara, Calif) and with a ray tracing device (Tracey Technologies, Houston, Tex). In mild cases of irregular astigmatism, treatment with waveprint has been done with successful and encouraging results (Figure 39-7). Although this use of new technology is still investigational, the future can be foreseen with the application of wavefront for mild cases of irregularities. In more severe irregularities, a topography-assisted treatment such as the CAP method will be used first to regulate the corneal contour. A second procedure with waveprint-guided ablation will refine the result.

The CAP method is still the first choice to correct the irregularities of a cornea with the help of topography.

References

1. Gibralter R, Trokel SL. Correction of irregular astigmatism with the excimer laser. *Ophthalmology.* 1994;101:1310-1315.
2. Snook R. Pachymetry and true topography using the Orbscan system. In: Gills J, Sanders D, Thornton S, eds. *Corneal Topography: The State of the Art.* Thorofare, NJ: SLACK Incorporated; 1995:89-103.
3. Tamayo G, Serrano M. Grid corneal marker. A new surgical approach for the treatment of irregular astigmatism. Poster presented at: the Panamerican Congress; May 1997; Cancun, Mexico .
4. Tamayo G, Serrano M. Early clinical experience using custom excimer laser ablations to treat irregular astigmatism. *J Cataract Refract Surg.* 2000;26:1442-1450.
5. Alio JL, Artola A, Claramonte PJ, et al. Complications of photorefractive keratectomy for myopia: two year follow up of 3000 cases. *J Cataract Refract Surg.* 2000;24:619-626.
6. Buzard KA, Fundingsland BR. Treatment of irregular astigmatism with a broad beam excimer laser. *J Cataract Refract Surg.* 1997;13:624-636.
7. Maeda N, Klyce SD, Tano Y. Detection and classification of mild irregular astigmatism in patients with good visual acuity. *Surv Ophthalmol.* 1998;43:53-58.
8. Friedlander MH, Granet MS. Non-placido disk corneal topography. In: Elander R, Rich L, Robin J, eds. *Principles and Practice of Refractive Surgery.* Philadelphia, Pa: WB Saunders; 1997.
9. Belin M, Litoff D, Stroods S, et al. The PAR technology corneal topography system. *Refract Corneal Surg.* 1992;8:88-96.
10. Sborgia C. Usefulness of the Orbscan machine in the management of photorefractive keratectomy. Paper presented at: ISRS/AAO Orbscan Clinical Topography Symposium; October 24-26, 1996; Chicago, Ill.
11. Andreassen T, Simonsen A, Oxlund H. Biomechanical properties of keratoconus and normal corneas. *Exp Eye Res.* 1980;31:435-444.
12. Bilgihan K, Ozdec SC, Konu KO, et al. Results of photorefractive keratectomy in keratoconus suspects at 4 years. *J Refract Surg.* 2000;16:438-443.
13. Bille J, Freischlad K, Jahn G, et al. Image restoration by adaptive optical phase conjugation. Paper presented at: the Proceedings of the 6th International Conference of Pattern Recognition; 1982; Munich, Germany.

Chapter 40

Surgeon-Guided Retreatment of Irregular Astigmatism and Aberrations

Gilles Lafond, MD, FRCS(C)

Corneal surface irregularities, decentration of the treatment zones, or inadequate treatment zone diameters are possible complications of excimer laser refractive surgery (laser in-situ keratomileusis [LASIK] or photorefractive keratectomy [PRK]). Such inadequate ablations are a source of irregular astigmatism and degrade the optical performance of the cornea. Consequences are loss of best-corrected vision, halos, glare, monocular diplopia, or residual ametropia.[1-9] In the future, new customized ablation technologies (topo-link- or wavefront-based) will probably be available to correct those types of complications. However, such technologies are not likely to be widely available for several years. Patients who are experiencing significant vision difficulties after an initial excimer laser surgery are usually motivated by a short-term solution to their problem. With the current laser technology, it is possible to improve the quality of vision for several of these patients.

In this chapter, we describe techniques to retreat cases of initial corneal surface irregularities or inadequate ablations by using combinations of small diameter or decentered ablations. The first technique describes the use of decentered small diameter myopic ablations to decrease irregular astigmatism due to corneal irregularities. The second technique involves a combination of decentered myopic and hyperopic standard wide diameter ablations to correct cases of previous decentered treatment. The third technique, used to enlarge previous small diameter ablation zones, also involves a combination of myopic and hyperopic ablations but without decentration. A summary of these three retreatment techniques is presented in Table 40-1.

The retreatment parameters, dioptric value, diameter, axis, and distance of decentration were determined using measurements from topographical maps taken after the initial surgery. Defining optimal retreatment parameters is difficult due to the multiple variables that must be considered: initial and residual ametropia, diameter, elevation of the irregular zone, distance and axis of decentration, etc. Therefore, each case has to be analyzed individually. Some cases need more than one retreatment session to achieve significant visual improvement. In these more complex cases, an initial conservative retreatment with limited parameters is probably more appropriate than an aggressive retreatment with results that are difficult to predict, although this course of action implies several retreatment sessions. This multi-step approach is easier with LASIK cases because of the short healing time and the little pain associated with this technique. For this reason, LASIK was preferred for the retreatment of decentration and for the enlargement of an initial small ablation treatment zone, even if PRK was used for the initial surgery. However, cases of irregular astigmatism due to localized small irregular zones were retreated with the same technique that was used in the initial surgery. It seemed logical to correct these irregularities where they are located, either on the stromal surface or under the flap.

The laser used for all these retreatments was the Technolas 217Z (Bausch & Lomb, Rochester, NY), which is a scanning laser using a 2.00 millimeter (mm) flying spot and an active tracking system. This instrument is equipped with two diode lasers: one is the fixation light, while the other coincides with the center of the 2.00 mm spot of the excimer beam. After the tracker has been activated and locked on the eye's visual axis, it is possible to decenter the treatment beam from the fixation light by using the compatible laser program. The swivel scale integrated into the ocular of the laser microscope was used to align the treatment at the planned axis and distance from the eye's optical center.

Editor's note:
This chapter reviews the well-planned efforts of correcting surgically-induced aberrations without a wavefront or topographic uplink. First, irregular steep areas are corrected with well-placed, decentered, small zone myopic ablations. Second, previous decentrations are corrected with a combination of decentered or inversely decentered hyperopic and myopic ablations. Finally, small zone ablations are corrected (enlarged) by a combination of myopic and hyperopic ablations without decentration.
R. Krueger, MD, MSE

Retreatment of Corneal Surface Irregularities

Irregular corneal surface, after excimer laser refractive surgery, can be the consequence of nonhomogeneous laser ablation; of a flap complication in LASIK surgery; or of a postoperative complication with resulting corneal tissue loss, such as infection, diffuse lamellar keratitis (DLK) or epithelial ingrowth.[10-14]

A small diameter myopic ablation can be used to flatten irregular steep areas to reduce the irregular astigmatism and aberrations that result as a complication after an initial excimer laser procedure. This technique is similar to a technique we have used to correct central islands.[15] However, for the correction of irreg-

Table 40-1
Summary of Retreatment Types

Type of Irregularity	Retreatment Technique	Retreatment Parameters	Refractive Effect
Corneal surface irregularities	Very small diameter Decentered myopic ablations	-2.00 D to -3.00 D Diameter: 2.30 to 3.50 mm Delivered on steeper corneal areas	Induces some myopic correction
Decentration	Combination of decentered standard wide diameter myopic and hyperopic ablations	+2.00 D to -2.75 D Diameter: 8.00 to 9.50 mm Decentration: 1.00 to 2.00 mm	No refractive change
Small zone ablation	Combination of standard wide diameter myopic and hyperopic ablations without decentration	+1.75 D to -2.00 D Diameter: 8.30 to 9.60 mm	No refractive change

ular astigmatism, this previous technique was modified by decentering the retreatment from the visual axis. It was decentered to correspond to the location of the irregularity to be corrected. In our experience, this retreatment technique achieved a better corneal surface regularity and better vision in most of the retreated cases, although the irregular astigmatism correction was only partial in several cases. In some cases, a standard myopic or hyperopic large diameter ablation was added to the small diameter ablation in order to correct some residual ametropia. The following examples describe the retreatment parameters used and illustrate the results obtained.

A small diameter myopic ablation can be used to flatten irregular steep areas to reduce the irregular astigmatism and aberrations that result as a complication after an initial excimer laser procedure.

The following five examples (see p. 342) describe cases of irregular astigmatism due to a localized steeper or flatter corneal area, in relation to the surrounding ablated cornea. These areas were decentered in relation to the central papillary axis. Except for the last example, the retreatments consisted of a small diameter myopic ablation delivered to the localized steep cornea area. Cases initially treated with PRK were retreated with PRK, and LASIK cases were retreated with LASIK. For PRK cases, the epithelium was removed with the laser. This transepithelial approach with the laser has the advantage of using the epithelium as a masking agent, which helps to decrease the underlying stromal surface irregularities. For LASIK cases, the surgical approach was always to lift the previous flap. The diameter, curvature, distance, and axis of decentration of the steep corneal zone to be treated were evaluated on topographical maps taken prior to the retreatment. Immediately before the laser ablation, an ink mark was placed under slit lamp visualization at 6:00 and 12:00 to rule out a possible cyclotorsion during the laser treatment when the patient is lying down.

In our experience of 10 initially myopic eyes retreated with this technique, best-corrected visual acuity (BCVA) lines were recovered in nine cases and significant subjective improvement was also described by the patients in these nine cases. These results showed that this technique is effective in reducing the irregular astigmatism present as a complication of a previous excimer laser myopic treatment. Also, this technique was found to be safe: no complications were encountered, no eyes lost lines of vision, and no patients experienced any subjective worsening of vision. The main difficulty with this technique was aligning the retreatment exactly over the area to be retreated; there is risk that a misalignment could worsen the corneal surface regularity instead of improving it. The same technique was also used in four cases of irregular ablation present after initial excimer treatment to correct hyperopia. A good result was obtained in only two cases (Example 4). In the other two cases, no significant improvement was noted; however, no deterioration was induced.

Defining optimal parameters is difficult, as our experience is limited to several cases and there are multiple variables to consider. These variables are the initial and residual ametropia, distance from the optical corneal center, and the axis of the steep zone to be retreated (ie, its curvature, its diameter, and its regular or irregular contour). Therefore, each case is different from the other and has to be analyzed individually. In general, wider ablation diameters and higher dioptric values were used for the retreatment of wider and steeper corneal irregularities. The retreatment diameters used for small localized irregularities, as in Examples 1 and 2, were between 2.30 and 3 mm. For a wider irregular zone, as in Example 3, a 3.50 mm zone was preferred. Retreatment dioptric value was usually between 2 and 3 D. Total ablation thicknesses were between 9 and 14 microns (μm). One point to emphasize is that the laser used for these retreatments, the Technolas 217Z laser, is a scanning laser that automatically creates a transition zone. In contrast to the same treatment diameter without such transition zone, the ablation thickness is greater if a transition zone is added. Consequently, if this small diameter ablation technique is performed with a broadbeam laser without transition zones, slightly larger diameter or higher dioptric values should be used to respect this range of 9 to 14 µm of localized tissue removal. We have no experience with an initially more aggressive retreatment. Considering our limited experience and the inherent difficulties of this type of retreatment, we believe that in more complicated cases it is probably safer to use limited retreatment parameters. Although doing so may imply more than one retreatment session, this conservative approach decreases the risk of inducing undesirable effects resulting from excessive tissue removal.

> One point to emphasize is that the laser used for these retreatments, the Technolas 217Z laser, is a scanning laser that automatically creates a transition zone. In contrast to the same treatment diameter without such transition zone, the ablation thickness is greater if a transition zone is added.

We found that these very small diameter myopic ablations induced some myopic correction, but this correction is significantly less than the retreatment dioptric value (ie, less than the same myopic ablation value delivered on a standard wide diameter). In our experience, the average refractive correction obtained per diopter of retreatment, delivered at a mean 3 mm diameter zone, was -0.27 D. For example, a -3 D ablation delivered on this 3 mm diameter zone should induce a final refractive change of -0.81 D. Therefore, when a minimal residual myopia is present prior to the retreatment of a localized irregular steeper area, this retreatment by itself should correct this myopia (Examples 3 and 4). However, when some hyperopia is present, the retreatment should increase this hyperopia. To correct for the residual ametropia one might expect after a small diameter myopic treatment, a standard large diameter ablation (myopic or hyperopic) can be added in the retreatment process (Examples 1 and 2).

> We found that these very small diameter myopic ablations induced some myopic correction, but this correction is significantly less than the retreatment dioptric value. In our experience, the average refractive correction obtained per diopter of retreatment, delivered at a mean 3.00 mm diameter zone, was -0.27 D.

Another particular point to emphasize is the correction of residual or induced astigmatism. An irregular corneal surface resulting from the initial treatment is often the source of some astigmatism. The process of flattening the irregular steep area with the small diameter spherical myopic ablation should by itself decrease the astigmatism. Therefore, when some induced astigmatism is present after the initial surgery, the full correction of this astigmatism with a standard wide diameter treatment zone should not be added to the small diameter myopic ablation. In Example 2, a partial correction of the induced astigmatism delivered at a standard wide diameter was included in the retreatment process. The residual astigmatism, with a 90 degree axis shift, shows that this astigmatism correction—although partial—was slightly excessive.

> The process of flattening the irregular steep area with the small diameter spherical myopic ablation should by itself decrease the astigmatism. Therefore, when some induced astigmatism is present after the initial surgery, the full correction of this astigmatism with a standard wide diameter treatment zone should not be added to the small diameter myopic ablation.

This retreatment technique can improve some cases of irregular astigmatism that developed as a complication from a previous excimer laser procedure. The retreatment uses very small diameter regular myopic ablations. However, because corneal irregularities are obviously irregular, the retreatment cannot correspond exactly to the contour of the steep zone to be treated and can only decrease its overall elevation. Also, it is difficult to achieve a precise retreatment alignment on the area to be retreated. Therefore, this technique does have limitations and does not completely correct the irregular astigmatism. Although the correction can be only partial, it may significantly improve the visual symptoms of some patients.

Example 5 is completely different from the others. In this case, the irregular astigmatism is not due to a localized steep area, but is rather due to a localized flat area, being the consequence of a corneal melt after severe DLK. In association with the irregular astigmatism, a marked overcorrection was present. In this case, the retreatment was done with the use of a decentered hyperopic ablation. The treatment zone diameter was a standard wide diameter. We believe that there is probably a greater limitation in decentering a hyperopic ablation than a myopic ablation, and that hyperopic ablation should be used only with a standard wide diameter zone. The main reason for these concerns is the ablation profile in the hyperopic transition zone, which is the inverse of the central zone. The central treatment zone induces a steepening of the treated corneal area, whereas the transition zone induces a flattening of the cornea. The overlapping of the transition zone in the visual axis could induce an unpredictable result with an increase of the irregular astigmatism. Our experience with decentered hyperopic ablation for the retreatment of such cases of irregular astigmatism is limited to two eyes. In both cases, marked improvement was achieved. However, as described in the following pages, we have used more extensively decentered hyperopic ablations for the correction of previous treatment decentration.

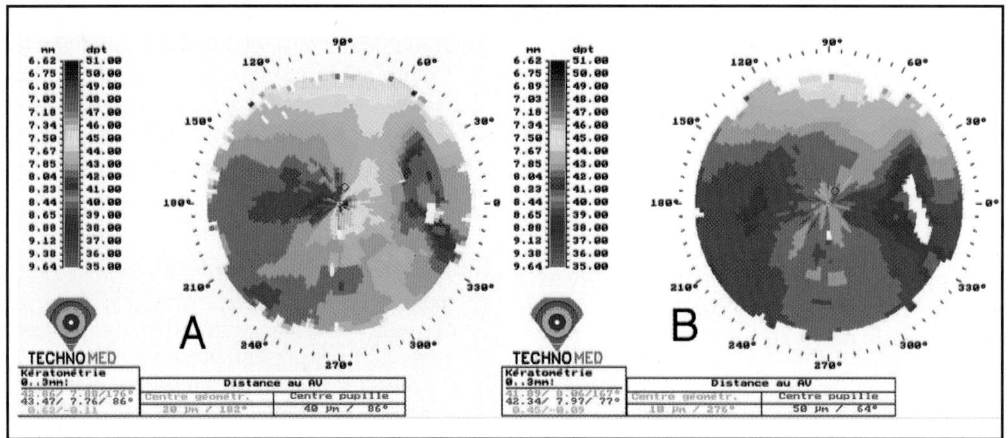

EXAMPLE 1

A 37-year-old female had an initial myopic LASIK treatment of -3.25 + 1.00 x 170. This treatment induced an irregular corneal surface (map A) with a resulting three-line BCVA loss. Ablation over a wet corneal bed after the LASIK cut was believed by the referring surgeon to be the reason for this result. Residual ametropia was +0.50 + 0.25 x 65 for 20/40 vision. The initial LASIK flap was lifted and a -3.00 myopic retreatment was delivered within a 2.50 mm zone (transition zone extending to 5.50 mm) with a 1 mm decentration at 315 degrees. This resulted in a marked improvement of the surface regularity (map B), with two lines of vision recovery. However, this small diameter myopic ablation increased the hyperopia induced by the initial treatment, and the resulting refraction was +1.25. A second retreatment session was needed to correct this hyperopia. A standard wide diameter hyperopic ablation of +1.25 on a 5.80 mm zone with a transition zone extending to 9.30 mm was added 2 months after the first retreatment. Final refractive outcome was plano, resulting in 20/20 vision.

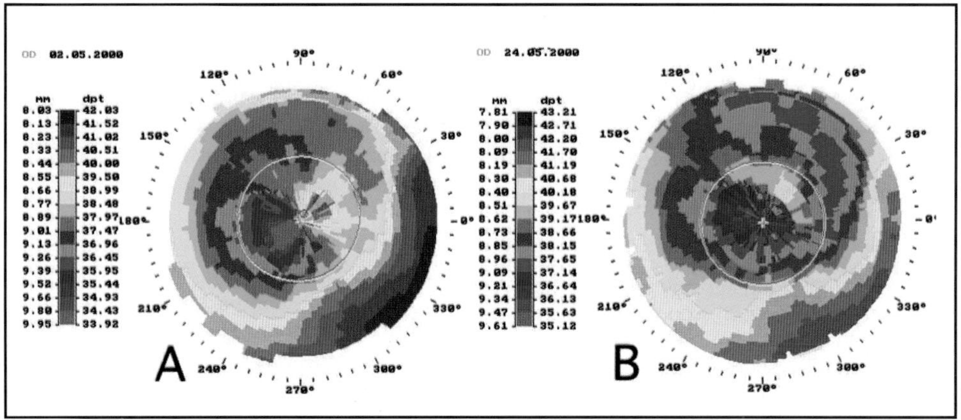

EXAMPLE 2

This 48-year-old male had LASIK for -6.00 D of myopia. Three months after this initial surgery, because of a minor undercorrection, the surgeon performed a touch-up. Instead of lifting the initial flap, a new cut was done with the microkeratome. The result was a corneal surface irregularity (map A), probably the consequence of the intersection of the two cuts with the resulting displacement or loss of microlayers of corneal tissue. In addition to a three-line BCVA loss, the patient was complaining of very disturbing monocular diplopia. Refractive result was +0.50 + 1.00 x 0.5 for 20/40 vision. When the initial LASIK flap was lifted for the retreatment, the two different cut layers were visible. The retreatment profile, used to flatten the steep irregular area, was -2.00 D within a 3 mm diameter zone (tapering zone extending to 6 mm) with a 2 mm decentration at 35 degrees. Because this patient was already overcorrected after the initial treatment, it was expected that such further myopic ablation would increase this hyperopia. Therefore, during the same retreatment session, a standard wide diameter hyperopic ablation was also included. The value of this ablation was +1.00 + 0.75 x 0.5 delivered centrally within a 5.80 mm zone with a transition zone extending to 9.30 mm. Final refractive outcome was plano + 0.50 x 97 for a 20/25 vision. Although some surface irregularities are still present after retreatment, a significant improvement is visible (map B). Two BCVA lines were recovered, and the patient's subjective symptoms were markedly reduced.

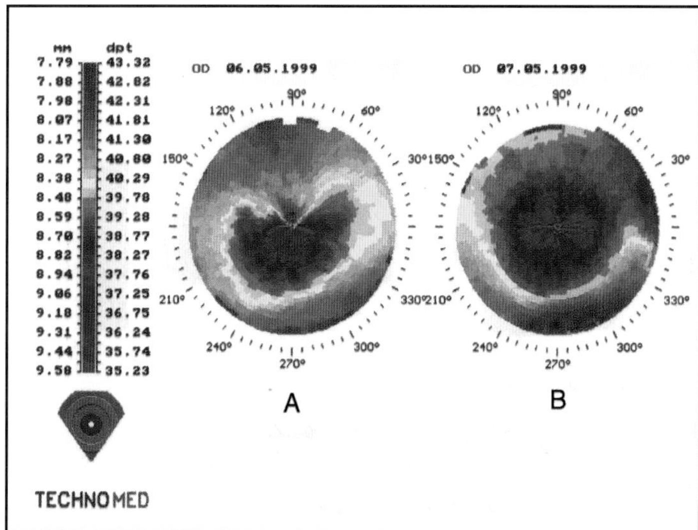

Example 3

This 38-year-old female presented an incomplete ablation in the superior part of the treatment zone (map A) after an initial LASIK for -4.75 D of myopia. It was the source of irregular astigmatism, ghost images, and a one-line loss of BCVA. Initial myopia was -4.75 for 20/20 vision. Refraction after this initial LASIK was -1.00 + 0.25 x 105, resulting in 20/25 vision. Retreatment consisted of a -2.00 D myopic ablation delivered within a 3.50 mm zone (transition zone extending to 6.30 mm) with a superior 2 mm decentration. Topographical map taken after retreatment (map B) shows a regular ablation zone. Final refractive outcome was plano + 0.25 x 90 resulting in 20/20 vision, and there was a complete regression of the patient's subjective symptoms. Compared to the two previous examples, the irregular steeper area to be flattened was wider; consequently, a wider retreatment diameter was used. The retreatment diopter value exceeded the residual myopia measured after the initial treatment. However, because these retreatments were decentered and within a small diameter, their refractive effect was much less than their standard zone dioptric value.

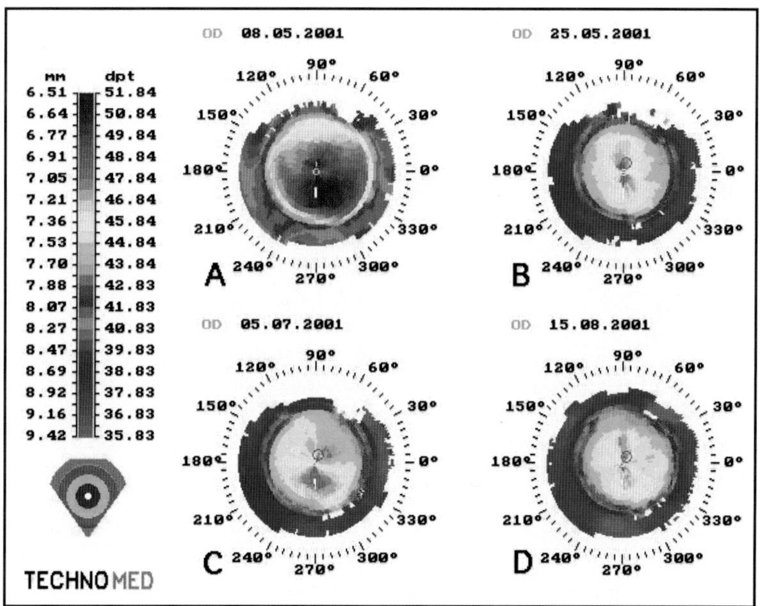

Example 4

A 49-year-old male had initial hyperopic PRK treatment of +3.25 + 1.00 x 170 D, which induced an inferior steepening (map A). Initial vision was 20/20. The refractive outcome was -1.25, resulting in 20/50 vision. At first, a -2.50 D retreatment was performed within a small 2.60 mm ablation zone (transition zone of 5.60 mm), with a 1.50 mm inferior decentration at 270 degrees. This was used to flatten the steep zone and resulted in an initially good result (map B). However, some of this irregularity recurred in the following months (map C). A second treatment, using identical ablation parameters, succeeded in producing a stable result with a regular corneal surface (map D). Final result was -1.25 + 1.00 x 140 for 20/25 vision.

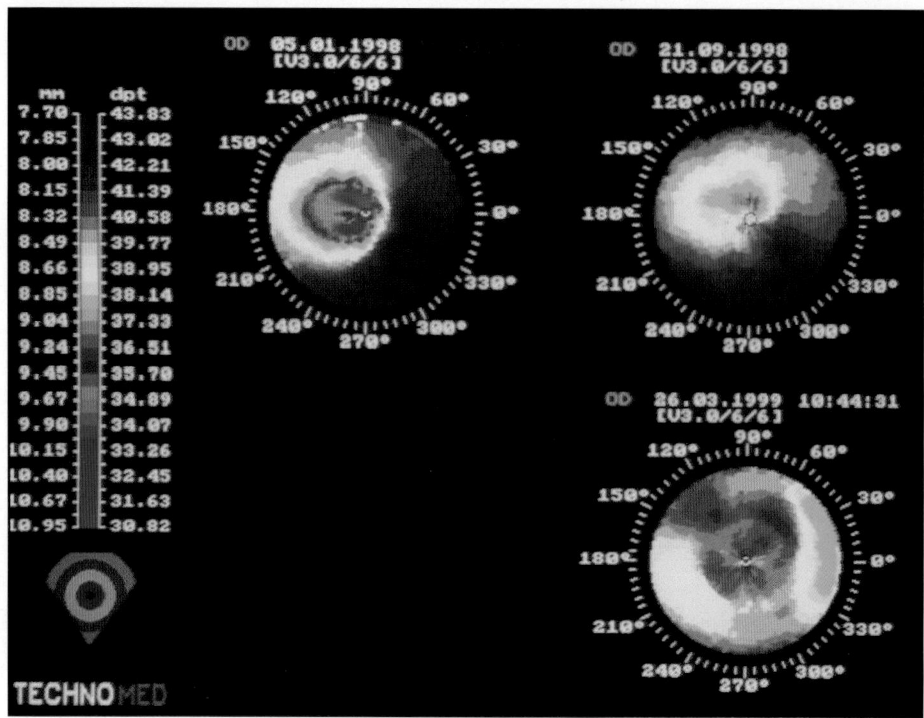

Example 5

Following LASIK for -4.50 D of myopia, this 47-year-old male developed severe diffuse lamellar keratitis (DLK) with corneal melting. Initial vision was 20/50-. The result 10 months postoperatively was approximately +2.50 D resulting in 20/50 vision. Marked irregular astigmatism was present. The topographical map (first map) showed an area of marked flattening, which corresponded to the zone of corneal melting. An initial retreatment was performed 10 months after the initial surgery. The surgical approach was to lift the initial flap followed by a retreatment of +1.75 D hyperopia within a 5.80 mm diameter with a transition zone extending to 9.30 mm. This ablation was decentered 1.50 mm at 180 degrees. Topography taken after the retreatment (second map) showed a significant improvement, although some surface irregularities persisted. The refractive result was +1.00 with a marked decrease of the irregular astigmatism. Four months later, the LASIK flap was lifted again for a second retreatment. A +1 hyperopic ablation within a 5.80 mm diameter (transition zone extending to 9.30 mm) was added with a 1.00 mm decentration at 130 degrees. The final result was -0.75 + 0.50 x 170 D resulting in 20/25- vision. Topographical map taken after this second retreatment (third map) showed a marked improvement of corneal surface.

Retreatment of Previous Decentered Ablation

Decentration can be a complication of excimer laser refractive surgery.[16-18] Causes for this complication are varied: poor patient fixation, inadequate laser beam centration on the cornea, poor performance of an eye tracker system, etc. Minor decentration can induce few symptoms, mostly halos in low light conditions. However, significant decentration can degrade the cornea's optical performance and result in decreased vision, monocular diplopia, constant halos, or induced astigmatism.[19-21] Several retreatment techniques have been proposed for decentration, including selective blocking of part of the retreatment to be delivered and decentration of a myopic ablation in the opposite direction from the first ablation.[21-28] However, these techniques, by increasing the total myopic ablation, are only indicated for decentration associated with significant undercorrection. In cases of decentration associated with a near plano refractive result, additional myopic treatment will result in overcorrection. In our experience, we have retreated cases with significant undercorrection by retreating with a decentration in the opposite direction of the initial decentered treatment (Example 6 [see p. 346]). However, the approach was different when the initial decentration is associated with a near plano or minimal residual ametropia (Examples 7 to 11 [see pp. 347 to 350]). Such cases are more complex, and the objective of a retreatment is to recenter the ablation zone without altering the refractive result obtained by the first surgery. This can be achieved with a combination of a decentered myopic and a decentered hyperopic ablation. In the same surgical session, the hyperopic ablation is first decentered in the same direction as the original off-center myopic treatment. A myopic ablation of a near equivalent dioptric power is then added, but in the opposite direction (ie, 180 degrees apart). These hyperopic and myopic ablations are of near equivalent dioptric value so that their respective refractive effects are neutralized, and the eye's refractive status should not be altered significantly.

The initial decentration can be classified as mild, moderate, or marked. When, as measured on topographical maps, the distance between the center of the ablation and the optical center of the

When the initial decentration is associated with a near plano or minimal residual ametropia, the hyperopic ablation is first decentered in the same direction as the original off-center myopic treatment. A myopic ablation of a near equivalent dioptric power is then added, but in the opposite direction (ie, 180 degrees apart).

eye was less than 1 mm, it was classified as mild. It was classified as moderate when this distance was between 1 and 2 mm and as marked for distance greater than 2 mm. Example 6 illustrates the retreatment of a marked decentration case with marked undercorrection by using a decentered myopic ablation. Although our experience is limited to few such cases, this retreatment technique was simple and effective. The other examples illustrate moderate and marked decentrations, but without such undercorrection. The technique, using a combination of myopic and hyperopic ablations, was used in the retreatment of 16 such cases. Prior to retreatment, all of these patients complained of various symptoms such as halos, glare, or ghost images, and BCVA loss was present in five cases. This technique was very effective in recentering the ablation zone and has a predictable refractive outcome. The efficacy of this technique is readily visible after comparing topographical maps before and after retreatment in the following examples. After the retreatment, all but one patient acknowledged a reduction of the presenting symptoms. Five eyes with BCVA loss after the initial surgery recovered lines of vision. Results can be improved even further with additional retreatment as seen in Examples 10 and 11. In our experience, ablations used for the retreatment of these cases were delivered with decentration distances ranging from 1 to 2 mm from the visual axis, 2 mm being the maximum distance used. This 2 mm decentration was used for the retreatment of marked decentration. For cases of initial moderate decentration, retreatment decentration was between 1 and 1.50 mm. The hyperopic and myopic ablation values were usually between 1 and 2 D. However, in cases in which some residual ametropia was present, these values can be set smaller or higher to correct this ametropia. These ablations were performed within a large diameter. The hyperopic ablation diameter used for retreatment is usually 6 mm with a transition zone extending to 9.60 mm. The myopic ablation was usually 6 mm with transition zone to 9 mm. However, smaller diameters were used in cases of limited residual corneal thickness, or small LASIK flap diameters.

Our analysis of the results showed that final refractive outcomes were predictable. The final refractive results were within ±0.50 D (spherical equivalent) in 11 of these 16 eyes. No significant astigmatism was induced by the retreatment. A second retreatment session was needed to correct some residual ametropia in only three cases. Concerning the safety of this technique, the only complication encountered is illustrated in Example 6, where the retreatment induced an inadvertent new decentration in the opposite direction of the initial treated one, resulting in a one-line BCVA loss. However, a second retreatment session improved the centration and recovered the visual loss.

In most cases of decentration, some induced or residual astigmatism is present. Usually moderate decentrations induce minor astigmatism, but marked decentration can induced a significant amount of astigmatism, as observed in Examples 6, 9, 10, and 11. Recentering the ablation zone, with spherical ablation, by itself should correct some of the induced astigmatism. In Example 6, which illustrates a decentration with marked undercorrection and induced astigmatism, less than half of the induced astigmatism value was included in the myopic ablation retreatment. The result was its complete correction. In Examples 7 and 9, no toric ablation at all was included in the retreatment protocol. Results show that the induced astigmatism was also corrected by the decentration of this combination of myopic and hyperopic ablations. In one of our first cases retreated with the technique of combined decentered ablations, the full value of the residual astigmatism was included in the retreatment parameters, and the final result was an unexpected residual astigmatism that shifted 60 degrees from its previous axis. Therefore these results suggest that, in the retreatment of decentrations, the retreatment protocol should not include the total amount of astigmatism induced by the initial decentered treatment.

In a decentration with marked undercorrection and induced astigmatism, less than half of the induced astigmatism value was included in the myopic ablation retreatment. The result was its complete correction.

What should be the optimal retreatment parameters? Each case of decentration differs from the others in the following ways: the initial correction delivered, the amplitude and axis of decentration, the regularity or irregularity of the initial ablation, and the presence or absence of a residual ametropia or an induced astigmatism. Therefore, ideal standard retreatment nomograms would be difficult to define precisely. In our experience of moderate to marked decentration retreatment, retreatment decentration ranged from 1 to 2 mm and retreatment dioptric values were relatively small, usually between 1 and 2 D. Those parameters proved adequate for most cases. However, for some severe cases, such as Example 10, these retreatment parameters were insufficient, and several retreatment sessions were needed. For such extreme cases, retreatment parameters are very difficult to estimate. Aggressive retreatment could induce unpredictable results. A conservative approach with limited parameters was preferred, knowing that probably more than one retreatment session would be needed to restore good vision quality.

There is probably a greater limitation in the use of a decentered hyperopic ablation than the equivalent decentered myopic ablation. The main reason for this concern is the ablation profile in the hyperopic transition zone. For example, with the laser used for these retreatments, the Technolas 217Z, a 6 mm myopic treatment has a transition zone extending to 9 mm. The myopic treatment profile is a convex ablation with a regular curve in the central 6 mm zone and then flattens progressively in the transition zone. A 6 mm hyperopic treatment has a transition zone extending to 9.60 mm. The ablation has a concave profile in the 6 mm central zone; however, in the transition zone, the ablation changes for a convex profile. A myopic ablation flattens the corneal curvature in the central zone and also in the transition zone, but to a lesser extent. A hyperopic ablation steepens the corneal curvature in the central zone, but flattens the corneal curvature in the transition zone. For example, using 6 mm myopic and hyperopic ablations, with each one decentered 1.50 mm from the eye's optical center, but in opposite directions, the total distance between the centers of each of these ablations is 3 mm. Therefore, these two 6 mm ablations overlap in a central 3 mm zone and their respective refractive effects are neutralized. Outside this central 3 mm zone, on the side of the hyperopic ablation, 3 mm of the hyperopic central ablation zone juxtapose the myopic transition zone, but the hyperopic refractive effect exceeds the myopic correction effect and the result is a steepening of this part of the cornea. In the hyperopic transition zone, the ablation profile changes from a concave to a convex profile. However, considering the 6 mm zone ablation and the 1.50 mm decentration, this hyperopic transition zone is located 4.50 mm from the optical center and therefore has little effect on the final refractive result. In the other direction, on the side of the myopic ablation but outside the central 3 mm zone, the myopic correction juxtaposes the hyperopic transition zone, which starts at this level. Unlike the myopic transition zone, which has an ablation profile similar to the myopic central ablation zone but with a decreasing curve, the hyperopic transition zone has an ablation curve that is inverted compared to the central hyperopic zone. The effect of the hyperopic transition zone is to flatten the corneal curvature in this area; therefore, this effect is additive to the concurrent myopic ablation that also flattens the cornea. In light of these considerations on the hyperopic transition zone profile, we think that there is a greater limitation in decentering the hyperopic ablation than the myopic ablation in order to keep this transition zone outside of the eye's optical center. Also, the largest hyperopic ablation diameter possible should probably be used.

In our experience, the maximum decentration distance used for the retreatment of severe decentration cases was 2 mm.

We think that there is a greater limitation in decentering the hyperopic ablation than the myopic ablation in order to keep this transition zone outside of the eye's optical center. Also, the largest hyperopic ablation diameter possible should probably be used.

In conclusion, cases of moderate and marked decentration, after an initial excimer laser refractive surgery, can be corrected or markedly improved with the current laser technology. The decentration retreatment techniques, using a decentered myopic ablation or a combination of myopic and hyperopic ablation, were successful in recentering the treatment zone with predictable refractive results. The retreatment parameters used seem adequate for moderate cases of decentration but are probably not optimal for all cases. However, repeated retreatments are possible, and this is surely a good option for difficult cases.

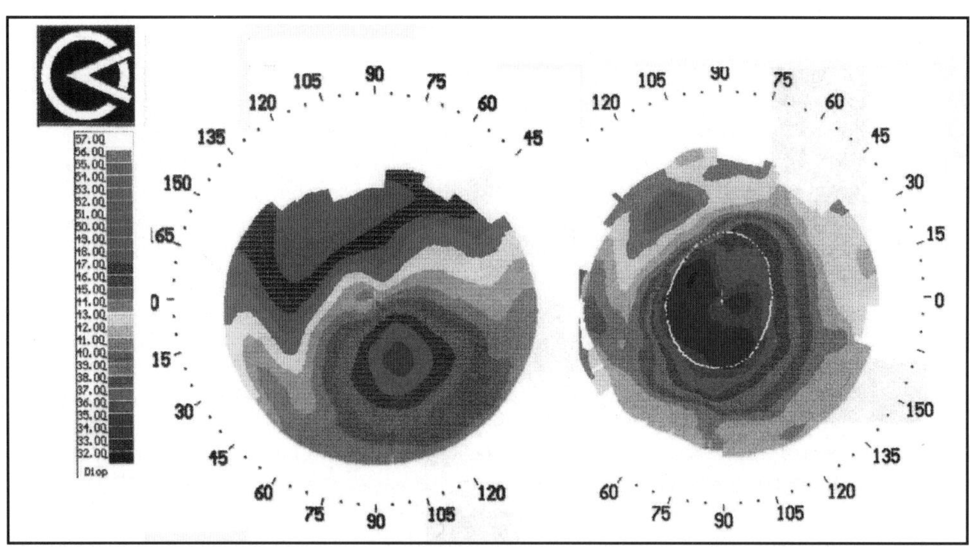

EXAMPLE 6

This 52-year-old female had keratomileusis in 1991. Initial refraction was -13.75 + 1.25 x 95, yielding 20/30 vision. A significant decentration was present postoperatively and visible on topography (left map). Refractive result was -7.75 + 3.25 x 25, resulting in 20/50 vision. In addition to undercorrection, induced astigmatism, and a two-line BCVA loss, the patient complained of marked halos around lights. A retreatment with LASIK was performed 6 years after the initial surgery. In order to recenter the ablation zone, the retreatment was decentered 2 mm from the optical center in the opposite direction from the first decentered ablation. It was estimated that the decentration of this ablation, by itself, should neutralize some of the induced astigmatism. Therefore, less than half of this astigmatism was included in the retreatment, but the retreatment was calculated to correspond to the spherical equivalent of the undercorrection. The retreatment parameters were -6.75 + 1.50 x 25, delivered with a 2 mm decentration from the optical center at 110. The retreatment diameter was 4.30 mm with a transition zone extending to 7.30 mm. The decision was made not to use a larger diameter ablation in order to limit the ablation thickness. The map on the right shows a marked centration improvement. Final refractive result was -0.50, resulting in 20/30 vision and a marked decrease of halos.

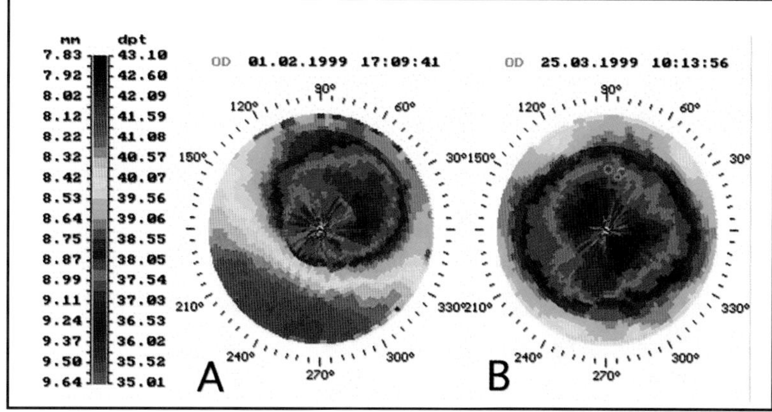

EXAMPLE 7

This 40-year-old engineer had an initial myopic PRK performed with a broadbeam laser for -6.50 + 0.25 x 145 myopia (20/15) in his right eye. The refractive result was -0.50 + 0.75 x 120, resulting in 20/20 vision. The patient had good vision in daylight but he complained of marked halos in dim illumination that made night driving difficult. A moderate decentration (map A) was believed to be the cause of these symptoms.

The retreatment with LASIK consisted of a +1 D hyperopic ablation using a 6 mm diameter zone with a transition zone extending to 9.60 mm. This ablation was decentered 1.50 mm at 60 degrees. Then a -1.25 myopic ablation using a 5.80 mm zone with a transition extending to 8.80 mm was added with a 1.50 mm decentration at 240. Because the refractive spherical equivalent prior to the retreatment was minimally myopic, the myopic correction exceeded the hyperopic correction by -0.25 D. No toric ablation was included in this retreatment. It was supposed that the astigmatism observed after the first surgery was a result of the decentration, and recentering the ablation should by itself correct this astigmatism. The result of this retreatment was a refraction of -0.25 D, yielding 20/20 vision and an almost complete disappearance of halos. Map B shows topographic maps after retreatment. A recentration and an enlargement of the ablation zone, without significant central corneal curvature modification, can be observed on this post-retreatment map.

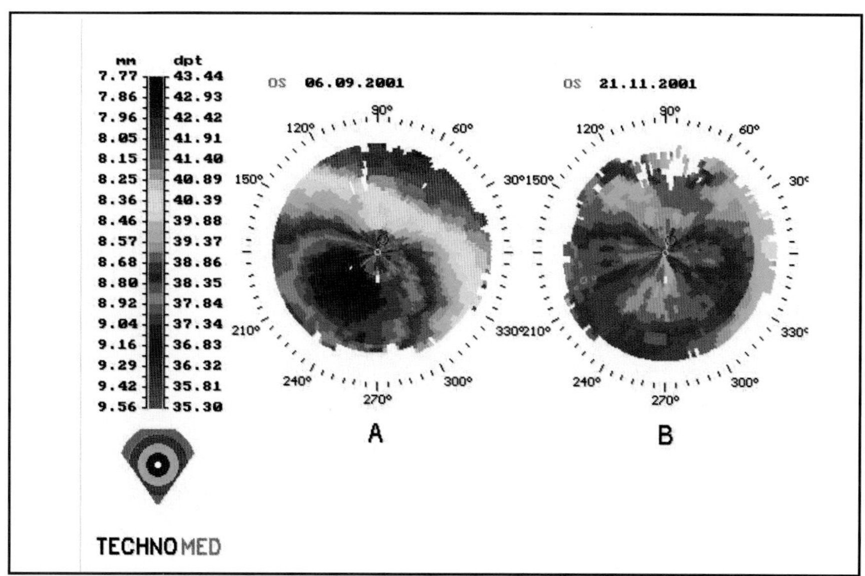

EXAMPLE 8

This 44-year-old male had myopic LASIK for -5.00 myopia (20/20). The result was a marked decentration as noted on map A. Postoperative refraction was +0.50 + 0.25 x 90, resulting in 20/30 vision. In addition to a decreased vision, the patient was experiencing disturbing glare and halos. Three months after the initial surgery, a retreatment was performed. The LASIK flap was relifted and the retreatment parameters consisted of a +1.50 D hyperopic ablation within a 5.80 mm zone (transition zone extending to 9.30 mm) with a 1.50 mm decentration at 235, and a myopic ablation of -1 D within a 5.50 mm diameter zone (transition zone extending to 8.5 mm) with a 2 mm decentration at 55 degrees. Refractive results were plano + 0.50 X 100, yielding 20/20 vision. Post-retreatment topography, on map B, confirmed a well-centered ablation zone, which correlated with recovery of the patient's symptoms.

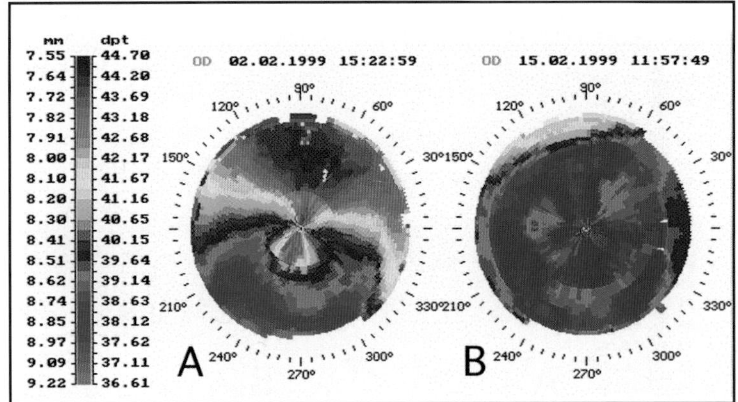

Example 9

This 22-year-old patient had myopic LASIK for -3.50 D (20/15), with resulting decentration. Consequences of this marked decentration were undercorrection, induced astigmatism, monocular diplopia, and a two-line BCVA loss. Postoperative refraction was plano -2.50 x 165 degrees, yielding 20/25- vision. The topographical map (map A) shows a marked inferior decentration. It was estimated that treating only the undercorrection would not be sufficient to achieve an adequate centration. The approach chosen for this patient was combined myopic and hyperopic ablations. The retreatment was performed only 1 week after the initial surgery, and the surgical approach chosen was to lift the LASIK flap. The patient was undercorrected (spherical equivalent -1.25); therefore, the myopic ablation value exceeded the hyperopic ablation. Also, because of the patient's young age, a slight overcorrection of +0.50 D was planned. A -2.75 D treatment using a 5.50 mm zone with a transition zone extending to 8.50 mm was delivered with a 2 mm superior decentration from the optical center. Then a +1 D hyperopic treatment using a 6 mm zone with a transition zone extending to 9.60 mm was added with a 2 mm inferior decentration. Although the ametropia present after the initial treatment was induced myopic astigmatism, the retreatment consisted of pure spherical ablations. No toric ablation was included in this retreatment protocol; the correction of the cylinder was achieved by the decentration of these spherical myopic and hyperopic ablations. An excellent result was obtained. The postoperative topography (map B) shows a large and well-centered final ablation zone. The refraction is plano + 0.75 x 15 degrees for a 20/20 vision. This small residual astigmatism showed a 60-degree shift from the astigmatism axis measured before the retreatment.

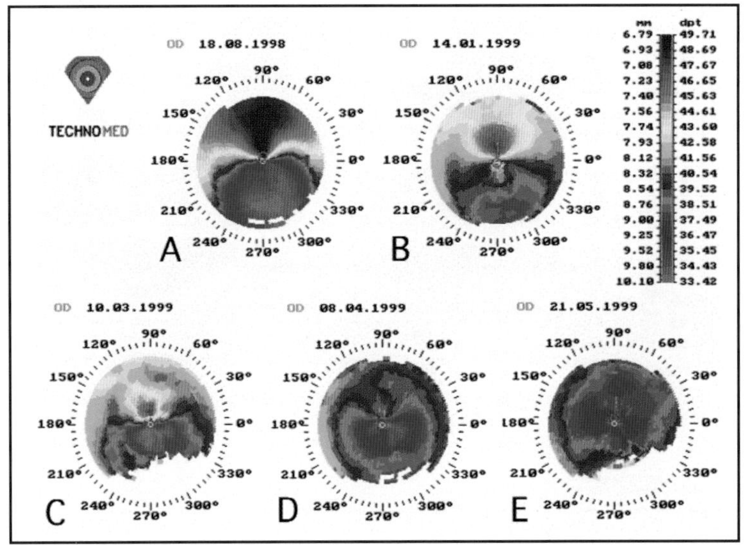

Example 10

This 53-year-old man consulted for a severe treatment decentration after an initial myopic LASIK surgery of -11.50 D (20/25). Postoperative refraction was very inaccurate, due to a marked irregular astigmatism. Best subjective result was +0.50 + 0.75 x 180 for 20/60- vision. On the topographical map, a 15.00 D difference was present between corneal curvature measurement taken 2.00 mm superior and 2.00 mm inferior to the optical center (map A). The astigmatism measurement on this map was 5.82 D. The approach for the retreatment was to lift the flap and deliver a combination of myopic and hyperopic ablations. The retreatment parameters consisted of a 2.50 D hyperopic ablation within a 5.70 mm zone (transition zone extending to 9.30) with a 2.00 mm inferior decentration, and a -1.25 D myopic ablation within a 5.5 mm zone (transition zone extending to 8.50) with a 2.00 mm superior decentration. With no experience in retreating higher parameters (decentration distance or dioptric values), a conservative approach was preferred to the risk of unpredictable result that could be the consequence of a more aggressive retreatment. A decrease of the corneal irregularity was obtained by this first retreatment (map B); however, the refractive result was unexpected. Refraction measured after the retreatment was -2.50 for 20/50 vision. Before this retreatment, the patient seemed overcorrected by 0.87 D (spherical equivalent). The myopic ablation was -1.25 D and hyperopic ablation was +2.75 D; therefore, a resulting refractive value of -0.67 D was expected instead of the -2.50 D obtained.

Two months after the first retreatment, a second retreatment was performed. A small diameter myopic ablation technique (as described previously to correct surface irregularities) was used. A -4 D myopic ablation within a 4 mm zone (transition zone extending to 6 mm) was performed. This retreatment was delivered with a 1.50 mm superior decentration at 100 degrees. The third topography (map C), taken 20 minutes after this retreatment, showed the persistence of a localized steep zone superior to the optical center. The corneal flap was than immediately lifted again and an additional -3 D ablation was delivered with the same 1.50 mm decentration at 100 degrees, but within a 3 mm zone (transition zone extending to 5 mm). The value of these retreatments exceeded the residual myopia; however, no resulting marked hyperopia was expected. It was learned from previous experience that an off-center ablation within a small diameter gives less refractive effect than the same dioptric value treatment delivered centered and within a standard wider diameter.[15] On another map, taken 1 month later (map D), a marked improvement was visible. The refraction after these retreatments was plano + 1.75 x 83, yielding 20/40 vision.

One month after the second retreatment session, a third retreatment was performed. An additional -3 myopic ablation within a small 3 mm diameter was delivered with a 1.50 mm decentration at 100 degrees to flatten the persisting steep zone. Because this ablation was decentered and within a small diameter, it was estimated that the effect on the final refraction should be less than 1 D. Then a +1.00 + 0.50 x 83 hyperopic ablation within a 5.50 mm zone (with a transition extending to 9.10 mm) was added with a 1.00 mm inferior decentration at 270 degrees. The cylinder correction was only +0.50 D, much less than the +1.75 to be corrected. This undercorrection was chosen based on the belief that the astigmatism is secondary to the corneal irregularity and the combined decentered retreatments, by decreasing this irregularity, should correct at least partly this astigmatism. The final result was +0.50 + 0.50 x 80 for 20/25 vision. Topo-graphical map taken after this final retreatment (map E) shows a much more regular and centered ablation. Monocular diplopia disappeared and the four-line BCVA loss was recovered.

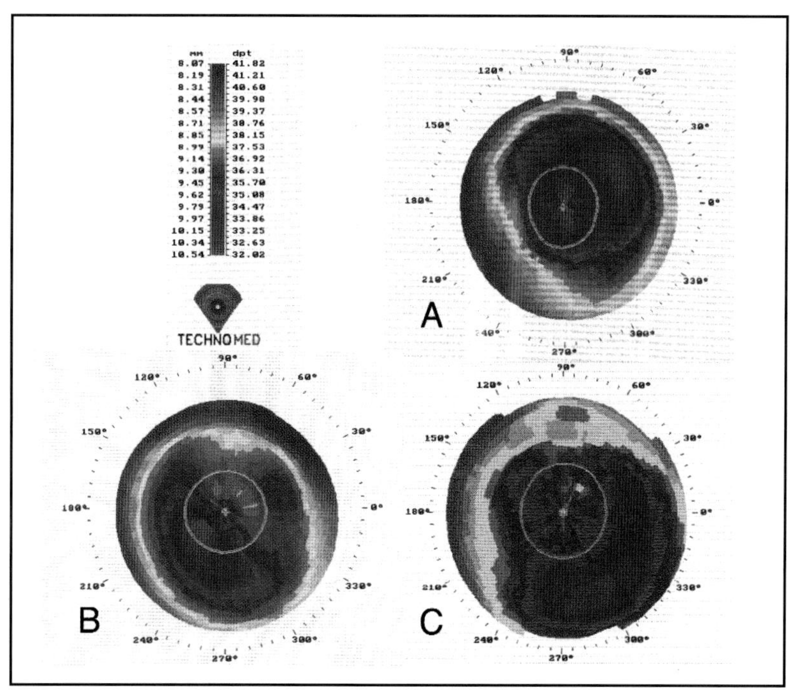

EXAMPLE 11

This example shows the only case of "over-retreatment" we observed with this combined myopic and hyperopic retreatment technique. A first retreatment was performed to correct a problem with halos, believed to be the consequence of a moderate decentration. This retreatment resulted with a decentration worse and in the opposite direction from the initial one. Also, it induced one line of visual loss. A second retreatment session succeeded in improving the final outcome.

The first map (A) shows the decentration present after the initial treatment. The myopia was -9.50 + 1.50 x 7 for 20/20 vision. The surgical result was +0.75 + 1.75 x 168, yielding 20/20 vision. The first retreatment parameters consisted of a +1.50 + 1.25 x 168 hyperopic ablation with a 1.5 mm decentration at 30 degrees using a 5.50 mm diameter zone (with a transition zone extending to 9.10 mm) and a -1.00 myopic ablation with a 1.50 mm decentration at 210 degrees using a 5.50 mm diameter zone (with a transition zone extending to 8.50 mm). Result of this retreatment was +0.50 + 2.50 x 155, yielding 20/25 vision. The second map (B), taken after this retreatment, shows a decentration that has shifted 180 degrees in the opposite direction. A second retreatment session consisted of a decentered hyperopic ablation of +1.00 + 2.00 x 155 within a 5.80 mm diameter zone (transition zone 9.3 mm). Decentration distance was 1.30 mm at 220 degrees. The third map (C) was taken after this second retreatment and shows better centration. Final refractive result was +0.25 + 0.25 x 105, yielding 20/20 vision. In this particular case, the initial retreatment diameters and decentration distances were not much different from those used for the other cases. However, this case had the highest induced hyperopia value prior to the retreatment, and a higher hyperopic astigmatic correction was delivered. Given the moderate decentration, the initial retreatment should have been performed with lesser distance decentration or with lesser dioptric values.

Enlargement of Previous Small Diameter Ablations

Small treatment zones can be a cause of halos and glare after an excimer laser refractive procedure. These symptoms are more commonly experienced in lowlight situations. Despite good UCVA in daylight conditions, some patients are substantially incapacitated with night driving.[29-33] The reasons for these halos and glare sometimes can be complex. They can result from a small diameter treatment zone or a large pupil diameter in relation to the treatment zone diameter. They also can be the consequence of aberrations due to a large curvature difference between the treated and the nontreated cornea or the consequences of higher-order aberrations.[34-37] These symptoms were more common with treatments performed using first-generation broadbeam lasers. These lasers had a smaller treatment diameter and a less regular ablation pattern, as compared to more recent scanning lasers. However, halos can still be encountered, even with the most recent instrumentation. Enlargement of the optical zone can be effective in reducing halos and glare.[38,39]

With the current laser technology, it is possible to enlarge the ablation zone without significantly altering the refractive effect obtained by the initial surgery. The retreatment technique consists of a combination of myopic and hyperopic ablations, both delivered during the same operative session. These two ablations are delivered on the visual axis. Because their relative power—negative and positive—are nearly equivalent (eg, a -1.00 D ablation and +1.00 D ablation), they should neutralize one another. Consequently, they should not significantly alter the cornea's refractive power.

We have retreated eight eyes from six patients with this technique. In all cases, the patient's main presenting complaints were halos, diminished vision in low light situations, and night driving difficulties. In all cases, the initial ablation was regular and well-centered, and any minimal residual ametropia was measured. Eyes initially treated with PRK were retreated with LASIK. Eyes initially treated with LASIK had the initial flap lifted.

The diopter value of the retreatment, myopic and hyperopic, was between 1 D and 1.50 D. Wide myopic and hyperopic ablation diameters were used. The myopic ablation diameter ranged from 5.50 mm (with a transition zone extending to 8.50 mm) to 6.50 mm (with a transition zone extending to 9.50 mm). The hyperopic ablation diameter ranged from 5.80 mm (with a transition zone extending to 9.30 mm) to 6 mm (with a transition zone extending to 9.60 mm). Factors influencing the choice of ablation diameter were residual corneal thickness and LASIK flap diameter. Smaller diameters were preferred in case of limited residual corneal thickness or smaller LASIK flaps.

Although our experience is limited, this technique seems very effective; it achieved good results in most treated cases. In six out of eight cases, a moderate or marked decrease of the symptoms was achieved, and these patients were satisfied with the retreatment result. Only one patient (two eyes) did not notice significant change. In all cases, topographical maps showed a larger ablation zone after retreatment. The improvement was less noticeable in cases in which the initial treatment was for the correction of higher myopia. It is possible that for these cases, higher retreatment values would be more effective and lead to a better result; however, more aggressive retreatment parameters possibly have a higher risk of inducing irregular astigmatism. We do not have experience using this retreatment technique with dioptric value combinations higher than 1.50 D. Another consideration is that in cases of initial deep ablations, residual corneal thickness is often limited. Therefore, in order to respect a safe minimal residual corneal thickness, it is often not possible to use more aggressive retreatment parameters. Thus, this above-mentioned technique has more limitations for the patients who were initially in the higher myopic group, and these patients are precisely those types who are more at risk for experiencing symptoms after an initial surgery and who would benefit more from this technique. Furthermore, in some cases, it is possible that other higher-order aberrations can also contribute to the halo symptoms and yet are not corrected by an enlargement of the treatment zone.[40-44]

This technique is safe and has predictable refractive outcomes. In our experience, no visual loss or other complication was observed. Results show that after the retreatment all eight eyes were in a -0.50 to +0.50 range (spherical equivalent). Induced astigmatism did not exceed 0.50 D in any case.

In conclusion, enlargement of previous small diameter myopic ablations, without altering the refractive effect of the initial surgery, is possible with a combination of large diameter myopic and hyperopic treatments. Although our experience is limited, this technique seems to be effective and safe in selected cases.

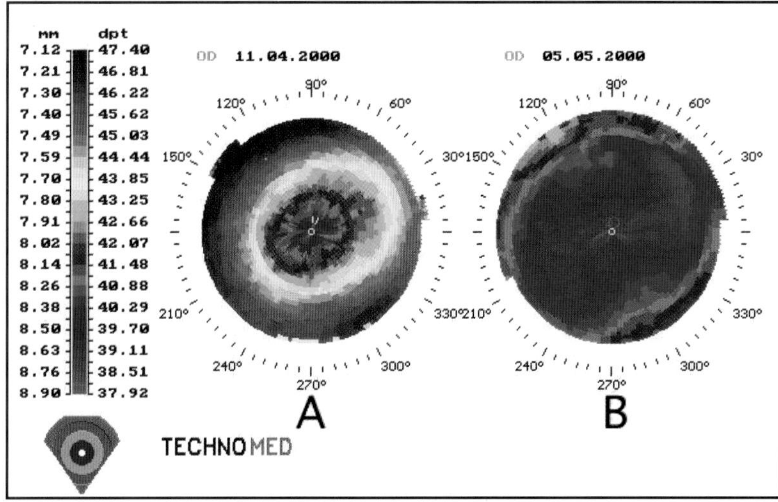

EXAMPLE 12

This example shows the topographical maps before and after a retreatment performed to enlarge a previous small diameter myopic ablation zone. Four years earlier, this 24-year-old female had PRK performed within 4 and 5 mm diameter zones for -5.75 D myopia. The refractive result was -0.25 + 0.75 x 155, yielding 20/20 vision. She had good vision in daylight conditions, but with dim light conditions she complained of halos, decreased vision, and marked difficulties with driving. Retreatment consisted of an enlargement of the ablation zone with a combination of +1.25 D hyperopic treatment and -1.75 D myopic treatment. Both ablations were delivered on the visual axis. An additional plano +0.75 x 155 astigmatism treatment was included as a retreatment of residual astigmatism. A final +0.25 refractive result was planned. The hyperopic treatment zone diameter was 5.80 mm with a transition zone extending to 9.30 mm, and the myopic treatment zone diameter was 5.50 mm with a transition zone extending to 8.50 mm. As noted on map B, a marked enlargement of the optical zone was achieved by this retreatment. The patient experienced an almost complete disappearance of her symptoms. Final refraction was +0.25 D, yielding 20/15 vision.

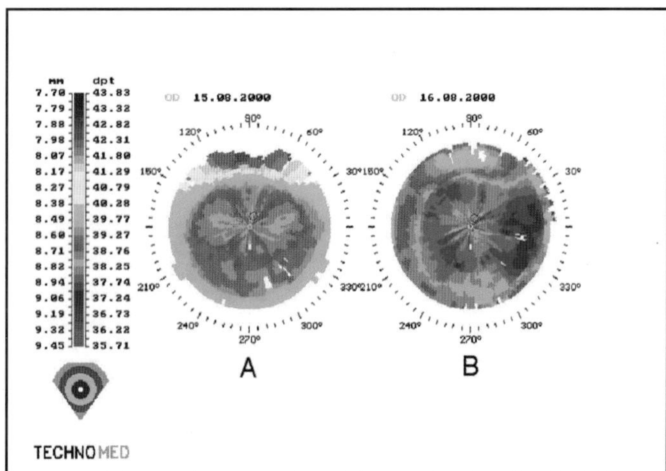

EXAMPLE 13

These topographical maps illustrate another example of enlargement of the treatment zone. This 26-year-old patient was complaining of halos at night and marked night-driving difficulties. These symptoms were not corrected by the use of glasses for a small residual myopic astigmatism of -1.00 + 0.75 x 88 (20/20). In the retreatment protocol, in addition to a -1.00 + 0.75 x 88 ablation for the correction of this small residual myopic astigmatism, a combination of -1.25 D and +1.00 D ablations was included to enlarge the treatment zone. The myopic treatment exceeded the hyperopic treatment by 0.25 D because a final refraction of +0.25 was planned. The hyperopic treatment zone diameter was 6 mm with a transition zone extending to 9.50 mm, and the myopic treatment zone diameter was 6 mm with a transition zone extending to 9 mm. As noted on map B, a marked enlargement of the treatment zone was present after the retreatment. Final refraction was plano + 0.25 x 50, resulting in 20/20 vision. A very significant diminution of halos under low light conditions was experienced by the patient, although some mild residual symptoms were still experienced.

References

1. Alpins NA. Treatment of irregular astigmatism. *J Cataract Refract Surg.* 1998;24:634-646.
2. Borderie V, Laroche L. Measurement of irregular astigmatism using semi-meridian data from videokeratographs. *J Refract Surg.* 1996;12: 595-600.
3. Endl MJ, Martinez CE, Klyce SD, et al. Irregular astigmatism after photorefractive keratectomy. *J Refract Surg.* 1999;15:S249-S251.
4. Gilbralter R, Trokel S. Correction of irregular astigmatism with the excimer laser. *Ophthalmology.* 1994;101:1310-1315.
5. Adamsons I, et al. Corneal clarity, irregular astigmatism, and visual function in patients undergoing phototherapeutic keratectomy (PTK). *Invest Ophthalmol Vis Sci.* 1993;34:S893.
6. Cantera I, et al. Qualitative topographic evaluation after excimer laser photorefractive keratectomy. *Invest Ophthalmol Vis Sci.* 1994;35:1739.
7. Kim JH, Sah WJ, Hahn TW, Lee YC. Some problems after photorefractive keratectomy. *J Refract Corneal Surg.* 1994;10:S226-S230.
8. Oshika T, Tomidokoro A, Maruo K, et al. Quantitative evaluation of irregular astigmatism by Fourier series harmonic analysis of videokeratography data. *Invest Ophthalmol Vis Sci.* 1998;39:705-709.
9. Raasch T. Corneal topography and irregular astigmatism. *Optom Vis Sci.* 1995;72:809-815.
10. Probst LE, Machat JJ. Removal of flap striae following laser in-situ keratomileusis. *J Cataract Refract Surg.* 1998;24:153-155.
11. Lin RT, Maloney RK. Flap complications associated with lamellar refractive surgery. *Am J Ophthalmol.* 1999;127:129-136.
12. Tham VMB, Maloney R. Microkeratome complications of laser in-situ keratomileusis. *Ophthalmology.* 2000;107:920-924.
13. Smith RJ, Maloney RK. Diffuse lamellar keratitis: a new syndrome in lamellar refractive surgery. *Ophthalmology.* 1998;105:1721-1726.
14. Wang M, Maloney R. Epithelial ingrowth after laser in-situ keratomileusis. *Am J Ophthalmol.* 2000;129:746-751.
15. Lafond G, Solomon L. Retreatment of central islands after photorefractive keratectomy. *J Cataract Refract Surg.* 1999;25:188-196.
16. Seiler T. Photorefractive keratectomy: European experience. In: Thompson FM, McDonnell PJ, eds. *Color Atlas: The Cornea.* New York: Igaku-Shain Medical Publishers; 1993:53-62.
17. Seiler T, McDonnell PJ. Excimer laser photorefractive keratectomy. *Surv Ophthalmol.* 1995;40,2:100-101.
18. Probst LE. Optical aberration following PRK: starburst, halos and decentration. In: Machat JJ, ed. *Excimer Laser Refractive Surgery.* Thorofare, NJ: SLACK Incorporated; 1996:188-189.
19. Wilson SE, Klyce SD. Quantitative descriptors of corneal topography: a clinical study. *Arch Ophthalmol.* 1991;109:349-353.
20. Seiler T, Reckman NW, Maloney RK. Effective spherical aberration of the cornea as a quantitative descriptor in corneal topography. *J Cataract Refract Surg.* 1993;19(Suppl):155-165.
21. O'Brart DP, Corbett MC, Verma S, et al. Effect of ablation diameter, depth, and edge contour on the outcome of photorefractive keratectomy. *J Refract Surg.* 1996;12(1):50-60.
22. Deitz MR, Piebenga LW, Matta CS, et al. Ablation zone centration after photorefractive keratectomy and its effect on visual outcome. *J Cataract Refract Surg.* 1996;22(6):696-701.
23. Gauthier-Fournet L. LASIK results. In: Pallikaris IG, Siganos DS, eds. *LASIK.* Thorofare, NJ: SLACK Incorporated; 1998:235-236.
24. Mendez-Noble A, Mendez AG. LASIK: the Latin experience. In: Pallikaris IG, Siganos DS, eds. *LASIK.* Thorofare, NJ: SLACK Incorporated; 1998:207.
25. Machat JJ. Lasik complications and their management. In: Machat JJ, ed. *Excimer Laser Refractive Surgery.* Thorofare, NJ: SLACK Incorporated; 1996:233-234:380-381.
26. Seiler T, Schmidt-Petersen H, Wollensuk J. Complications after myopic photorefractive keratectomy, primarily with the Summit excimer laser. In: Salz JJ, McDonnell PJ, McDonald MB, eds. *Corneal Laser Surgery.* St. Louis, Mo: Mosby; 1995.
27. Eggink FA, Houdijn Beekhuis W, Trockel SL, den Boon JM. Enlargement of the photorefractive optical zone. *J Cataract Refract Surg.* 1996;22(9):1159-1164.
28. Knorz MC, Jendritza B. Topographically-guided laser in-situ keratomileusis to treat corneal irregularities. *Ophthalmology.* 2000;107(6):1138-1143.
29. Holladay JT, Dudeja DR, Chang J. Functional vision and corneal changes after laser in-situ keratomileusis determined by contrast sensitivity, glare testing and corneal topography. *J Cataract Refract Surg.* 1999;25:663-669.
30. Jain S, Khoury JM, Chamon W, Azar DT. Corneal light scattering after laser in-situ keratomileusis and photorefractive keratectomy. *Am J Ophthalmol.* 1995;120:532-534.
31. Melki SA, Proano CE, Azar DT. Optical disturbances and their management after myopic laser in-situ keratomileusis. *Int Ophthalmol Clin.* 2000;40:45-56.
32. Pallikaris IG. Quality of vision in refractive surgery. *J Refract Surg.* 1998;14:551-558.
33. Casson EJ, Racette L. Vision standards for driving in Canada and the United States. A review for the Canadian Ophthalmological Society. *Can J Ophthalmol.* 2000;35:192-203.
34. Melki SA, Azar DT. Lasik complications: etiology, management, and prevention. *Surv Ophthalmol.* 2001;46:95-116.
35. Hersh PS, Abbassi R. Surgically induced astigmatism after photorefractive keratectomy and laser in-situ keratomileusis. Summit PRK-LASIK study group. *J Cataract Refract Surg.* 1999;25:389-398.
36. O'Brart DP, Corbett MC, Verma S, et al. Effects of ablation diameter, depth, and edge contour on the outcome of photorefractive keratectomy. *J Refract Surg.* 1996;12(1):50-60.
37. Haw WW, Manche EE. Effect of preoperative pupil measurements on glare, halos, and visual function after photoastigmatic refractive keratectomy. *J Cataract Refract Surg.* 2001;27(6):907-916.
38. Eggink FA, Houdijn Beekhuis W, Trokel SL, den Boon JM. Enlargement of the photorefractive keratectomy optical zone. *J Cataract Refract Surg.* 1996;22(9):1159-1164.
39. Lafond G. Treatment of halos after photorefractive keratectomy. *J Refract Surg.* 1997;13(1):83-88.
40. Liang J, Williams DR. Effect of higher-order aberrations on image quality in the human eye. Vision Science and its applications, OSA technical digest series. *Optical Society of America.* 1995;1:70-73.
41. Oliver KM, Hemenger RP, Corbett MC, et al. Corneal, optical aberrations induced by photorefractive keratectomy. *J Refract Surg.* 1997;13:246-254.
42. Applegate RA. Limits to vision: can we do better than nature? *J Refract Surg.* 2000;16:S547-S551.
43. Oshika T, Klyce SD, Applegate RA, et al. Comparison of corneal wavefront aberrations after photorefractive keratectomy and laser in situ keratomileusis. *Am J Ophthalmol.* 1999;127:1-7.
44. Seiler T, Kaemmerer M, Mierdel P, Krinke HE. Ocular optical aberrations after photorefractive keratectomy for myopia and myopic astigmatism. *Arch Ophthalmol.* 2000;118:17-21.

Chapter 41

Customized Visual Correction of Presbyopia

Fabrice Manns, PhD; Arthur Ho, MOptom, PhD; and Ronald R. Krueger, MD, MSE

If the term *super vision* is taken literally to mean vision of a quality or performance exceeding the norm, then one could argue that by definition, any technique correcting presbyopia achieves super vision since presbyopia is a part of the normal aging process. More ambitiously, the quest for the correction of presbyopia ideally will lead to a technique that will restore the normal accommodative function of the eye: a continuously variable and active focusing system.

Customization of the visual correction of presbyopia adds another dimension to the problem at hand. In addition to restoring accommodation, a wavefront-guided customized correction of presbyopia could simultaneously correct ametropia and higher-order aberrations and perhaps optimize the focusing range and visual quality according to the patient's individual needs. Comparing the visual outcomes of current clinical techniques for the correction of presbyopia with these ideal goals clearly indicates that the quest for the customized correction of presbyopia is very much in its infancy.

The accommodation response of the eye involves intricate dynamic optomechanical interactions. Developing successful technology to restore lost accommodation in the presbyope, as well as to customize the correction, poses formidable challenges. Compared to wavefront-guided customized correction of myopia, hyperopia, or even astigmatism, the dynamic aspect of accommodation adds an additional dimension and level of complexity to the issues at hand. Currently, the first and fundamental hurdle is the absence of a definite and complete description of the mechanism of accommodation and its degradation leading to presbyopia. Today, the quest for the customized correction of presbyopia still relies on the acceptance of either a century-old theory some regard as dogma, or on other quasi-theories ill-supported by objective data relating to accommodation and presbyopia.

Accommodation and Presbyopia

Accommodation can be defined as the ability of the eye to change its refractive power in response to a stimulus. Accommodation provides the eye with a continuously variable focusing ability, which affords a clearly focused image to the eye regardless of the reading distance. The accommodation mechanism is a complex process that involves the lens, lens capsule, zonules, ciliary muscles, ciliary body, choroid, and vitreous mounted on the mechanical framework of the cornea and sclera. The contribution of each of these elements to the accommodation response is still not fully understood, but most experimental studies[1] support the principles of Helmholtz's theory of accommodation.[2] According to this theory, the ciliary muscles of the eye contract in response to a stimulus to accommodation bringing about a relaxation of the zonules suspending the crystalline lens. This relaxation of the zonules permits the elastic crystalline lens to adopt a more curved shape, thereby increasing its refractive power (Figure 41-1).

A number of alternate or modified theories of the accommodation mechanism have been proposed. In his "catenary theory," Coleman suggests that the vitreous plays an active role in the accommodation mechanism by providing support to the lens.[3-5] According to this theory, ciliary muscle contraction during accommodation causes a forward movement of the choroid and vitreous. Together with relaxation of the zonules and vitreous support, this motion induces an anterior protrusion of the lens accompanied by steepening of the lens surfaces. More recently, Schachar proposed a controversial theory of accommodation in which relaxation of the ciliary muscle relieves tension in the anterior and posterior zonules, but increases the tension of equatorial zonules. According to the Schachar theory, this tension increases the lens equatorial diameter and steepens the central optical zone of the lens.[6]

The paucity of solid information relating to the accommodation mechanism extends to presbyopia. There is currently no definitive explanation for the age-related changes in the eye leading to presbyopia. Most likely, presbyopia results from a combination of factors affecting several of the anatomical structures involved in the accommodation response.[7] However, there is strong evidence that a substantial amount of the accommodative loss with presbyopia can be explained by the inability of the aging crystalline lens to change shape[7,8] in concordance with Helmholtz's theory.

> According to Helmholtz's theory,[9] the age-related loss of accommodation is caused by a gradual loss of elasticity of the crystalline lens with age, which prevents the lens from changing shape. Substantial evidence also suggests that in addition to a change in the mechanical properties of the crystalline lens, there are accompanying changes in the gradient distribution and magnitude of the refractive index of the crystalline lens with presbyopia.[10-12]

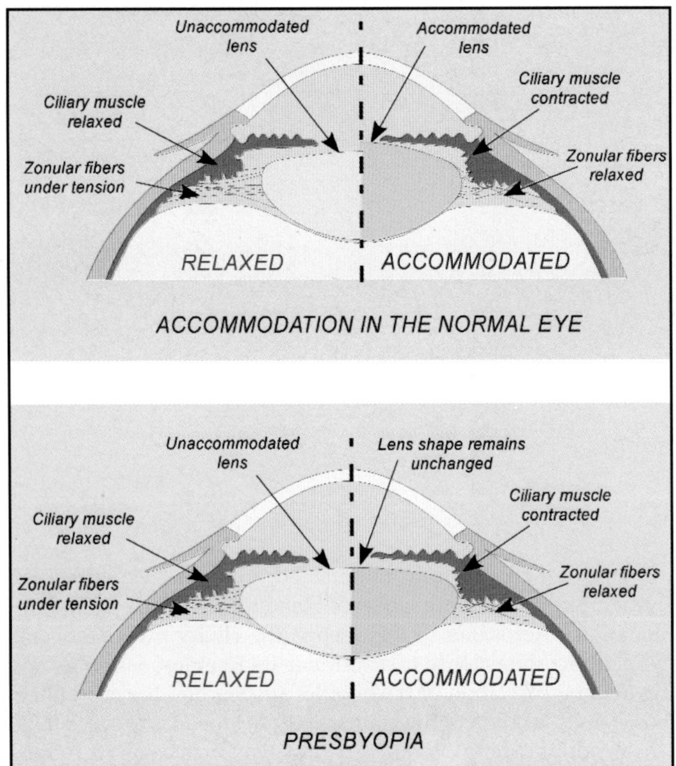

Figure 41-1. Helmholtz's theory of accommodation and presbyopia.

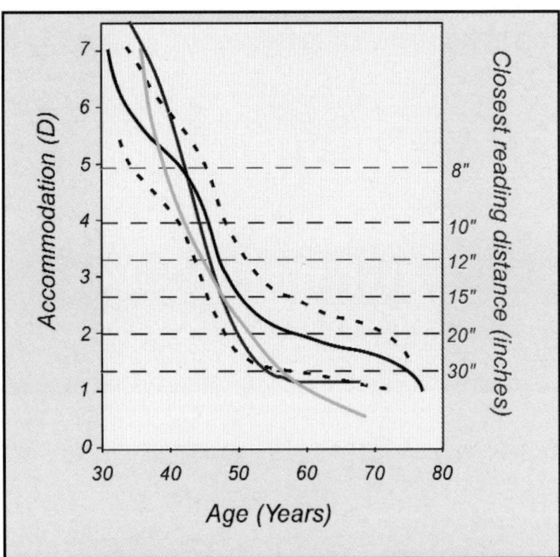

Figure 41-2. The decrease in amplitude of accommodation with age causes nearest unaided reading distance to increase. Some form of reading correction is required for virtually everyone by the age of 50. Graph shows combined data from Duane (1912)[13] (in red), data from The Ayreshire Group with standard deviation (in black), and textbook curve (in green) as reported in Borish (1949).[14]

According to Helmholtz's theory,[9] the age-related loss of accommodation is caused by a gradual loss of elasticity of the crystalline lens with age, which prevents the lens from changing shape. Although the ciliary muscles and zonules remain intact and operational during near vision, the more rigid crystalline lens of the presbyopic eye is unable to change shape to facilitate an increase in refractive power. Substantial evidence also suggests that in addition to a change in the mechanical properties of the crystalline lens, there are accompanying changes in the gradient distribution and magnitude of the refractive index of the crystalline lens with presbyopia.[10-12]

> Of the global population of 6 billion, there are currently over 1.3 billion presbyopes in the United States. More than 40% of the population will be presbyopic over the next decade.

Regardless of the cause, the effect to presbyopes is a gradual decrease in their amplitude of accommodation with age (Figure 41-2), eventually leading to the loss of the ability of the eye to focus on near objects. With symptoms commencing around the age of 40, virtually everyone requires optical aids for reading and other close work by the age of 50. Of the global population of 6 billion, there are currently over 1.3 billion presbyopes. In the United States, due to improved health care and life expectancy, the percentage of presbyopes is higher, at around 35%. The US Bureau of Census's International Database (IDB)[15] predicts that over the next 10 years (by the year 2012), over 40% of people in the United States will be in the presbyopic age group. Thus, presbyopia is an extensive issue in vision correction and vision care delivery. The enormity of the presbyopia population and the associated size of the potential market for vision correction products in this sector are driving many developments in this area.

The Correction of Presbyopia

> Editor's note:
> A number of strategies have been developed to treat presbyopia, including diffractive optics, multifocal lenses, and monovision. They have resulted in mixed success with trade-offs in distance and near vision. A promising strategy is the removal of the human lens and replacement with a flexible gel that allows accommodative movement. This option presents a different set of technical and biologic challenges for success.
> S. MacRae, MD

A number of techniques for the correction of presbyopia are currently available or under development. These include what may be called the conventional correction devices currently regularly prescribed, such as spectacles, contact lenses, or intraocular lenses (IOLs), as well as more recent innovations such as laser surgery of the cornea or lens and scleral surgery. Except for scleral surgery, these devices and techniques rely on a variety of optical designs or treatment approaches, including monovision, bifocal, multifocal, progressive, or accommodative corrections. Table 41-1 categorizes these devices and techniques according to how a change in refractive power is effected from distance to near viewing. It can be seen, generally, that all conventional devices compromise on some aspect of optical performance for the near power. Consequently, all of these devices suffer some form of visual performance reduction, as will be discussed further. Only those techniques that can deliver continuously variable power from distance to near precisely when needed truly restore the accommodative ability of the prepresbyopic eyes. These techniques include a few surgical techniques currently under development and will be discussed in later sections.

Table 41-1
Presbyopia Correction Devices and Techniques

Change in Power effected by	**Discrete Power Change:** Disadvantage of dead spots between powers	**Continuous Power Change:** Replicates accommodative system
Division across field of view: Disadvantage of restricted field of view	Conventional bifocal, trifocal, multifocal spectacles	Progressive aspheric spectacle lenses (PAL)
Division across aperture stop: Disadvantage of contrast-related problems (eg, ghosting, halos)	Simultaneous vision bifocal contact lenses, IOLs, PRK, LASIK, LTK, etc. Diffractive contact lenses and IOLs	Aspheric ("progressive") contact lenses, IOLs, PRK, LASIK, LTK, etc.
Division between eyes: Disadvantage of binocular functions (eg, stereopsis)	Monovision	
Change in power: Just in time as required, replicates accommodative system	Reading glasses Alternating viewing (translating) bifocal contact lenses	Accommodating and "pseudoaccommodating" IOLs Lens refilling: Phaco-Ersatz, intracapsular "balloons" Phacomodulation Scleral expansion surgery (controversial)

Presbyopia correction devices and technology may be loosely categorized according to how they bring about a change in power during reading, and whether that power change is discrete or continuously variable. Devices and techniques that sacrifice field of view, aperture stop, or binocularity (top three rows) inherently introduce some form of visual performance reduction, while those that provide only discrete power changes (middle column) do not restore the continuously focusing capability of the natural accommodative system.

Spectacles and Contact Lenses

The most basic technique to correct (or perhaps more appropriately "relieve") presbyopia is the wear of simple reading glasses or bi- or multifocal spectacles.[16] While simple and inexpensive, these optical devices possess only discrete power steps. There are distances at which the eye cannot achieve sharp focus—the optical "dead spots"—resulting in blurred vision at certain viewing distances. Limited options exist for continuously variable focusing. Progressive aspheric spectacle lenses (PALs) overcome some of the limitations of the discretely powered devices and have taken over as the primary means for correcting presbyopia. However, these types of spectacles sacrifice the field of view in order to provide continuous power, while their complex optical surfaces necessarily introduce significant distortion and other aberrations. Clinically, these disadvantages are tolerated by the majority of wearers, as evidenced by the popularity of this mode of correction. However, they fall short of the full field of view, continuously variable system of natural accommodation.

Contact lens options available for correction of presbyopia include the simultaneous vision and the alternating vision bifocal/multifocals and can be either soft or rigid gas permeable (RGP).[17] The most common of these are the simultaneous vision soft contact lenses, of which over five individual models and types are currently available around the world. Simultaneous vision contact lenses (and IOLs, discussed later in this chapter) divide their optic zone into a near and a distance focusing portion. Typically, these portions consist of a circular central optic zone and an annular peripheral optic zone (termed "concentric" bifocals) although other configurations have been attempted. In such an arrangement, light from both the distance and the near visual object are admitted simultaneously to the eye (Figure 41-3). The result is a superimposition of a blurred distance (or near) image over a sharp near (or distance) image that produces visual symptoms relating to contrast loss as well as ghosting and halos.[18,19] A variation on the concentric simultaneous vision contact lens are designs that make use of diffractive optics to provide a near and distance image simultaneously, and with similar visual outcome.

An alternative exists to the simultaneous vision bifocal contact lenses that could potentially offer good field of view at full aperture with near power and only when required. This is the alternating vision, or "translating," bifocal modality. In these types of contact lenses, the optic zones are situated such that only the distance optic zone lies substantially over the pupil during distance gaze. During near viewing, when the wearer's gaze tends to be depressed, the lens is translated upwards due to its interaction with the eyelids. This puts the near optic zone in position directly over the pupil. Due to the alternating nature of this design approach, translating bifocals can potentially offer excellent vision at both distance and near.[20] However, with one exception*, all such types currently available are RGP contact lenses, which suffer the problems of poor initial comfort that is worsened by the need to ensure lens movement. Hence, they generally have poor acceptance rates by patients. Nevertheless, given the potential optical benefits, this modality merits further investigation and development.

Bifocal and aspheric (progressive) contact lenses are generally more difficult to fit than standard contact lenses. For reason of simplicity, among other advantages, the majority of contact lens fittings for presbyopes are currently achieved with the monovision principle, in which one eye of the patient is corrected for far vision and the other eye is corrected for near vision.[21,22] Not all patients tolerate monovision corrections, and there are a number of adverse visual effects,[23] including a potential deficit in binocular function[24] and a significant degradation of visual performance at night or under scotopic conditions. The relative acceptability and clinical success of this modality is not so much an indication of their acceptable performance as it is a reflection of the poor performance of current forms of bifocal and aspheric contact lenses.

Yet, from the point of view of super vision, contact lenses do have potential advantages for the presbyope. They remain relatively concentric with the axis of the eye, providing the possibility of optimized, aberration-corrected designs at all directions of gaze, while offering the benefits of simple replacement or change in design/prescription that is unlike many surgical approaches, as they are irreversible. Some implementation issues have been studied, demonstrating that wavefront aberration-corrected or controlled contact lenses can return useful visual benefits.[25] With the availability of sophisticated lens design software and multi-axis, numerically controlled contact lens lathes that can produce nonaxisymmetric designs, we should expect further developments in the area of aberration optimized multifocal contact lenses.

In summary of the above discussion, while the near focus that is required for reading can be achieved optically with bifocal spectacles or monovision contact lenses, these methods do not truly restore the accommodative function of the eye.

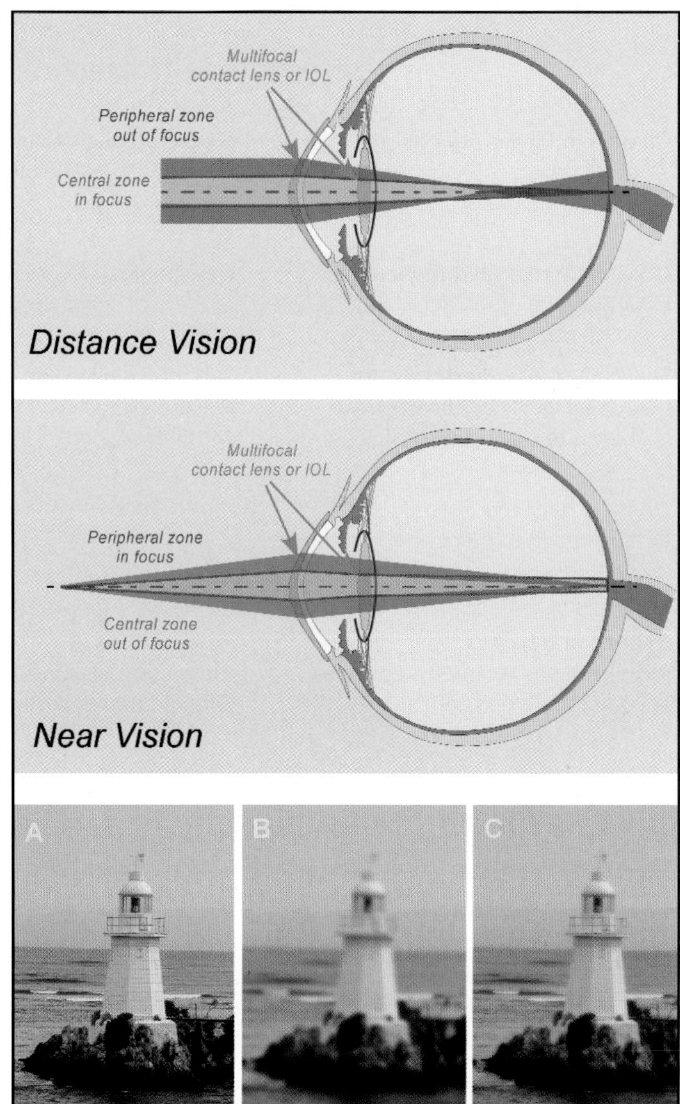

Figure 41-3. The principle of presbyopia correction using a simultaneous vision-type multifocal contact lens or multifocal IOL. *Top*: distance vision; *center*: near vision; *bottom*: simulated views of a distant object as seen clearly through the peripheral/annular distance vision zone (A), out of focus through the central near vision zone (B), and the resulting blurred retinal image (C).

Multifocal and Accommodating IOLs

Conventional IOLs implanted following cataract surgery are designed to provide clear distance vision. Patients implanted with these traditional IOLs must wear corrective glasses for near vision. Several multifocal IOLs designed to provide a clear image at both near and far distance are currently available on the market. In general, multifocal IOLs are designed with a central optical zone of lowest power that provides clear distance vision, surrounded by two or more concentric zones of higher optical power that allow near distance vision (see Figure 41-3). Other designs use diffractive surfaces to provide multifocality.

In general, multifocal IOLs are designed with a central optical zone of lowest power that provides clear distance vision, surrounded by two or more concentric zones of higher optical power that allow near distance vision.

Similar to the simultaneous vision bifocal contact lenses, the retinal image produced by multifocal IOLs is the superposition of the individual images produced by each of the optical zones. In principle, these implants can be tolerated as long as the patient can suppress the unwanted image. A number of clinical studies have shown that multifocal IOLs provide a significant improvement of near vision acuity when compared to conventional IOLs. However, patients with multifocal IOLs generally have lower contrast sensitivity and often report ghosting and halos, especially during scotopic conditions.[26-29]

*At the time of publication, a soft contact lens translating bifocal was recently introduced. Early clinical experience suggested good visual performance at distance and near, but reduced comfort was reported by wearers. Given the customizable design of this lens, we could anticipate improvements in comfort and overall performance in subsequent releases.

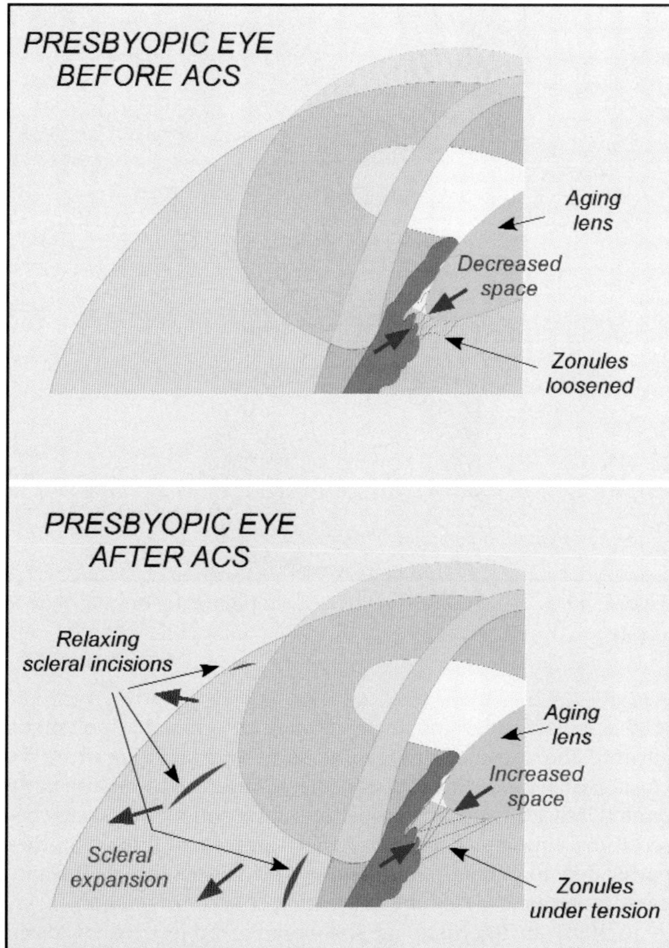

Figure 41-4. The theory and principle of ACS.

A number of clinical studies have shown that multifocal IOLs provide a significant improvement of near vision acuity when compared to conventional IOLs. However, patients with multifocal IOLs generally have lower contrast sensitivity, and often report ghosting and halos, especially during scotopic conditions.[26-29]

The current trend in the search for a technique to correct presbyopia is the design of accommodating IOLs. A number of ingenious, and sometimes complex, accommodating IOL designs have recently been patented or are currently under clinical investigation.[30-34] Today, the most common type of accommodating IOL is a design that provides pseudoaccommodation by translation of the implant along the optical axis of the eye. A displacement of the implant toward the anterior chamber increases the total power of the cornea-IOL system and simulates the increase of power provided by accommodation in the normal eye. Several implants have been designed according to this principle, using mechanical forces of the ciliary muscle, capsule, vitreous, or even magnets to displace the implant.

These implants generally provide a low amplitude of accommodation, typically 1.00 to 2.00 D, and their long-term safety and efficacy remains to be demonstrated.

Presbyopic Laser Corneal Surgery (PRK, LASIK, LTK)

A number of modified ablation algorithms have been developed and tested for the combined correction of myopia or hyperopia and presbyopia.[35-37] These include bi- or multifocal ablation patterns that mimic the optical design of spectacles, contact lenses, or IOLs, or even decentered ablations. These treatments are generally more complex to deliver than traditional PRK or LASIK treatment and their safety and efficacy remains to be demonstrated. Most commonly, laser correction of presbyopia is achieved by using traditional treatment algorithms of PRK, LASIK, or laser thermokeratoplasty (LTK), but with a monovision prescription.[35] Naturally, visual outcome and patient satisfaction are comparable to what is obtained with traditional monovision correction using contact lenses.

Phacomodulation

Recently Myers, Krueger, and colleagues[38,39] proposed an original concept for the correction of presbyopia using lasers. They suggested that photodisruption of the crystalline lens with a Q-switched Nd:YAG laser can either reduce the lens volume (photophako reduction [PPR]) or soften the lens nucleus (photophako modulation [PPM]). Preliminary experimental studies of PPM on cadaver eyes demonstrated that application of laser pulses at energies above the threshold for cavitation bubble formation in an annular pattern increased the elasticity of lenses from old donors. Additional studies are needed to confirm these findings and to demonstrate the feasibility of these procedures.

Scleral Expansion Surgery

In the early 1990s, Thornton proposed anterior ciliary sclerotomy (ACS) as a procedure to reverse presbyopia.[40] ACS relies on the hypothesis that accommodation is caused by a forward movement of the lens when the ciliary muscle contracts, instead of a change in lens shape. According to this theory, presbyopia results from continuous lens growth with age, rather than lens hardening. Due to lens growth, the space between the lens and ciliary body progressively decreases with age, which loosens zonular tension. In the presbyopic eye, the decrease in zonular tension is such that ciliary muscle contraction and relaxation can no longer stretch the zonules and produce anterior lens displacement (Figure 41-4).

ACS is a purely incisional technique. A series of equally-spaced radial incisions are performed in the sclera near the limbus to increase the circumference of the globe at the level of the ciliary body. Due to expansion of the globe, the space between the ciliary body and lens increases, and normal zonular tension and ciliary body action is restored (see Figure 41-4). ACS has been used as a treatment for both presbyopia and glaucoma.[41]

According to some reports, the procedure provides 2 to 3 D of accommodation postoperatively, but the effect is temporary due to wound closure and loss of the expansion effect, with a return to the initial state 4 to 8 months after surgery. To avoid regression, the procedure has been modified to include insertion of silicone implants (ie, scleral expansion plugs, or SEPs) to avoid wound closure.[41] The effectiveness of the modified ACS procedure in maintaining globe expansion and the measured accommodative effect remains to be demonstrated.

In recent years, Schachar introduced and developed another concept for scleral expansion surgery (ie, surgical reversal of presbyopia, or SRP) that relies on his controversial (and disputed) theory of accommodation.[42] The underlying hypothesis of SRP is the

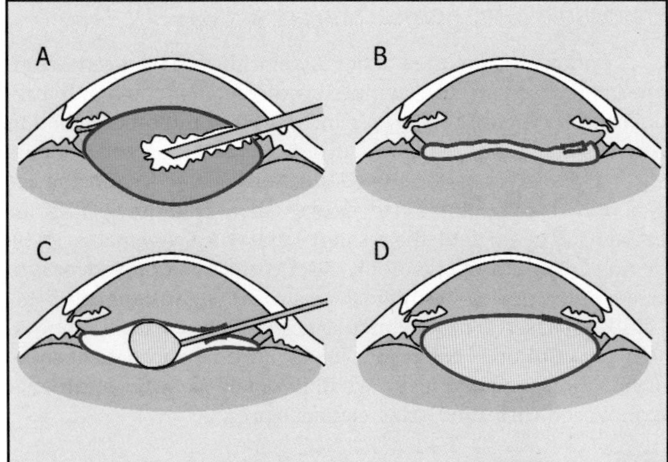

Figure 41-5. The key steps for restoring accommodative function to the crystalline lens using the surgical technique of phaco-ersatz include the extraction of the nucleus and cortex through a small hole (minicapsulorrhexis) in the capsule while leaving the capsule intact.

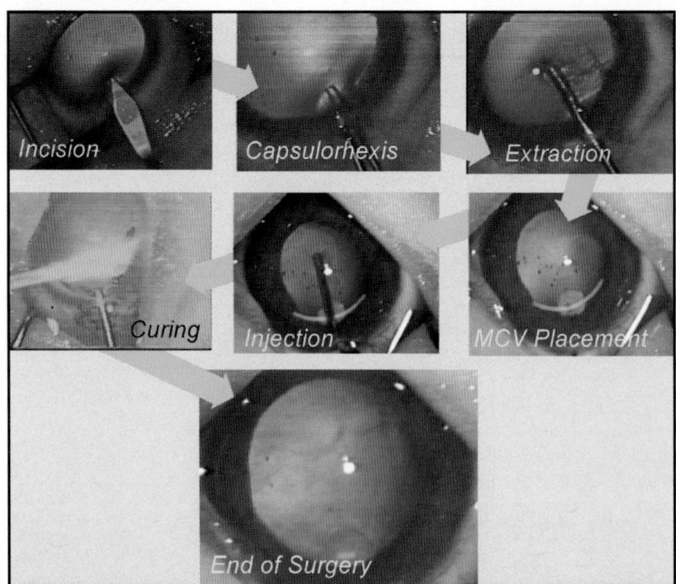

Figure 41-6. The current preferred implementation of phaco-ersatz.

same as for ACS: an increase in space between the ciliary body and lens will restore sufficient accommodation range for near vision. In the current version of this procedure, the globe is expanded at the level of the ciliary body by inserting four polymethyl methacrylate (PMMA) implants (ie, scleral expansion bands, or SEBs) in the sclera near the limbus. According to some undocumented or unreviewed reports, the procedure is capable of restoring 3.00 D to 8.00 D of accommodation.[43,44] The validity of these outcomes has been contested[45] and contradicted by several other clinical studies that found no gain in accommodation.[46-48]

Lens Refilling: Phaco-Ersatz

Given our understanding of the mechanism of accommodation and the origin of presbyopia, it seems appropriate that a most direct strategy for restoring accommodation in presbyopia is to restore the elasticity of the crystalline lens. Early work by Kessler[49] and Agarwal and colleagues[50] suggested the feasibility of removing the lens contents and refilling the empty capsule with an optically similar substance. Since then, there have been several attempts made to restore accommodation using this approach.

The most notable series of work is from the group led by Nishi, who fabricated an injectable balloon that could be inserted into the crystalline lens capsule following extraction of the nucleus and cortex.[51,52] This balloon is then filled with a viscous material such as silicone oil. Using a rabbit model, Nishi and colleagues demonstrated that an average of 1.1 D of refractive accommodation can be observed after pilocarpine injection.[51] Another study using primates resulted in an even greater result: accommodation amplitude ranging from 1 D to 4.50 D.[52] However, due to problems associated with biocompatibility and the leakage of silicone oil into the anterior chamber, the studies using this approach have been discontinued. Nevertheless, Nishi's studies demonstrated the relative merits of restoring accommodation by restoring the mechanical properties of the crystalline lens.

A group led by Jean-Marie Parel introduced the surgical technique of phaco-ersatz in 1979.[53,54] Phaco-ersatz is a direct lens refilling procedure that involves removal of the lens material (ie, nucleus and cortex) through a small opening in the capsule (a minicapsulorrhexis) and then injection of a suitable polymeric gel into the capsule through the same opening (Figure 41-5). During this procedure the capsule, zonules, and ciliary body remain intact. Ideally, the properties of the polymeric gel are chosen to be equivalent to that of the young natural lens. Studies performed in young[53] and senile[54] primates with a siloxane-based polymer showed the restoration of accommodation.

In 1997, an international collaborative project led by Brien Holden's group at the Cooperative Research Centre for Eye Research and Technology (CRCERT) in Sydney and by Jean-Marie Parel's group at Bascom Palmer Eye Institute's Ophthalmic Biophysics Center in Miami was established to further develop a surgical realization of the phaco-ersatz technique. This project led to the development of a refined surgical approach (Figure 41-6), and currently addresses some of the remaining issues of the phaco-ersatz procedure, including the development of a material with the required optical and mechanical characteristics, prevention of secondary cataract, and intraoperative control of the shape of the phaco-ersatz implant.

Wavefront-Guided Customized Presbyopia Correction

In their current state, none of the clinical techniques for the correction of presbyopia is of sufficient predictability or flexibility to be suitable for wavefront-guided customization. Of the techniques discussed in this chapter, most likely only diffractive lenses, laser corneal reshaping, and lens refilling may eventually allow wavefront-guided correction of presbyopia with simultaneous correction of ametropia and higher-order aberrations.

Wavefront-Guided Presbyopic Laser Corneal Surgery

In theory, wavefront-guided treatment algorithms could be calculated for presbyopic LASIK or PRK. For instance, in monovision treatments, the ablation pattern for each eye could be optimized based on wavefront measurements. Wavefront analysis could perhaps also help reduce some of the common undesired

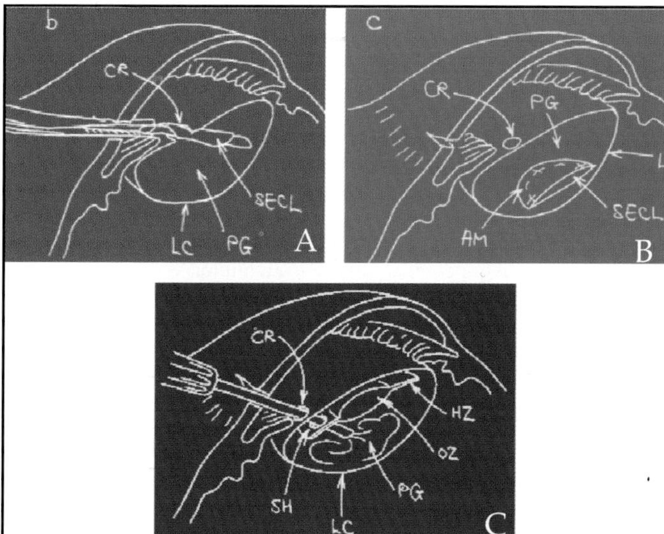

Figure 41-7. Addition of a supplemental endocapsular lens (SECL) during phaco-ersatz surgery for simultaneous correction of presbyopia, ametropia, and higher-order aberrations. (A) Insertion of the SECL. (B) The SECL in place before polymer injection. (C) Injection of the polymer.

visual effects of multifocal ablations. In the end, however, optical effects inherent to multifocality (reduced contrast) and monovision (binocular effects) will limit potential improvements.

Wavefront-Guided Diffractive Lens Design

Within practical limits, diffractive lenses can be designed to produce any desired type of monofocal or multifocal aberration pattern in the image plane. In theory, diffractive contact lenses or IOLs could therefore be patient customized using ocular wavefront aberrometry. However, the feasibility of tailored diffractive lenses will eventually be determined by the cost of fabrication of custom diffractive optics and by the required fitting and/or positioning accuracy of the contact lens or implant. Many implementation issues need to be resolved. For example, especially in the case of contact lenses but also in IOLs, biofouling over time of the diffractive echellettes that provide the diffractive performance will need to be either eliminated or compensated. In addition, even if customized, diffractive optics will not restore true dynamic accommodation.

Wavefront-Guided Lens Refilling

The ultimate goal of the phaco-ersatz procedure is not only to restore the normal opto-mechanical response of the lens during accommodation in the presbyopic eye, but also to optimize the visual outcome of the procedure, including ametropia correction and control of ocular aberrations.[55]

In principle, direct lens refilling is an adjustable procedure. Early studies by Parel and colleagues[56] have already demonstrated that the shape of the implant can be modulated by controlling the injected volume of polymer. The refractive index of the lens refilling material can also be modulated, within limits, to adjust the optical power of the implant. A number of materials with different refractive indices could thus be made available to the surgeon to adjust postoperative refraction. At least in theory, a phaco-ersatz procedure with preoperative selection of the refractive index and intraoperative wavefront-guided volume control could be envisioned. Such a procedure would provide the adjustability required to control postoperative ametropia and aberrations. However, optical modeling studies[55] have shown that the precision on volume or refractive index required to control ametropia during phaco-ersatz is not achievable in practice.

The concept of an adjustable supplemental endocapsular lens (SECL) has been introduced to address this issue. The SECL would be a thin implant that can be placed in the capsular bag to adjust the refractive power and aberrations of the lens refilling implant. Preliminary animal experiments (in unpublished reports) have demonstrated the feasibility of phaco-ersatz surgery with addition of a SECL (Figure 41-7). Another feasible, although arguably less desirable, option to adjust the outcome of phaco-ersatz surgery would be wavefront-guided laser corneal reshaping to correct residual ametropia and wavefront aberrations.

Conclusions

The correction of presbyopia is considered to be "the last frontier of refractive surgery."[57] The ideal technique for presbyopia correction is one that would restore the accommodation function of the normal, young eye. Most of the techniques available today do not truly correct presbyopia, but attempt to compensate for the loss of accommodation by using monovision or multifocal approaches, or pseudoaccommodation. The current trend is the development of accommodating IOLs, as well as lens refilling or lens modifying procedures.

Since the current technologies for correction of presbyopia are still in their infancy, it appears unlikely that techniques to restore accommodation will be ready for a customized wavefront-guided approach before 2010. If successfully developed at that time, given the demographics of presbyopia, wavefront-guided presbyopia correction could well become the main driving force of wavefront technology.

References

1. Glasser A, Kaufmann PL. The mechanism of accommodation in primates. *Ophthalmology.* 1999;106:863-872.
2. Helmholtz von HH. Handbuch der Physiologishen Optik (1909). In: Southall JPC (Translator). *Helmholtz's treatise on physiological optics.* New York: Dover; 1962:143-172.
3. Coleman DJ. Unified model for accommodative mechanism. *Am J Ophthalmol.* 1970;69:1063-1079.
4. Coleman DJ. On the hydraulic suspension theory of accommodation. *Trans Am Soc Ophthalmol.* 1986;84: 846-868.
5. Coleman DJ, Fish SK. Presbyopia, accommodation and the mature catenary. *Ophthalmology.* 2001;108:1544-1551.
6. Schachar RA, Cudmore DP, Black TD. Experimental support for Schachar's hypothesis on accommodation. *Ann Ophthalmol.* 1993; 25:404-409.
7. Atchison DA. Review of accommodation and presbyopia. *Ophthalmic Physiol Opt.* 1995;15:255-272.
8. Glasser A, Campbell MCW. Presbyopia and the optical changes in the human crystalline lens with age. *Vision Res.* 1998;38:209-229.
9. Duke-Elder S, Abrams D. Ophthalmic optics and refraction. In: *System of Ophthalmology.* Vol 5. St Louis, Mo: CV Mosby Company; 1970:180-182.
10. Smith G, Atchison DA, Pierscionek BK. Modeling the power of the aging human eye. *J Optic Soc Am.* 1992;9:2111-2117.

11. Koretz JF, Cook CA, Kaufman PL. Aging of the human lens: changes in lens shape upon accommodation and with accommodative loss. *J Opt Soc Am A*. 2002;19:144-151.
12. Moffat BA, Atchison DA, Pope JM. Explanation of the lens paradox. *Optom Vis Sci*. 2002;79:148-150.
13. Duane A. Normal values of the accommodation at all ages. *Tr Ophthalmol AMA*. 1912;383.
14. Borish IM. *Clinical refraction*. 3rd ed. Chicago, Ill: The Professional Press; 1949:171.
15. US Census Bureau. International Program Center, Population Division (2000). International Database (IDB) Version 2000/05.
16. Barker FM. The effectiveness of multifocal correction upon presbyopic near and intermediate visual resolution performance. *Journal of the American Optometric Association*. 1984;55:753-757.
17. Woods C, Ruston D, Hough T, Efron N. Clinical performance of an innovative back surface multifocal contact lens in correcting presbyopia. *The CLAO Journal*. 1999;25:176-181.
18. Back A, Holden B, Hine NA. Correction of presbyopia with contact lenses: comparative success rates with three systems. *Optom Vis Sci*. 1989;66:518-525.
19. Back A, Grant T, Hine N. Comparative visual performance of three contact lens corrections. *Optom Vis Sci*. 1992;69:474-480.
20. Hansen DW. Problem solving for RGP alternating multifocal lenses. *Optometry Today*. 1999;Feb 12:36-38.
21. Gauthier CA, Holden BA, Grant T, Chong MS. Interest of presbyopes in contact lens correction and their success with monovision. *Optom Vis Sci*. 1992;69:858-862.
22. Erickson P, McGill EC. Role of visual acuity, stereoacuity, and ocular dominance in monovision patient success. *Optom Vis Sci*. 1992;69:761-764.
23. Josephson JE, Erickson P, Back A, Holden BA, Harris M, Tomlinson A, Caffrey BE, Finnemore V, Silbert J. Monovision. *Journal of the American Optometric Association*. 1990;61:820-826.
24. Harris M, Sheedy J, Gan C. Vision and task performance with monovision and bifocal contact lenses. *Optom Vis Sci*. 1992;69:609-614.
25. Guirao A, Williams DR, Cox IG. Effect of rotation and translation on the expected benefit of an ideal method to correct the eye's higher-order aberrations. *J Opt Soc Am A*. 2001;18:1003-1015.
26. Goes F. Personal results with the 3M diffractive multifocal intraocular lens. *J Cataract Refract Surg*. 1991;17:577-582.
27. Gimbel HV, Snaders DR, Gold Ranaan M. Visual and refractive results of multifocal intraocular lenses. *Ophthalmology*. 1991;98:881-888.
28. Holladay JT, van Dijk H, Lang A, et al. Optical performance of multifocal intraocular lenses. *J Cataract Refract Surg*. 1990;16:413-422.
29. Hunold W, Auffarth G, Wesendahl T, Mehdorn E, Kuck G. Pseudoakkommodation diffraktiver multifokallinsen und monofokallinsen. *Klinische Monatsblatter der Augenheilkunde*. 1993;202:19-23.
30. Küchle M, Langenbucher A, Gusek-Schneider GC, Seitz B, Hanna KD. Erste ergebnisse der implantation einer neuen, potenziell akkommodierbaren hinterkammer linse—eine prospektive sicherheitsstudie. *Klinische Monatsblatter der Augenheilkunde*. 2001;218:603-608.
31. Hara T, Hara T, Yasuda A, Yamada Y. Accommodative intraocular lens with spring action. Part 1: design and placement in an excised animal eye. *Ophthalmic Surgery*. 1990;21:128-133.
32. Cumming JS, Slade SG, Chayet A, AT45 Study Group. Clinical evaluation of the model AT-45 silicone accommodating intraocular lens: results of feasibility and the initial phase of a Food and Drug Administration clinical trial. *Ophthalmology*. 2001;108:2005-2009.
33. Skottun BC. Encapsulated accommodating intraocular lens. US Patent No. 6,117,171; 2000.
34. Preussner PR, Wahl J, Gerl R, Kreiner C, Serester A. Akkommodatives linsenimplantat. *Der Ophthalmologe*. 2001;98:97-102.
35. Epstein D, Vinciguerra P, Frueh BE. Correction of presbyopia with the excimer laser. *Int Ophthalmol Clin*. 2001;41:103-111.
36. Anschutz T. Laser correction of hyperopia and presbyopia. *Int Ophthalmol Clin*. 1994;34:107-137.
37. Bauerberg JM. Centered versus inferior off-center ablation to correct hyperopia and presbyopia. *J Refract Surg*. 1999;15:66-69.
38. Krueger RR, Sun XK, Stroh J, Myers M. Experimental increase in accommodative potential after Neodymium:Yttrium-Aluminum-Garnet laser photodisruption of paired cadaver lenses. *Ophthalmology*. 2001;108:2122-2129.
39. Myers RI, Krueger RR. Novel approaches to correction of presbyopia with laser modification of the crystalline lens. *Journal of Refractive Surgery* 1998;14:136-139.
40. Thornton SP. Anterior ciliary sclerotomy (ACS): a procedure to reverse presbyopia. In: Sher N, ed. *Surgery for Hyperopia and Presbyopia*. Baltimore, Md: Williams and Wilkins; 1997:33-36.
41. Fukasaku H. Marron JA. Anterior ciliary sclerotomy with silicone expansion plug implantation: effect on presbyopia and intraocular pressure. *Int Ophthalmol Clin*. 2001;41:133-141.
42. Schachar RA. The correction of presbyopia. *Int Ophthalmol Clin*. 2001;41:53-70.
43. Cross W. Theory behind surgical correction of presbyopia. *Ophthalmol Clin North Am*. 2001;14:315-333.
44. Marmer RH. The surgical reversal of presbyopia: a new procedure to restore accommodation. *Int Ophthalmol Clin*. 2001;41:123-132
45. Kaufman PL. Scleral expansion surgery for presbyopia (letter). *Ophthalmology*. 2001;108:2161-2162.
46. Matthews S. Scleral expansion surgery does not restore accommodation in human presbyopia. *Ophthalmology*. 1999;106:873-877.
47. Malecaze FJ, Gazagne CS, Tarroux MC, Gorrand JM. Scleral expansion bands for presbyopia. *Ophthalmology*. 2001;108:2165-2171.
48. Singh G, Chalfin S. A complication of scleral expansion surgery for treatment of presbyopia. *Am J Ophthalmol*. 2000;130:521-523.
49. Kessler J. Experiments in refilling the lens. *Arch Ophthal*. 1964;71:412-417.
50. Agarwal LP, Narsimhan EC, Mohan M. Experimental lens refilling. *Oriental Arch Ophthalmol*. 1967;5:205-212.
51. Nishi O, Nishi K, Mano C, Ichihara M, Honda T. Lens refilling with injectable silicone in rabbit eyes. *J Cataract Refract Surg*. 1998;24:975-982.
52. Nishi O, Nishi K. Accommodation amplitude after lens refilling with injectable silicone by sealing the capsule with a plug in primates. *Arch Ophthalmol*. 1998;116:1358-1361.
53. Haefliger E, Parel, J-M, Fantes, F, Norton EWD, Anderson DR, Forster RK, Hernandez E, Feuer WJ. Accommodation of an endocapsular silicone lens (phaco-ersatz) in the nonhuman primate. *Ophthalmology*. 1987;94:471-477.
54. Haefliger E, Parel JM. Accommodation of an endocapsular silicone lens (phaco-ersatz) in the aging rhesus monkey. *J Refract Corneal Surg*. 1994;10:550-555.
55. Ho A, Erickson P, Pham T, Manns F, Parel J. Theoretical analysis of accommodation amplitude and ametropia correction by varying refractive index in phaco-ersatz. *Optom Vis Sci*. 2001;78:405-410.
56. Parel J-M, Treffers WF, Gelender H, Norton EWD. Phaco-ersatz: cataract surgery designed to preserve accommodation. *Graefes Arch Clin Exp Ophthalmol*. 1986;224:165-173.
57. Waring GO. Presbyopia and accommodative intraocular lenses—the next frontier in refractive surgery? *Refractive and Corneal Surgery*. 1992;8:421-423.

Section VI

The Future of Customization

Chapter 42

The Future of Customization

Ronald R. Krueger, MD, MSE; Scott M. MacRae, MD; and Raymond A. Applegate, OD, PhD

In looking to the future, a great challenge exists: a challenge to forecast a realistic view of how our field may change with wavefront technology. A challenge to be bold and pursue innovative concepts beyond the status quo. Sometimes in dreaming big dreams, one can actually change the future by being actively involved in the process of innovation. Yet, innovation requires a certain aspect of realism, which is predicated on the stepping stones of science. We look to the future of customization through the prism of science and technology with cautious optimism. The quest for super vision is not about visual perfection; it is accepting the challenge of continuously improving the technologies that optimize our patient's vision. Building blocks we have currently established may allow us to step into new areas as we move into the future.

> Sometimes in dreaming big dreams, one can actually change the future by being actively involved in the process of innovation.

The Quest for Super Vision

Beside the stepping stones of science required for us to move from our first book, *Customized Corneal Ablation*, to the second book, *Wavefront Customized Visual Correction*, one resounding theme ties both books together: the quest for super vision. As our field continues to advance, so will our concept and knowledge of customization. Even though the various customized titles that we use in subsequent editions of this book will likely change, the subtitle—"The Quest for Super Vision"—will remain the same.

Customization will continue to play a central role in this quest. In order to achieve super vision, which is defined as "exceptionally good quality of vision beyond that represented by the normal population," we will need to understand the visual needs, perceptions, and expectations of the individual patient within that normal population. Hence, customization takes on the goal to meet specific needs of an individual patient, as outlined in Chapter 1: functional vs anatomical. The functional needs of the patient include outcomes based on age, occupational vs recreational needs, and psychological acceptance of the current correction and resulting residual optical defects. Anatomical needs include corneal thickness limitations, ocular surface issues, pupil size, corneal curvature's influence on ablation efficiency, microkeratome safety, and anterior chamber depth when considering implants. Although these are rather specific, customization in the quest of super vision could also take on a more general optical and neural focus, as can be seen in the following sections.

The Quest for Super Vision in Diagnostics

Optical Limitations of Super Vision

In meeting all of the functional needs noted above, we will certainly encounter limitations. Only by understanding these limitations and trade-off and incorporating them into our custom designs will we truly optimize our wave aberration corrections. For example, did the human optical system evolve to have aberrations to provide biological advantages? That is, do we have optical systems optimized for modulation transfer in specific bands of spatial frequencies important to survival at the expense of others? Do we have optical aberrations like mild amounts of positive spherical aberration to increase the range of functional vision (depth of field) at the sacrifice of contrast at high frequencies? Will we be creating new classes of amblyopia by improving retinal image quality? Will aliasing be a problem? How big a role do individual differences play in designing optimized optical corrections?

Moving these and other questions aside for the moment, an accurate measurement and diagnostic representation of the wave aberration needs to be first obtained before an optical design can be generated. Further, it is crucial that wave aberration metrics be developed that can predict reliably the likely visual function resulting from treatment.[1] Current wavefront devices and aberrometers can measure wave aberration to the sixth and eighth Zernike order and higher (depending on the device). However, errors in capturing, sampling, and wave aberration representation, as well as errors intrinsic with wavefront variability over time and in differing environments, make the challenge of wavefront customization a matter of achieving a proper wavefront measurement to be used in designing an optimal correction.

To this end, the future of wavefront customization will employ better ways of measuring and expressing the whole eye wave aberration as well as the corneal wave aberration and surface shapes. It is likely that these calculations will become increasingly invisible to the clinician by becoming internal to wave aberration correction system. Expressing a complex wave aberration in terms of the Zernike expansion works well for normal eyes where the

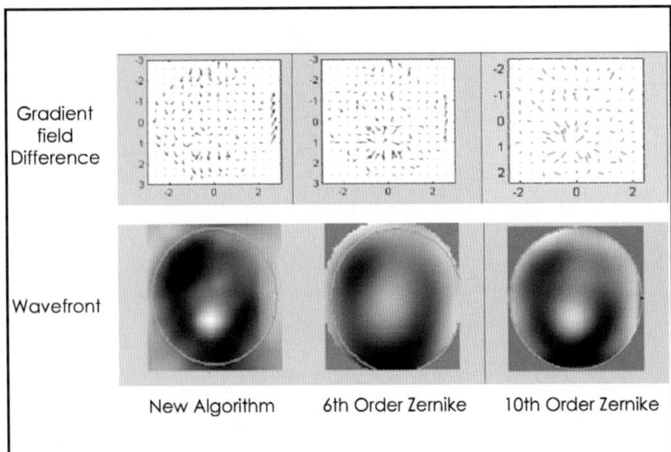

Figure 42-1. Complex wavefront shape of a highly aberrated eye expressed in sixth- and 10th-order Zernike modes as well as in a new reconstruction algorithm developed by VISX. The location of centroids back calculated from these representations and compared with the actual centroids are seen in the gradient field difference maps. These demonstrate the relative failures of Zernike expansion in a complex eye and improvements achieved with zonal reconstruction. (Courtesy of Doug Koch, MD.)

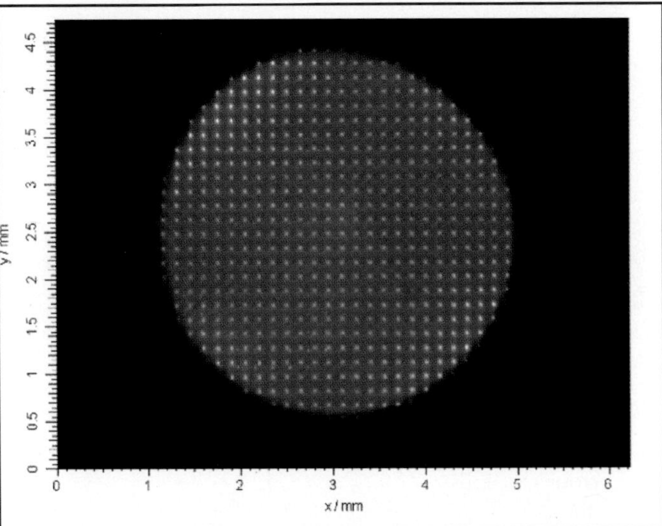

Figure 42-2. High density centroid pattern (600 lenslets in 3.50 mm pupil area) in an experimental Shack-Hartmann device, which also has multiple samplings over time (12 captures per second) and adaptive correction using a deformable mirror. (Courtesy of Michael Mrochen, PhD.)

wave aberration is well represented by the underlying Zernike modes. In fact, there is a distinct advantage to using a smoothing function to reduce noise in the fundamental data from erroneously influencing the representation of the wave aberration.

However, in cases where the wave aberration is particularly complex, and the underlying modes of the expansion do not represent the actual small details in the wave aberration, then a Zernike approach that is limited in the available modes to fit the error can, and will, fail to properly represent the wave aberration. Such a failure can be seen in Figure 42-1, where a complex wavefront shape is expressed in sixth- and 10th-order Zernike modes and the location of the centroids back calculated from these two Zernike representations reveal significant differences between the actual data samples and its Zernike representation by the gradient field difference maps. This is in contrast to alternative, non-Zernike algorithms proposed by VISX and others, also seen in this figure. To minimize adverse consequences of using a Zernike representation that does not accurately reflect the underlying measurement, we anticipate the inclusion of "fit error" limits in measurement devices to warn the user when the underlying data set is not being well-represented by the Zernike, or for that matter any selected basis, function expansion.

In clinically abnormal eyes (eg, penetrating keratoplasty, keratoconus, bad refractive surgery outcomes), the fit error can be high. To solve this potential problem, several commercial devices (VISX and Wavefront Sciences, Albuquerque, NM) are beginning to address these fitting errors using zonal reconstruction. Zonal reconstruction, as well as other methods, can provide an accurate representation of the underlying data set. The liability is that one has to believe that each point in the underlying data set accurately represents the actual wave aberration. Typically, as complexity of the measurement increases, so does the noise in the measurement. Said differently, one has to be careful to prevent measurement noise from overly influencing the wave aberration representation. A strategy to minimize noise in the underlying data prior to a zonal reconstruction is to take multiple measurements and determine an average location for each data point (eg, individual centroids in Shack-Hartmann wavefront sensing).

Optimizing our ability to measure the wavefront error at any one moment in time is only a first step. Variability of the ocular tear film and accommodation cause ocular wave aberration to vary from one measurement to the next, suggesting that some form of temporal averaging will likely be important in determining the ideal wave aberration correction. Consequently, future research efforts will likely seek to develop an even more sophisticated clinical aberrometer with a great density of lenslets; multiple samplings over time; adaptive optic capabilities for high resolution, dynamic sampling with adaptive correction to verify the accuracy of wavefront representation; and potential refractive surgical outcome. Figure 42-2 demonstrates the centroid pattern of an experimental Shack-Hartmann device with 600 lenslets within a 3.50 mm pupil that captures 12 times per second, and has a deformable mirror for adaptive correction to demonstrate optimal visual performance in real time.

> Future research efforts will likely seek to develop an even more sophisticated clinical aberrometer with a great density of lenslets, multiple samplings over time, and adaptive optic capabilities.

Another limitation in the representation of optical aberrations is whether we target a perfectly flat wavefront shape for high fidelity or a compensated, adjusted shape to enhance the dynamic range of vision in presbyopic patients. Although this limitation is not fundamental to adequate wavefront measurement and representation, it does impact visual correction and will certainly be involved in customization of the patients' individual optical and visual needs. As any refractive surgeon knows, there are tradeoffs to treating presbyopic patients fully for distance vision or giving them monovision. Future research may well focus scientifically on the various functional advantages and disadvantages of these and other strategies.

Neural Limitations of Super Vision

The fundamental limiting factor in the quest for super vision is dependent on the integrity and spacing of retinal photoreceptors, cortical processing of the image, and the brains plasticity in order to accept it.[2] The current limit of super vision acuity achieved under ideal optical conditions is ~20/8 based on the photoreceptor spacing. In the quest for super vision, a fundamental question that arises is that of refractive amblyopia: Will an eye that has never seen better than 20/20 be correctable to 20/8 or 20/10 if the ocular aberrations were adequately corrected and the pupil large enough to pass finer spatial detail? This question extends past the retina into the area of cortical processing. Although amblyopia has always been considered a limitation to visual rehabilitation, refractive amblyopia has been demonstrated to be age dependent and less dense when refractive errors are not excessive. The younger the patient, the more likely the eye is to recover some if not all of its processing ability.

In this regard, recent evidence from Seiler and associates has shown that multifactorial analysis in over 800 myopic eyes treated with conventional laser in-situ keratomileusis (LASIK) reveals a two-line improvement of best spectacle-corrected vision in 170 eyes being statistically associated with preoperative anisometropia of 3 diopters (D) or more seen after 1 year and preoperative astigmatism greater than 2 D, seen 2 to 3 years following surgery (personal communication, Theo Seiler, September 2003). Seeing a delayed improvement suggests that refractive amblyopia is being reversed as the brain begins to adjust to the higher fidelity retinal image. A further question of cortical adaptation that arises is whether an ideal optical (customized) correction would be acceptable to patients who have adapted to their ocular aberrations, or would they psychologically find this to be unacceptable because of a cortical inability to readapt? Like the adaptation to new glasses or a presbyopic prescription, such adaptation is patient specific. However, as with the adaptation to new glasses or a presbyopic correction, it is anticipated that if the correction provides quality vision, the patient is likely to adapt.

The Quest for Super Vision in Corneal Ablation

The current clinical proliferation of laser vision correction and customized corneal ablation demonstrates a high level of acceptance of customization in the area of corneal ablation. Besides needed improvements in the fidelity of wavefront devices, the future will likely hold further improvements in spot delivery, as well as tracking and registration of the delivery devices associated with corneal laser ablation.

LASIK vs Surface Ablation

One of the biggest questions in our field is that of LASIK vs surface ablation. Will the limitations of biomechanical predictability associated with LASIK and flap creation be adequately overcome, or will a form of surface laser ablation be adapted because of improvements and predictability in corneal wound healing? Efforts are being investigated in both areas, with the former seeking to find a level of predictability in flap induced aberrations with specific microkeratomes and flap diameter and thickness parameters.[3,4] In a recent, yet unpublished study by Krueger et al, a statistically significant shift toward hyperopia was noticed when creating a "flap only" in 12 eyes using the Moria M2 microkeratome (Moria, Antony, France), while a "flap only" using the SKBM microkeratome (Alcon Surgical, Fort Worth, Tex) showed no such shift and even larger variability in the standard deviation of the spherical term. As previously confirmed in the other studies,[3,4] this suggests that some level of predictability may be achieved with certain microkeratomes and will require larger studies and more detailed analysis of flap-induced aberrations in the future. Finally, in another unpublished study by MacRae et al, they found virtually no increase in higher order aberration when a flap was simply cut and not lifted. This, at first glance, seems not surprising, yet the finding raises the possibility that if the flap can be returned reproducibly to its native position using meticulous or more sophisticated future techniques, the low level of flap-induced, higher-order aberrations might continue to keep LASIK on the forefront of customized vision correction.

In the investigation of surface ablation, wound healing studies following photorefractive keratectomy (PRK), laser epithelial keratomileusis (LASEK), and epiLASIK are beginning to demonstrate predictable changes of cellular and biochemical markers of healing that might be better understood and even controlled with immunomodulating drugs.[5] Current clinical use of mitomycin C 0.02% in topical application following surface ablation has minimized the haze and regression effects often seen with surface ablation of high refractive correction.[6] This suggests that newer drugs might also be introduced to better regulate wound healing and refractive outcome. Future investigations into gene therapy of wound healing will likely also be pursued. Finding a gene that could be pharmacologically or interventionally turned on and off in an effort to better control the postlaser activation of keratocytes and other wound healing mediators would go a step beyond immunomodulation for wound healing to that of gene modulation. Recent advances in suppressing a proto-oncogene called C-fos in a knock-out mouse model of retinal degeneration to prevent light-induced apoptotic cell death of photoreceptors has demonstrated an exciting precedent into the role of gene therapy in treating eye disease, and suggests it may have an eventual role in corneal wound healing.[7]

Finding a gene that could be pharmacologically or interventionally turned on and off in an effort to better control the postlaser activation of keratocytes and other wound healing mediators would go a step beyond immunomodulation for wound healing to that of gene modulation.

Multifocal Ablation

In the quest for super vision, customization in an effort to correct presbyopia in addressing a patient's functional needs has also been investigated in multifocal corneal ablation. It may seem counter-intuitive to induce aberrations in order to create multifocality because of the potential loss of contrast sensitivity and quality of visual function. Yet, because of the functional needs of the patient, attempts are being made at steepening the central or inferior cornea in order to induce a level of multifocality. Previous attempts were unsuccessful, but they did not have the help of sophisticated eye trackers, corneal registration, and wavefront mapping to determine the best multifocal profile.[8,9] In the future, we will likely see wavefront mapping and adaptive optics simulation of multifocality to demonstrate to the patient how certain aberrations might expand the physiologic range of vision without significant loss of contrast and visual function. One group that is actively working in this area is the Emory

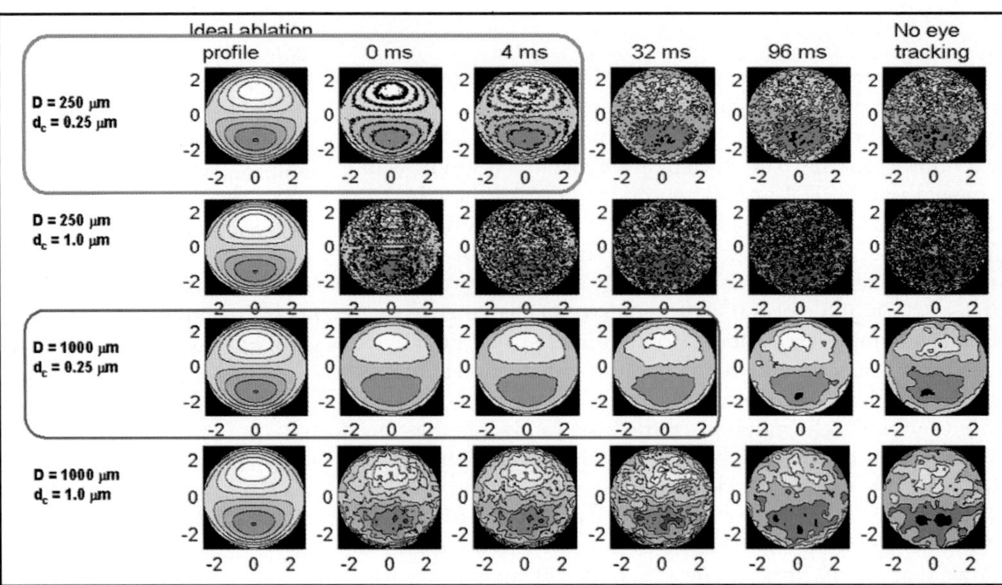

Figure 42-3. Array of computer simulated ablation profiles comparing two ablation depths and two spot diameters against five different eye tracker latencies and the referenced ideal profile. It demonstrates that tracker latencies less that 4 msec are required for adequately correcting higher-order aberrations when using a small laser spot (~0.25 mm). Using a larger laser spot (1.0 mm) is less dependent on tracker latency but is less effective in correcting detailed higher order aberrations. (Courtesy of Michael Bueeler, PhD.)

Vision Correction Group (Atlanta, Ga) using the spatially resolved refractometer (InterWave Unit) to subjectively determine the patient's aberrations in relation to the acceptability of a multifocal corneal shape (see Chapter 20).

Laser Delivery Refinements

Over the past decade, excimer laser delivery refinements have continued to move the field toward smaller spot delivery and faster eye tracking. A decade ago the excimer laser was basically a broad beam delivery system with no tracking device to provide for purely spherical and cylindrical correction of refractive errors in a rapid fashion. Although small spot scanning was introduced with eye tracking in an effort to deliver a more homogeneous beam, the advent of customized corneal ablation for the treatment of higher-order aberrations made the refinement of a smaller beam essential to achieve these corrections. With the reduction of spot size, the need for eye tracking became obvious. Over the course of this past decade, nearly every company providing laser vision correction platforms has now adapted eye tracking into its excimer laser systems. In two recently published studies, mathematically correlating the scanning spot size with the expected resolution of correction, a beam diameter of less $\leq$1.00 mm was found essential to correct up to fourth- and fifth-order aberrations.[10,11] Furthermore, correction of higher-order aberrations beyond the fifth order would require even smaller spot delivery on the order of 0.60 to 0.80 mm full width at half maximum (FWHM) using a Gaussian shape.[10] As the spot size gets smaller, the need for faster tracking gets greater. Currently, the LADAR 4000 Excimer Laser System (Alcon Surgical, Fort Worth, Tex) utilizes closed-loop laser radar tracking at a 4000 hertz (Hz) detection frequency, which essentially reduces the tracker response latency to less than to 1 millisecond (ms) (see Chapter 23). Other videocamera-based trackers sampling at a rate between 60 to 400 Hz have an intrinsic delay due to their sampling rate and method of open loop tracking, which leads to a latency of 8 to 40 milliseconds.[12]

A recent analysis by Bueeler and Mrochen at the Swiss Federal Institute of Technology in Zurich demonstrates the simulated efficacy of scanning spot correction of higher-order aberrations (vertical coma with an error magnitude of 0.60 microns [μm] at 5.70 millimeter [mm] pupil) using spot diameters of 0.25 and 1.0 mm; ablation depths of 0.25 and 1.0 μm/pulse; and tracker latencies varying from 0 ms, 4 ms, 32 ms, 96 ms, and no eye tracking. Figure 42-3 shows the array of profiles of differing spot diameter and ablation depth vs tracker latency in correcting this third-order coma. One can see in the figure that the clear contour lines of an ideal coma profile become increasingly distorted with increasing tracker latency. Even in the case of a perfect ablation without tracker latency, contour lines are distorted as a result of the overlap of a finite number of laser pulses. As one might expect, the case of a small spot diameter with a small ablation depth per pulse provides the best approximation to the ideal correction profile if all eye movements are completely compensated for by the tracker (0 ms latency). A more stable ablation, however, is achieved with a larger spot (approximately 1 mm) together with a small ablation depth per pulse, such that even long tracker latencies on the order of 32 ms and beyond might still be acceptable. However, the maximum detail in fully correcting a profile of coma is only achieved with the smaller spot diameter (250 μm) for which a very fast tracker is essential (0 to 4 milliseconds). One can assume from this data that scanning spot delivery and eye tracking will continue to be refined in the future in an effort to further enhance the predictability and outcome of customized corneal ablations.

The case of a small spot diameter with a small ablation depth per pulse provides the best approximation to the ideal correction profile if all eye movements are completely compensated for by the tracker (0 ms latency).

Most recently, Katena Products Inc (Denville, NJ) has developed a solid state excimer laser with a very small spot and rapid laser delivery rate as an alternative to the relatively larger spot and slower rate found with current excimer laser delivery systems. Although not yet coupled with customized ablation, the future may hold a greater involvement of solid state laser technology in refining our ablation profiles.

One final refinement in laser delivery has to do with proper registration and alignment of the wavefront pattern to the eye. Currently, registration is achieved translationally and rotationally with the Alcon LADARVision system. Similar registration

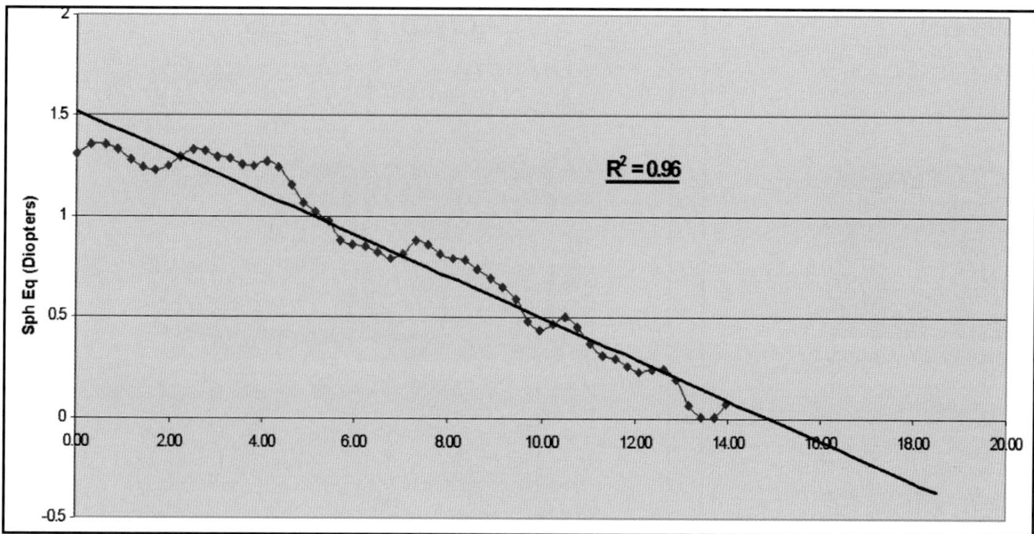

Figure 42-4. Real-time intraoperative wavefront monitoring (10 captures/second; spherical equivalent term) during a low energy laser thermal keratoplasty (LTK) procedure to correct +1.50 D of hyperopia (treatment time = 15 sec; R^2 = 0.96). (Reprinted with permission from Krueger RR, Gomez P, Kerekar S. Intraoperative wavefront monitoring during laser thermal keratoplasty. *J Refract Surg.* 2003;19(5):S602-S607.)

attempts are now being adapted internationally with the Bausch & Lomb system (Rochester, NY) (Bausch & Lomb has a 250 Hz rotational eye tracker outside the United States) as well as the new iris tracking provided by VISX (Santa Clara, Calif) and NIDEK (Gamagori, Japan). (Note: Neither are commercially available at the time of publication.) Further refinements in registration will certainly need to be pursued by the various custom ablation platforms, including those who currently provide registration. This registration when coupled with very fast tracking will provide a space-stabilized image for effective treatment of complex higher-order aberrations.

Environmental/Interface On-Line Control

Beside adequate registration, scanning spot delivery, and tracking issues, an additional technology requirement for precision customized corneal ablation is that of the environmental interface of the laser to the cornea during ablation. Environmental issues such as temperature, humidity, and physical variables of the cornea (such as pachymetry and topography) all have an impact on how accurately customized corneal ablation can be performed. Attempts at controlling temperature and humidity are already being made by many surgeons who have sophisticated environmental controls in their operating suite. But beyond this control of room temperature and humidity, the microenvironment around the cornea is the most essential for predictability of outcomes. Reproducible techniques, such as maintaining the same time of flap exposure, drying or lack of drying of the stromal bed before treatment, and plume evacuation, all have an impact on the depth of corneal ablation with each pulse. One device that helps control the microenvironment is the Mastel Clean Room (Mastel Precision Inc, Rapid City, SD), a suction ring evacuation system for the removal of particulate debris and maintenance of uniform hydration, giving a predictable ablation response. However, wide spread acceptance of this device has not been established, perhaps because of the cumbersomeness of its use with certain laser systems.

Control of anatomical factors may be of even greater importance, and new devices allowing for on-line measurement of corneal pachymetry during ablation can allow one to stop before going beyond the safety threshold of residual stroma. On-line topography control has also been proposed,[13] and this can allow one to see the changes that are being made as they occur. Nevertheless, none of these on-line devices has yet been able to adaptively modify the treatment during its analysis so as to improve the refractive outcome.

Adaptive Corneal Correction

The concept of intraoperative measurement of wavefront error goes a step beyond that of intraoperative pachymetry and topography to give real-time information about the change in the refractive and aberration profile of the eye. Although this would be virtually impossible to do with LASIK or surface laser treatment due to the scatter of the surface during ablation, it can be performed with other modalities such as laser thermal keratoplasty (LTK) (Figure 42-4).[14] Adaptive LTK has recently been proposed after success was demonstrated in the real-time measurement of wavefront error during a refractive procedure (Holmium LTK).[14] In an ideal situation, scanning spot delivery of Holmium laser energy coupled with a tracking system and registration might allow for real-time wavefront measurement and feedback to adapt the laser pulses to the dynamically changing wavefront during correction. Although adaptive LTK may be a more futuristic procedure, real-time wavefront monitoring during LTK procedures is currently being investigated and can also be useful in influencing the refractive outcome by developing thresholds beyond which treatment would stop (ie, certain value of induced astigmatism or passing a certain refractive spherical outcome). With further adaptation, perhaps even corneal ablation could be linked with real-time wavefront measurement and adaptive corneal correction. This would further refine wavefront corneal ablation by allowing the surgeon to measure the effectiveness of treatment and compensate for treatment variability in real time.

The concept of intraoperative measurement of wavefront error goes a step beyond that of intraoperative pachymetry and topography to give real-time information about the change in the refractive and aberration profile of the eye.

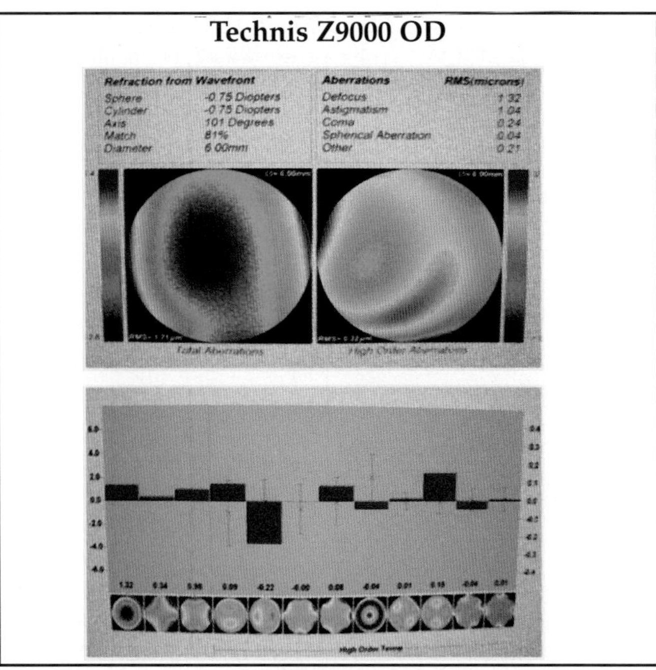

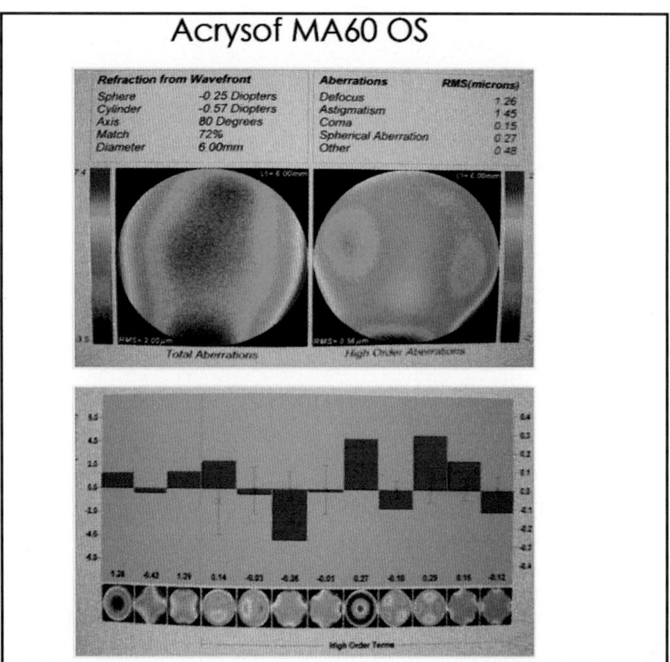

Figure 42-5. LADARWave aberration profile maps of a 3-month postoperative cataract surgery patient who received a Technis Z9000 IOL in the right eye (coma = 0.24 μm, spherical aberration = 0.04 μm) and an AcrySof MA 60 IOL (Alcon Surgical, Fort Worth, Tex) in the left eye (coma = 0.15 μm, spherical aberration = 0.27 μm). Although the Technis lens is effective in reducing postoperative spherical aberration, it often has higher values of coma due to the greater sensitivity of subtle decentration when using an aspheric prolate IOL.

The Quest for Super Vision in Refractive Implants

When considering the future of customization, one has to consider whether refractive surgery will mitigate toward refractive implants with a particular attention toward intraocular lenses (IOLs). Recent attention has been drawn toward a variety of specialized refractive IOLs that are currently under investigation and being applied with variable levels of success.[15-19] When considering wavefront customization of IOLs, the attention narrows somewhat but still holds broad ranging possibilities.

Optimized IOLs (Technis)

One of the most recently adapted specialized IOLs is the Technis aspherical lens, which is specifically designed to reduce spherical aberrations in patients following cataract surgery.[15,16] By analyzing a large population of cataract surgery patients regarding the asphericity they experience both pre- and postoperatively, an optimized aspheric IOL has been designed that will minimize the positive spherical aberrations often noted by these patients following surgery. The Technis lens (Pfizer, New York, NY) has enjoyed some success in its adoption into the field. Yet because it has a population-based optimized lens profile rather than a customized profile (individual-based), it still has errors due to the variability of spherical aberrations seen among individuals. Since approximately 10% of the population has negative spherical aberrations when examined by corneal wavefront sensing, further negative spherical aberration would be conveyed to these patients with implantation of this lens. Additionally, an aspheric lens with greater correction of spherical aberration has greater sensitivity to proper centration and alignment. A decentration of the Technis lens by as much as 0.40 mm or 7 degrees of tilt might induce new aberrations (eg, coma) that could negate the visual benefit of its asphericity (Figure 42-5).[16] Although this amount of decentration or tilt may be unlikely in a well-executed phacoemulsification with implantation procedure, when the surgery is less than optimal, implantation of this lens may not be recommended.

Customized IOLs Preinsertion

Just as the Technis aspheric IOL compensates for spherical aberration based on the mean values of a population, one could also consider correction of patient specific spherical aberration based on corneal topography. This is in contrast to utilizing wavefront-based measurements of preoperative spherical aberration as the unpredictable size and aspheric shape of the aging crystalline lens would make a postoperative spherical aberration less predictable. One could also conceptualize customizing the implant for the total ocular aberrations after cataract extraction but this would require a way of assuring proper alignment of the IOL during its implantation. Phacoemulsification of the crystalline lens with insertion of an IOL scaffold, giving a platform to anchor and align an IOL at a later date, might be one way to customize the IOL preinsertion. This, however, introduces the need to consider a two-step procedure of 1) initial cataract removal and scaffold implantation with subsequent whole wavefront measurements when the eye is stable, followed by 2) a secondary implantation of the customized IOL. Customized phakic IOLs might also be considered in this way. The implantation of a scaffold-anchoring element beforehand might be the most ideal way to assure proper alignment and registration of an IOL that is customized prior to its insertion.

Phacoemulsification of the crystalline lens with insertion of an IOL scaffold, giving a platform to anchor and align an IOL at a later date, might be one way to customize the IOL preinsertion.

Customized IOLs Postinsertion

One way of solving the problem of accurate alignment and registration of a wavefront customized implant is to customize it after it has been implanted inside the eye. This concept has been recently introduced and popularized by the new Calhoun Laser Adjustable Lens (LAL) (Calhoun Vision Inc, Pasadena, Calif).[17] This IOL is customized inside the eye by the radiation of a specific frequency of blue light on a silicone-based material with monomers that can migrate within the lens according to differences in the concentration gradient. By irradiating the lens in a specific location (ie, centrally), existing monomers can be polymerized into the underlying structure of the silicone and the remaining peripheral monomers can migrate centrally in order to re-establish the concentration gradient. This has the effect of increasing the central thickness of the lens, increasing its overall refractive power (ie, correcting residual hyperopia). Using this technology, higher-order aberrations can also be customized postinsertion by placement of the polymerizing light to the specific areas required for customization to improve wavefront error (see Chapter 35). With a predictable change on the order of 10s of microns, this kind of postinsertion customization should be able to eliminate nearly all significant higher-order aberrations.

With new biocompatible implant materials, alternative methods of customization after insertion might also be conceptualized and adapted. Although it is unlikely for laser ablation of an IOL to occur once it is inside the eye because of the ablation by-products, other novel ideas will presumably be proposed for implant customization in the future.

Customized Adaptive Correction

As suggested previously in this chapter, the concept of adaptive correction of corneal ablation could also be applied inside the eye for the adaptive correction of IOLs. The Calhoun LAL may not be ideal for this type of adaptive real-time wavefront correction due to the slower response of migrating monomers based on a concentration gradient. Newer concepts of rapidly modifying IOLs after they have been implanted could certainly allow one to rapidly monitor the changes as they are induced and with the proper closed-loop feedback mechanisms be able to control the further modification in real time. In the quest for super vision using refractive implants, herein lies perhaps the most promising concept for reproducibly achieving super vision corrections. Real-time, wavefront-adapted correction would allow an ideal refractive outcome to be achieved, especially when using refractive implants, which are not subject to wound healing.

In the quest for super vision using refractive implants, herein lies perhaps the most promising concept for reproducibly achieving super vision corrections. Real-time wavefront-adapted correction would allow an ideal refractive outcome to be achieved, especially when using refractive implants, which are not subject to wound healing.

Accommodating IOL Customization

Going one step further, implantation of an accommodating IOL that can be customized either pre- or postinsertion with proper registration and may give the patient optimized visual performance with the dynamic range enjoyed by nonpresbyopes.[18-20] One potential difficulty with this consideration is the fact that aberrations do change with typical accommodation and would likely also change with the pseudoaccommodation seen in accommodating IOLs. Matching this dynamic aberration change may be difficult in the near future, but may be achievable someday as technology evolves.

Capsular Filling Customization

The next step beyond an accommodating rigid implant is refilling of the capsular bag with a viscoelastic material. A deformed implant allows for accommodation. This could be accompanied by the removal of the lens[21] (see Chapter 41). Although there are many potential limitations to capsule refilling, its great promise is to restore a fully accommodating refractive lens to the eye following cataract surgery. The concept of postinsertion customization, as with the laser adjustable IOL, could also potentially be applied to the visco-elastic material injected into the capsular bag. In this way, it may be possible to restore accommodation, similar to a young healthy lens, and at the same time customize the refractive power of the lens to an emmetropic outcome with minimal aberrations.

Customized Corneal Inlay/Onlays

Finally, when considering a refractive implant that can be customized for super vision, one needs to also consider not only intraocular implants, but intracorneal implants as well as onlays. Although research investigations have been focused predominantly on intracorneal lenses, including recent efforts using the PermaVision lens (Anamed Inc, Lake Forest, Calif), difficulty with biocompatibility of an intrastromal implant has been observed due to poor nutrient transport from the aqueous to the anterior corneal structures. What may be more likely than a corneal implant is a corneal onlay. Recent work by Deborah Sweeney and colleagues at Comparative Research Centre for Eye Research and Technology (CRCERT) in Australia has demonstrated progress with an onlay material that conceptually could be applied as a permanent contact lens.[22] Many of the issues involved with customized contact lenses could be eliminated with a customized permanent contact lens, since movement of the lens would not be a factor. Additionally, ocular aberrations could be corrected right on the surface of the lens after its application and positional fixation. It may even be possible to use excimer laser photoablation on the synthetic surface implant, which would overcome potential limitations in the development of newer energy sources and delivery systems for customization. A similar concept was proposed over a decade ago by investigators at Emory Vision Correction Group using a synthetic collagen type IV copolymer in a procedure called *laser adjustable synthetic epikeratoplasty* (LASE).[23] However, primarily due to biocompatibility issues, this work was never fully commercially accepted. Newer synthetic polymers, as those being investigated by the CRCERT Group, show promise and suggest that some of these limitations may be overcome in the future.

Many of the issues involved with customized contact lenses could be eliminated with a customized permanent contact lens, since movement of the lens would not be a factor. Additionally, ocular aberrations could be corrected right on the surface of the lens after its application and positional fixation.

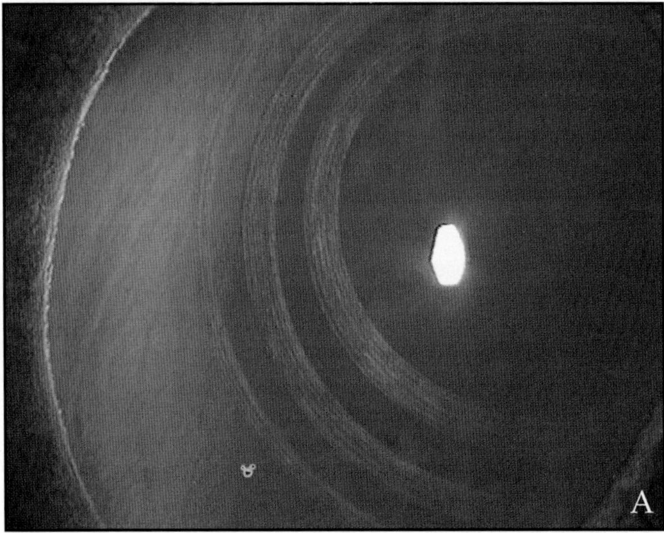

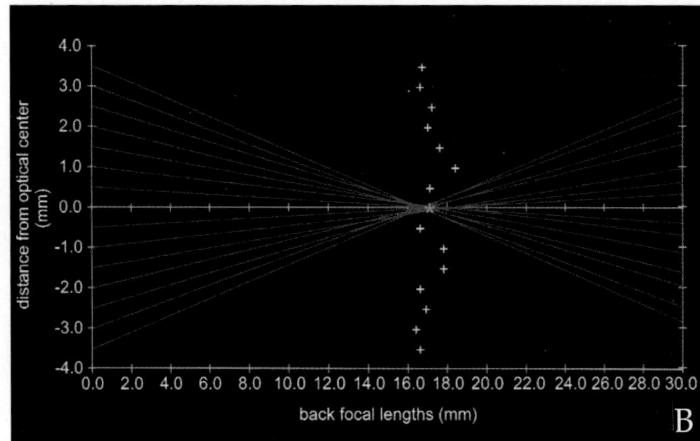

Figure 42-6. (A) Rabbit crystalline lens experimentally lasered with a femtosecond laser (Ti:sapphire amplified erbium fiber laser) demonstrating an annular pattern of several hundred thousand pulses. (B) HeNe laser scanning analysis 3 months later demonstrating the test of optical quality, which is similar in both the treated and the fellow control eye.

The Quest for Super Vision In Lenticular Modification

Although a somewhat new concept that has yet only been experimentally proposed, lenticular modification opens a new paradigm within refractive surgery, beyond the field of keratorefractive surgery (corneal reshaping), to that of lenticular refractive surgery (natural crystalline lens reshaping and modification).

Can the Lens be Modified Without Forming a Cataract?

In the mid-1980s, an important paradigm shift in ophthalmology occurred when the excimer laser was introduced for corneal ablation.[24] Prior to the introduction of the excimer laser, corneal injury and surgery penetrating beyond Bowman's layer was known to be associated with the formation of an anterior stromal scar. Therefore, it was a long-held belief that one should never operate on the optical center of the cornea. The early investigational work with excimer laser phototherapeutic keratectomy (PTK) and PRK violated this principle by asking the question, "Can one operate on the optical center of the cornea without creating a scar?" This paradigm shift introduced a new technology and way of thinking about corneal surgery, which led to the birth of a new subspecialty.

In a similar fashion, we are now only beginning to consider the question, "Can the natural crystalline lens be structurally modified without forming a cataract?" Recent investigation by Krueger and associates using femtosecond lasers has demonstrated that rabbit eyes can be irradiated with several hundred thousand pulses within the epinuclear lens tissue without the formation of a visible cataract or increase in lens light scatter (Figure 42-6A).[25] Rabbit lenses lasered using a titanium sapphire amplified erbium fiber laser in one eye, with the other eye serving as a control, demonstrated similar or less light scatter in six paired eyes after three postoperative months, when using helium-neon (HeNe) laser scanning studies (Figure 42-6B). The ultrastructural morphology of these lenses demonstrated only a 0.50 to 1.00 μm electron dense change adjacent to the laser disrupted lens fibers. Despite the electron-dense border, the surrounding hexagonal lens fibers appear essentially normal.

Photophaco Reduction

Once you can successfully deliver laser energy into the crystalline lens without causing a cataract, you can potentially modify the lens to change its shape or flexural properties. Photophaco reduction (PPR) is a process by which a femtosecond laser or alternative energy source actually reduces the volume of the crystalline lens to change it into a new shape for the correction of refractive error.[26] Although this is a concept that has not yet been experimentally demonstrated, PPR proposes to remove lens tissue more peripherally to induce greater refractive lens power or centrally to lessen the refractive power of the crystalline lens. In a similar way, this energy deposition can be customized because of the fine precision of femtosecond laser tissue ablation. However, because such a small volume of lens tissue is ablated with each laser pulse, the efficacy of PPR in changing the lens shape may make it impractical. Experimental and investigational studies need to be performed to realize its full potential.

Photophaco Modulation

The concept of depositing femtosecond laser energy, or energy from an alternative source, into the crystalline lens can also be used to separate lens tissue to increase its flexibility. Photophaco modulation (PPM) is a procedure whereby femtosecond laser pulses can separate lens fibers that are covalently bound during the process of aging, so as to modify the lens' modulus of elasticity for the correction of presbyopia. In the 1970s, Ronald Fisher demonstrated that one could measure the relative elasticity of human crystalline lenses by placing them on a pedestal that could be rotated at 1000 revolutions per minute (rpm), creating a centrifugal force simulating that of the zonules.[27] As a result, the anterior to posterior dimensions of the lens were reduced by the spinning (polar strain), and the amount of this reduction was found to be dependent on the lens' age, with younger lenses demonstrating a greater polar strain. To verify this observation,

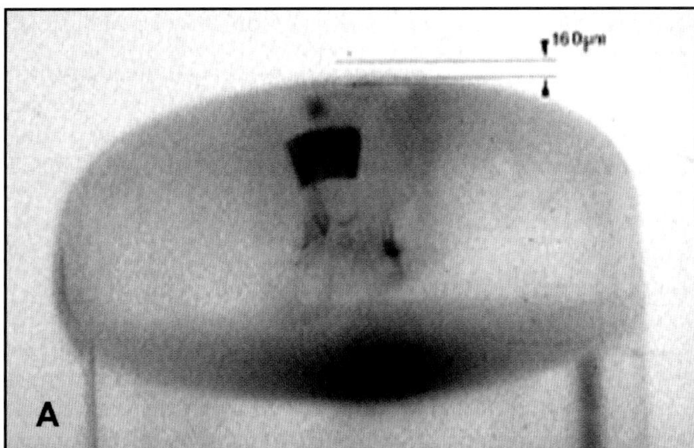

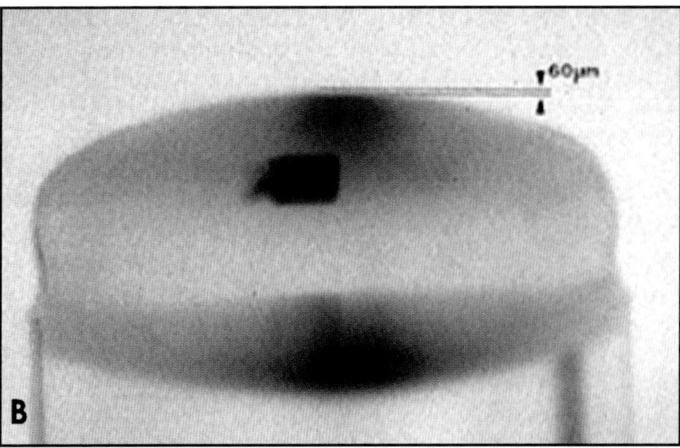

Figure 42-7. Rotational deformation of a pair of 54-year-old human cadaver lenses, demonstrating greater polar strain in the lasered lens (A) than in the unlasered control lens (B). A polar strain of 160 μm is consistent with that seen in a 35-year-old lens, compared to 60 μm in the unlasered 54-year-old lens.

Krueger and associates reproduced this experiment using 40 cadaver lenses, demonstrating a similar age-dependent polar strain as Fisher, using both direct measurement (viewed with a microscopic reticle) and photographic projection (high-speed camera film projected to a magnified view and referenced to a known calibration target).[28] Going one step further, 100 pulses of neodymium:yttrium-aluminum-garnet (Nd:YAG) laser energy were then placed within the lens nucleus/epinucleus in an annular fashion in 11 cadaver lenses of various ages, with the fellow eye's lens remaining as a control. Both the treated and control lenses were subjected to the rotational deformation experiments, demonstrating a statistically significantly greater polar strain in the treated lenses (Figure 42-7). The concept of modulating the elastic properties of the crystalline lens using an external energy source, such as a laser, could provide a simple means of presbyopia correction by restoring the age-dependent loss of accommodation. Further safety and efficacy experiments using femtosecond laser pulses will be required and are under investigation. There will likely be other concepts for customization of vision in presbyopia correction proposed in the future.

> Photophaco modulation (PPM) is a procedure whereby femtosecond laser pulses can separate lens fibers that are covalently bound during the process of aging, so as to modify the lens' modulus of elasticity for the correction of presbyopia.

The Quest for Super Vision in Neural Processing and Perception

Thus far, the quest for super vision in customized visual correction has dealt with an optical modification of ocular aberrations to improve the quality of the image placed on the retina. Since the limitations of super vision are not only optical but also neural, can we go beyond optics and also improve the retinal and neural processing or cortical perception?

Optical Solution to a Retinal Problem

Although customization in patients with retinal disease will likely be quite difficult, one recently proposed optical solution may provide a unique benefit to patients with focal lesions of the fovea. In a yet unpublished report by Seiler and associates, a patient with central areolar foveal dystrophy and a best-corrected visual acuity (BCVA) of 20/100 underwent a wavefront-guided LASIK procedure to correct not only a small refractive error, but to induce 3.50 degrees of horizontal tilt (personal communication, Theo Seiler, September 2003). Tilt, which is considered a first-order aberration, is best understood by its prismatic effect, which at the level of the cornea might cause the light rays to focus onto the parafoveal retina rather than the central fovea where the focal lesion is present. In this patient, the BCVA and uncorrected visual acuity (UCVA) improved to 20/40, which suggests that prismatic displacement of a foveal image may induce an eccentric fixation to help some patient's with focal retinal disease.

Photoreceptor Transplantation and/or Redistribution

Many may remember the television series in the late 1970s and 1980s about the "Six Million Dollar Man", who was rebuilt to be stronger, faster, and have better senses, including super vision. Although we are a long way off from rebuilding the complex visual system with which we are born, efforts in photoreceptor transplantation research of macular degeneration does lead us to wonder whether photoreceptor transplantation might be performed some day to increase the resolution of retinal image size to levels beyond the current limitations of nature. Perhaps customization of vision will someday find a solution for patients with macular degeneration to customize their visual correction at the retinal level. Retinal translocation surgery has also shown some benefit in transferring the functional photoreceptors in the macula to an area away from an underlying subretinal pathology. Although this has not resulted in super vision, it does represent a form of customization for visual correction.

Neural Adaptation and Amblyopia Correction

The question about neural limitations posed earlier in this chapter ("Would an eye that has never seen better than 20/20 be correctable to 20/8 or 20/10, if the ocular aberrations were sufficiently corrected?") is again important to ask when considering the quest for super vision in neural adaptation and amblyopia correction. Are we limited by our previous best spectacle-corrected vision, following an ideal optical correction, or is there a period of adaptation in which improvement in best-corrected vision can be achieved? Many of these questions, although currently unanswered, will likely be more definitively answered as we continue investigating customized corneal ablation of unique cases in which some level of refractive- or aberration-induced amblyopia exists. The previously mentioned work of Seiler and associates, regarding the correction of anisometropia and high astigmatism, respectively gaining two lines of best-corrected visual acuity 1 or 3 years later, suggests that neural adaptation and the correction of refractive amblyopia is possible. Reports of using magnets for amblyopia correction in several Fyodorov clinics in Russia also introduces the possibility of an external influence to encourage neural adaptation, which has yet been unsubstantiated in the Western world (personal communication, Nick Pastaev, MD, 1997).

The Quest for Super Vision is Here to Stay

Although ophthalmology has seen a number of novel concepts reach the realm of clinical practice, many of these have only been an evolutionary step or have been unsuccessful due to a lack of wide spread acceptance. This is especially true in refractive surgery in which dozens of procedures have been proposed and introduced for the correction of refractive error, yet only a handful are commonly used today as part of routine clinical practice. Most of the currently acceptable procedures today will be obsolete in a decade. So we ask this question about customized corneal ablation, wavefront customized visual correction, and the quest for super vision: Will these novel concepts that we are discussing today be here to stay, or will they slip from the scene as so many refractive procedures have done before? Let us take a moment to consider each of these three mentioned concepts in the following subsections.

Customized Corneal Ablation

Just as LASIK has dominated the refractive market in the United States for the past 5 or so years, so will customized LASIK and PRK come to dominate the refractive market for the next 5 years. This is because customized laser vision correction procedures are providing everything that conventional LASIK and PRK provide and more. Satisfactory visual outcomes with speedy recovery and good quality of vision in a safe and relatively simple procedure have been the mainstay of current, conventional laser vision correction. The disadvantage of conventional refractive surgery is that it increases higher-order aberrations and reduces visual quality in some patients.[29] Since the introduction of customized corneal ablation, we have seen superior visual outcomes, sharper contrast, and reduction of higher order aberrations, which has created more patient satisfaction and a reduced likelihood of dissatisfied patients. Consequently, customized corneal ablation is taking a widely-accepted procedure and making it better. Hence, customized corneal ablation is here to stay.

What about after 5 years have passed? Will customized corneal ablation continue to be the mainstay of refractive surgery in 10, 15, or 20 years? Although it is likely to remain an option for the next two decades, other forms of customized visual correction may take on a more dominant role.

Wavefront Customized Visual Correction

In looking to the future, other forms of wavefront customization, such as IOLs, onlays, and other synthetic implants, will take on an ever increasing role in the methods of visual correction and customization. Ocular wavefront sensing, as a method of determining refractive error, will increasingly be employed in vision assessment and refractive testing and will likely become routine in the refractive ophthalmic exam, similar to corneal topography. Since wavefront sensing will play such a large role in clinical practice, wavefront customization in visual correction will also continue to play an increasing role. Whatever procedure we choose to use for refractive surgical correction, we will want to employ wavefront customization to optimize this procedure. Hence, we believe some form of wavefront customized visual correction will be here to stay for as long as we are offering refractive surgical procedures, or at least until there is a better technology to optimize the human visual system.

We believe some form of wavefront customized visual correction will be here to stay for as long as we are offering refractive surgical procedures, or at least until there is a better technology to optimize the human visual system.

Quest for Super Vision

Finally, if there is ever a suspicion that customized corneal ablation will be displaced by an alternative method of vision correction or if wavefront customization will somehow be replaced by a superior method of customization, the quest for super vision will never be replaced because patients will always desire to have the best, sharpest vision obtainable. In conclusion, when all other things pass because of superior technology, the quest for super vision will ever be present. Hence, if we continue with subsequent volumes of this book, the titles may change; however, the subtitle—"The Quest for Super Vision"—will remain the same.

References

1. Cheng X, Thibos LN, Bradley A. Estimating visual quality from wavefront aberration measurements. *J Refract Surg*. 2003;19:S570-S584.
2. Wilson SE. Wavefront analysis: are we missing something? *Am J Ophthalmol*. 2003;136:340-342.
3. Pallikaris IG, Kymionis GD, Panagopoulou SI, et al. Induced optical aberrations following formation of a laser in-situ keratomileusis flap. *J Cataract Refract Surg*. 2002;28:2088-2095.
4. Porter J, MacRae S, Yoon G, et al. Separate effects of the microkeratome incision and laser ablation on the eye's wave aberration. *Am J Ophthalmol*. 2003;136(2):327-337.
5. Wilson SE, Mohan RR, Hong JW, et al. The wound healing response after laser in situ keratomileusis and photorefractive keratectomy . *Arch Ophthalmol*. 2001;119:889-896.
6. Carones F, Vigo L, Scandola E, Vacchini L. Evaluation of the prophylactic use of Mitomycin-C to inhibit haze formation after photorefractive keratectomy. *J Cataract Refract Surg*. 2002;28:2088-2095.
7. Hafezi F, Steinbach JP, Marti A, et al. The absence of C-fos prevents light-induced apoptotic cell death of photoreceptors in retinal degeneration in vivo. *Nat Med*. 1997;3:346-349.
8. Vinciguerra P, Nizzola GM, Bailo G, et al. Excimer laser photorefractive keratectomy for presbyopia: 24 month follow-up in three eyes. *J Refract Surg*. 1998;14(1):66-69.

9. Baverberg JM. Centered vs inferior off center ablation to correct hyperopia and presbyopia. *J Refract Surg.* 1999;15(1):66-69.
10. Huang D, Arif M. Spot size and quality of scanning laser correction of higher order wavefront aberrations. *J Cataract Refract Surg.* 2002; 28:407-416.
11. Guirao A, Williams DR, MacRae SM. Effect of beam size on the expected benefit of customized laser refractive surgery. *J Refract Surg.* 2003;19(1):15-23.
12. Huppertz M, Schmidt E, Teiwes W. Eye tracking and refractive surgery. In: MacRae SM, Krueger RR, Applegate RA, eds. *Customized Corneal Ablation: The Quest for Super Vision.* Thorofare, NJ: SLACK Incorporated; 2001:149-160.
13. Schruender SA, Fuchs H, Spasovski S, Dankert A. Intraoperative corneal topography for image registration. *J Refract Surg.* 2002; 18(5):S624-S629.
14. Krueger RR, Gomez P, Herekar S. Intraoperative wavefront monitoring during laser thermal keratoplasty. *J Refract Surg.* 2003; 19:S602-S607.
15. Holladay JT, Piers PA, Koranyi G, et al. A new intraocular lens design to reduce spherical aberration of pseudophakic eyes. *J Refract Surg.* 2002;18(6):683-691.
16. Packer M, Fine IH, Hoffman RS, Piers PA. Prospective randomized trial of an anterior surface modified prolate intraocular lens. *J Refract Surg.* 2002;18(6):692-696.
17. Sandstedt CA, Chang S, Schwartz DM. The light adjustable lens: A novel method for the correction of refractive error. In: Krueger RR, Applegate RA, MacRae SM, eds. *Wavefront Customized Visual Correction: The Quest for Super Vision.* Thorofare, NJ: SLACK Incorporated; 2001.
18. Steinert RF, Aker BL, Trentacost DJ, et al. A prospective study of the AMO array zonal progressive multifocal silicone intraocular lens and a monofocal intraocular lens. *Ophthalmology.* 1999;106:1243-1255.
19. Cummings JS, Slade SG, Chayet A. Clinical evaluation of the model AT-45 silicone accommodating intraocular lens: Results of feasibility and initial phase of a FDA clinical trial. *Ophthalmology.* 2001; 108:2005-2010.
20. Kuchle M, Nguyen NX, Langenbucher A, et al. Implantation of a new accommodative posterior chamber intraocular lens. *J Refract Surg.* 2002;18(3):208-216.
21. Haefliger E, Parel JM. Accommodation of an endocapsular silicone lens (Phaco-Ersatz) in the aging Rhesus monkey. *J Refract Corneal Surg.* 1994;10(5):550-555.
22. Evans MDM, McLean KM, Hughes TC, Sweeney DF. A review of the development of a synthetic corneal onlay for refractive correction. *Biomaterials.* 2001;22:3319-3328.
23. Thompson KP, Hanna K, Waring GO III, et al. Current status of synthetic epikeratoplasty. *Refract Corneal Surg.* 1991;7:240-248.
24. Trokel SL, Srinivasan R, Braren B. Excimer laser surgery of the cornea. *Am J Ophthalmol.* 1983;96:710-715.
25. Krueger RR, Kuszak J, Lubatschowski H, et al. The safety of femtosecond laser photodisruption in animal lenses: Tissue morphology and cataractogenesis. *Ophthalmology.* In press.
26. Myers RI, Krueger RR. Novel approaches to correction of a presbyopia with laser modification of the crystalline lens. *J Refract Surg.* 1998;14:136-139.
27. Fisher RF. The elastic constants of the human lens. *J Physiol.* 1971; 212:147-180.
28. Krueger RR, Sun XK, Stroh J, Myers R. Experimental increase in accommodative potential after Neodymium:YAG laser photodisruption of paired cadaver lenses. *Ophthalmology.* 2001;108:2122-2128.
29. Chalita MR, Xu M, Krueger RR. Correlation of aberrations with visual symptoms in post-LASIK eyes using wavefront analysis. *J Refract Surg.* 2003;19(6):S682-S686.

Appendix 1

Optical Society of America Wavefront Standards

Reprinted with permission from the Optical Society of America

Standards for Reporting the Optical Aberrations of Eyes

Larry N. Thibos,[1] Raymond A. Applegate,[2] James T. Schwiegerling,[3] Robert Webb[4], and VSIA Standards Taskforce Members

[1]School of Optometry, Indiana University, Bloomington, IN 47405, [2]Department of Ophthalmology, University of Texas Health Science Center at San Antonio, San Antonio, TX 78284, [3]Department of Ophthalmology, University of Arizona, Tucson, AZ 85721, [4]Schepens Research Institute, Boston, MA 02114
thibos@indiana.edu, Applegate@uthscsa.edu, jschwieg@u.arizona.edu, webb@helix.mgh.harvard.edu

Abstract: In response to a perceived need in the vision community, an OSA taskforce was formed at the 1999 topical meeting on vision science and its applications (VSIA-99) and charged with developing consensus recommendations on definitions, conventions, and standards for reporting of optical aberrations of human eyes. Progress reports were presented at the 1999 OSA annual meeting and at VSIA-2000 by the chairs of three taskforce subcommittees on (1) reference axes, (2) describing functions, and (3) model eyes. The following summary of the committee's recommendations is available also in portable document format (PDF) on OSA Optics Net at http://www.osa.org/.
OCIS codes: (330.0330) Vision and color; (330.5370) Physiological optics

Background

The recent resurgence of activity in visual optics research and related clinical disciplines (e.g. refractive surgery, ophthalmic lens design, ametropia diagnosis) demands that the vision community establish common metrics, terminology, and other reporting standards for the specification of optical imperfections of eyes. Currently there exists a plethora of methods for analyzing and representing the aberration structure of the eye but no agreement exists within the vision community on a common, universal method for reporting results. In theory, the various methods currently in use by different groups of investigators all describe the same underlying phenomena and therefore it should be possible to reliably convert results from one representational scheme to another. However, the practical implementation of these conversion methods is computationally challenging, is subject to error, and reliable computer software is not widely available. All of these problems suggest the need for operational standards for reporting aberration data and to specify test procedures for evaluating the accuracy of data collection and data analysis methods.

Following a call for participation [1], approximately 20 people met at VSIA-99 to discuss the proposal to form a taskforce that would recommend standards for reporting optical aberrations of eyes. The group agreed to form three working parties that would take responsibility for developing consensus recommendations on definitions, conventions and standards for the following three topics: (1) reference axes, (2) describing functions, and (3) model eyes. It was decided that the strategy for Phase I of this project would be to concentrate on articulating definitions, conventions, and standards for those issues which are not empirical in nature. For example, several schemes for enumerating the Zernike polynomials have been proposed in the literature. Selecting one to be the standard is a matter of choice, not empirical investigation, and therefore was included in the charge to the taskforce. On the other hand, issues such as the maximum number of Zernike orders needed to describe ocular aberrations adequately is an empirical question which was avoided for the present, although the taskforce may choose to formulate recommendations on such issues at a later time. Phase I concluded at the VSIA-2000 meeting.

Reference Axis Selection

Summary

It is the committee's recommendation that the ophthalmic community use the line-of-sight as the reference axis for the purposes of calculating and measuring the optical aberrations of the eye. The rationale is that the line-of-sight in the normal eye is the path of the chief ray from the fixation point to the retinal fovea. Therefore, aberrations measured with respect to this axis will have the pupil center as the origin of a Cartesian reference frame. Secondary lines-of-sight may be similarly constructed for object points in the peripheral visual field. Because the exit pupil is not readily accessible in the living eye whereas the entrance pupil is, the committee recommends that calculations for specifying the optical aberration of the eye be referenced to the plane of the entrance pupil.

Background

Optical aberration measurements of the eye from various laboratories or within the same laboratory are not comparable unless they are calculated with respect to the same reference axis and expressed in the same manner. This requirement is complicated by the fact that, unlike a camera, the eye is a decentered optical system with non-rotationally symmetric components (Fig. 1). The principle elements of the eye's optical system are the cornea, pupil, and the crystalline lens. Each can be decentered and tilted with respect to other components, thus rendering an optical system that is typically dominated by coma at the foveola.

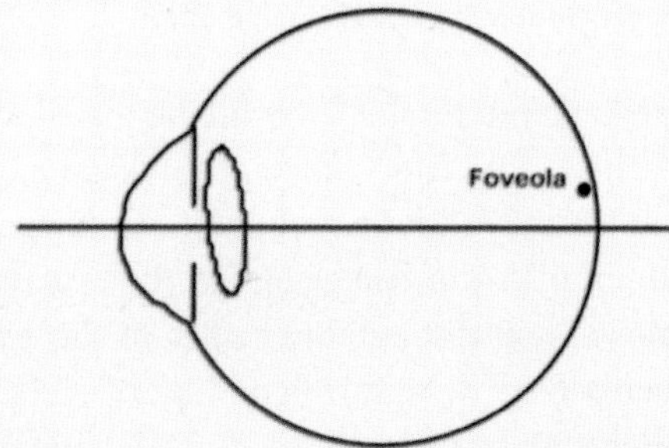

Fig. 1. The cornea, pupil, and crystalline lens are decentered and tilted with respect to each other, rendering the eye a decentered optical system that is different between individuals and eyes within the same individual.

The optics discipline has a long tradition of specifying the aberration of optical systems with respect to the center of the exit pupil. In a centered optical system (e.g., a camera, or telescope) using the center of the exit pupil as a reference for measurement of on-axis aberration is the same as measuring the optical aberrations with respect to the chief ray from an axial object point. However, because the exit pupil is not readily accessible in the living eye, it is more practical to reference aberrations to the entrance pupil. This is the natural choice for objective aberrometers which analyze light reflected from the eye.

Like a camera, the eye is an imaging device designed to form an in-focus inverted image on a screen. In the case of the eye, the imaging screen is the retina. However, unlike film, the "grain" of the retina is not uniform over its extent. Instead, the grain is finest at the foveola and falls off quickly as the distance from the foveola increases. Consequently, when viewing fine detail, we rotate our eye such that the object of regard falls on the foveola (Fig. 2). Thus, aberrations at the foveola have the greatest impact on an individual's ability to see fine details.

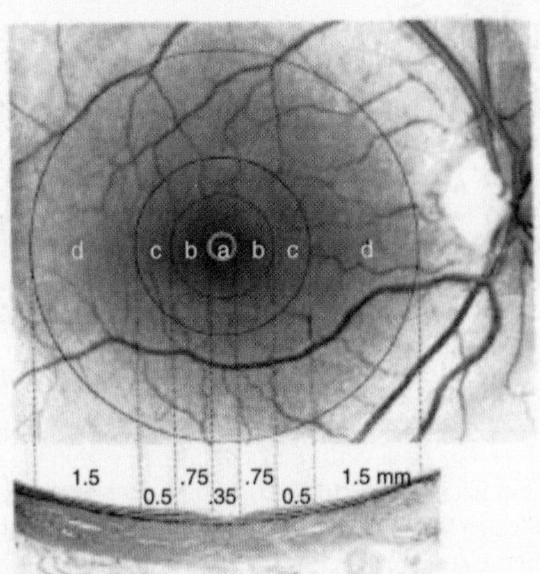

Fig. 2. An anatomical view of the macular region as viewed from the front and in cross section (below). a: foveola, b: fovea, c: parafoveal area, d: perifoveal area. From *Histology of the Human Eye* by Hogan. Alvarado Weddell, W.B. Sauders Company publishers, 1971, page 491.

Two traditional axes of the eye are centered on the foveola, the visual axis and the line-of-sight, but only the latter passes through the pupil center. In object space, the visual axis is typically defined as the line connecting the fixation object point to the eye's first nodal point. In image space, the visual axis is the parallel line connecting the second nodal point to the center of the foveola (Fig. 3, left). In contrast, the line-of-sight is defined as the (broken) line passing through the center of the eye's entrance and exit pupils connecting the object of regard to the foveola (Fig. 3, right). The line-of-sight is equivalent to the path of the foveal chief ray and therefore is the axis which conforms to optical standards. The visual axis and the line of sight are not the same and in some eyes the difference can have a large impact on retinal image quality [2]. For a review of the axes of the eye see [3]. (To avoid confusion, we note that Bennett and Rabbetts [4] re-define the visual axis to match the traditional definition of the line of sight. The Bennett and Rabbetts definition is counter to the majority of the literature and is not used here.)

When measuring the optical properties of the eye for objects which fall on the peripheral retina outside the central fovea, a secondary line-of-sight may be constructed as the broken line from object point to center of the entrance pupil and from the center of the exit pupil to the retinal location of the image. This axis represents the path of the chief ray from the object of interest and therefore is the appropriate reference for describing aberrations of the peripheral visual field.

Methods for aligning the eye during measurement.

Summary

The committee recommends that instruments designed to measure the optical properties of the eye and its aberrations be aligned co-axially with the eye's line-of-sight.

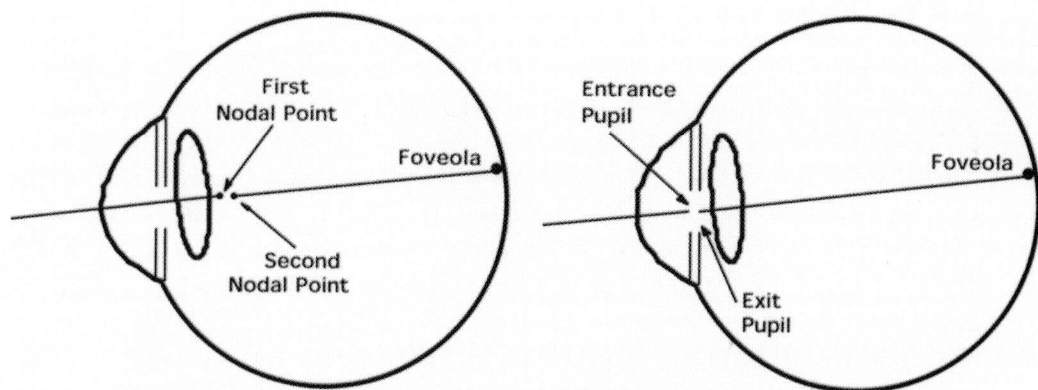

Fig. 3. Left panel illustrates the visual axis and panel right illustrates the line of sight.

Background

There are numerous ways to align the line of sight to the optical axis of the measuring instrument. Here we present simple examples of an objective method and a subjective method to achieve proper alignment.

Objective method

In the objective alignment method schematically diagramed in Fig. 4, the experimenter aligns the subject's eye (which is fixating a small distant target on the optical axis of the measurement system) to the measurement system. Alignment is achieved by centering the subject's pupil (by adjusting a bite bar) on an alignment ring (e.g., an adjustable diameter circle) which is co-axial with the optical axis of the measurement system. This strategy forces the optical axis of the measurement device to pass through the center of the entrance pupil. Since the fixation target is on the optical axis of the measurement device, once the entrance pupil is centered with respect to the alignment ring, the line-of-sight is co-axial with the optical axis of the measurement system.

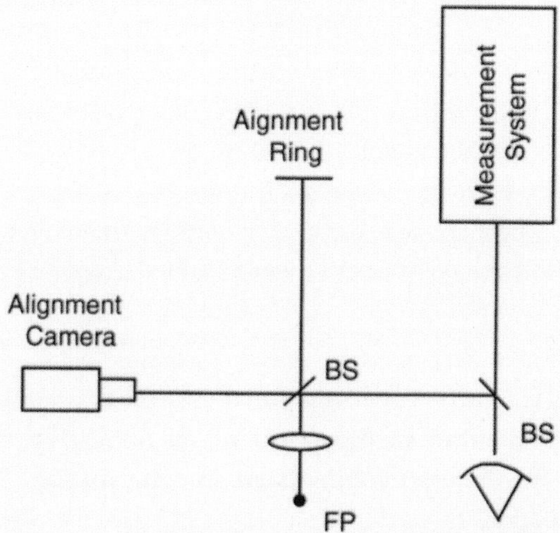

Fig. 4. Schematic of a generic objective alignment system designed to place the line of sight on the optical axis of the measurement system. BS: beam splitter, FP: on axis fixation point.

Subjective method

In the subjective alignment method schematically diagramed in Figure 5, the subject adjusts the position of their own pupil (using a bite bar) until two alignment fixation points at different optical distances along and co-axial to the optical axis of the measurement device are superimposed (similar to aligning the sights on rifle to a target). Note that one or both of the alignment targets will be defocused on the retina. Thus the subject's task is to align the centers of the blur circles. Assuming the chief ray defines the centers of the blur circles for each fixation point, this strategy forces the line of sight to be co-axial with the optical axis of the measurement system. In a system with significant amounts of asymmetric aberration (e.g., coma), the chief ray may not define the center of the blur circle. In practice, it can be useful to use the subjective strategy for preliminary alignment and the objective method for final alignment.

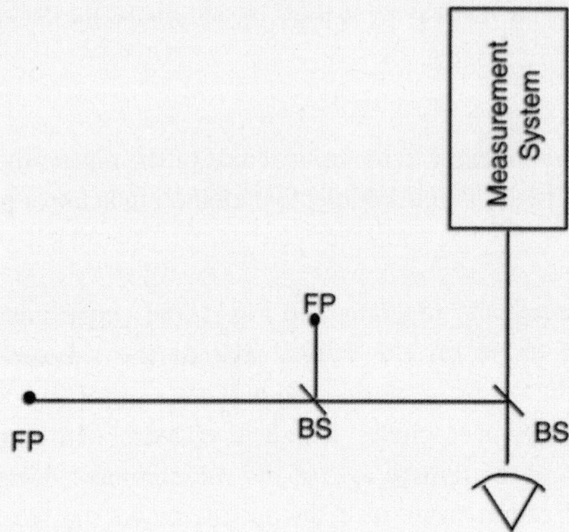

Fig. 5. Schematic of a generic subjective alignment system designed to place the line of sight on the optical axis of the measurement system. BS: beam splitter, FP: fixation point source.

Conversion between reference axes

If optical aberration measurements are made with respect to some other reference axis, the data must be converted to the standard reference axis (see the tools developed by Susana Marcos at our temporary web site: //color.eri.harvard/standardization). However, since such conversions involve measurement and/or estimation errors for two reference axes (the alignment error of the measurement and the error in estimating the new reference axis), it is preferable to have the measurement axis be the same as the line-of-sight.

Description of Zernike Polynomials

The Zernike polynomials are a set of functions that are orthogonal over the unit circle. They are useful for describing the shape of an aberrated wavefront in the pupil of an optical system. Several different normalization and numbering schemes for these polynomials are in common use. Below we describe the different schemes and make recommendations towards developing a standard for presenting Zernike data as it relates to aberration theory of the eye.

Double Indexing Scheme

The Zernike polynomials are usually defined in polar coordinates (ρ,θ), where ρ is the radial coordinate ranging from 0 to 1 and θ is the azimuthal component ranging from 0 to 2π. Each of the Zernike polynomials consists of three components: a normalization factor, a radial-dependent component and an azimuthal-dependent component. The radial component is a polynomial, whereas the azimuthal component is sinusoidal. A double indexing scheme is useful for unambiguously describing these functions, with the index n describing the highest power (order) of the radial polynomial and the index m describing the azimuthal frequency of the sinusoidal component. By this scheme the Zernike polynomials are defined as

$$Z_n^m(\rho,\theta) = \begin{Bmatrix} N_n^m R_n^{|m|}(\rho)\cos m\theta \,;\ for\ m \geq 0 \\ -N_n^m R_n^{|m|}(\rho)\sin m\theta \,;\ for\ m < 0 \end{Bmatrix} \tag{1}$$

where N_n^m is the normalization factor described in more detail below and $R_n^{|m|}(\rho)$ is given by

$$R_n^{|m|}(\rho) = \sum_{s=0}^{(n-|m|)/2} \frac{(-1)^s (n-s)!}{s!\left[0.5(n+|m|-s\right]!\left[0.5(n-|m|-s\right]!}\rho^{n-2s} \tag{2}$$

This definition uniquely describes the Zernike polynomials except for the normalization constant. The normalization is given by

$$N_n^m = \sqrt{\frac{2(n+1)}{1+\delta_{m0}}} \tag{3}$$

where δ_{m0} is the Kronecker delta function (i.e . $\delta_{m0} = 1$ for $m = 0$, and $\delta_{m0} = 0$ for $m \neq 0$). Note that the value of n is a positive integer or zero. For a given n, m can only take on values -n, -n + 2, -n +4, ...n.

When describing individual Zernike terms, the two index scheme should always be used. Below are some examples.

Good:

"The values of $Z_3^{-1}(\rho,\theta)$ and $Z_4^2(\rho,\theta)$ are 0.041 and -0.121, respectively."

"Comparing the astigmatism terms, $Z_2^{-2}(\rho,\theta)$ and $Z_2^2(\rho,\theta)$ ..."

Bad

"The values of $Z_7(\rho,\theta)$ and $Z_{12}(\rho,\theta)$ are 0.041 and -0.121, respectively."

"Comparing the astigmatism terms, $Z_5(\rho,\theta)$ and $Z_6(\rho,\theta)$ ..."

Single Indexing Scheme

Occasionally, a single indexing scheme is useful for describing Zernike expansion coefficients. Since the polynomials actually depend on two parameters, n and m, ordering of a single indexing scheme is arbitrary. To avoid confusion, a standard single indexing scheme should be used, and this scheme should only be used for bar plots of expansion coefficients (Fig. 6). To obtain the single index, j, it is convenient to lay out the polynomials in a pyramid with row number n and column number m as shown in Table 1.

Table 1. Zernike pyramid. Row number is polynomial order n, column number is sinusoidal frequency m, table entry is the single-index j.

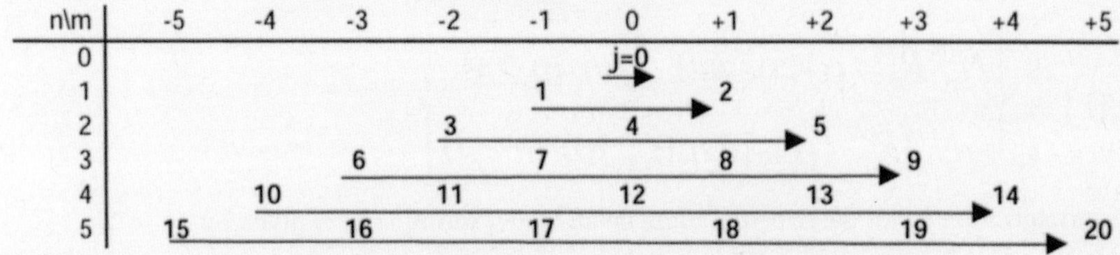

n\m	-5	-4	-3	-2	-1	0	+1	+2	+3	+4	+5
0						j=0					
1					1		2				
2				3		4		5			
3			6		7		8		9		
4		10		11		12		13		14	
5	15		16		17		18		19		20

The single index, j, starts at the top of the pyramid and steps down from left to right. To convert between j and the values of n and m, the following relationships can be used:

$$j = \frac{n(n+2)+m}{2} \qquad \text{(mode number)} \qquad (4)$$

$$n = roundup\left[\frac{-3+\sqrt{9+8j}}{2}\right] \qquad \text{(radial order)} \qquad (5)$$

$$m = 2j - n(n+2) \qquad \text{(angular frequency)} \qquad (6)$$

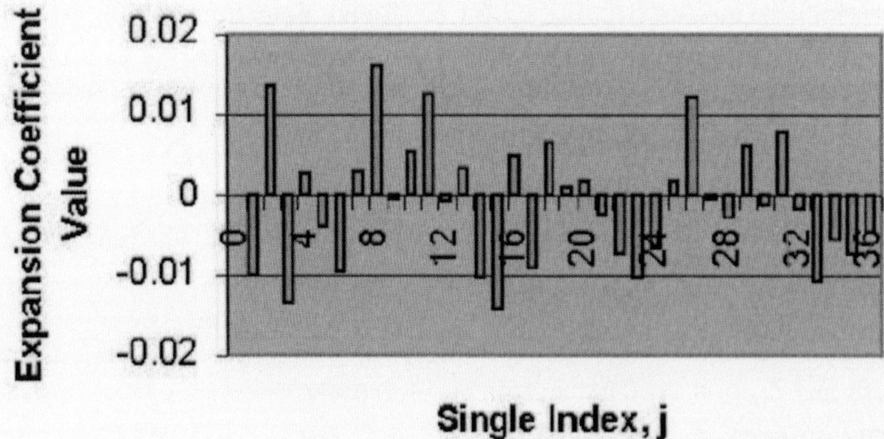

Fig. 6. Example of a bar plot using the single index scheme for Zernike coefficients.

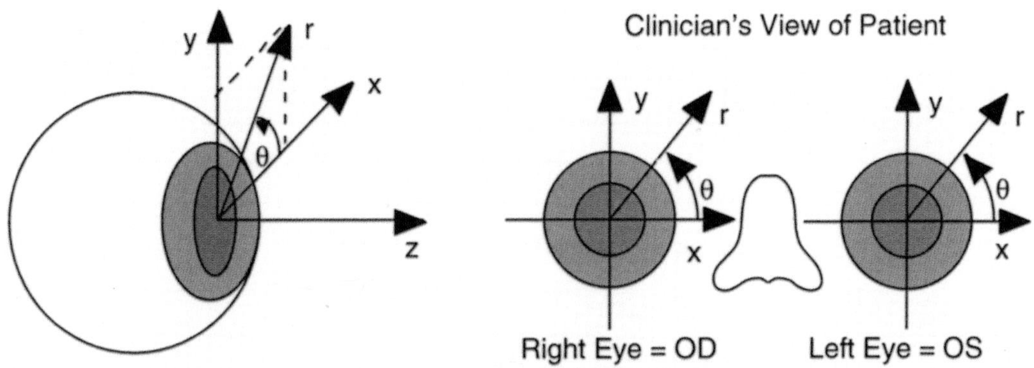

Fig. 7. Conventional right-handed coordinate system for the eye in Cartesian and polar forms.

Coordinate System

Typically, a right-handed coordinate system is used in scientific applications as shown in Fig. 7. For the eye, the coordinate origin is at the center of the eye's entrance pupil, the +x axis is horizontal pointing to the right, the +y axis is vertical pointing up, and the +z Cartesian axis points out of the eye and coincides with the foveal line-of-sight in object space, as defined by a chief ray emitted by a fixation spot. Also shown are conventional definitions of the polar coordinates $r = \sqrt{x^2 + y^2}$ and $\theta = \tan^{-1}(y/x)$. This definition gives $x = r\cos\theta$ and $y = r\sin\theta$. We note that Malacara [5] uses a polar coordinate system in which $x = r\sin\theta$ and $y = r\cos\theta$. In other words, θ is measured clockwise from the +y axis (Figure 1b), instead of counterclockwise from the +x axis (Figure 1a). Malacara's definition stems from early (pre-computer) aberration theory and is not recommended. In ophthalmic optics, angle θ is called the "meridian" and the same coordinate system applies to both eyes.

Because of the inaccessibility of the eye's image space, the aberration function of eyes are usually defined and measured in object space. For example, objective measures of ocular aberrations use light reflected out of the eye from a point source on the retina. Light reflected out of an aberration-free eye will form a plane-wave propagating in the positive z-direction and therefore the (x,y) plane serves as a natural reference surface. In this case the wavefront aberration function W(x,y) equals the z-coordinate of the reflected wavefront and may be interpreted as the shape of the reflected wavefront. By these conventions, $W > 0$ means the wavefront is phase-advanced relative to the chief ray. An example would be the wavefront reflected from a myopic eye, converging to the eye's far-point. A closely related quantity is the optical path-length difference (OPD) between a ray passing through the pupil at (x,y) and the chief ray point passing through the origin. In the case of a myopic eye, the path length is shorter for marginal rays than for the chief ray, so $OPD < 0$. Thus, by the recommended sign conventions, $OPD(x,y) = -W(x,y)$.

Bilateral symmetry in the aberration structure of eyes would make W(x,y) for the left eye the same as W(-x,y) for the right eye. If W is expressed as a Zernike series, then bilateral symmetry would cause the Zernike coefficients for the two eyes to be of opposite sign for all those modes with odd symmetry about the y-axis (e.g. mode Z_2^{-2}). Thus, to facilitate direct comparison of the two eyes, a vector R of Zernike coefficients for the right eye can be converted to a symmetric vector L for the left eye by the linear transformation L=M*R, where M is a diagonal matrix with elements +1 (no sign change) or –1 (with sign change). For example, matrix M for Zernike vectors representing the first 4 orders (15 modes) would have the diagonal elements [+1, +1, -1, -1, +1, +1, +1, +1, -1, -1, -1, -1, +1, +1, +1]

Table 2. Listing of Zernike Polynomials up to 7th order (36 terms)

j = index	n = order	m = frequency	$Z_n^m(\rho,\theta)$
0	0	0	1
1	1	-1	$2\ \rho \sin\theta$
2	1	1	$2\ \rho \cos\theta$
3	2	-2	$\sqrt{6}\ \rho^2 \sin 2\theta$
4	2	0	$\sqrt{3}\ (2\rho^2-1)$
5	2	2	$\sqrt{6}\ \rho^2 \cos 2\theta$
6	3	-3	$\sqrt{8}\ \rho^3 \sin 3\theta$
7	3	-1	$\sqrt{8}\ (3\rho^3-2\rho) \sin\theta$
8	3	1	$\sqrt{8}\ (3\rho^3-2\rho) \cos\theta$
9	3	3	$\sqrt{8}\ \rho^3 \cos 3\theta$
10	4	-4	$\sqrt{10}\ \rho^4 \sin 4\theta$
11	4	-2	$\sqrt{10}\ (4\rho^4-3\rho^2) \sin 2\theta$
12	4	0	$\sqrt{5}\ (6\rho^4-6\rho^2+1)$
13	4	2	$\sqrt{10}\ (4\rho^4-3\rho^2) \cos 2\theta$
14	4	4	$\sqrt{10}\ \rho^4 \cos 4\theta$
15	5	-5	$\sqrt{12}\ \rho^5 \sin 5\theta$
16	5	-3	$\sqrt{12}\ (5\rho^5-4\rho^3) \sin 3\theta$
17	5	-1	$\sqrt{12}\ (10\rho^5-12\rho^3+3\rho) \sin\theta$
18	5	1	$\sqrt{12}\ (10\rho^5-12\rho^3+3\rho) \cos\theta$
19	5	3	$\sqrt{12}\ (5\rho^5-4\rho^3) \cos 3\theta$
20	5	5	$\sqrt{12}\ \rho^5 \cos 5\theta$
21	6	-6	$\sqrt{14}\ \rho^6 \sin 6\theta$
22	6	-4	$\sqrt{14}\ (6\rho^6-5\rho^4) \sin 4\theta$
23	6	-2	$\sqrt{14}\ (15\rho^6-20\rho^4+6\rho^2) \sin 2\theta$
24	6	0	$\sqrt{7}\ (20\rho^6-30\rho^4+12\rho^2-1)$
25	6	2	$\sqrt{14}\ (15\rho^6-20\rho^4+6\rho^2) \cos 2\theta$
26	6	4	$\sqrt{14}\ (6\rho^6-5\rho^4) \cos 4\theta$
27	6	6	$\sqrt{14}\ \rho^6 \cos 6\theta$
28	7	-7	$4\ \rho^7 \sin 7\theta$
29	7	-5	$4\ (7\rho^7-6\rho^5) \sin 5\theta$
30	7	-3	$4\ (21\rho^7-30\rho^5+10\rho^3) \sin 3\theta$
31	7	-1	$4\ (35\rho^7-60\rho^5+30\rho^3-4\rho) \sin\theta$

32	7	1	$4\ (35\rho^7-60\rho^5+30\rho^3-4\rho)\cos\theta$
33	7	3	$4\ (21\rho^7-30\rho^5+10\rho^3)\cos 3\theta$
34	7	5	$4\ (7\rho^7-6\rho^5)\cos 5\theta$
35	7	7	$4\ \rho^7\cos 7\theta$

A standard aberrator for calibration

The original goal was to design a device that could be passed around or mass-produced to calibrate aberrometers at various laboratories. We first thought of this as an aberrated model eye, but that later seemed too elaborate. One problem is that the subjective aberrometers needed a sensory retina in their model eye, while the objective ones needed a reflective retina of perhaps known reflectivity. We decided instead to design an aberrator that could be used with any current or future aberrometers, with whatever was the appropriate model eye.

The first effort was with a pair of lenses that nearly cancelled spherical power, but when displaced sideways would give a known aberration. That scheme worked, but was very sensitive to tilt, and required careful control of displacement. The second design was a trefoil phase plate (OPD = $Z_3^3 = \kappa\, r^3\sin 3\theta$) loaned by Ed Dowski of CDM Optics, Inc. This 3rd order aberration is similar to coma, but with three lobes instead of one, hence the common name "trefoil". Simulation of the aberration function for this plate in ZEMAX® is shown in Figs. 8, 9. Figure 8 is a graph of the Zernike coefficients showing a small amount of defocus and 3rd order spherical aberration, but primarily C_3^3. Figure 9 shows the wavefront, only half a micron (one wave) peak to peak, but that value depends on κ, above.

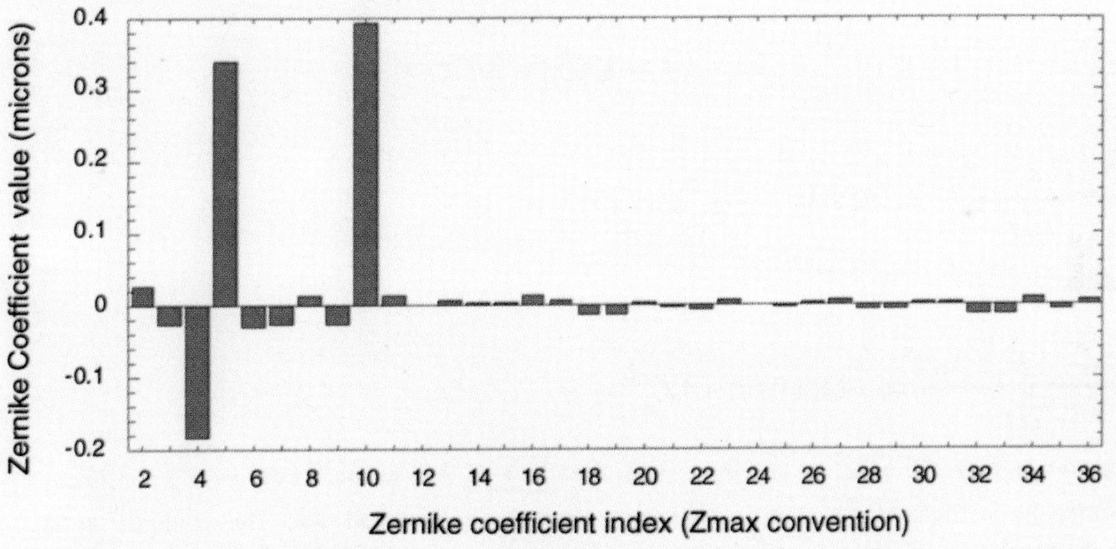

Fig. 8: Zernike coefficients of trefoil phase plate from ZEMAX® model (note different numbering convention from that recommended above for eyes).

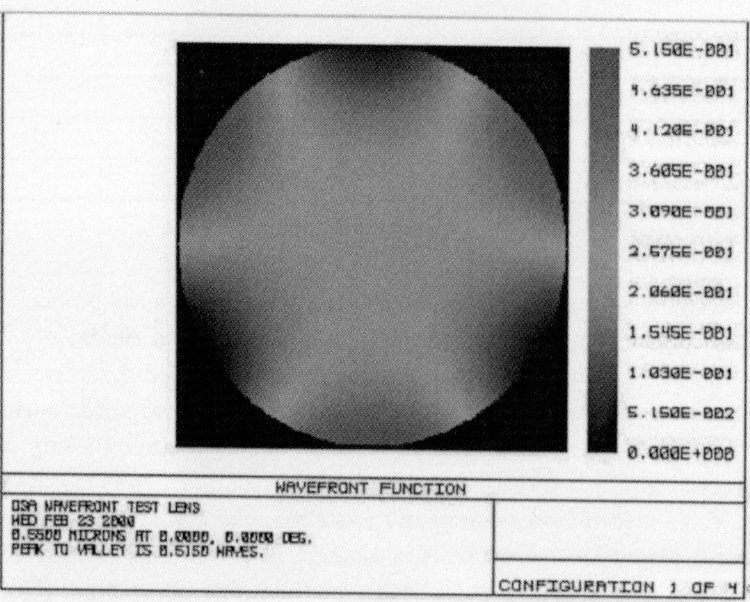

Fig. 9: Wavefront map for trefoil phase plate from the ZEMAX® model

We mounted the actual plate and found that it had even more useful qualities: As the phase plate is translated across the pupil, it adds some C_2^2, horizontal astigmatism. When the plate is perfectly centered, that coefficient is zero. Further, the slope of C_2^2 (Δx) measures the actual pupil.

$$Z_3^3(x-x_0) = \kappa\,(r-x_0)\sin 3\theta = \kappa\,(3xy^2 - x^3) \tag{7}$$

so

$$\frac{\partial Z_3^3(x-x_0)}{\partial x} = 3\kappa\,(3y^2 - x^2) = 3Z_2^2 \tag{8}$$

and similarly

$$\frac{\partial Z_3^{-3}(x-x_0)}{\partial x} = -6\kappa xy = -3Z_2^{-2} \tag{9}$$

This means that $\Delta Z_3^3 = 3Z_2^2\Delta x$ and then, since $W = \sum\sum C_n^m Z_n^m$, we get a new term proportional to Δx. Plotting the coefficient C_2^2 against Δx, we need to normalize to the pupil size. That could be useful as a check on whether the aberrator is really at the pupil, or whether some smoothing has changed the real pupil size, as measured. Figures 10-13 confirm this behavior and the expected variation with rotation (3θ).

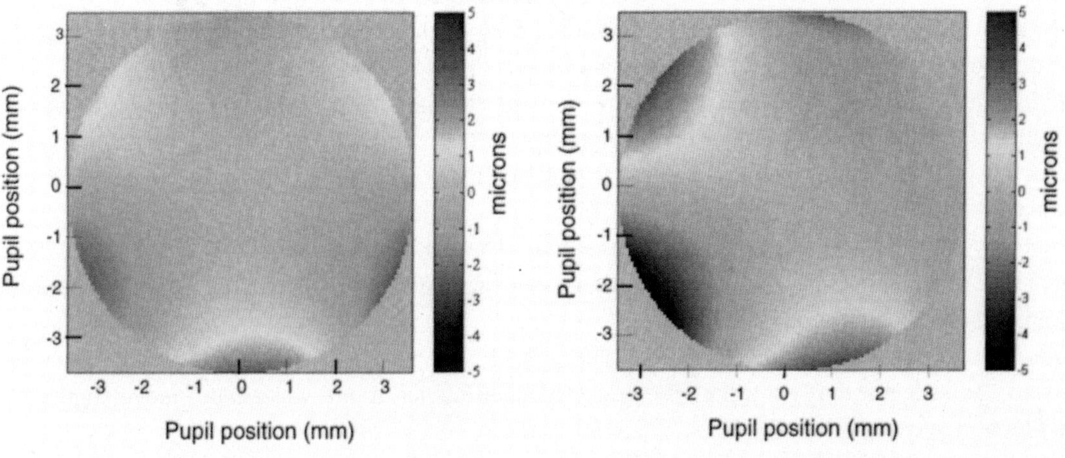

Fig. 10: Wavefront map from the aberrator, using the SRR aberrometer.

Fig. 11: The phase plate of Figure 10 has been moved horizontally 4 mm.

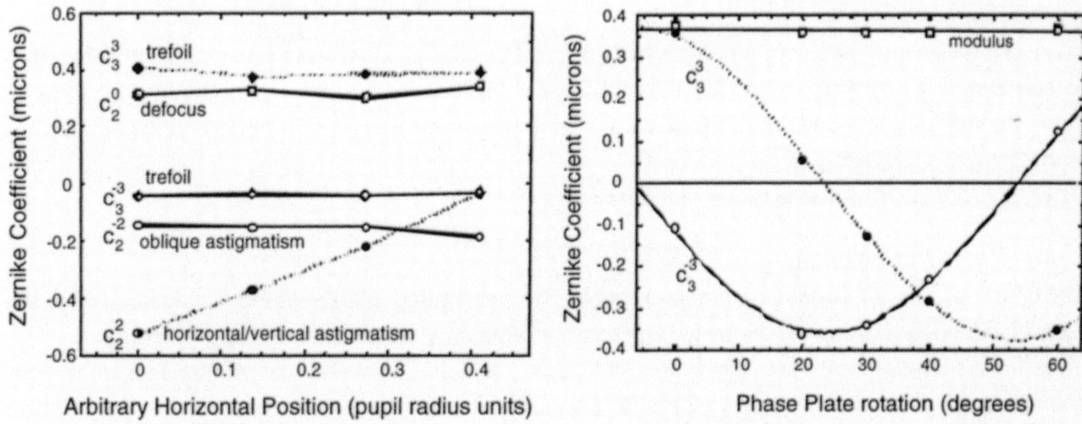

Fig. 12: Zerike coefficients are stable against horizontal displacement, except for C_3^3.

Fig. 13: Zernike coefficients C_3^3 and C_3^{-3} as a function of rotation of the phase plate about the optic axis.

Although the phase plate aberrator works independently of position in a collimated beam, some aberrometers may want to use a converging or diverging beam. Then it should be placed in a pupil conjugate plane. We have not yet built the mount for the phase plate, and would appreciate suggestions for that. Probably we need a simple barrel mount that fits into standard lens holders – say 30 mm outside diameter. We expect to use a standard pupil, but the phase plate(s) should have 10 mm clear aperture before restriction. The workshop seemed to feel that a standard pupil should be chosen. Should that be 7.5 mm?

We have tested the Z_3^3 aberrator, but it may be a good idea to have a few others. We borrowed this one, and it is somewhat fragile. Bill Plummer of Polaroid thinks he could generate this and other plates in plastic for "a few thousand dollars" for each design. Please send suggestions as to whether other designs are advisable (webb@helix.mgh.Harvard.edu), and as to whether we will want to stack them or use them independently. That has some implications for the mount design, but not severe ones. We suggest two Z_3^3 plates like this one, and perhaps a Z_6^0, fifth order spherical.

At this time, then, our intent is to have one or more standard aberrators that can be inserted into any aberrometer. When centered, and with a standard pupil, all aberrometers should report the same Zernike coefficients. We do not intend to include positioners in the mount, assuming that will be different for each aberrometer.

Another parameter of the design is the value of κ. That comes from the actual physical thickness and the index of refraction. Suggestions are welcome here, but we assume we want coefficients that are robust compared to a diopter or so of defocus.

The index will be whatever it will be. We will report it, but again any chromaticity will depend on how it's used. We suggest that we report the expected coefficients at a few standard wavelengths and leave interpolation to users.

Plans for Phase II

Reference Axes Sub-committee

- develop a shareware library of software tools needed to convert data from one ocular reference axis to another (e.g., convert a wavefront aberration for the corneal surface measured by topography along the instrument's optical axis into a wavefront aberration specified in the eye's exit pupil plane along the eye's fixation axis.)
- generate test datasets for evaluating software tools

Describing functions subcommittee

- develop a shareware library of software tools for generating, manipulating, evaluating, etc. the recommended describing functions for wavefront aberrations and pupil apodizing functions.
- develop additional software tools for converting results between describing functions (e.g. converting Taylor polynomials to Zernike polynomials, or converting single-index Zernikes to double-index Zernikes, etc.)
- generate test datasets for evaluating software tools

Model eyes subcommittee

- build a physical model eye that can be used to calibrate experimental apparatus for measuring the aberrations of eyes
- circulate the physical model to all interested parties for evaluation, with results to be presented for discussion at a future VSIA meeting.

Acknowledgements

The authors wish to thank the numerous committee members who contributed to this project.

References

1. L. N. Thibos, R. A. Applegate, H. C. Howland, D. R. Williams, P. Artal, R. Navarro, M. C. Campbell, J. E. Greivenkamp, J. T. Schwiegerling, S. A. Burns, D. A. Atchison, G. Smith, and E. J. Sarver, "A VSIA-sponsored effort to develop methods and standards for the comparison of the wavefront aberration structure of the eye between devices and laboratories.," in *Vision Science and Its Applications*, (Optical Society of America, Washington, D.C., 1999) pp 236-239.
2. L. N. Thibos, A. Bradley, D. L. Still, X. Zhang, and P. A. Howarth, "Theory and measurement of ocular chromatic aberration," Vision Research **30**, 33-49 (1990).
3. A. Bradley and L. N. Thibos (Presentation 5) at http://www.opt.indiana.edu/lthibos/ABLNTOSA95
4. A. G. Bennett and R. B. Rabbetts, *Clinical Visual Optics*, 2nd ed., (Butterworth, 1989).
5. D. Malacara, *Optical Shop Testing*, 2nd ed., (John Wiley & Sons, Inc., New York, 1992).

Index